Limb Preservation for the Vascular Specialist

Sreekumar Madassery • Aesha Patel

Editors

Limb Preservation for the Vascular Specialist

From Wound Care to Wound Closure

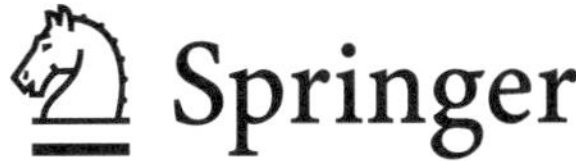 Springer

Editor
Sreekumar Madassery
Rush University Medical Center
Chicago, IL, USA

Assistant Editor
Aesha Patel
Rush University Medical Center
Chicago, IL, USA

ISBN 978-3-031-36482-2   ISBN 978-3-031-36480-8   (eBook)
https://doi.org/10.1007/978-3-031-36480-8

This Springer imprint is published by the registered company Springer Nature Switzerland AG
The registered company address is: Gewerbestrasse 11, 6330 Cham, Switzerland

Preface

I have dedicated much of my career to CLTI limb salvage/limb preservation, and as those involved know, it is an immense effort to manage and effectively help these patients. Nothing brings more personal satisfaction than helping a patient continue to walk on their own limbs, especially when they were told the only option is to have a major amputation. This is not always possible for many reasons, rightfully or wrongfully.

The contributing comorbidities, patient access to care, disparities in management and collaboration, as well as the lack of complete understanding of how to properly treat these patients, all make this a herculean effort.

In my training, and still to this day, what I have found most disheartening in this space is the vast piecemeal nature of resources and information, disagreements and politics between specialties for patient ownership and management, and the lack of standards in revascularization outcomes. We are a far cry away from having a proper system in place with global guidelines and standards to give all patients the right to a safe and good outcome, and to be armed with all the right information. While we are slowly seeing changes with a few large-scale trails, we are still left with many unanswered questions, with many people utilizing them to claim ownership of disease processes; nonetheless there is hope. I also realized that when I tell a trainee to look up a topic regarding an upcoming case or clinic patient, there is no sound starting point to get an overall global perspective of the topic and disease process, after which then they can further go onto exploring the minutia when desired.

So, with all this in mind, I envisioned this book as a single source of pearls, examples, and explanations of everything from A to Z related to limb preservation in CLTI, from global experts that I have had the pleasure of meeting and interacting with, as a jump off point for anyone interested. By including endovascular and surgical revascularization specialists from all disciplines, as well as experts in podiatry, vascular medicine, infectious disease, and plastic surgery, I intended to demonstrate the collaborative nature that must exist if we intend to give our best to all patients. In the end, no one person or specialty can help all patients dealing with PAD and CLTI, but together, we can impact a much larger population.

My sincerest thanks to my mentors and friends that have supported me in the past and on this endeavor. This also would not have been possible without the impressive work by Dr. Aesha Patel, who as a current resident managed to organize, edit, and help facilitate its formulation. It is truly inspiring to see that there is a bright future ahead with trainees that can carry the torch that we all hopefully have, and still preserve what is pure and innocent about healthcare. To my family, my biggest cheerleaders in life and trusted source of motivation, hopefully always know my undying love and thanks.

Chicago, IL, USA
Chicago, IL, USA

Sreekumar Madassery
Aesha Patel

Contents

Introduction

1

Sreekumar Madassery and Aesha Patel

Peripheral vascular disease (PVD) is a progressive circulation disorder caused by narrowing, occlusion, or otherwise abnormal flow in the peripheral blood vessels, most commonly affecting the legs and feet. The affected vessels include the arteries, veins, and/or lymphatic system. In the arterial system, the progression is part of the Peripheral Arterial Disease (PAD) spectrum, and in the Venous system, part of Venous Insufficiency. PVD presents with a multitude of symptoms, often leading to poor quality of life, exacerbation of a patient's comorbidities such as coronary artery disease and stroke, and unfortunately can result in amputations.

PAD affects more than 200 million people worldwide and has become increasingly recognized as an important cause of cardiovascular morbidity and mortality with rising prevalence throughout the world [1]. It is a manifestation of atherosclerotic disease, defined as plaque buildup and loss of elasticity of the arterial walls, leading to narrowing and stenosis of the vasculature. Other etiologies can be from acute embolic disease or vasculitis. The most common risk factors include smoking, diabetes, hypertension, hyperlipidemia, chronic kidney disease, obesity, and age. There is a broad spectrum of clinical presentation, ranging from asymptomatic to intermittent claudication, to rest pain and tissue loss. The most severe presentation is Critical Limb Ischemia (CLI) or Chronic Limb Threatening Ischemia (CLTI), which is defined as PAD with rest pain or tissue loss for greater than 2 weeks. CLTI has a mortality risk of 24% over the first year and 60% over 5 years [2]. After lung cancer, CLTI is responsible for the most deaths over 5 years in the United States [3]. This is why we, along with many operators refer to this as "arterial cancer," so as to raise the appropriate level of concern within the medical community and in the public. Historically, PAD has been understated compared to coronary artery disease and cerebrovascular disease. However, with substantial evidence showing its direct links to heart attack and stroke, its high morbidity and mortality rates, as well as the significant functional decline and disability of patients suffering from CLI/CLTI, it has become of increasing importance in recent years.

Similarly, chronic venous disease, referred to as Venous Insufficiency, and Lymphedema have long-term deleterious effects on the lower extremities of patients. They are some of the biggest contributors to healthcare costs due to the prolonged and progressively debilitating nature of their processes, which relies often on continuous wound care. Pain, numerous surgeries, hospitalizations due to recurrent VenoThromboembolism (VTE) and infections also plague this population. Additionally, many

S. Madassery (✉) · A. Patel
Department of Vascular and Interventional Radiology,
Rush University Medical Center, Chicago, IL, USA
e-mail: aesha_d_patel@rush.edu

S. Madassery, A. Patel (eds.), *Limb Preservation for the Vascular Specialist*,
https://doi.org/10.1007/978-3-031-36480-8_1

1

patients with non-healing wounds of the lower extremities may have a mixed disease pattern of PAD and Venous Insufficiency with or without lymphedema, which can make management incredibly difficult for providers, as well as for patients and their families.

To succeed, Limb Preservation requires a multidisciplinary approach, that can direct patient treatment with a combination of wound care, reconstructive surgery, medical optimization, and revascularization. In recent years, with rising awareness, limb preservation programs have been increasing across the country. These programs offer a multidisciplinary approach to care for patients at risk for amputation with the combined goal of limb salvage. This is still few and far between to make a significant impact as of yet. Many reasons exist for this, including institutional, financial, political, specialty-based societal and other external factors, which detract from the main goal we should all be pursuing, which is to improve the quality of life of our patients. Additionally, the vast quantity of topics related to managing PVD patients and Limb Preservation can be daunting for anyone, particularly for trainees of all specialties involved in or interested in this space to learn. It has been difficult to find credible sources of information in one place, in order to jump start their understanding of the vital topics that need to be grasped. This is one of the main reasons this book was formulated, to bring together many of the leading experts in Limb Preservation, particularly those who actually perform the types of cases they speak of, which carry the highest merit, and develop an abbreviated, up-to-date source of guidance for all involved.

In this handbook, we discuss all aspects of peripheral vascular disease and limb preservation. With a diverse authors list from across the globe, consisting of endovascular specialists, surgeons, podiatrists, vascular medicine, and infectious disease specialists, this handbook will serve as a guideline to the comprehensive care and management of limb preservation for all disciplines. We begin with understanding the different wound types and evaluating the underlying causes that have been typically underdiagnosed and undermanaged in these patients, as well as the management of those underlying causes. We then further elaborate on wound care management as well as proper diagnosis with various non-invasive imaging modalities. From there, we dive deep into the treatment of arterial, venous, and lymphatic therapies. This includes treatment algorithms, unique and complex approaches, technique tips and tricks, possible complications and how to manage them, as well as cutting-edge options. We conclude by covering how to continue evaluating the wounds post-procedurally and in long-term follow-up, when reintervention or surgery is needed, and how to tackle the highly involved medication management of these patients.

All these aspects will play a significant role in saving these patients' limbs. It has been well demonstrated that succeeding in limb preservation and keeping these patients alive longer requires a multidisciplinary effort, and long-term management of these complex patients. Not all major amputations can be prevented, and some are needed to save a patient's life (such as grossly infected/wet gangrene), however far too many limbs are lost due to inadequate prevention, management, and intervention. By providing a multidisciplinary comprehensive review of the evaluation, management, and treatment of peripheral vascular disease for limb preservation, we hope to empower the physician with the knowledge and tools needed to treat this important disease.

We hope this can be the essential go-to handbook for all those involved in limb preservation, from wound care to wound closure.

References

1. Adaw AW, Matsushita K. Epidemiology of peripheral artery disease and polyvascular disease. Circ Res. 2021;128(12):1818–32. https://doi.org/10.1161/circresaha.121.318535.
2. Mustapha JA, Katzen BT, Neville RF, Loostein RA, Zeller T, Miller LE, Jaff MR. Disease burden and clinical outcomes following initial diagnosis of critical limb ischemia in the Medicare population. JACC Cardiovasc Interv. 2018;11:1011–2.
3. Armstrong DG, Swerdlow MA, Armstrong AA, Conte MS, Pdula WV, Bus SA. Five year mortality and direct costs of care for people with diabetic foot complications are comparable to cancer. J Foot Ankle Res. 2020;13:16.

Nicholas Alianello, David G. Armstrong,
Amir Dorafshar, J. Karim Ead, David Kurlander,
Sreekumar Madassery, Hannah K. Park,
and Idanis Perez-Alvarez

2.1 Mastering the Wound Care Physical Exam

Nicholas Alianello

Not unlike any other illness, the appropriate wound diagnosis can only be made after a thorough physical exam is performed. A wound exam should be quick and concise. Proper and timely assessment is critical in healing all wounds. The first, and most critical step in wound evaluation is assessment of the vascularity to the wound site. The next step should be assessing for wound contamination or infection. Following these two important assessments, evaluation of mechanical foot/extremity deformities should be performed. Lastly, a complete evaluation of the quality of the wound itself is performed [1].

2.1.1 Vascular Exam

It is common knowledge that a wound requires oxygenation from arterial perfusion to heal. Perfusion to the skin and surrounding structures of the wound can be monitored by these simple exam findings.

1. Skin color (pallor), hyperpigmentation, and shiny skin.
2. Elevation pallor or dependent rubor.
3. Distribution of hair growth on the digits.
4. Skin atrophy.
5. Decreased temperature gradient compared with contralateral limb.
6. History of claudication or rest pain.

Next, one must assess perfusion.

1. Palpate Dorsalis Pedis and Posterior Tibial Pulse.
2. Evaluate capillary fill time (normal <5 s) to the digits.

If one or both pedal arteries are non-palpable or the capillary fill time is visibly delayed, a hand-held Doppler should be used to evaluate the pha-

N. Alianello · H. K. Park
Weil Foot and Ankle Institute, Chicago, IL, USA
e-mail: hpark@weil4feet.com

D. G. Armstrong · J. K. Ead
Keck School of Medicine, University of Southern California, Los Angeles, CA, USA

A. Dorafshar · D. Kurlander · I. Perez-Alvarez
Department of Surgery, Division of Plastic and Reconstructive Surgery, Rush University Medical Center, Chicago, IL, USA
e-mail: Amir_Dorafshar@rush.edu;
David_Kurlander@rush.edu;
Idanis_M_Perez-Alvarez@rush.edu

S. Madassery (✉)
Department of Vascular and Interventional Radiology, Rush University Medical Center, Chicago, IL, USA

S. Madassery, A. Patel (eds.), *Limb Preservation for the Vascular Specialist*,
https://doi.org/10.1007/978-3-031-36480-8_2

sic nature of the arterial flow. Confirming adequate perfusion is essential to wound healing and is the most important step. If the blood flow is deemed inadequat by exam or additional non-invasive testing, a more in-depth, invasive vascular workup should be immediately performed [1].

2.1.2 Infection

Immediate assessment for infection is paramount in limb salvage. No credible amount of wound healing will occur in the presence of acute or chronic infection. The classic signs of local infection to the surrounding wound include redness, swelling, pain, and warmth. An evaluation for streaking cellulitis should be made at this time and, if present, should be marked with a dark line at its most proximal extension. Next, the wound should be palpated, and manual force should be used in an attempt to express purulent drainage from the wound. If present, the purulent drainage should be sent for culture. The surrounding area of the wound and deep structures should be palpated and checked for crepitus that could represent an underlying abscess or subcutaneous gas. Any foul odor should be documented. Finally, if the patient should report symptoms including nausea, vomiting, chills, loss of appetite, malaise, and/or diarrhea—concern for systemic infection would be high [1].

2.1.3 Foot Deformity and Soft Tissue Breakdown

Areas of the foot and ankle that present as large bony prominences pose an immediate threat to skin breakdown. Deformities like hammer toes, bunions, and Charcot plantar foot collapse all contribute to increased foot pressure and ulcer development [2]. If previous digital or partial foot amputations have been performed, this too must be examined. It is not uncommon for wounds to form at amputation sites. Assessing the foot deformity and ulceration site has a direct impact on understanding the wound etiology and

one's ability to properly offload the wound, both of which will be discussed later in the chapter.

2.1.4 Direct Assessment of the Wound

1. Location: Location of wound on the extremity. Plantar versus dorsal foot. Proximity to bony prominence.
2. Shape: Wounds present in a variety of shapes, but it should be documented for completeness.
3. Border: Majority of neuropathic wounds present with a hyperkeratotic border, unlike ischemic wounds that have a punched out border.
4. Base: Granular vs Fibrotic vs necrotic. It should be quantified in percent as to how much the wound base is granular vs fibrotic vs necrotic. A granular base is composed of vascular buds and indicates positive healing potential. Fibrotic base consists of disorganized collagen commonly found in more chronic, less vascularized wounds. Necrotic base consists of diseased, infected tissue that requires immediate removal. Description of tissue type at the base of the wound is also essential (wound probe to subcutaneous tissue, tendon, muscle, or bone).
5. Undermining: Wound undermining refers to the pocket of space beneath the skin around the wound's edge. The position and area of the undermining should be documented and measured.
6. Drainage: Clear vs serous vs hemorrhagic vs purulent. Drainage should be cultured when necessary.
7. Size: Wound dimensions include length, width, and depth.

The ease and availability of digital photography with the immediate ability to document the picture in the electronic health record adds to the descriptive nature of the above exam and should be performed at each wound examination [1]. Overall wound classification can be monitored through well-established systems such as the Bates-Jensen wound assessment tool.

2.2 How to Classify the Wound

Nicholas Alianello

Information obtained from the wound exam in combination with information obtained from a total body history and physical will allow for adequate classification of wound etiology.

There are four main etiologies that one should be familiar with:

1. Neuropathic Wound (diabetic ulceration).
2. Ischemic Wound.
3. Decubitus Wound.
4. Venous Wound.

Neuropathic Wound: Neuropathic wounds are commonly found on the plantar surface of the foot or weight-bearing structure/extremity, usually at the area of increased pressure or bony prominence (Fig. 2.1). These are mostly seen in patients with advanced peripheral neuropathy secondary to uncontrolled diabetes, however, other causes for neuropathy exist. Whatever the cause for neuropathy, it is the loss of protective sensation that prohibits one from sensing the plantar pressures at the foot, ultimately leading to skin breakdown and wound formation. These wounds will present as granular ulcerations with thick hyperkeratotic borders. If left untreated or managed poorly, they tend to probe very deep often to muscle tendon and bone. The Wagner and Meggitt classification system is widely accepted in classifying diabetic and neuropathic ulcerations (Table 2.1) [3, 4].

Ischemic Wound: Formed as a direct result of poor perfusion followed by tissue breakdown, ischemic wounds commonly present in two forms: Gangrenous Digits or Punched out lesions (Fig. 2.2). Unlike the granular wounds seen in neuropathic ulcerations, ischemic wounds present mostly with thick eschar to the periphery and center and are fibrotic in appearance. The mixed fibrous/eschar base is the byproduct of the lack of perfusion to the underlying tissue. In isolated instances of acute ischemia, these wounds typically are very painful. In the most severe case,

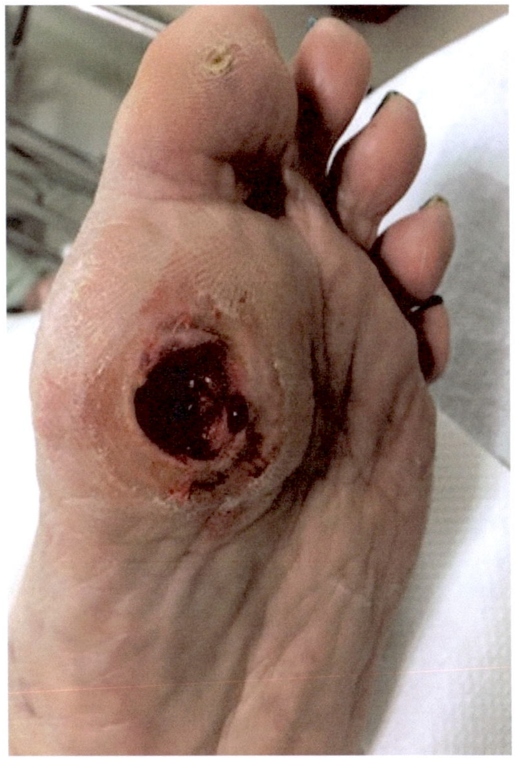

Fig. 2.1 Neuropathic ulcer

Table 2.1 Diabetic foot classification by Wagner and Meggitt

Grade 0	Intact skin, hyperkeratotic lesion around or under bony deformity
Grade 1	Superficial ulcer, base may be necrotic or viable with early granulation tissue
Grade 2	Deeper lesion extending to bone, ligament, tendon, joint capsule, or deep fascia; no abscess or osteomyelitis
Grade 3	Deep abscess, osteitis, or osteomyelitis
Grade 4	Portion of the toes or forefoot is gangrenous
Grade 5	Complete involvement of the foot, no foot healing or local procedure is possible

necrotic tissue will be present throughout the entirety of the wound.

Decubitus Wound: Decubitus wounds present in areas of the body most susceptible to cutaneous pressure. In the lower extremity the most common areas of skin breakdown include the posterior heel, lateral malleolus, and medial mal-

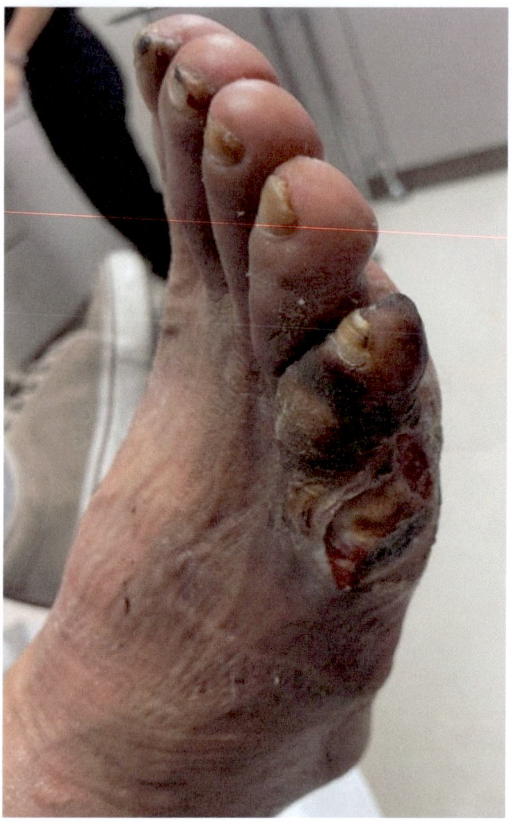

Fig. 2.2 Ischemic ulcer

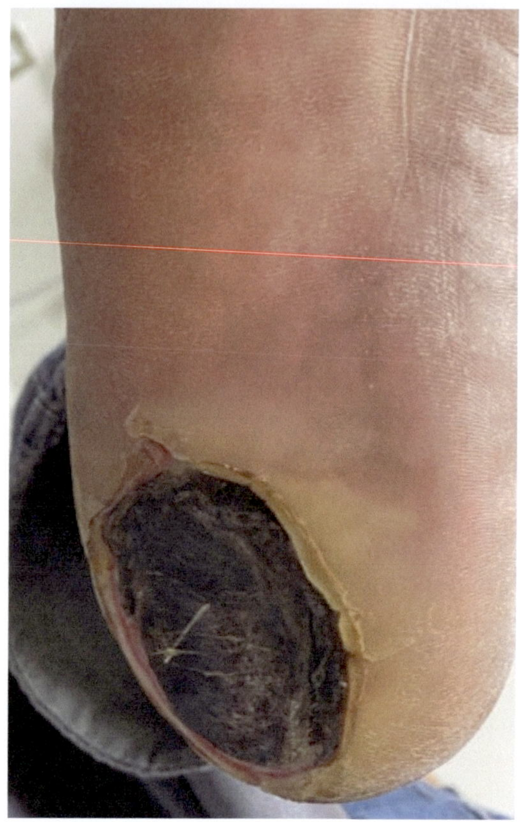

Fig. 2.3 Decubitus ulcer of heel

leolus (Fig. 2.3). Dry, stable decubitus wounds present first as a blister or area of non-blanchable erythema. Once tissue death continues, eschar formation eventually forms, and skin slough occurs. These wounds tend to be difficult to treat given their proximity to underlying bony structures. When infected, it is not uncommon for bone to become exposed, most notably at the posterior heel of the foot. Classification and staging by the National Pressure Ulcer Advisory Panel (NPUAP) can be found in Table 2.2 [5].

Venous Wound: Venous leg ulcerations are commonly found on the medial ankle, lateral ankle, or pre-tibial region of the lower leg (Fig. 2.4). Typical presentation involves significant pitting edema within the leg secondary to severe venous insufficiency. These wounds present with punched out borders with mixed granular/fibrotic bases and drain heavy serous fluid. They are typically very irregular in shape and are extremely painful, most notably during

Table 2.2 National Pressure Ulcer Advisory Panel, Staging System 2007

Stage 1	Intact skin with non-blanchable redness of localized area
Stage 2	Partial thickness loss of dermis presenting as a shallow open ulcer with red, pink wound bed
Stage 3	Full-thickness tissue loss. Subcutaneous fat may be visible but tendon, muscle, bone NOT exposed
Stage 4	Full-thickness tissue loss WITH exposed tendon, muscle, and bone
Unstageable	Full-thickness tissue loss covered by eschar or necrotic tissue, unable to determine depth

debridement. Edema, varicose veins, reticular/spider veins, and thickened hyperpigmented lower extremities are also commonly seen in these patients. A history of deep vein thrombosis, prior IVC filter usage, and undiagnosed May Thurner Syndrome may also be discovered.

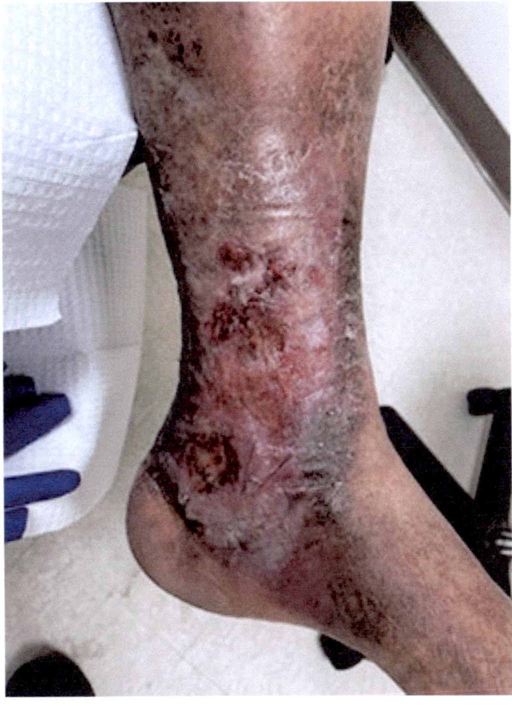

Fig. 2.4 Venous leg ulcer

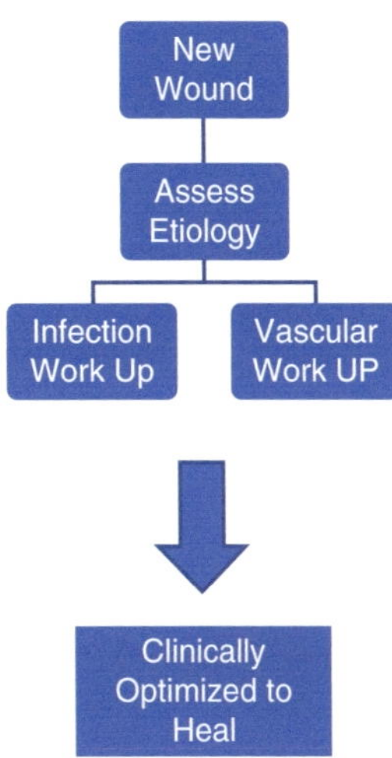

Fig. 2.5 Flowchart for assessing and optimizing a wound's healing potential

2.2.1 When Should I Consider Venous or Mixed Wounds?

Above, we have briefly discussed the four most common wound types seen in the lower extremity. It is important to note that the four classifications are not mutually exclusive. A complete and thorough work up for advanced neuropathy, peripheral arterial disease, and venous disease needs to be performed prior to determining treatment. As an example, it is common for a patient with diabetic neuropathy to develop a neuropathic ulcer with adjacent gangrenous changes to surrounding tissue and digits. It is also common for patients to develop mixed venous and arterial ulcerations. A thorough evaluation and recognition of characteristics of all types of wounds present in a single wound should raise clinical suspicion and lead to further evaluation.

A true understanding of the above principles will allow you to assess the etiology of the wound in a quick and concise manner. Following a thorough vascular and infection work up, one

can ensure the wound is optimized to heal (Fig. 2.5).

2.2.2 Managing Neuropathic Wounds

The purpose of determining the wound etiology and proper classification along with quick infection work up and vascular exam is to ensure that the wound is clinically optimized to heal.

Once optimized, three principles of wound care are performed:

1. Debridement
2. Offloading
3. Moist wound environment

These three principles are most important in the management of diabetic neuropathic ulcerations:

1. **Debridement:** Fundamental first step in treatment. It involves removing the necrotic and fibrotic tissues to increase granulation tissue and removal of bioburden [6].
   (a) Sharp Debridement: Use of a scalpel and curette to sharply remove tissue is the most common, fundamental form of debridement. This is performed both in

the outpatient and OR setting. It is of critical importance to not debride a necrotic heel ulcer without confirming adequate perfusion, unless it is an unstable, boggy wound in which case debridement may be needed immediately.

(b) Enzymatic debridement: Collagenase, an ointment formulation that works to break down collagen, fibrin, and eschar formation. Used in small wounds or in larger wounds in conjunction with sharp debridement.

(c) Mechanical: Wet to dry dressing, hydrotherapy.

(d) Biologic debridement: Maggot therapy.

2. **Offloading:** Peak plantar pressures have been measured and proven to be elevated in areas of ulceration. This in combination with areas of bony prominence serves as compromised areas of the extremity prone to develop ulcers. Once the ulcer forms, it is paramount to remove the source of peak pressure with the use of an offloading device. No matter the modality of choice, offloading should be maintained throughout the duration of the wound healing until closed [1].

(a) Non-weight bearing: Ideal form of offloading but often not ideal for the patient. Can be performed with the use of crutches or knee scooter.

(b) Total contact cast.

(c) Removable cast walker.

(d) Wedge offloading shoes.

(e) Extra-depth shoes with plastazote inserts and offloading pads.

3. **Maintain Moist Wound Environment:**

(a) Rule of thumb: Always attempt to maintain a moist wound environment. If the wound is too wet, dry it. If the wound is too dry, wet it.

(b) The wound dressing market includes a vast array of collagens, gels, foams, hydrocolloids alginates, and gauze. Each dressing of choice should be carefully chosen for the correct function in either drying or moistening the wound.

(c) Combination of dressing strategies in conjunction with weekly wound assessment is of paramount to maintain the ideal moisture balance of the wound bed.

If clinically optimized to heal, treated weekly with debridement, as well as offloading and moisture balance, a neuropathic wound should heal (decrease in surface area) by 50% in 4 weeks (Fig. 2.6) [7].

If 50% healing is not achieved one should:

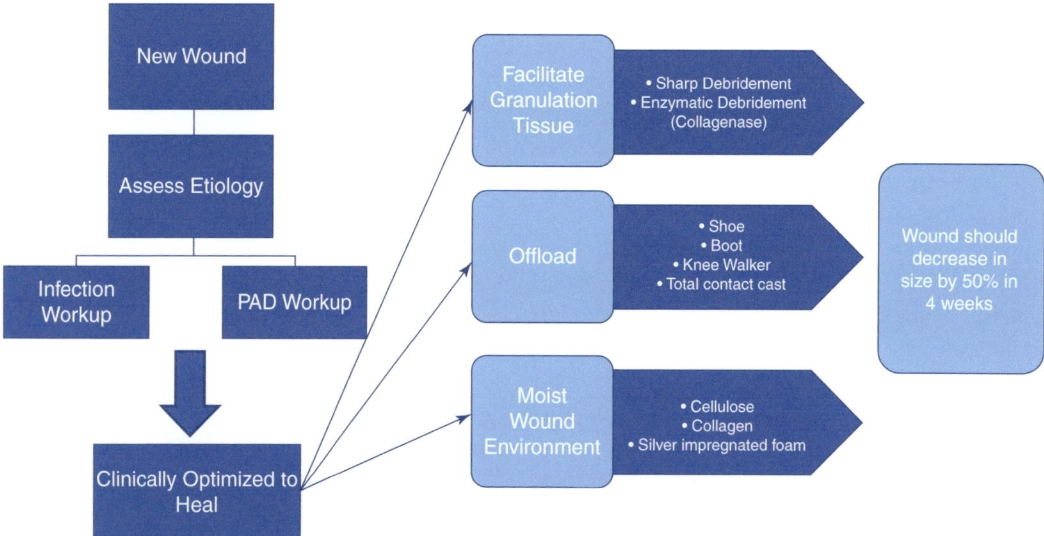

Fig. 2.6 Flowchart demonstrating the expected course of healing if a wound is clinically optimized to heal and treated weekly with debridement, offloading, and moisture balance

1. Re-evaluate for infection.
2. Re-evaluate perfusion to the wound site.
3. Consider biologic wound dressing (skin substitutes and advanced biologics).

2.3 Mixed Wounds: How to Manage?

Sreekumar Madassery

When a mixed wound is suspected, referral to a vascular specialist should be made. Based on definitive diagnosis of both arterial and venous insufficiency by way of a thorough history, physical exam, as well as confirmatory non-invasive studies (i.e., Abi, duplex, and venous insufficiency studies), a proper plan can be made. It is recommended to address the arterial revascularization first to allow tissue oxygenation to commence. This is also imperative as the standard long-term treatment for venous insufficiency is compression therapy, which cannot be maximized in the presence of arterial insufficiency. Generally, a reliable minimum ABI of 0.7 should be present for aggressive compression therapy. Therefore, if the arterial perfusion is optimized first, then the appropriate level of compression wraps/dressings can be used to improve the wound.

For the venous insufficiency component, after the arterial perfusion is addressed, this can start with aggressive compression therapy along with appropriate wound care dressings based on the wound characteristics. Based on the findings within non-invasive tests such as the duplex insufficiency study, or others such as CTV/MRV scans, the vascular specialist may consider venous interventions such as percutaneous superficial vein closure (thermal ablation, liquid-based closure) of the greater saphenous vein and/or the small saphenous vein, along with perforators if deemed necessary. While in general, these interventions are commonly used for cosmetic and symptomatic purposes, comprehensive wound care has incorporated these approaches to improve wound closure success. In patients without incompetent superficial veins or with previously closed veins, peri-wound varices can sometimes be discovered, that once treated with percutaneous sclerotherapy, can potentially increase wound closure. It is important to consider multi-disciplinary consideration whether or not the superficial vein is needed for potential bypass.

2.4 Basics of Debridement of Wounds

Hannah K. Park

Wound debridement is essential to wound care as prepping the wound bed is a vital step to remove chronic biofilm. It stimulates the wound bed that has been stalled and not healing, into an inflammatory phase, which then promotes growth factors, granulation tissue, and epithelization for wound healing.

The presence of biofilm indicates a bacterial layer with devitalized unhealthy tissue that needs to be debrided sharply to reduce the risk of infection and even remove the source of infection that is delaying the wound from healing. The presence of devitalized tissue and biofilm is a source of nutrients for bacteria as well as a physical barrier that reduces epithelization and wound healing.

Debriding a wound first is necessary to obtain accurate cultures for antibiotic therapy and reduce the probability of antibiotic resistance. Debriding a wound will also allow for the wound dressings to work more effectively.

There are several types of wound debridement dependent on the skill level of the physician and the patient's wound needs:

- **Sharp/Surgical:** The removal of the biofilm and nonviable tissue with a blade or sharp curette. It can be painful (even with topical analgesic use) if the patient is sensate, but it is the fastest way to clean a wound bed.
- **Enzymatic:** The removal of devitalized tissue with chemical proteolytic enzymes such as collagenase.
- **Autolytic:** The use of the body's own enzymes, WBCs and bacteria to break down the devitalized tissue.

   – Performed by use of hydrocolloids, hydrogels, alginates, etc. in order to support a proper moist environment in the wound.
- **Biologic:** The use of sterile bottle fly larvae (aka maggots) that eat away the devitalized tissue and leave healthy tissue intact. This can be used to clean substantial amounts of necrosis without inflicting pain.
- **Mechanical:** The use of gauze, wet-to-dry dressings, irrigation, and other dressings to remove biofilm and devitalized tissue with mechanical force.

2.4.1 Debridement of What Exactly?

It is important to know what part of the wound should be debrided:

1. Necrotic nonviable tissue that is gray, black, and even white in discoloration is dead from injury, infection, and underlying disease process.
   (a) Gangrenous
   (b) Macerated
   (c) Fibronecrotic (Fig. 2.7)
2. Slough, which is a byproduct of inflammation, is stringy yellow tan in color, and is made of fibrin, leukocytes, and dead and living cells. This slough also attracts bacteria to the wound surface (Fig. 2.8).
3. Biofilm (Viscous and shiny coating).

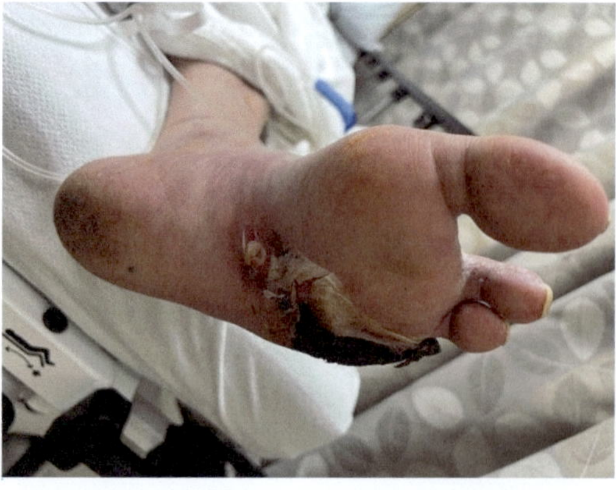

Fig. 2.7 Fibronecrotic plug extending to the osteomyelitic bone with dry gangrene

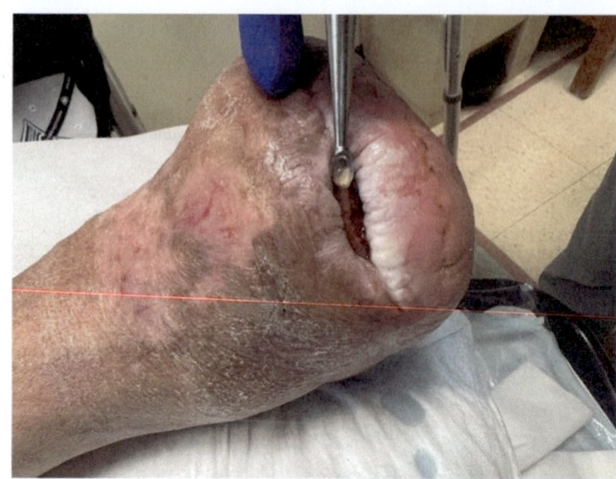

Fig. 2.8 Slough picked up with curette instrument

2.5 Basics of Dressings and When to Make a Change

Hannah K. Park

Wound dressings, originally used as a protective barrier made of cotton/linen gauze and bandages, commonly get attached as the wound would grow hypergranular tissue, and cause damage during removal of the dressings.

Ideal wound dressings should:

1. 1.Be able to manage exudate, retain moisture for the wound, as well as have mechanical properties to reduce bacterial load, and the right pore density and pore size for oxygen permeability.
2. Dressings should be able to be removed without increasing the wound.
3. There are numerous types of wound dressings, and it will be up to the provider to find the best dressing regimen for the specific type of wound as the requirements of wound healing would vastly differ based on the wound's needs [8].

Dressings 101: What does the wound need? Does it have the basic building structures for wound healing?

1. **Collagen** is an unbranched fibrous protein synthesized from animal fibroblasts helping to provide the scaffold of wound healing as

many diabetics are deficient in collagen production. It can be derived from animal tendons, ligaments, cartilage, and other skin connective tissues and it can be easily extracted, biodegraded, and absorbed.
   (a) Examples of various collagen powders: Prisma Ag, Endoform.
2. **Chitin and Chitosan** are biotype dressings found in bones of some mollusks, crustaceans, and cell walls of fungi. This is degraded into N-acetylglucosamine on the wound surface and is then absorbed by epidermal cells and essential for maintenance of growth and production of epidermal cells. It increases the scaffold structure of wounds and wound tensile strength. It also has air permeability and increases the production of macrophages and can also be anti-inflammatory and aid in hemostasis.
3. **Alginate** is made from insoluble alginate (seaweed) that is made from methyl sodium carbide cellulose and calcium alginate. It is characterized by high hygroscopicity, glue forming, and hemostatic properties. This is used in dressing with heavy exudate. It turns the insoluble calcium alginate into a soluble sodium alginate absorbing the exudate that is double its weight. It also releases calcium ions into the wound that increases platelet activation and promotes wound healing as it absorbs the bacteria from the wound increasing the release of macrophages for autolysis debridement.
   (a) Example: Urgosorb, Sorsbsan.
4. **Hydrogel** is a water insoluble colloidal substance made by water soluble polymer material which has a 96% water content providing moisture into the wound. It can also promote autolysis of debrided necrotic tissue and can be applied without disrupting the wound bed while removed. It should not be used on highly exudative wounds.
5. **Hydrocolloids** are elastic polymeric hydrogels with synthetic rubber and mucilage which can be used for low-exudating wounds. Due to its thick occlusive dressing, it holds moisture at the wound surface which can promote autolysis of fibrin and necrotic tissue but also may cause maceration and infection due to the lack of oxygen.
   (a) Example: Aquacel

Dressing 102: Presence of Exudate Drainage

1. Exudative drainage is fluid that leaks out of blood vessels when wound is present. This occurs due to localized inflammation that releases mediators and enzymes causing increased interstitial fluid that leads to exudate.
   (a) It can be helpful for wound healing in acute wounds by providing a moist environment.
   (b) It helps with autolytic debridement by separating the dead and damaged tissues.
   (c) It helps with migration of tissue repairing cells and immune mediators and growth factors.
   (d) It supplies essential nutrients for wound healing.
2. However, if the wound is chronic the exudate drainage is alkaline and can impede healing.
3. Too much exudative drainage can cause maceration (soggy, white/pale areas) to the wound borders making wounds enlarge and painful [9].
4. Classifying wound exudate based on color and consistency.
   (a) Serous: Clear and watery from blood and serous membranes of body.
   (b) Serosanguinous: Thin and pink made of serum and RBCs.
   (c) Sanguineous: Thin and bright red.
   (d) Purulent: Thick or thin, tan and yellow made of leukocytes, dead tissue debris, and dead and living bacteria.
   (e) Slough: Thin, yellow, and stringy that is adhered to the wound, cannot be washed away like pus.
5. Factors that affect exudate production:
   (a) Local factors:
      • Infection
      • Foreign body
      • Edema
      • Tumor
      • Fistula

- Presence of eschar/ischemia
- Positioning (not elevating)

(b) Systemic factors:
  - CHF
  - Renal failure
  - Fluid overload
  - Malnutrition
  - Systemic medications
  - Endocrine disease
  - Advanced age
  - Inflammatory markers: CRP elevation
  - Hypovolemic shock

6. Absorbent dressings and superabsorbent dressings.
   (a) It is important to reduce the amount of maceration in the wound by absorbing exudative drainage.
   (b) Helps to sequester and retain the bacteria and metalloproteinases from the wound to reduce infection.
   (c) Examples: Calcium Alginate, Drawtex, Acquacel Ag.

7. Polymers and foams.
   (a) These pads/films absorb fluids, keep out bacteria and can have antibiotic agent impregnation.

8. Negative pressure wound therapy (wound vacs):
   (a) Help to reduce the size of a wound, reduce exudate, increase blood flow to the wound bed, and increase the production of granulation tissue as well as reduce the risk of infection while maintaining a moist environment for wound healing.

Dressings 103: Reduce adherence to dressings to minimize trauma when changing the dressings.

1. Low to non-adherent dressings are useful on fragile skin and reduce the chances of causing trauma to the wound.
   (a) Examples: Adaptic, UrgoTUL, Xeroform.

Dressings 104: Presence of infection:

1. Iodine is an antiseptic and helps to manage infection.
   (a) Examples: Iodoflex, Iodosorb, Oxyzyme

2. Medihoney is a medical-grade honey that has antimicrobial and anti-inflammatory properties which also provide a moist environment to promote autolysis and reduce odor.

3. Silver (Ag) can be used in alginates, collagen, foams, and hydrocolloids to reduce infection.

Dressings 105: Presence of depth, gapping, and spacing:

1. Moist gauze packing
2. Calcium alginate
3. Gelling fiber
4. Super absorber
5. Negative Pressure Therapy (wound vac)

When should I change the dressings and plan of treatment?

1. Wound bed has not improved in its size and depth with standard of care after 4 weeks.
2. Wound bed becomes infected with physical exam findings of malodor, discoloration, hypergranulation, +/− erythema, edema, and purulence.
3. Wound bed becomes necrotic.
4. Wound bed has increased in exudate.

2.6 When Should I Culture?

Hannah K. Park

Why has not the wound healed for the past 4 weeks with standard wound care? The bioburden may not only need wound debridement but a short oral (or sometimes long-term intravenous) course of broad-spectrum antibiotics, to kick-start wound healing.

Any wounds with signs of infection, or signs of chronic infection in an open wound, should be cultured to help select the best antibiotic treatment. Signs of chronic wound infection may be a malodor, discoloration (green or blue), abnormal uneven level of hypergranular tissue, or drainage and tracking to deeper tissues like the bone. Any time bone is exposed, cultures should be taken by sending pieces of bone along with

infectious disease referral and surgical debridement should be considered. Depending on the wound care specialist's discretion, patients may be started on an empiric antibiotic or wait for a microbiologic diagnosis. A swab culture allows the physician to identify the underlying cause of the chronic wound [10].

Site of Cultures: Should be the area of infection in the wound base that may be discolored or hypertrophic with drainage. Wounds should first be washed with sterile water so that the wound swabs are not taken from heavily contaminated areas that may give false culture results. Once resulted, culture-directed antibiotic therapy can be started or adjusted [10].

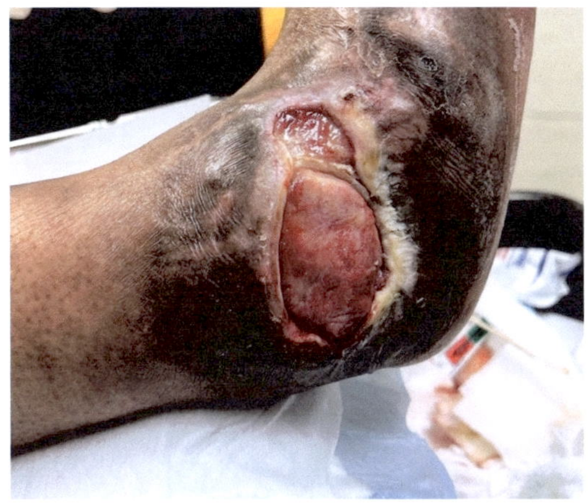

Fig. 2.9 Chronic wound with bone and joint exposed is highly suspicious for chronic osteomyelitis

2.7 When Should I Biopsy?

Hannah K. Park

Bone biopsy is necessary if there is suspicion of bone infection. This can be done with:

1. Ronguer
2. Jamshidi needle
3. Trephine
4. Craig needle

When assessing wound infection, wound biopsy was not shown to assess wound infection differently from wound cultures taken with a wound swab. Assessments did not significantly differ when specific microorganisms were cultured nor for different wound types. It is recommended to perform a wound swab initially as there is less burden on the patient of enlarging the wound or creating pain/fear compared to a wound biopsy.

However, if the chronic wound is not healing with standard methods, and there are clinical signs of possible skin malignancy, wound biopsy should be performed. Clinical signs to look out for are abnormal wound borders, bleeding, abnormal discoloration (black or blue), changing shape and size, and various levels of thickness (Fig. 2.9).

1. Excisional biopsy
2. Incisional biopsy
3. Punch biopsy

2.8 How Do I Biopsy a Wound?

Nicholas Alianello

Most lower extremity wounds can be classified by etiology, the majority being in patients with diabetes in conjunction with peripheral neuropathy, ischemia, and sometimes both. A foot and ankle deformity and/or area of increased pressure lends itself to wound formation in the above-mentioned patient.

When to biopsy a wound?

1. When a wound presents in atypical anatomical site (e.g., Dorsum of the foot).
2. Etiology and appearance of wound are atypical and do not fall into normal classification.
3. When a wound fails to improve despite strict adherence to standard wound healing principles.

How to biopsy the wound:

Cleanse wounds with sterile saline. Anesthetize the wound with local anesthesia if needed. Remove full-thickness sample of tissue from center of lesion/ulcer. It is okay to take samples from multiple areas of the wound if the lesion is big enough. Use a camera and picture to document the wound appearance and location of biopsy to assist pathology in diagnosis.

Incision biopsy: Use a 15-blade and take a full-thickness section of the ulceration. Send the sample in formalin to pathology.

Punch biopsy: Type of incisional biopsy by use of cylindrical blade. Creates full-thickness sample. Comes in multiple sizes – 4 mm and 6 mm are most commonly used for lower extremity wounds. This is also sent in formalin to pathology.

2.9 When Should I Not Debride?

Nicholas Alianello

1. In ischemic wounds with dry/stable eschars (Fig. 2.10) prior to vascular intervention.
   (a) Debridement will only lead to worsening tissue death and likely expose bone.

   (b) Always await vascular intervention to ensure level of debridement and tissue removal will be adequate to heal.
2. All pressure ulcers with dry stable eschars. Even when these ulcers have adequate perfusion you should avoid removing the dry stable eschar. Removing the dry eschar will likely expose bone as these pressure injuries occur at boney prominences of the extremity.
   (a) One should focus on **enzymatic** debridement and avoid sharp debridement until the periphery of the eschar begins to lift from the wound base and becomes mobile. When the eschar breaks down or is loose, then it is adequate to debride (Figs. 2.11, 2.12, 2.13, and 2.14).

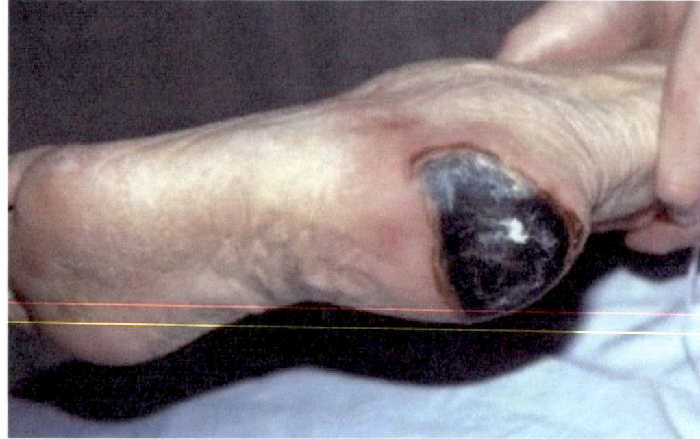

Fig. 2.11 Dry eschar along the heel. DO NOT debride lesion. Begin Enzymatic debridement with collagenase application to wound base daily

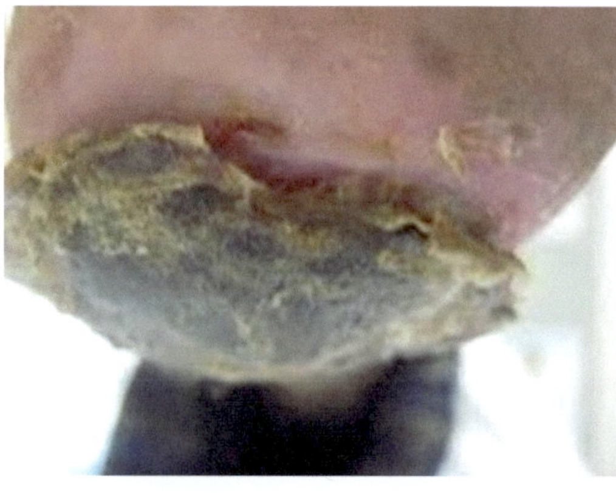

Fig. 2.12 Heel eschar after collagenase application. Eschar begins to loosen from peripheral of wound base and becomes mobile

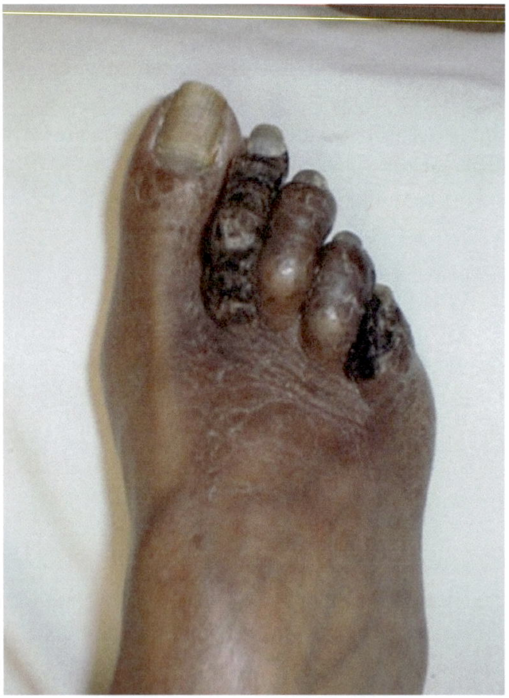

Fig. 2.10 Dry eschar of second and fifth toe

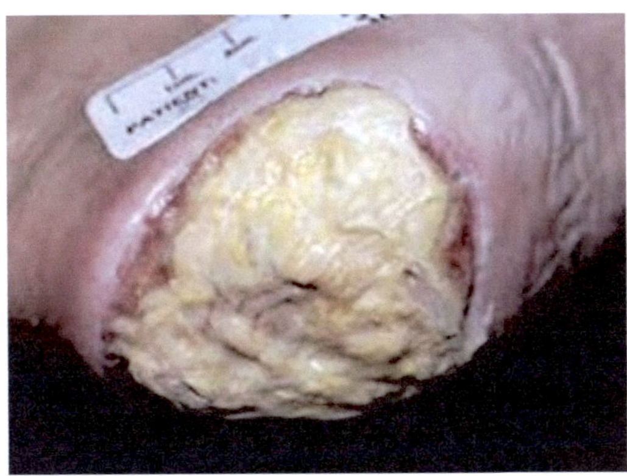

Fig. 2.13 Heel eschar is now mobile enough to remove without exposing bone. Continue collagenase application to assist in fibrotic tissue removal

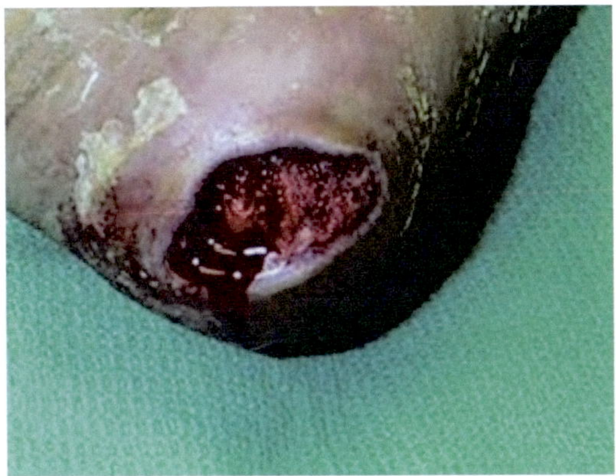

Fig. 2.14 Heel eschar with wound base now granular with no exposed bone. It is now ok to return to sharp debridement

3. Pyoderma gangrenosum wounds: Wound management should focus on pathergy avoidance. NO debridement, dressing management, and overall disease management with systemic medications are mainstay treatment.

2.10   Identifying and Managing Calciphylaxis

Nicholas Alianello

Identification: Start off as small plaques/eschar that worsen and form larger lesions. They form a lacy appearance and are acutely painful (Fig. 2.15). Eventually, the plaques form deep,

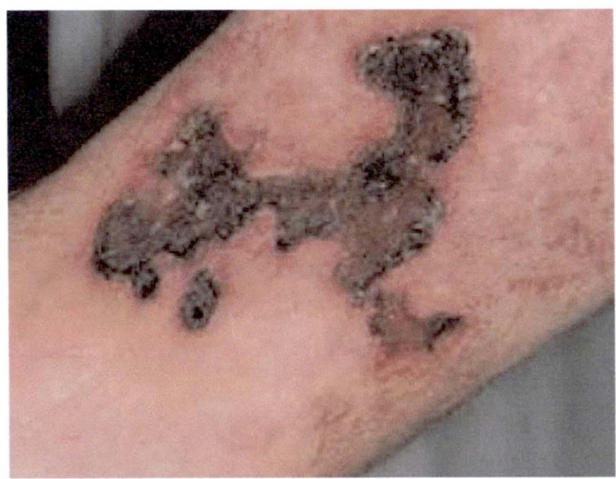

Fig. 2.15 Calciphylaxis of lower extremity

ischemic ulcers. Normally found on areas of body with high amounts of adipose tissue (trunk and thighs).

Wound Management: Due to intense pain associated with wounds, sharp debridement is difficult. Enzymatic debridement of fibrous tissue and eschar is best performed with "collagenase" applied during daily dressing changes. Proper wound dressings are paramount to control moisture balance. Hyperbaric oxygen therapy should be used when wound healing stalls.

The complexity of the diagnosis calls for a total team approach to treat underlying systemic disease.

2.11   When Do I Wound Vac?

Nicholas Alianello

A wound vac should be used in wounds with depth that need assistance in increasing granulation tissue within the wound base.

In most cases, the wound vac is used as adjunctive therapy after aggressive surgical debridement that leaves a wound with a deep deficit (Figs. 2.16 and 2.17).

To allow for epidermal growth, a wound base must be granular and must be at the level of the skin. A wound vac uses negative pressure therapy to promote granulation through capillary budding at the wound site. The goal is to increase granulation tissue to eliminate wound depth.

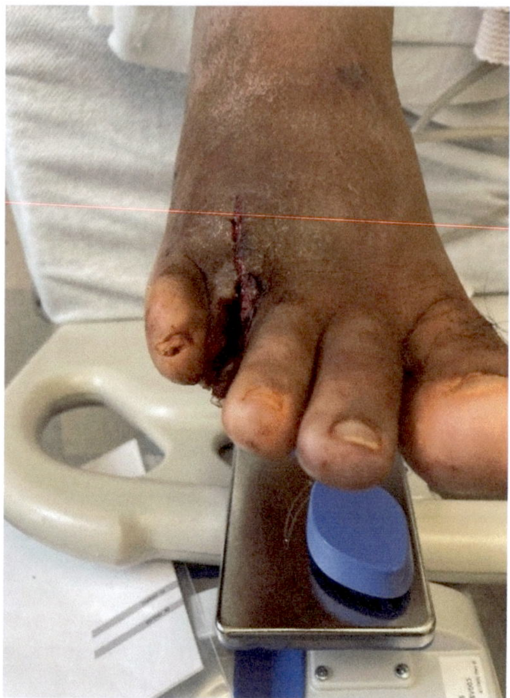

Fig. 2.16 Deep wound after fourth digit amputation

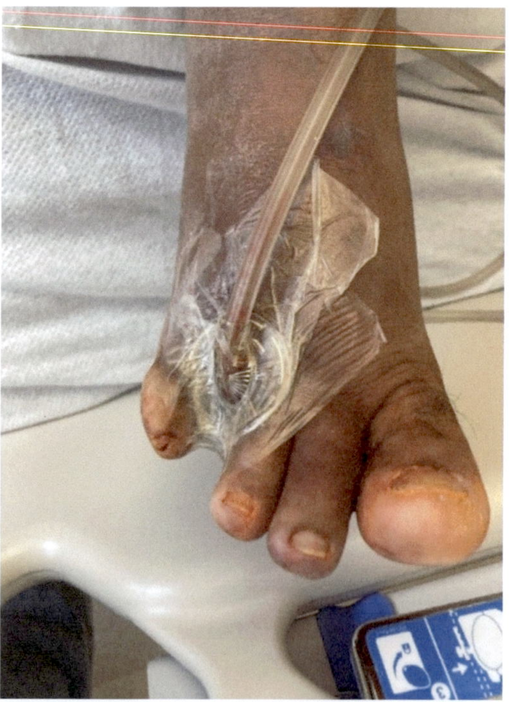

Fig. 2.17 Wound vac placement along wound base of fourth digit amputation

Standard treatment protocol calls for pressure to be set at 125 mmHg with oscillation between continuous and intermittent suction.

2.12 Offloading

Nicholas Alianello

When to offload: When wounds occur on the plantar surface of the foot, there is a need to eliminate the vertical plantar peak pressure associated with walking (diabetic neuropathic foot ulcers).

2.12.1 Options for Offloading

1. Total Non-weight Bearing: Crutches, Wheelchair, Knee Scooter.
2. Total Contact Cast: Gold standard for offloading DFUs.
3. Wedge Shoes (Half shoes).
4. Removable Cam Walker with offloading pad.
5. Felt/foam pads and donut pads were applied to surgical shoe.
6. Extra-depth shoe with custom cut-out tri-laminate insert.

2.12.2 When to Make a Change?

The issue with aggressive offloading is the impractical nature of requesting a patient to remain off the foot for the lifetime of the wound. Non-compliance is high. The recommendation is that you aggressively offload immediately when a wound forms. Recommend strict non-weight bearing (NWB) or Total Contact Cast during the initial treatment plan. As the wound heals and becomes smaller, you can transition to the wedge shoe or offloading pads (Figs. 2.18, 2.19, 2.20, and 2.21).

Large deep wounds: Strict NWB, Total Contact Cast, Wedge Shoes.

Small, shallow wounds: Felt/Foam Pads, Removable Cam walker, Extra-depth shoe.

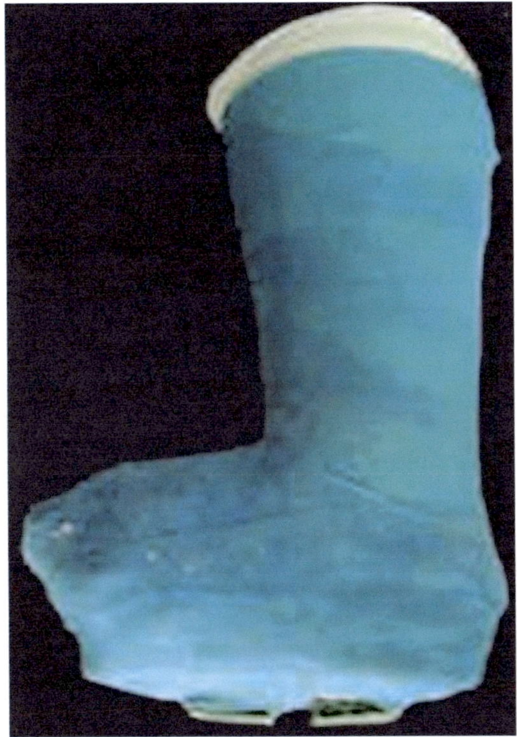

Fig. 2.18 Total contact cast

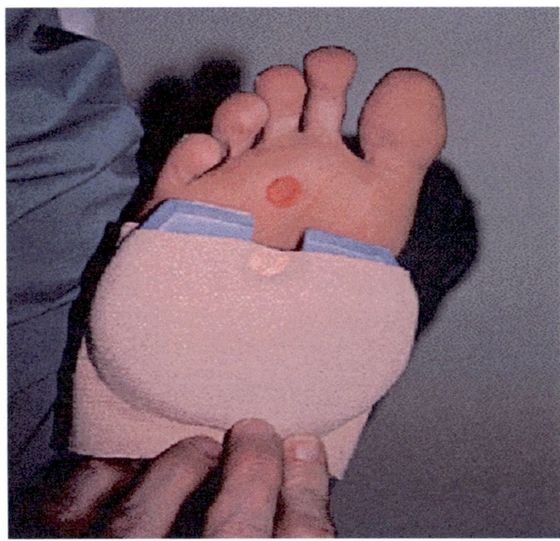

Fig. 2.20 Offloading pads

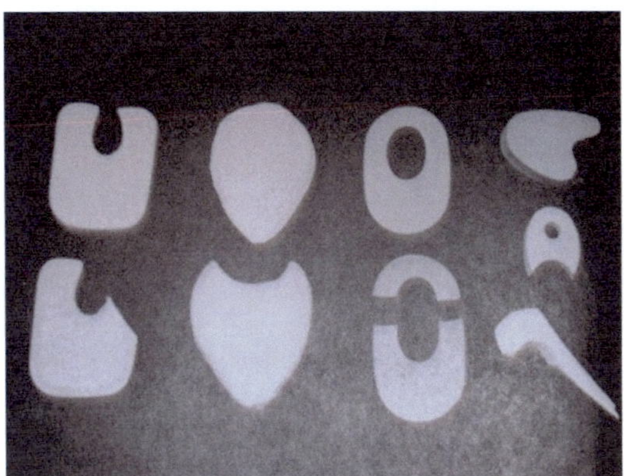

Fig. 2.21 Accommodative padding

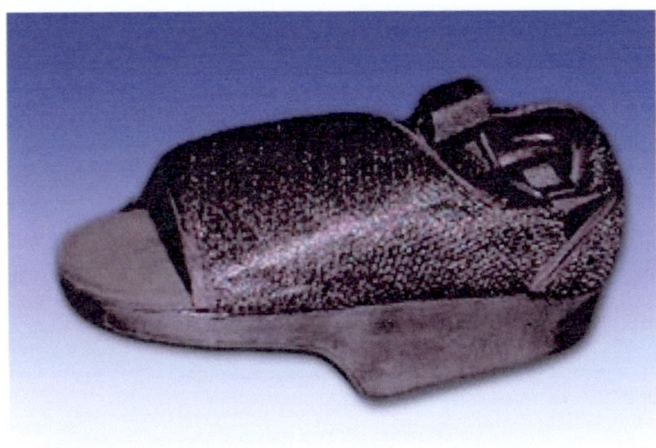

Fig. 2.19 Wedge shoe

2.13 Oxygen Therapy in the Treatment of Chronic Wounds

J. Karim Ead and David G. Armstrong

Wound healing represents a comprehensive series of well-orchestrated physiological reactions that create an orderly healing cascade [11]. This process theoretically includes four key overlapping phases: hemostasis, inflammation, proliferation, and remodeling. It progresses along a continuum that should result in the restoration of anatomical and functional integrity [12]. Acute wounds in a relatively healthy host will continue through the wound healing cascade quickly due to the robust utilization of intrinsic growth factors, cytokines, and matrix proteins that keep the wound on a well-regulated trajectory [11].

In contrast, chronic wounds manifest when the normal healing cascade is interrupted at one or more points during the phases of wound healing (often stagnating in the inflammatory or proliferative phases [13]. Various theories have been proposed to explain why some wounds become chronic and non-healing. Despite the etiological differences in chronic wounds, they often share common pathogenic features. Common causes for chronic inflammation include various inflammatory-based comorbidities, infection, an externally induced pressure injury, devitalized tissue that has been incom-pletely debrided, mechanical insults from retained foreign body, and hypoxia secondary to ischemia [14]. Initial efforts should focus on correcting or ruling out these causes of wound chronicity. Normal tissue repair is a dynamic process that balances deficient and excessive healing (Fig. 2.22).

2.13.1 The Simple SALSA Wound Treatment Guideline: Vertical and Horizontal Approach

- If a wound does not reduce in size by 40% or more after 4 weeks of standard-of-care treatment, consider the utilization of alternative advanced therapies [15, 16].
  - The *"Vertical"* approach is to fill/provide coverage for vital structures using negative pressure wound therapy (NPWT).
    NPWT promotes localized perfusion, increased granulation tissue formation, and facilitates wound closure.
  - The *"Horizontal"* component is achieved via skin grafting (bioengineered or autologous split-thickness skin grafts).
    Offloading is a vital component of wound healing that should be integrated in any treatment algorithm.
- If the wound is older than 3–4 months or not responsive after 4 weeks of therapy; consider *biopsy* to rule out malignancy).

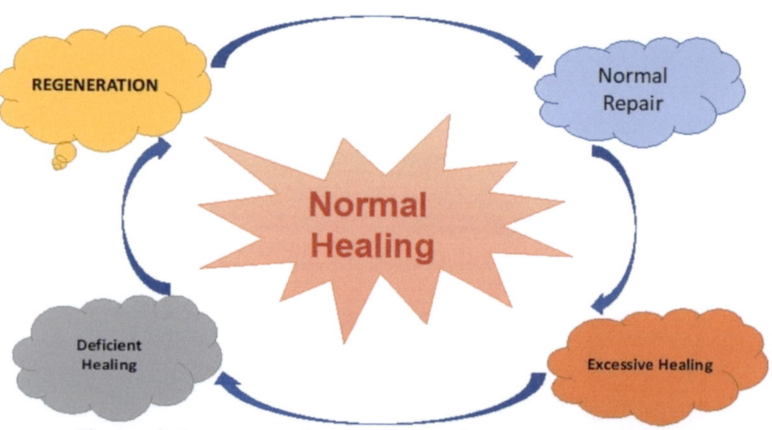

Fig. 2.22 Wound healing is a balance

*SALSA = The Southwestern Academic Limb Salvage Alliance (SALSA).

Chronic wounds are comprised of pro-inflammatory cytokines and proteases that disrupt extracellular matrix communication with other cells in the wound [16]. During these inflammatory states, there is increased oxygen consumption and vascular dysfunction within the wound environment causing hypoxic tissue formation [17]. Oxygen is recognizably essential for life itself, and it is no less essential for wound healing and tissue repair. It is a necessary co-factor for several oxygen-dependent biochemical processes that are vital in the wound healing cascade. The two main oxygen-based therapies include hyperbaric oxygen and topically based oxygen therapies.

2.13.2 Hyperbaric Oxygen Therapy

Hyperbaric oxygen therapy (HBOT) might be considered in situations of chronic wounds that have not responded to the standard of care. Today there are several approved applications and indications/contraindications for HBOT [18]. HBOT mechanism of action on chronic wounds includes localized vascular modulation, angiogenesis, leukocyte oxidative killing, growth factor proliferation, and immune cell revitalization (Fig. 2.23) [19]. Treatment protocols for HBOT vary depending on the suspected pathophysiology.

Simply put, HBOT is utilized to help restore abnormal tissue oxygen tension by applying basic physical gas laws. In certain circumstances, hyperbaric oxygen therapy represents the primary treatment modality, while in others it is an adjunct to surgical or pharmacologic interventions. Treatment is typically performed in either a mono- or a multi-place chamber. In a monoplace chamber, a single patient occupies an entire chamber and is pressurized with 100% oxygen. The patient breathes the ambient chamber oxygen directly. Whereas a multi-place chamber holds two or more people and is pressurized with compressed air while patients breathe 100% oxygen (with masks, head hoods, or endotracheal tubes) [20]. It should be noted that HBOT studies have been ridiculed for significant bias and large numbers of dropouts or adverse events. There will likely be a decline in the use of HBOT therapy without robust evidence regarding optimal therapy for specific wounds.

2.13.3 Topical Oxygen Therapy

Over the years, there has been some controversy as to whether topical oxygen therapy (TOT) can be utilized as a wound healing agent (Fig. 2.24). TOT has been in clinical use for over 50 years with encouraging pre-clinical and clinical studies [21]. However, early studies were observational, including several comparative cohort studies. Even when conducted prospectively, lack of randomized (blinded) studies have led many to suspect its efficacy in the treatment of chronic wounds [22].

There are three general types of delivery systems for TOT:

1. Continuous delivery of oxygen (CDO) at negligible pressures.
2. Low constant pressure delivery in a contained chamber.
3. Higher cyclically pressurized (humidified delivery in a contained extremity chamber).

As previously mentioned, chronic wounds are typically hypoxic, in that the partial pressure of

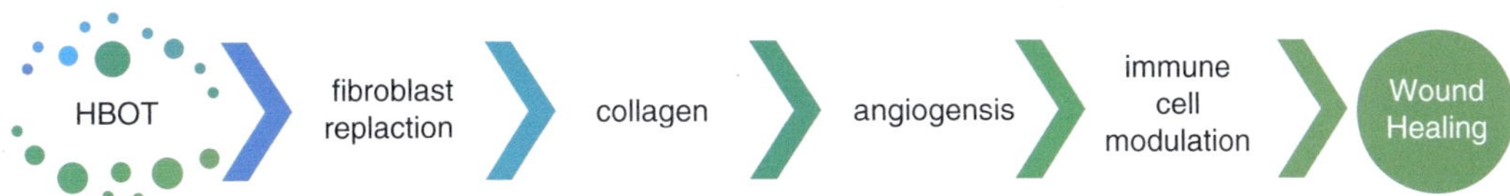

Fig. 2.23 Oxygen and its potential effects on wound healing

O2 Modality	Indications	Relative Cost	Level of evidence	Problems w/ evidence
Topical O2 Therapy	VLU, DFU (Neuro/Neuro ischemic)	+++	Several RCTs, observational, meta-analysis positive results	Numerous devices difficult to compare
HBOT	Neuropathic, ischemic ulcers	+++	Few RCT's showing efficacy	Observer bias, high drop out rates/ adverse events

Fig. 2.24 Head-to-head HBOT vs TOT

oxygen (pO_2) at the central aspect of the wound is often insufficient to support vital biochemical processes required for wound healing and tissue repair. Providing localized topical oxygen can potentially raise pO_2 levels to better optimize enzymatic/cellular function. It should be emphasized that on a molecular level, oxygen is the rate limiting substrate for many vital biochemical reactions in cellular metabolism. Molecular oxygen is, of course, also necessary for the synthesis of nitric oxide (NO) that regulates vasodilation [22].

Oxygen-dependent processes, relevant to wound healing, include the following:

- Mitochondrial-driven adenosine triphosphate (ATP).
  - Production for chemical/cellular energy.
- Nicotinamide adenine dinucleotide phosphate (NADPH) oxidase.
  - Production of ROS ("respiratory burst") involved in signal transduction of growth factors, cellular recruitment, and bacterial killing.

In animal models, TOT mechanism of action has been demonstrated to increase/improve the following:

- Central wound pO_2 from a baseline of 5–7 mmHg to levels of >40 mmHg 4 min into treatment.

- Vascular endothelial growth factor (VEGF) levels.
- Angiogenesis.
- Enhance collagen deposition.

Three recent systematic reviews with meta-analyses focused on the clinical effectiveness of TOT for healing chronic diabetic foot ulcers (DFUs) [22–24]. All three studies indicated that TOT (using CDO and cyclically pressurized devices) can significantly improve wound healing among people with chronic DFUs [23, 25].

2.14 Skin Substitutes and Matrixes Demystified

J. Karim Ead and David G. Armstrong

Advances in cell biology and tissue engineering have led to an increase in the quantity and quality of biological wound dressings, also referred to as biologics, skin substitutes, or matrixes [26]. Skin substitutes are a diverse group of biologics or biosynthetic materials that can provide temporary or permanent coverage of open or ulcerated skin lesions (Fig. 2.25) [27]. These advanced modalities can be a combination of cellular or acellular tissue products, both human and animal derived such as from human placenta, foreskin allografts, fish scales, and other sources. It is

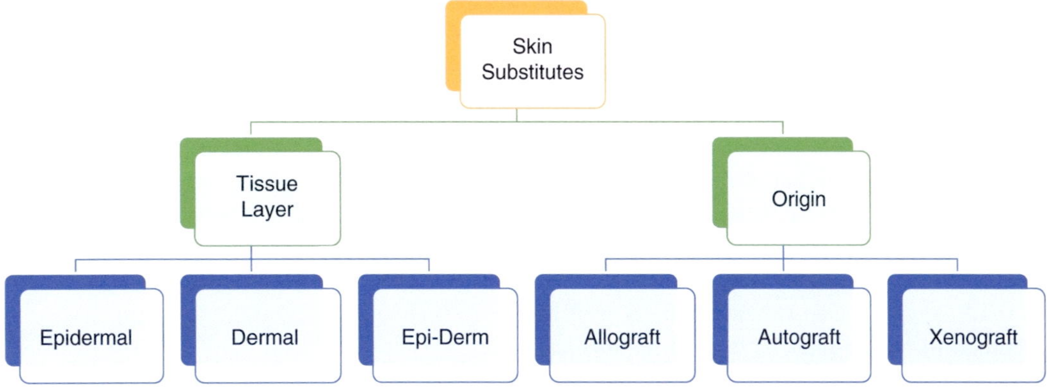

Fig. 2.25 Skin substitutes

essential purpose is to stimulate the host to regenerate lost tissue and replace the wound with functional skin.

Cellular-based therapies, also called bioengineered cellular therapies are comprised of skin cells (fibroblasts, keratinocytes, or both) that create a new source of growth factors, cytokines, and enzymes that promote wound healing and tissue regeneration. For example, one possible treatment option for non-healing ulcers is the use of platelet-rich plasma or platelet-rich fibrin, which have recently been developed into multilayered patches comprising autologous leucocytes, platelets, and fibrin. These patches can be made at the bedside without adding any reagents. This autologous therapy can potentially aid in the release of several key cytokines and growth factors involved in tissue repair, angiogenesis, and inflammation [27].

Goals for treating acute and chronic wounds with skin substitutes are to:

- Provide temporary coverage or permanent wound closure.
- Reduce healing time.
- Reduce post-operative contracture.
- Improve function.
- To decrease morbidity from more invasive treatments such as skin grafting.

Chronic non-healing wounds are often secondary to systemic pathological processes, it is critical that skilled medical personnel encompass a holistic approach in their treatment pathways. In 2019, Samsell et al. conducted a cost-effectiveness study on eight skin substitutes, they found that the costs of a skin substitute itself did not necessarily correlate with its healing efficacy. Snyder et al. conducted a follow-up head-to-head comparative analysis on five skin substitutes and found that an autologous-based graft was more cost-efficient as an advanced therapy in the treatment of diabetic foot ulcers when compared to four other advanced cellular-based tissue products [28].

Armstrong et al. retrospectively analyzed data from the Medicare Limited Dataset [29]. They took a close look at patients receiving care for lower extremity diabetic foot ulcerations treated with advanced treatment (AT) versus no advanced treatment (NAT). The advanced treatment included patients receiving skin substitutes (cellular and acellular dermal grafts) derived mostly from human placental membranes and animal tissue sources [22].

Key variables in the study included major and minor amputations, emergency department (ED) visits, and hospital readmissions. It was discovered that AT for diabetic ulcers resulted in fewer Major and Minor amputations, ED visits, and Re-Admissions when compared to NAT.

These findings emphasize the importance of choosing the appropriate advanced skin substitutes that are both effective and cost efficient when considering a treatment plan for patients with non-healing lower extremity wounds.

2.15 This Patient Needs to be Admitted Now

J. Karim Ead and David G. Armstrong

The incidence of skin and soft tissue infections (SSTI) in the general population has been increasing in recent years. Consequently, increasing the number of patients being seen and treated in the Emergency Department (ED), as well as admitted to the hospital. It is vital for medical personnel to utilize evidence-based consensus guidelines for the management of suspected SSTI [30]. These conditions are subdivided into specific categories (non-purulent, purulent, ulcerative, and recurrent/refractory SSTI) (Fig. 2.26). Recent data suggests that lower extremity-based ED visits generate 81.2% hospital admission rate with an annual bill of at least $1.2 billion in the United States alone [12].

The likelihood of hospital admission, amputation, and other subsequent adverse outcomes is associated with three key factors [31]:

1. Wound severity (degree of tissue loss)
2. Ischemia
3. Foot infection

The Infectious Diseases Society of America (IDSA) recommends clinicians to consider the possibility of infection occurring in any foot/lower extremity wound (especially in the diabetic patient) [29]. If an in-office patient presents with significant tissue loss, a thorough history and physical exam should be performed. If there are obvious signs of either infection or ischemia, hospital admission should be advised (Fig. 2.27).

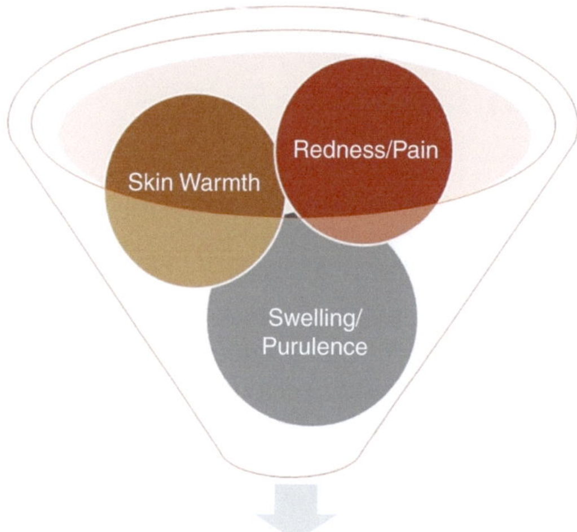

Fig. 2.27 Evidence of infection includes classic signs of inflammation

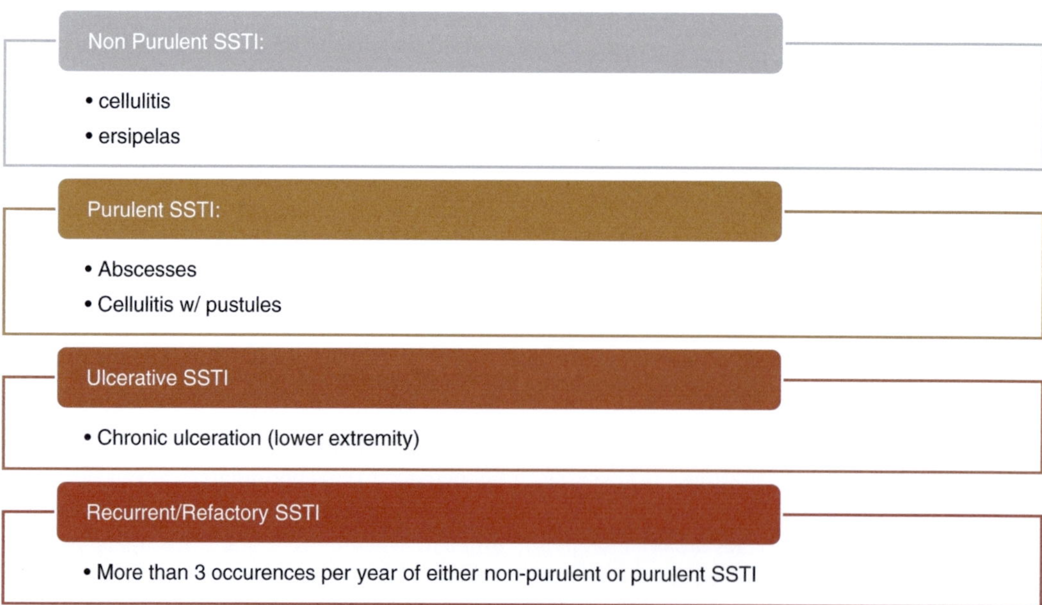

Fig. 2.26 SSTI definitions

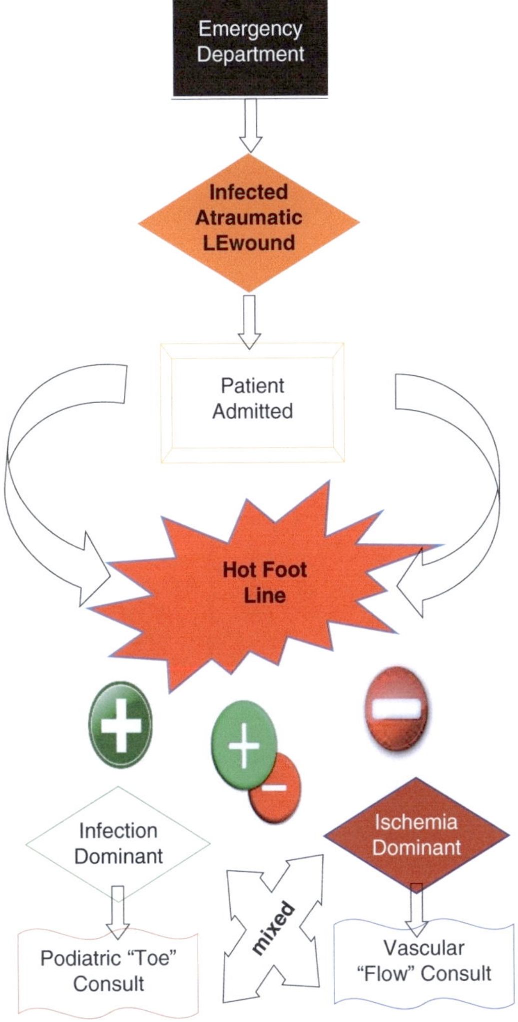

Fig. 2.28 Inpatient "Hot Foot Line" Algorithm

Upon further workup in the ED, plain film radiographs and a complete blood count with differential should be ordered. Once the patient is admitted to the hospital, the Hot Foot Line (if established), or a wound care vascular specialist ideally should be consulted for further workup (Fig. 2.28). Suspicion of osteomyelitis or presence of soft tissue gas on plain film radiographs alone indicates the need for immediate hot foot line consultation. Once this process has been initiated, the members will evaluate the dominant clinical findings of ischemia and/or infection.

This comprehensive workup may then be used to guide the course of both short- and long-term managements (Fig. 2.29) [32].

Patients that are immunocompromised may present with secondary signs that include:

- Non-purulent secretions
- Friable or discolored granulation tissue
- Undermining of wound edges
- Foul odor

It should be emphasized that the most important therapy for an SSTI is to open the incision, evacuate the infected material, and continue dressing changes until the wound heals by secondary intention. A decision to hospitalize, administer antibiotics directed against *S. aureus* as an adjunct to incision and drainage should be made based on clinical presentation and with presence or absence of systemic inflammatory response syndrome (SIRS) features such as:

- Temperature >38 °C or <36 °C
- Tachypnea >24 breaths per minute
- Tachycardia >90 beats per minute
- White blood cell count >12,000 or <400 cells/μL

Deep infections that include the fascial and/or muscle compartments could potentially lead to significant tissue destruction and death. Necrotizing infections typically develop from an initial break in the skin secondary to trauma or surgery. There is a plethora of bacterial species that instigate these necrotizing infections. The initial approach to diagnosis, antibiotic therapy, and surgical intervention is similar for all forms and is more important than determining the specific variant [19]. The IDSA/PEDIS guideline should be referenced when assessing/stratifying the severity of infection (Fig. 2.30) [33].

Surgical intervention is the primary therapeutic modality in cases of necrotizing fasciitis or severe soft tissue infections. Features suggestive of necrotizing fasciitis include:

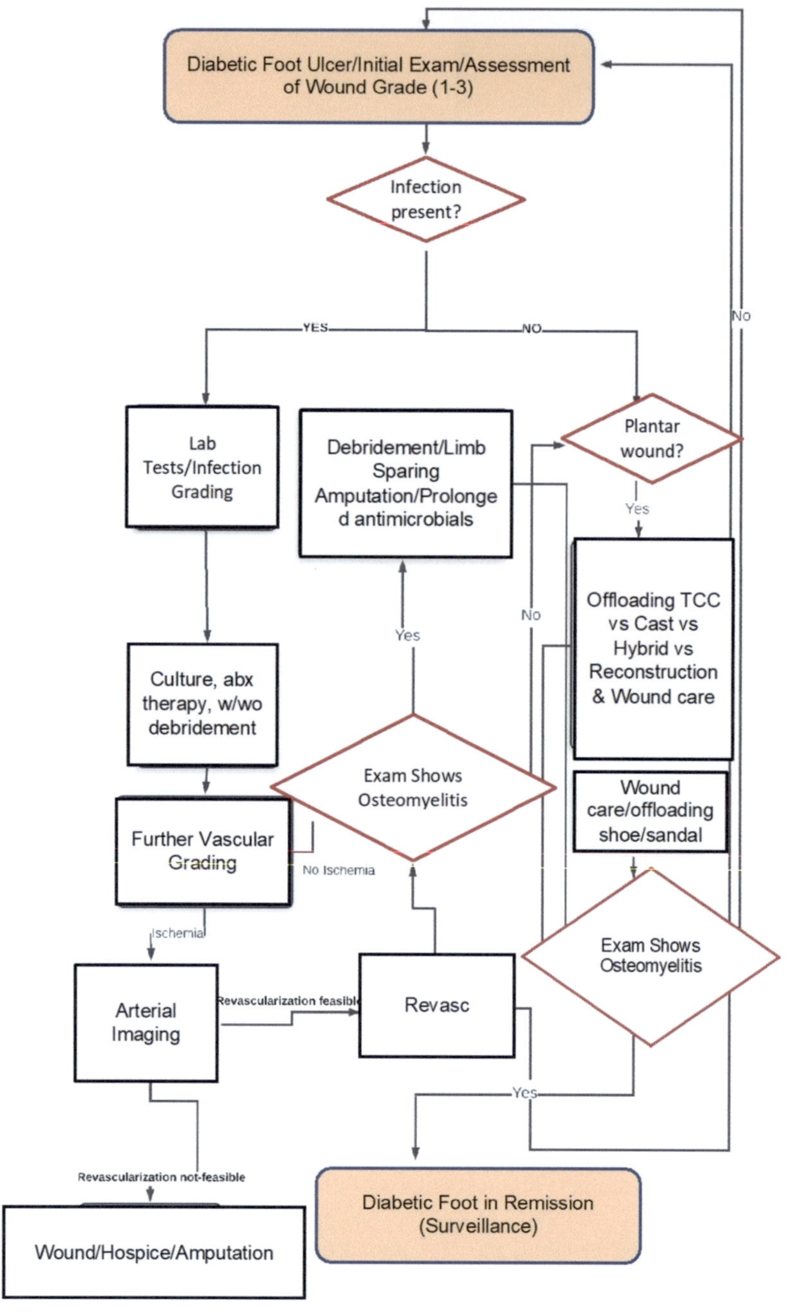

Fig. 2.29 Assessment of the diabetic foot decision tree—adapted from Armstrong et al.

- Infectious processes include superficial and deep muscle compartments.
- Failure of uncomplicated cellulitis to respond to antibiotics after a reasonable trial.
- Profound toxicity: Fever, hypotension, or advancement of the SSTI during antibiotic therapy.

- Skin necrosis with easy dissection along the fascia by a blunt instrument; or presence of gas in the soft tissues.

These conditions warrant immediate surgical intervention (deep cultures), hospitalization,

foot Infection		
Grade	**Clinical manifestation of infection**	**IDSA/PEDIS infection severity**
0	No symptoms or signs of infection	Uninfected
1	Infection present, as defined by the presence of at least two of the following items: • Local swelling or induration • Erythema >0.5 to ≤2 cm around the ulcer • Local tenderness or pain • Local warmth • Purulent discharge (thick, opaque to white, or sanguineous secretion)	Mild
	Local infection involving only the skin and the subcutaneous tissue (without systemic signs). Exclude other causes of an inflammatory response of the skin (e.g., trauma, gout, acute Charcot Neuro-osteoarthropathy, fracture, thrombosis, venous stasis)	
2	Local infection (as described above) with erythema >2 cm, or involving structures deeper than skin and subcutaneous tissues (e.g., abscess, osteomyelitis, septic arthritis, fasciitis)	Moderate
	No systemic inflammatory response signs (as described below)	
3	Local infection (as described above) with the signs of SIRS as manifested by two or more of the following: • Temperature >38° or <36°C • Heart rate >90 beats/min • Respiratory, rate >20 breaths/min or $PaCO_2$ <32 mmHg • White blood cell count >12,000 or <4000 cu/mm or 10% immature (band) forms	Severe[a]
$PaCO_2$, Partial pressure of arterial carbon dioxide; *SIRS,* systemic inflammatory response syndrome		
[a]Ischaemia may complicate and increase the severity of any infection. Systemic infection may sometimes manifest with other clinical findings, such as hypotension, confusion, vomiting, or evidence of metabolic disturbances, such as acidosis, severe hyperglycaemia, new-onset azotaemia.		

Fig. 2.30 IDSA/SVS WIfI Wound Severity Classification Clinical manifestation of infection SVS WIfI IDSA Infection Severity

aggressive broad-spectrum IV antibiotic therapy, and continuous medical observation.

2.16 Soft Tissue Reconstruction Options

Idanis Perez-Alvarez, David Kurlander, and Amir Dorafshar

An array of non-surgical and surgical options exists for reconstruction of lower extremity wounds in patients with peripheral vascular disease. Local wound factors including size, location, exposed structures, infection, contamination, and blood flow may dictate the means of reconstruction. Additionally, patient factors including medical comorbidities, nutritional status, compliance, function, and expectations may influence the surgical plan [34, 35].

Successful outcomes for reconstruction rely on aggressive patient and wound optimization. Often this requires serial debridement and prolonged wound care to remove all devitalized tissue and infection as pre-requisite for definitive reconstruction. Patients must be counselled regarding the journey required for reconstruction, associated risks of interventions, and potential for failure that may result in major amputation.

2.16.1 Reconstructive Options

After the decision is made to proceed with limb salvage, and the patient and wound have been optimized, realistic goals must be agreed upon with the patient. Most commonly this includes durable weight-bearing bony support, restoring stable soft tissue coverage, adequate wound healing, and achieving pain-free mobility [36]. The "reconstructive ladder" provides a systematic approach to wound reconstruction. At the bottom of the ladder are simpler techniques traditionally used for simpler wounds. At the top of the ladder are more complex techniques required to treat more complex wounds (Fig. 2.31).

As one starts from the bottom of the ladder, simple techniques are utilized for wound management. Moving up the ladder, more complex wounds require more involved techniques

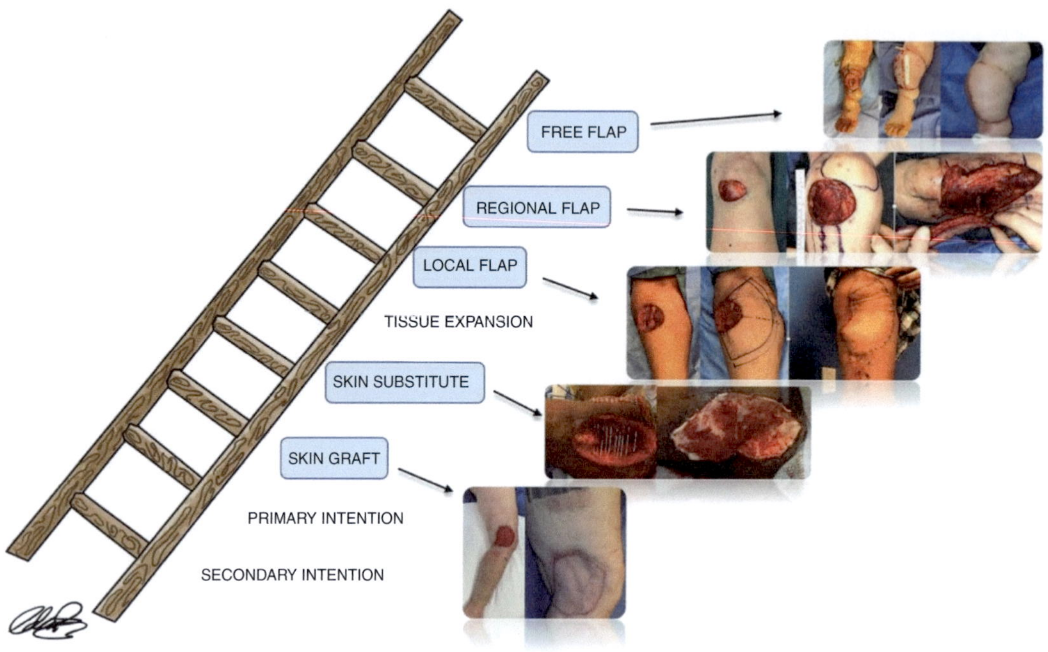

Fig. 2.31 Reconstructive ladder for lower extremity reconstruction

such as flaps. Case examples of a few of the techniques are shown to the right. Images from D. Kurlander MD.

2.16.1.1 Primary Intention

Primary intention refers to approximating the wound edges with suture. This is infrequently the ideal option for patients with vascular disease and chronic wounds either because there are concerns for wound healing when blood supply is compromised, or tension prevents adequate wound edge opposition. An example of primary closure in patients with vascular disease is layered repair of a fasciotomy wound.

2.16.1.2 Secondary Intention

Secondary intention refers to spontaneous wound healing using local wound care products to facilitate wound contraction and epithelialization. Skin substitutes may also facilitate wound closure by secondary intention and reduce fibrosis. Secondary intention is indicated for small wounds and for patients unable to tolerate more advanced reconstructive techniques.

2.16.1.3 Skin Grafts

A split thickness skin graft (STSG) involves harvest of the epidermis and partial dermis. Secondary intention healing occurs at the donor site. A full-thickness skin graft (FTSG) includes harvest of the epidermis and full thickness of dermis. Primary donor site closure is performed. The full or split thickness skin graft is secured to a healthy, well-vascularized wound bed. Skin grafts heal by plasmatic imbibition of nutrients from the wound bed, inosculation (aligning of the skin graft and wound bed capillaries), and revascularization. Skin graft healing takes about 5 days and can be compromised by sheering, infection, fluid collection, or an inadequately prepared wound bed. Exposed bone, tendon, nerve, and vessels are relative contraindications to skin graft.

For lower extremity reconstruction, STSGs are typically harvested from the thigh and can cover large wounds. FTSG are typically harvested from the groin for smaller wounds. Full-thickness skin grafts have less secondary contracture but are limited by ratio of donor site area to recipient wound size.

2.16.1.4 Adjacent Tissue Transfer

Adjacent tissue transfer implies rotation, advancement, or transposition of skin and subcutaneous tissue with unnamed (random) blood supply to close a wound. This is indicated when sufficient healthy tissue and laxity surround the wound. Adjacent tissue transfer can be used to cover wounds lacking a vascular bed, including those with exposed bone, tendon, and hardware. An example of adjacent tissue transfer includes V-Y advancement (term describing incision pattern) of tissue to close a plantar first metatarsal wound with exposed bone.

2.16.1.5 Regional Flaps

Flaps, unlike grafts, have blood supply from a named (axial) vessel allowing perfusion independent of the surrounding tissues. Flaps can also cover wounds lacking a vascular bed, including those with exposed bone, tendon, and hardware. Flaps can be comprised of muscle, skin, fascia, bone, or multiple tissue types supplied by a commonly named vessel. Examples of conventional regional flap use in lower extremity limb salvage include:

1. Gastrocnemius muscle flap for proximal third tibia wounds.
2. Soleus muscle flap for middle third tibia wounds.
3. Peroneus brevis muscle flap for lateral malleolus wounds.
4. Medial plantar artery flap for heel wounds.

2.16.1.6 Free Flaps

Free flaps are defined by harvest of tissue based on a named vessel, transfer to a distant location, and re-perfusion of the tissue by arterial and venous microvascular anastomosis. Free flaps are indicated when no regional flap option is sufficient or available, which is common for larger wounds with exposed bone or hardware of the distal third of the leg, ankle, and foot. Free flap success depends on arterial inflow and venous outflow. Recipient vessels most common in the leg are the posterior tibial and anterior tibial arteries. Microvascular arterial anastomosis is typically performed in an end-to-side manner to preserve distal perfusion, especially when less than three vessel runoff to the foot is present. Common free flaps used in the lower extremity include:

1. Latissimus muscle or myocutaneous flap
2. Rectus abdominis muscle flap
3. Gracilis muscle flap
4. Anterolateral thigh fasciocutaneous flap

2.16.2 Amputation Optimization

Some patients are not candidates for any of these reconstructive options and some patients fail wound reconstruction leading to amputation. As in patients who undergo limb salvage, the patient and the extremity should be optimized to maximize perfusion and wound healing for amputation. Should wounds of an amputated extremity occur, all options of the reconstructive ladder are available to preserve length, in addition to shortening of the amputation. The residual limb should have maximally preserved length, be suitable for a prosthetic, and be pain free.

Patients requiring major limb amputation may benefit from active nerve management to prevent phantom and neuroma pain with targeted muscle reinnervation (TMR) [37]. TMR involves coapting the ends of transected sensory or mixed nerves (e.g., tibial nerve) to redundant, expendable motor branches to minimize risk of chronic pain, otherwise seen in nearly two-thirds of patients who have vascular disease and amputation [38]. TMR is also indicated for treatment of chronic amputation-related phantom and residual limb pain.

References

1. Steinburg JS, Kim PJ. Evaluation and Management of the Diabetic foot wound. In: Southerland JT, Boberg JS, Downey MS, Nakra A, Rabjohn LV, editors. McGlamry's comprehensive textbook of foot and ankle surgery, vol. 2. 4th ed. Philadelphia, PA: Lippincott Williams & Wilkins; 2013. p. 986–1007.
2. Ledoux WR, Shofer JB, Smith DG. Relationship between foot type, foot deformity, and ulcer

occurrence in the high-risk diabetic foot. J Rehabil Res Dev. 2005;42(5):665–72.

3. Wagner FW. The diabetic foot. Orthopedics. 1987;10(1):163–72.

4. Meggit B. Surgical management of the diabetic foot. Br J Hosp Med. 1976;16:227–32.

5. National Pressure Sore Advisory Panel. Consensus Development Conference Staging System, February 2007. http://www.npuap.org/pr2.htm (Accessed August 7, 2011).

6. Bhrem H, Sheehan P, Boulton AJM. Protocol for treatment of diabetic foot ulcers. Am J Surg. 2004;187(Suppl):1S–10S.

7. Sheehan P, Jones P, Casselli A, et al. Percent change in wound area of diabetic foot ulcers over a 4 week period is a robust predictor of complete healing in a 12 week prospective trial. Diabetes Care. 2003;26(6):1879–82.

8. Holloway S, Harling KG. Wound dressings. Wound Manage. 2021;10:25–32.

9. Anderson K, Hamm RL. Factors that impair wound healing. J Am Coll Clin Wound Specialist. 2014;4:84–91.

10. Haalboom M, Blokhauis-Arkes MHE, Beuk RR, Meerwaldt R, Klont R, Schijffelen MJ, Bowler RB, Burnet M, Sigl E, van der Palen JAM. Culture results from wound biopsy verses swab: does it matter for the assessment of wound infection? Clin Microbiol Infect. 2019;25:629.e7–629.e12.

11. Snyder RJ, Driver V, Fife CE, Lantis J, Peirce B, Serena T, et al. Using a diagnostic tool to identify elevated protease activity levels in chronic and stalled wounds: a consensus panel discussion. Ostomy Wound Manage. 2011;57:36–46.

12. Eming SA, Martin P, Tomic-Canic M. Wound repair and regeneration: mechanisms, signaling, and translation. Sci Transl Med. 2014;6(265):265sr6. https://doi.org/10.1126/scitranslmed.3009337.

13. Schultz GS, Chin GA, Moldawer L, et al. Principles of wound healing. In: Fitridge R, Thompson M, editors. Mechanisms of vascular disease: a reference book for vascular specialists [Internet]. Adelaide (AU): University of Adelaide Press; 2011. p. 23. Available from: https://www.ncbi.nlm.nih.gov/books/NBK534261/.

14. Liu YF, Ni PW, Huang Y, Xie T. Therapeutic strategies for chronic wound infection. Chin J Traumatol. 2022;25(1):11–6. https://doi.org/10.1016/j.cjtee.2021.07.004.

15. Pappalardo J, Plemmons B, Armstrong D. wound healing simplification: a vertical and horizontal philosophy illustrated. J Wound Technol. 2013;19:38–9.

16. Snyder RJ, Kirsner RS, Warriner RA 3rd, Lavery LA, Hanft JR, Sheehan P. Consensus recommendations on advancing the standard of care for treating neuropathic foot ulcers in patients with diabetes. Ostomy Wound Manage. 2010;56:S1–S24.

17. Hong WX, Hu MS, Esquivel M, Liang GY, Rennert RC, McArdle A, Paik KJ, Duscher D, Gurtner GC, Lorenz HP, Longaker MT. The role of hypoxia-inducible factor in wound healing. Adv Wound Care. 2014;3(5):390–9. https://doi.org/10.1089/wound.2013.0520.

18. Gesell LB, editor. Hyperbaric oxygen therapy indications. 12th ed. Durham, NC: Undersea and Hyperbaric Medical Society; 2008.

19. Bhutani S, Vishwanath G. Hyperbaric oxygen and wound healing. Indian J Plastic Surg. 2012;45(2):316–24. https://doi.org/10.4103/0970-0358.101309.

20. Shah J. Hyperbaric oxygen therapy. J Am Coll Certified Wound Specialists. 2010;2(1):9–13. https://doi.org/10.1016/j.jcws.2010.04.001.

21. "New Evidence- Based Therapies for Complex Diabetic Foot Wounds - ADA Compendium Boulton Armstrong et Al 2022.pdf." n.d.

22. Nataraj M, Maiya AG, Karkada G, et al. Application of topical oxygen therapy in healing dynamics of diabetic foot ulcers: a systematic review. Rev Diabet Stud. 2019;15:74–82.

23. Connaghan F, Avsar P, Patton D, O'Connor T, Moore Z. Impact of topical oxygen therapy on diabetic foot ulcer healing rates: a systematic review. J Wound Care. 2021;30:823–9.

24. Armstrong DG, Boulton AJM, Bus SA. Diabetic foot ulcers and their recurrence. N Engl J Med. 2017;376(24):2367–75. https://doi.org/10.1056/NEJMra1615439.

25. Thanigaimani S, Singh T, Golledge J. Topical oxygen therapy for diabetes-related foot ulcers: a systematic review and meta-analysis. Diabet Med. 2021;38:e14585.

26. Ho J, Walsh C, Yue D, Dardik A, Cheema U. Current advancements and strategies in tissue engineering for wound healing: a comprehensive review. Adv Wound Care. 2017;6(6):191–209. https://doi.org/10.1089/wound.2016.0723.

27. Figus A, Leon-Villapalos J, Philp B, Dziewulski P. Severe multiple extensive postburn contractures: a simultaneous approach with total scar tissue excision and resurfacing with dermal regeneration template. J Burn Care Res. 2007 Nov-Dec;28(6):913–7. https://doi.org/10.1097/BCR.0b013e318159eb8c.

28. Snyder DL, Sullivan N, Schoelles KM. Skin substitutes for treating chronic wounds. Final report. Rockville (MD): Agency for Healthcare Research and Quality (AHRQ); 2012 Dec 18. 203 p. (Technology assessment report; Also available: http://www.ahrq.gov/research/findings/ta/skinsubs/HCPR0610_skinsubst-final.pdf.

29. Armstrong DG, Tettelbach WH, Chang TJ, De Jong JL, Glat PM, Hsu JH, Kelso MR, Niezgoda JA, Tucker TL, Labovitz JM. Observed impact of skin substitutes in lower extremity diabetic ulcers: lessons from the Medicare Database (2015–2018). J Wound Care. 2021;30(Sup7):S5–S16. https://doi.org/10.12968/jowc.2021.30.Sup7.S5.

30. Kaye KS, Petty LA, Shorr AF, Zilberberg MD. Current epidemiology, etiology, and burden of acute skin infections in the united states. Clin Infect Dis.

2019;68(Suppl 3):S193–9. https://doi.org/10.1093/cid/ciz002.

31. Stevens DL, Bisno AL, Chambers HF, Patchen Dellinger E, Goldstein EJC, Gorbach SL, Hirschmann JV, Kaplan SL, Montoya JG, Wade JC. Practice Guidelines for the diagnosis and management of skin and soft tissue infections: 2014 Update by the Infectious Diseases Society of America. Clin Infect Dis. 2014;59(2):e10–52. https://doi.org/10.1093/cid/ciu296.

32. Mills JL, Conte MS, Armstrong DG, Pomposelli FB, Schanzer A, Sidawy AN, Andros G, Society for Vascular Surgery Lower Extremity Guidelines Committee. The Society for Vascular Surgery lower extremity threatened limb classification system: risk stratification based on Wound, Ischemia, and foot Infection (WIfI). J Vasc Surg. 2014;59(1):220–34. based on Wound, Ischemia, and foot Infection (WIfI). Journal of Vascular Surgery. 2014;59(1):220–234.e2

33. Miller JD, Lew EJ, Giovinco NA, et al. How to create a hot foot line to prevent diabetes-related amputations: instant triage for emergency department and inpatient consultations. J Am Podiatr Med Assoc. 2019;109(2):174–9.

34. Black CK, Zolper EG, Ormiston LD, Schwitzer JA, Luvisa K, Attinger CE, et al. Free anterolateral thigh versus vastus lateralis muscle flaps for coverage of lower extremity defects in chronic wounds. Ann Plast Surg. 2020 Jul;85(S1):S54–9.

35. Hollenbeck ST, Toranto JD, Taylor BJ, Ho TQ, Zenn MR, Erdmann D, et al. Perineal and lower extremity reconstruction. Plast Reconstr Surg. 2011;128(5):551e–63e.

36. Wei FC, Mardini S. Flaps and reconstructive surgery; 2017.

37. Dumanian GA, Potter BK, Mioton LM, Ko JH, Cheesborough JE, Souza JM, et al. Targeted muscle reinnervation treats neuroma and phantom pain in major limb amputees: a randomized clinical trial. Ann Surg. 2019;270(2):238–46.

38. Chang BL, Mondshine J, Attinger CE, Kleiber GM. Targeted muscle reinnervation improves pain and ambulation outcomes in highly comorbid amputees. Plast Reconstr Surg. 2021;148(2):376–86.

Determining the Appropriate Workup

Mary Costantino, Faris Galambo, Ryan Lutz, Sreekumar Madassery, Nicholas Petruzzi, Jill Sommerset, David M. Tabriz, Desarom Teso, and Ulku C. Turba

3.1 When to Utilize ABI, Arterial Duplex, and Advanced Anatomical Imaging

Nicholas Petruzzi

Non-invasive imaging has utility in screening wounded patients for peripheral arterial disease (PAD) and venous disease, aiding with patient selection for intervention and outcome documentation/surveillance. Non-invasive arterial testing can be divided into two broad categories: functional tests and anatomic tests. Functional tests include the ankle-brachial index (ABI), segmental pressures and pulse volume recordings (PVRs), segmental Doppler waveforms, skin perfusion pressures (SPP), tissue oxygen testing (TcPO2), and venous insufficiency testing. This contrasts with anatomical testing, which includes duplex ultrasound (US), CT angiography (CTA), and Magnetic Resonance Imaging (MRI, MRA, MRV). The choice of appropriate testing can vary widely depending on the patient's symptomatology, presentation (acute vs chronic, gangrene, tissue loss or rest pain, venous stasis changes, etc.), and comorbidities.

3.1.1 When Should I Order ABI, Toe Pressures, or Arterial Duplex?

All patients presenting with lower extremity ulcers should be assessed for the presence of arterial disease including those with suspected venous etiology [1]. The specific test of choice, however, may vary depending on patient presentation and comorbidities among other factors.

The initial examination for a vascular specialist evaluating a wounded patient requires a thorough history, detailed pulse examination, and an ABI. For the CLI/CLTI patient, the ABI should be considered as one of the "vital signs of the limb." All patients with wounds should have an initial ABI calculated both to determine etiology, guide surgical/interventional therapy, and determine suitability for compression if warranted.

It is common to encounter mixed arterial/venous etiology of initially "venous appearing"

M. Costantino · J. Sommerset
Advanced Vascular Centers, Springfield, OR, USA
e-mail: m.costantino@advasc.com

F. Galambo · R. Lutz · S. Madassery (✉)
D. M. Tabriz · U. C. Turba
Department of Vascular and Interventional Radiology, Rush University Medical Center, Chicago, IL, USA
e-mail: Faris_Galambo@rush.edu;
Ryan_W_Lutz@rush.edu; David_M_Tabriz@rush.edu;
Ulku_C_Turba@rush.edu

N. Petruzzi
The Vascular Institute at AMI, Brick Township, NJ, USA
e-mail: Npetruzzi@aminj.com

D. Teso
Elson S. Floyd College of Medicine, Washington State University, Pullman, WA, USA

wounds, and as such, ABI testing and pulse examination remain crucial. If the initial ABI or pulse examination is abnormal then further testing is warranted.

The ABI, however, is not without its own significant limitations, and therefore it should be understood that this is a screening test. A systematic review showed a sensitivity ranging from 15% to 79% and specificity from 83% to 100% for detecting >50% vessel stenosis in the lower limb [2]. A significant portion of CLI/CLTI patients will have abnormally elevated ABIs or noncompressible vessels secondary to medial calcinosis, often seen in renal failure and diabetic patients. This can falsely underestimate disease or even "pseudo-normalize" the ABI value. These patients should be considered for more advanced functional or anatomical testing.

3.1.2 The Role of PVR and Segmental Pressure Studies

3.1.2.1 Segmental Pressures

Once PAD has been confirmed via an abnormal ABI measurement, segmental limb pressures can aid with identification of the anatomic location and severity. This is performed by comparing systolic blood pressure measurements at various sites, such as the thighs, calves, and ankles.

A pressure drop of >20 mmHg from one level to the next, or a lateral pressure difference of >20 mm Hg is typically considered indicative of significant disease [3]. In patients with ischemic ulceration an absolute ankle SBP of <50 mmHg is independently associated with poor ulcer healing [4, 5].

3.1.2.2 Pulse Volume Recordings

Similar to segmental pressure recordings, pulse volume recording (PVR) tracings provide additional physiological information and these two tests are typically combined. Volume changes that occur with pulsatility during diastole and systole correlate with the presence of arterial flow. Pressure transducers in the pneumatic cuffs can provide plethysmography tracings. Early changes of obstruction can be detected in the

arterial waveform by loss of a dicrotic notch on the downslope whereas blunting of the entire waveform can be seen in more severe PAD [6, 7].

3.1.3 Role of TBI, TCP02, or Skin Perfusion Pressures

3.1.3.1 Toe Brachial Index

Toe pressures and Toe Brachial Index (TBI) are valuable when the ABI value is elevated, inconclusive, or noncompressible, often seen in diabetic and renal failure patients with heavy medial artery calcifications. TBI is performed by measuring the highest systolic pressure in the toes on each foot and dividing by the highest systolic pressure of the brachial arteries.

A Photoplethysmograph (PPG) sensor is placed on the toe distally to a small blood pressure cuff to determine the systolic pressure at which the tracing returns. Toe Pressures have variability in what is considered normal, with consensus that <30 mmHg is indicative of poor healing in diabetic foot ulcers, and <70–96 mmHg may be indicative of PAD in patients where ABI may not be conclusive.

A normal TBI cutoff value is >0.70. Although this is not strictly evidence based and studies have shown variable sensitivities ranging from 0.60 to 0.75 cutoff [8, 9]. If the TBI is abnormal and revascularization is not being primarily considered, then a TcP02 or SPP can be considered to evaluate the likelihood of wound healing, which will be further discussed.

3.1.3.2 Tissue Oxygen Testing

Tissue oxygen testing (TcPO2) is a metabolic test that measures the oxygenation of tissues in the peri-wound tissues. However, it is not the equivalent of a pulse oximetry reading. Instead, it determines the actual partial pressure of oxygen in the tissue. An electrode is heated, and a sensor is attached to the skin via a gas permeable membrane. If the value is abnormal, then a "challenge" must be administered to determine the etiology, with arterial disease being only one of many factors that can reduce TcPO2. Interestingly, TcPO2 may also be abnormally depressed in chronic wounds of venous etiology with severe post-thrombotic syndrome [10].

In general, TcPO2 measurements <40 mmHg predicts poor wound healing potential [11].

3.1.3.3 Skin Perfusion Pressure

Skin Perfusion Pressure (SPP) is a noninvasive means to evaluate the pressure of capillary opening after occlusion. This is done by inflating a cuff to occlude flow and then slowly deflating the cuff to allow return of flow. A laser device senses the pressure at which the blood flow to skin is returned. SPP has advantages in that it is quicker to perform than TcPO2, can be used on more areas of skin including callous or digits, and is not as affected by vessel calcification. A cutoff value of 40 mmHg or greater is typically considered sufficient for wound healing.

Lo and colleagues compared SPP and TcPO2 in terms of ability to predict healing outcomes in 100 patients with lower extremity wounds. A threshold of <30 mmHg was selected as the cutoff below which the test was considered significantly abnormal and indicative of a wound unlikely to heal. SPP alone successfully predicted outcome in 87% of the patients compared to TcPO2 at a rate of 64% ($P < 0.0002$) [12].

In patients who cannot have toe pressures obtained, SPP can be a suitable alternative to predict wound healing potential.

3.1.4 When and Why Do I Need Cross-Sectional/Anatomic Imaging?

In modern-day practice, arterial duplex US, CTA, or MRA can be extremely beneficial for planning the method and approach of revascularization. This is especially true in CLI/CLTI where the findings can help direct initial access sites. This may also supplant the need for conventional arteriography in some patients that may be deemed candidates for open surgery such as bypass and/or endarterectomy. Arterial duplex is also a simple, inexpensive, and non-invasive means of monitoring stents or intervention site patency. Cross-sectional imaging with CTA can be critical in patients with extensive surgical history as well.

In the authors' practice, we perform a thorough vascular examination, and obtain ABI values and standard vital signs at every patient's initial visit and follow-up visits. If arterial etiology of the wound is suspected, more advanced testing can be obtained. This is typical via lower extremity arterial duplex or CTA/MRA with runoff. If inflow disease is suspected CTA is strongly preferred if renal function allows. Both modalities inform the operator of available access sites, enable the physician to better inform the patient as to the anatomic levels involved, as well as the associated anticipated success rates and long-term patency.

3.1.4.1 Arterial Duplex

Arterial duplex has several benefits over ABI, TBI, and PVR/segmental pressures. B-mode (grayscale) imaging provides anatomic detail as to the appearance of the artery, size, calcification, and length of occlusions. In addition to anatomic imaging, functional data such as the waveform appearance, upslope, and phasicity can be assessed.

Arterial duplex is used as the main method of continued surveillance post-intervention, especially in the infrainguinal distribution. When compared to the gold standard of digital subtraction angiography (DSA), agreement is best in the supragenicular segments than in the infragenicular segments [13].

Several criteria exist for categorizing stenosis. In general, velocity ratios greater than 2:1 when compared to the more proximal segment, correlates with a significant lesion of over 50%. Velocity ratios greater than this (i.e., 2.5:1, 3:1, and 3.5:1), signify increasing degrees of stenosis [14, 15].

Figures 3.1 and 3.2 demonstrate color and spectral Doppler evaluation of the common femoral artery and the dorsalis pedis.

High-resolution US images can be obtained in the distal runoff vessels both for confirming patency and pre-planning alternate access sites prior to intervention. However, duplex ultrasonography does have overall limited utility in providing the detail necessary for assessment of the smallest vessels, such as plantar arch and beyond, in the forefoot.

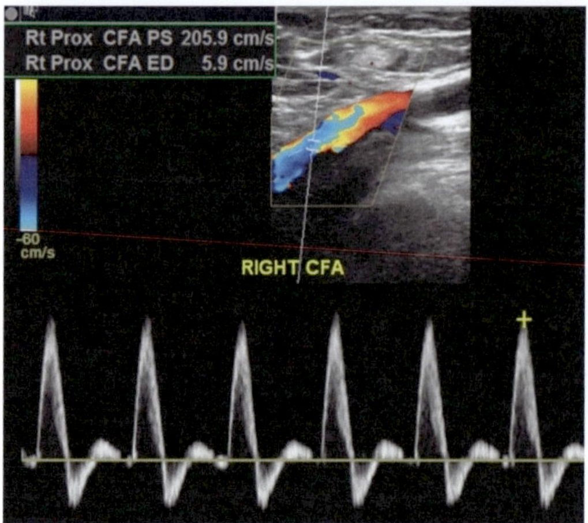

Fig. 3.1 Color and spectral arterial duplex showing patent common femoral artery with multiphasic waveform

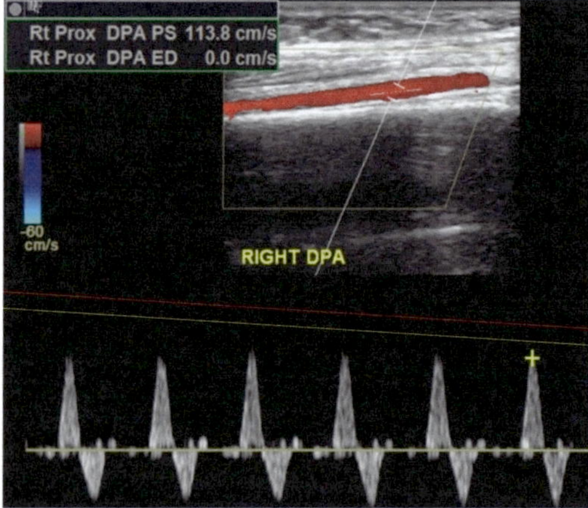

Fig. 3.2 Color and spectral arterial duplex showing patent dorsalis pedis artery runoff, which could serve as an alternative access site for intervention

3.1.4.2 CT Angiography

CT Angiography (CTA) with multidetector scanning provides a rapid non-invasive assessment of the peripheral arterial vasculature. With more modern equipment, the image quality, acquisition time, and thinner sections with multiplanar reconstruction result in very high sensitivity and specificity for PAD of 95% and 96%, respectively [16, 17].

This examination can be extremely useful when inflow / iliac disease is suspected by clinical examination such as with decreased femoral pulses, and when a patient has had extensive surgical revascularizations. It also has the added benefit of pre-planning multiple conventional and alternative access points for intervention such as femoral, pedal, popliteal, or radial approaches that might be necessary.

CTA does have some limitations. The use of ionizing radiation is one downside when compared to arterial duplex. Iodinated contrast bolus is also required which may be contraindicated in patients with existing chronic kidney disease (CKD) or severe contrast allergy. Other limitations are beam hardening resulting in overestimation of disease with calcified lesions, and poor resolution of the tibial vessels in patients with advanced medial calcinosis.

Figures 3.3 and 3.4 demonstrate maximal intensity projection (MIP) images reconstructed following raw data acquisition. A left proximal

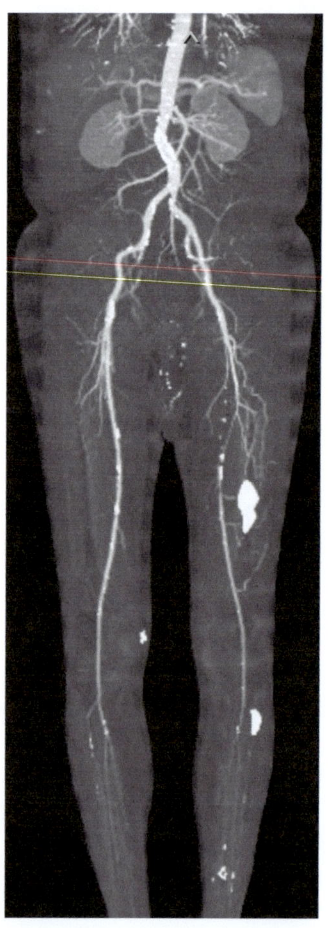

Fig. 3.3 Maximum Intensity Projection (MIP) demonstrates patent iliofemoral segment with proximal left SFA occlusion and scattered calcification

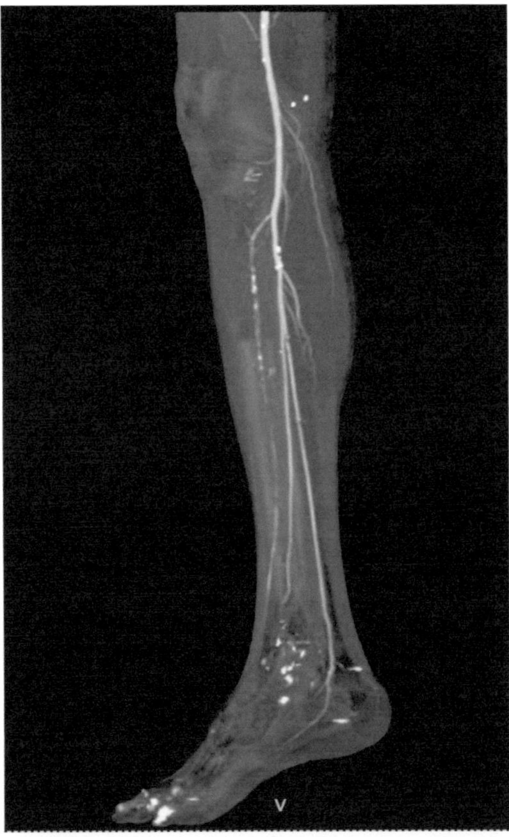

Fig. 3.4 Below the knee MIP demonstrates anterior tibial artery stenosis and occlusion with reconstitution distally

SFA occlusion with calcification is seen in Fig. 3.3. Figure 3.4 demonstrates a below-the-knee MIP showing anterior tibial occlusive disease with reconstitution distally.

3.1.4.3 Magnetic Resonance Angiography

Magnetic Resonance Angiography (MRA) may be performed with and/or without IV gadolinium contrast injection. Non-contrast MRA utilizes time-of-flight imaging whereby flowing blood into a radiofrequency pre-saturated field can be detected by the coil. With this technique, resolution of collateral or retrograde flow may be difficult. For this reason, MRA is typically combined with gadolinium contrast infusion. Contrast MRA when performed in experienced centers has been shown to have a sensitivity of 95% and specificity of up to 97% in detecting significant stenoses [18].

Limitations of MRA include time, cost, and contrast agent potential risk. Due to prolonged image acquisition times over CTA, MRA may suffer from venous contamination, especially in the tibial vessels. Time-resolved imaging can help overcome this by capturing multiple phases of enhancement in the distal vessels. Nephrogenic systemic fibrosis (NSF), a rare dermopathy involving the joints, skin, eyes, and internal organs, has been associated with linear gadolinium-based contrast agents. Newer, agents have not been associated with this complication. For this reason, the American College of Radiology (ACR) and the National Kidney Foundation (NKF) released a joint statement that since the risk of nephrogenic systemic fibrosis is so low with current agents, the potential harms of delaying or withholding MRI in a patient with acute kidney injury or estimated glomerular filtration rate less than 30 mL/min per 1.73 m^2 is likely to outweigh the risk in most clinical situations [19]. One additional limitation is that some patients may not be able to tolerate the MRI experience and require sedation/anesthesia, as well as may have contraindications such as non-MRI compatible metallic implants and cardiac devices.

3.1.5 Superficial and Deep Venous Imaging

Evaluating for venous stasis, insufficiency, or obstruction is of equal importance to evaluating the arterial circulation in patients with wounds. Many patients with calf or ankle wounds that have arterial insufficiency also have underlying venous insufficiency or stasis. This can lead to wounds with an "arterial appearance" but in a "venous distribution," and thus a mixed etiology. Correction of the underlying arterial insufficiency is typically undertaken first both to improve perfusion and allow for compression should this be necessary. There is a subset of patients that will require treating both the arterial and the venous circulations to achieve full healing.

Evaluation of the venous appearing wound begins with a thorough history and vascular examination. Patients should be examined with the legs in dependent position to see clinical signs of venous insufficiency such as bulging varicosities, peripheral venous pooling, and color change, as well as edema and calf/leg asymmetry.

3.1.5.1 Venous Insufficiency Ultrasound Testing

The workhorse of imaging evaluation for venous wounds is the venous insufficiency ultrasound. This is performed by having the patient in a standing position or dependent position on tilting table if unable to tolerate standing. Evaluation of the truncal superficial veins is then undertaken to look for "reflux" or blood flowing in the opposite direction following a squeeze or augmentation challenge distal to the segment. Imaging the distribution of malfunctioning segments as well as the understanding of superficial venous anatomy is crucial when planning for treatment. Figure 3.5 demonstrates insufficiency involving the thigh segment greater saphenous vein following augmentation.

3.1.6 When Should I Consider CT or MR Venography?

Non-invasive imaging of the central lower extremity veins may be obtained by performing CT Venography (CTV) or Magnetic Resonance Venography (MRV). This can be useful in multiple scenarios where evaluating the central veins beneath the diaphragm is necessary. For the patient with a chronic presentation (post-thrombotic syndrome, chronic DVT, venous stasis ulceration, etc.), anatomic imaging can assist in multiple areas. Specifically, CTV is excellent at evaluating IVC filters for possible retrieval, confirming patency of the IVC, excluding non-thrombotic and chronic/thrombotic May-Thurner syndrome, gonadal vein reflux, and ruling out additional nonvascular sources of pelvic pain or lower extremity swelling (Figs. 3.6 and 3.7).

CTV is typically accomplished utilizing a larger bolus of contrast and an imaging delay. Although CTV is cheaper, quicker, and widely available, ionizing radiation and contrast-induced nephropathy are a concern.

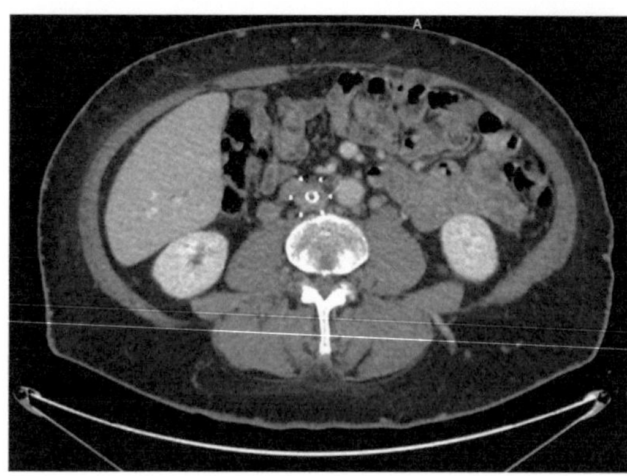

Fig. 3.6 CT Venogram demonstrates IVC occlusion at the level of an embedded IVC filter with atretic / chronically occluded bilateral common iliac veins

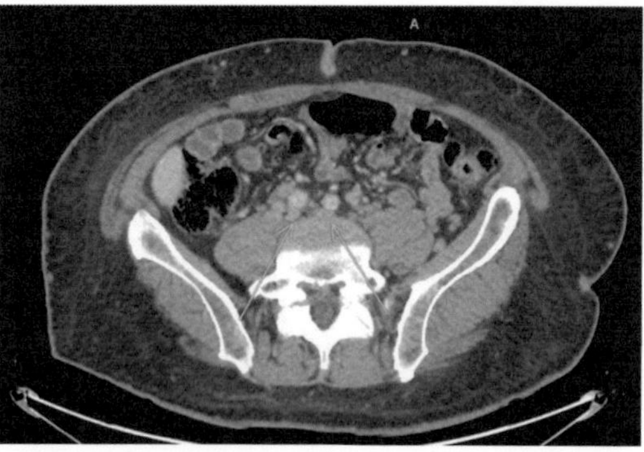

Fig. 3.7 CT Venogram demonstrates IVC occlusion at the level of an embedded IVC filter with atretic/chronically occluded bilateral common iliac veins

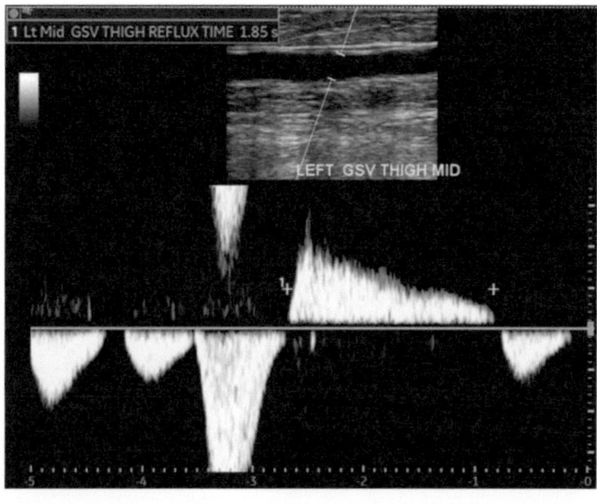

Fig. 3.5 Venous insufficiency US showing mid-thigh segment greater saphenous vein reflux following augmentation spike

Magnetic resonance venography (MRV) is an alternative imaging modality for detecting central venous disease. The main advantage over CT is the lack of ionizing radiation, which is desirable in younger patients and when serial investigations are required. Despite its excellent accuracy, MRV is underused in both acute and chronic situations, due to a combination of cost, protocol availability, and time.

In the authors' practice, we routinely perform CTV for those patients with adequate renal function and current or prior history of multiple left-sided DVT, active unilateral swelling with CEAP 4 or greater disease including those with active venous ulceration, and those with asymmetric left lower extremity varicosities or labial/scrotal superficial varicosities. For those patients with acute presentations of femoropopliteal DVT where the proximal extent of the thrombus is not well visualized by ultrasound, CTV is performed.

3.1.6.1 Putting it All Together

In the authors' practice, we typically follow an algorithmic approach to working up the patient presenting with lower extremity wounds or evidence of ischemic rest pain. All wound evaluations begin with ABI testing, thorough vascular examination and history, and examination of the wound (if present). Based on the initial visit additional testing may or may not be warranted.

Patients with abnormal ABI, abnormal vascular examination, or clinical evidence of arterial component to the wound are considered for advanced imaging and arteriography as indicated. Those with evidence of inflow/iliac or femoropopliteal occlusive disease are primarily considered for preprocedural CTA runoff. Those patients with suspected tibioperoneal occlusive disease by examination are considered for arterial duplex ultrasound. If the patient is diabetic and wound Wagner stage 3 or greater, then TcPO2 or SPP testing may be adjunctively considered to evaluate candidacy for hyperbaric oxygen therapy (HBOT).

Patients who present with sequelae of venous disease are stratified according to the severity of their disease and clinical appearance. Those with active venous ulceration and bilateral venous stasis changes are typically referred for venous insufficiency testing / venous reflux US testing. Those with unilateral disease or a history of multiple prior unilateral (typically left) deep venous thrombosis (DVT) are referred for central venous imaging (usually CTV) as well as superficial venous US testing.

3.2 Interpreting the ABI, TBI, and Toe Pressures: Know the Pitfalls

Ryan Lutz and Ulku C. Turba

3.2.1 Ankle-Brachial Index

- Determined by taking the higher pressure of the two arteries at the ankle (anterior tibial or posterior tibial) divided by the brachial artery systolic pressure (Table 3.1) [20].
  - It is important to look at each tibial ABI result as only the higher value is usually reported. This additional info has value depending on your wound-related angiosome, which may be in the non-reported territory.
- Quick and cost-effective examination to screen patients for PAD → if abnormal you can move on to non-invasive physiologic vascular studies such as segmental arterial pressures, pulse volume recordings, and Doppler waveforms.
- Level of disease is usually found just ABOVE the level of abnormality and can be determined by waveform changes (Table 3.2).

Table 3.1 Interpretation of ankle-brachial index class and waveform

Class	ABI	Waveform
Normal	0.95–1.0	Triphasic
Mild	0.80–0.94	Biphasic or Triphasic
Moderate	0.50–0.79	Biphasic
Severe	0.30–0.49	Biphasic
Critical	< 0.30	Monophasic

Table 3.2 Various levels of disease that can be determined by waveform analysis

Level of disease
Aortoiliac
Iliofemoral
SFA
Popliteal
Infra-popliteal
Pedal

Table 3.3 Interpretation of toe brachial index class

Class	TBI
Normal	> 0.70
Mild	0.60–0.69
Moderate	0.40–0.59
Severe	< 0.39
Critical	< 0.30

- It is critical to remember that in patients with Small Arterial Disease (SAD) pattern in the foot, which is a microvascular pattern seen in Diabetes and Renal Failure, patients can have normal ABIs but inadequate perfusion for wound healing or rest pain.
  - This can be distinguished with Toe Pressure/TBI/SPP and confirmed with direct angiograms.
- ABI additional considerations:
  - >0.15 change in ABI is considered significant.
  - >20 mmHg pressure gradient between segments considered significant.
  - Post-exercise ABI decrease by 0.15 is considered significant.

3.2.2 Toe Brachial Index

- Often used when the ABI is abnormally high (>1.4) due to calcifications [21].
  - Seen most often in diabetic and renal failure patients with medial artery calcifications (MAC), thus reducing reliability.
- Determined by taking the highest toe pressure divided by the brachial artery systolic pressure (Table 3.3).

- A normal Toe Pressure may be misleading in patients with severe hypertension.
  - May need to consider TcPO2 or SPP.

3.2.3 Toe Pressures/TcPO2

- Used as an adjunct of lower limb vascular function and often as a predictor of wound healing.
- Toe pressures <30 mmHg predictive of non-healing diabetic foot ulcers [21].
- Note that Toe Pressures and TcPO2 are different diagnostic tests, and commonly referred to incorrectly.
- These tests can be time consuming, highly technologist dependent, and the electrode cannot be placed on digits or on the wound itself.
- Both tests can have additional variability based on environment temperature and patient factors such as recent caffeine intake, exercise, and alcohol consumption.

3.2.4 Pitfalls When Interpreting ABIs

- Lower extremity calcifications.
  - Classically seen in diabetics, ESRD, etc.
  - Results in elevated ABI (>1.4) or pseudo-normalized ABI [22].
  - Solution: Utilize TBI and toe pressures.
- Severe aortic valve regurgitation.
  - Results in elevated ABI due to comparatively low brachial artery systolic pressure.
  - Always check echo and EKG if available.
- Upper limb arterial stenosis.
  - Classically seen in ESRD patients.
  - Results in elevated ABI due to comparatively low brachial artery systolic pressure.
- Narrow/loose cuff width for the ankle.
  - Ensure proper equipment is being used.

3.3 Interpreting the CT and MRI: Know the Limitations

Faris Galambo and David M. Tabriz

3.3.1 CT and MRI: Arterial Imaging

3.3.1.1 CT Arteriography (CTA)
Suggested Protocol:
- Patient positioning: Supine, feet first.
- Both extremities together and aligned to scanner isocenter.
- Avoid excessive dorsi/plantar flexion.
- Intravenous (IV) access for contrast administration.
- Contrast: 80–120 cc contrast with bolus tracking.
- Second acquisition from the knees to the toes after first scan is obtained.
  - Infra-popliteal arteries may not be adequately opacified on first acquisition.
- Small FOV reconstruction of each limb can be helpful.
  - Greater spatial resolution [23].

Additional Considerations:
- Dual-energy CT.
- Can be used to reconstruct virtual non-contrast images.
- Can be used to reduce contrast volume needed for diagnosis.
- Can use plaque removal functions to aid in heavy arterial disease.

Limitations:
- Requires ionizing radiation.
- Requires iodinated contrast.
  - The presence of dense atheromatous calcification compromises diagnostic accuracy and may exaggerate plaque and overestimate stenotic disease (especially problematic below the knee due to small caliber of vessels).

3.3.1.2 Contrast-Enhanced MR Arteriography (CE-MRA)
Suggested Protocol:
- Use of dedicated peripheral/surface coils, or a 3-station coil is preferred.

- Patient positioning: Supine, feet first.
  - Patient comfort is key to minimizing motion artifacts (i.e., if patient has rest pain, consider pre-procedure analgesia).
  - Breath holds are highly recommended. If breath holds are not possible, reduced scan time is recommended at the expense of resolution.
- Intravenous (IV) access for contrast administration.
  - Contrast: 15–10 mL, rate 5 mL/s, bolus tracking at the juxta-renal aorta.
- Sequences.
  - T1-weighted spoiled gradient echo (FSGRE).
  - Pre-contrast acquisition (for subtraction imaging) or Dixon fat suppression sequence.
  - High-resolution equilibrium-phase angiography (allows a second chance for arterial interrogation in case of poor timing).
  - Time-resolved (TR) is superior to the standard technique CE-MRA [23].

Limitations:
- Requires gadolinium-containing contrast agents.
- Decreased visualization of calcifications compared to CTA.
- Susceptible to artifacts from metallic stents/devices.

3.3.1.3 Non-Contrast MR Arteriography (NC-MRA)
Many PVD patients have concomitant kidney disease, which may prevent contrast use.

Suggested Protocol:
- Use of dedicated peripheral/surface coils, or a 3-station coil is preferred.
- Patient positioning: Supine, feet first.
  - Patient comfort is key to minimizing motion artifacts (i.e., if patient has rest pain, consider pre-procedure analgesia).
  - Breath holds are highly recommended. If breath holds are not possible, reduced scan time is recommended at the expense of resolution.

- Sequences.
  - Time-of-flight (TOF)—More widely available but with limited image quality in the peripheral vessels (below the knee).
  - Quiescent interval single-shot or slice selective (QISS).
    - Performs better in the peripheral vessels.
  - (3D) Turbo spin-echo (TSE) with STIR with cardiac triggering during systole.
  - Multiple other NC-MRA techniques are emerging but are not yet widely available [24].

Limitations:
- More sensitive to artifacts than CE-MRA.
- Decreased visualization of calcifications compared to CTA.
- Susceptible to artifacts from metallic implants and cardiac devices.

3.3.2 CT and MRI: Venous Imaging

3.3.2.1 CT Venography (CTV)
Suggested Protocol:
- Patient positioning: Supine, feet first.
- Both extremities together and aligned to scanner isocenter.
- Avoid excessive dorsi/plantar flexion.
- Intravenous (IV) access for contrast administration.
  - Contrast: 80–120 cc contrast, can have a saline chaser if desired.
- Scan timing: 180 second delay.
- Scan foot to diaphragm [23].

Limitations:
- Requires ionizing radiation.
- Requires iodinated contrast.
- Beam hardening artifacts from hardware or adjacent arterial calcifications can mimic filling defects [25].

3.3.2.2 Contrast-Enhanced MR Venography (MRV)
Suggested Protocol:
- Use of dedicated peripheral/surface coils, or a 3-station coil is preferred if available.

- Patient positioning: Supine, feet first.
  - Patient comfort is key to minimizing motion artifacts (i.e., if patient has rest pain, consider pre-procedure analgesia).
  - Breath holds are highly recommended. If breath holds are not possible, reduced scan time is recommended at the expense of resolution.
- Intravenous (IV) access for contrast administration.
  - Contrast: 15–10 mL, rate 5 mL/s, bolus tracking at the juxta-renal aorta.
- Sequences.
  - TOF Angiography: TO identify and isolate the arterial tree.
  - Pre-contrast T1-weighted acquisition (for substruction imaging) or Dixon fat suppression sequence.
  - 3D T1-weighted Gradient Echo sequences with contrast, starting at 5 minutes post-contrast administration.
  - T2 fast spin-echo (FSE) sequences [23].

Limitations:
- Susceptible to artifacts from metallic stents/devices.
- CT is superior if there is a concern for IVC filter complication.
- Gadolinium contrast-related risks.

3.3.2.3 Non-Contrast MR Venography (ncMRV)
Suggested Protocol:
- Use of dedicated peripheral/surface coils, or a 3-station coil is preferred if available.
- Patient positioning: Supine, feet first.
  - Patient comfort is key to minimizing motion artifact.
  - Breath holds are also highly recommended. If that is not possible, reduced scan time is recommended at the expense of resolution.
- Key sequence.
  - Non-contrast 3D turbo spin-echo (TSE) with STIR and cardiac triggering during systole.

Limitations:

- Susceptible to artifacts from metallic stents/devices.
- CT is superior if there is a concern for IVC filter complication.
- More sensitive to artifacts than CE-MRV [23].

3.4 Pedal Duplex Imaging and Advanced Intraoperative Ultrasound

Jill Sommerset, Desarom Teso, and Mary Costantino

Given the rise of diabetes mellitus (DM) and end-stage renal disease (ESRD) in chronic limb-threatening ischemia patients (CLTI), our current physiologic tests may not completely answer the question regarding lower extremity disease and more specifically pedal perfusion. Medial wall calcinosis precludes an accurate ankle pressure and in the setting of digital wounds or previous great toe amputation, TBI may not be obtainable (Fig. 3.8). As discussed previously, TCP02 and skin profusion testing (SPP) are alternative options to provide microvascular testing, however, these tests may also prove to be challenging due to edema and tissue loss. A simple waveform analysis at the ankles can still be obtained. However, in patients with dense calcific plaque, there is a loss in compliancy in the artery wall, resulting in abnormal waveform analysis [26].

Moreover, patients with foot ulcers require more in-depth evaluation of pedal flow. Pedal arch disease in diabetics and renal failure patients can be significant. Therefore, it is paramount that flow to the wound bed should be quantified and used in the decision-making process for these complex patients.

Up until 2016, standard arterial duplex imaging stopped at the level of the ankle. In 2017, the discovery of direct ultrasound interrogation of the pedal arch was developed and published, describing the techniques and criteria for patients with chronic limb-threatening ischemia [27].

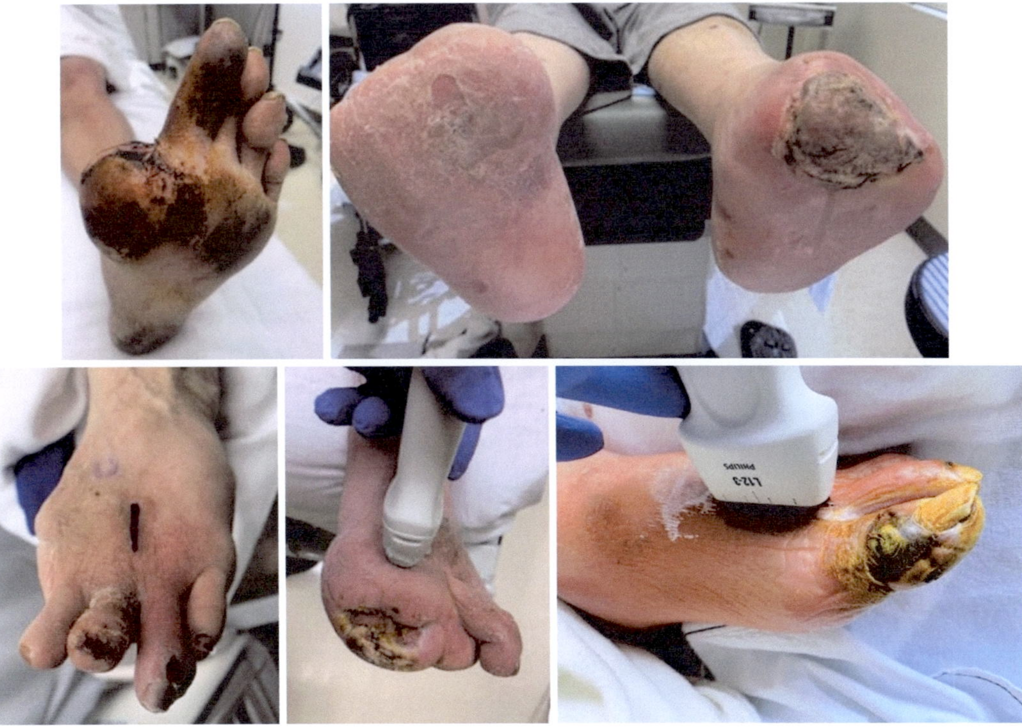

Fig. 3.8 Various types of wounds where standard physiologic testing may not provide adequate information

Pedal duplex imaging provides valuable information that includes understanding the pedal anatomy, obtaining reliable objective Pedal Acceleration Time (PAT), and comprehensive evaluation of pedal flow hemodynamics. This combination of valuable information provides an understanding of potential direct or indirect flow patterns to the wound bed.

3.4.1 Pedal Anatomy (Figs. 3.9 and 3.10)

Using a standard 8–12 MHz linear probe, the pedal anatomy can be evaluated. A high frequency of 12–18 mHz may be helpful when imaging smaller caliber, Dorsal Metatarsal Arteries to the digits. The technique for imaging the anterior pedal circulation is the cuneiform window, which is a soft tissue space where the bifurcation of the Arcuate Artery and first Dorsal Metatarsal Artery can be visualized. The Arcuate Artery will have a "waterfall" image, with the first Dorsal Metatarsal Artery visualized more superficially (Fig. 3.11).

The posterior circulation can initially be evaluated with the probe in transverse on the midfoot. With probe compressions, the Lateral Plantar Veins can be easily compressed and used as a landmark to locate the Lateral Plantar Artery (LPA) (Fig. 3.12). Once identified, the probe can be turned in a long axis, color applied with a low scale (below 12 cm/s), and the LPA visualized. With a slight angle of the probe to the medal foot the Medial Plantar Artery (MPA) can be identified as it lies more superficial with no metatarsal bony landmark. The MPA is typically smaller in caliber and can be challenging to image in patients with no disease. However, if the LPA is occluded or atretic, the MPA will be the dominant pedal artery and should be imaged in CLT patients.

In regard to non-healing foot wounds, care should be taken to place the ultrasound probe at the edge of the wound bed to obtain anatomical

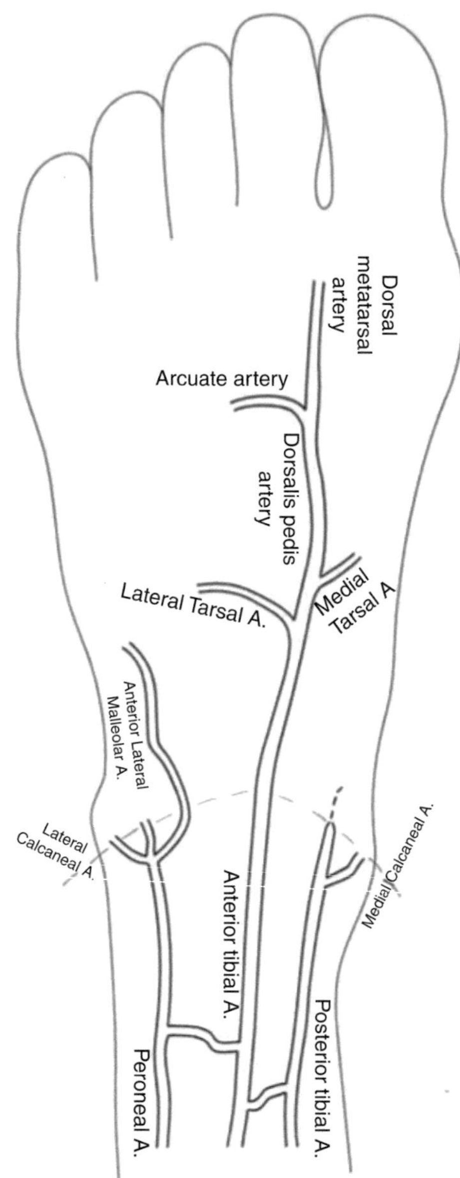

Fig. 3.9 Pedal diagram highlighting the typical anterior and posterior pedal anatomy

pathways to the wound bed. To further assist in decision-making, tracing the artery near the wound, to the pedal arch as well as the supplying tibial artery can result in improved targeted interventions.

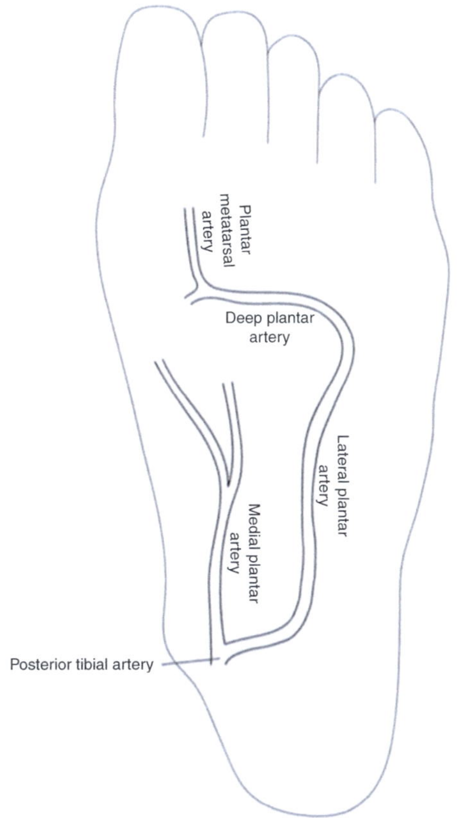

Fig. 3.10 Pedal diagram highlighting the typical anterior and posterior pedal anatomy

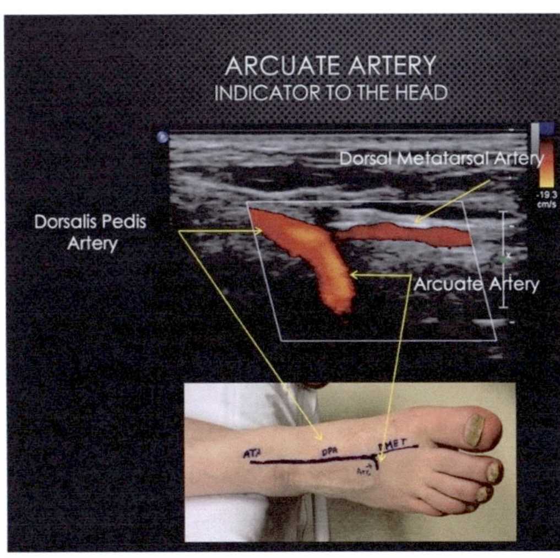

Fig. 3.11 Duplex imaging in the cuneiform window visualizing the Arcuate Artery and first Dorsal Metatarsal Artery

3.4.2 Pedal Acceleration Time (PAT)

Applying Acceleration Time to the pedal arteries provides an understanding of foot perfusion based on previously published work [28]. For reliability and accuracy, the PAT must be measured properly. Proper technique includes lowering the baseline, increasing the sweep speed to appreciate 3–4 cardiac cycles, and decreasing the Doppler scale so the waveform takes up three-fourth of the spectrum. Then, precisely measure the onset of systole to the peak of systole, to obtain a PAT.

PAT criteria consist of four published classifications. Class 1 is normal to Class 4 being consistent with tissue loss and rest pain. PAT not only correlates with reliable ABI but also correlates with clinical symptoms. This can be helpful in patients with claudication in need of an exercise program to build collaterals, as PAT reflects the proximal collateral flow.

3.4.3 Pedal Flow Hemodynamics

Flow direction in the pedal arch depends on anatomy, proximal disease, and if the pedal arch is intact. Figure 3.13 illustrates antegrade and retrograde flow in the Arcuate Artery. Knowledge of pedal flow direction may be helpful if the only way to revascularize is through an indirect route.

1. If the Arcuate Artery is retrograde, this indirectly suggests the pedal arch is intact, and flow in the posterior circulation is supplying the anterior circulation.
2. If the Lateral or Deep Plantar Artery is retrograde, this indirectly suggests the pedal arch is intact, and flow from the anterior circulation is supplying the posterior circulation [29].

Pedal artery duplex is a novel technique that provides real-time, hemodynamic information in complex patients and should be considered an integral part of the perioperative care in patients with CLTI (Fig. 3.14).

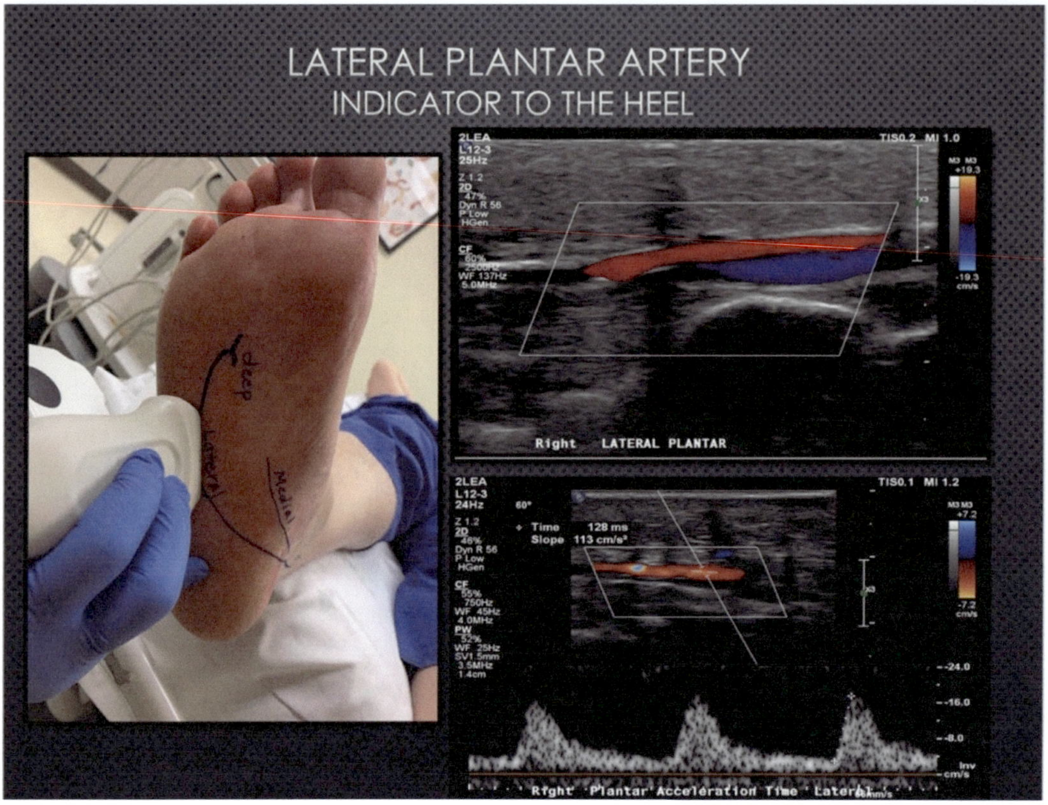

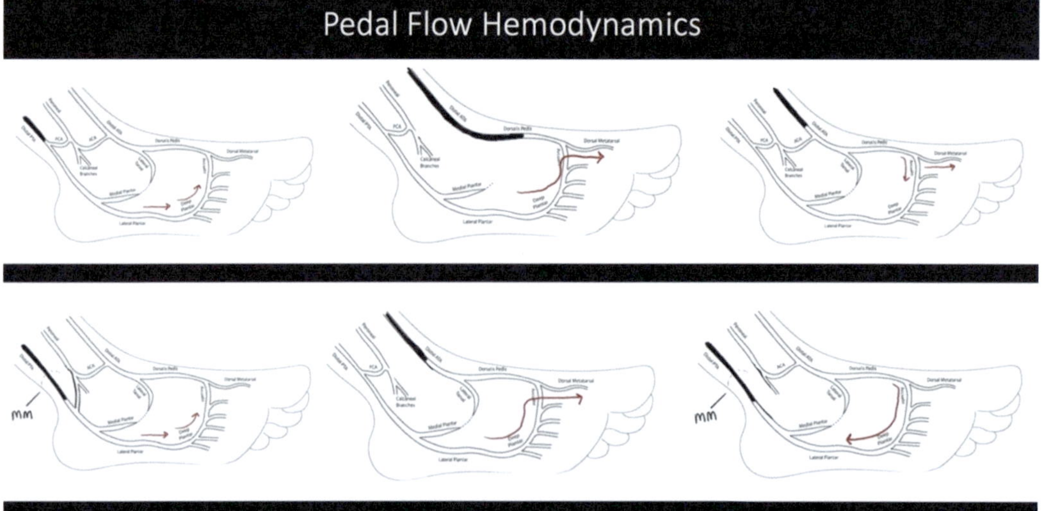

Fig. 3.12 Duplex imaging in the cuneiform window visualizing the Lateral Plantar Artery using the Lateral Plantar Vein as a landmark

Fig. 3.13 Various pedal flow directions based on proximal disease patterns (*MM:* medial malleolus)

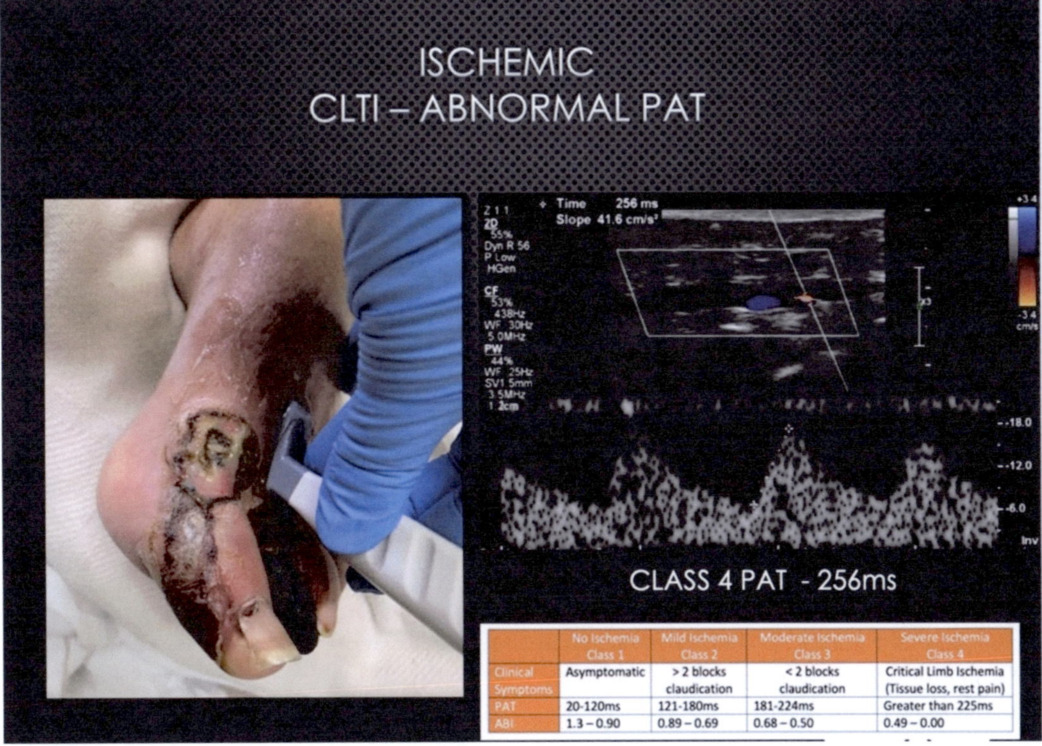

	No Ischemia Class 1	Mild Ischemia Class 2	Moderate Ischemia Class 3	Severe Ischemia Class 4
Clinical Symptoms	Asymptomatic	> 2 blocks claudication	< 2 blocks claudication	Critical Limb Ischemia (Tissue loss, rest pain)
PAT	20-120ms	121-180ms	181-224ms	Greater than 225ms
ABI	1.3 – 0.90	0.89 – 0.69	0.68 – 0.50	0.49 – 0.00

Fig. 3.14 Class 4 PAT illustrating the severity of peripheral arterial disease

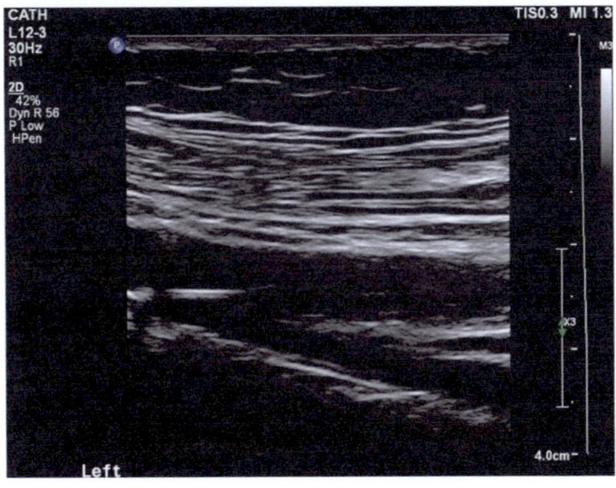

Fig. 3.15 Wire tip engaging a chronic total occlusion in the Superficial Femoral Artery

3.4.4 Advanced Intraoperative Duplex Ultrasound

Intraoperative ultrasound is underutilized in the endovascular suite. The benefit of intraoperative ultrasound includes real-time objective evidence of a procedural endpoint. The endpoint is a PAT of less than 180 ms [30]. Additional benefits of intraoperative ultrasound include guidance through chronic total occlusions (CTO), challenging stenoses, and confirmation of intraluminal position.

Real-time intraoperative ultrasound allows the operator to know which disease burden needs to be addressed before there is successful reperfusion of the foot utilizing PAT. With a highly skilled ultrasound technologist performing intermittent pedal ultrasound throughout the case, the operator will know if single or multiple lesions need to be treated to relieve rest pain or heal ulcers. This has significant benefits in reducing the number of staged procedures and more importantly, eliminating a subjective opinion about improved perfusion based on angiography. PAT is an objective number that is quantifiable and reproducible. For example, in a patient with diffuse Superficial Femoral Artery, Popliteal, and significant Tibial disease, a real-time objective endpoint allows the operator to know whether a femoropopliteal intervention is adequate (based on the PAT number), or whether further intervention into the tibial territory must be performed in the same setting.

Guidance through chronic total occlusions (CTO) is extremely helpful in selective patients. The operator can be more aggressive with wires and catheters, knowing that the intraluminal position is maintained (Fig. 3.15). Ultrasound is also used to detail the location of the calcifications with softer channels to help guide the direction of catheters and wires toward the small channels, which can improve successful crossing. If the artery is densely calcified, then intraoperative ultrasound may not be beneficial. Confirmation of intraluminal position can be used many times throughout the case. This saves significant time when ultrasound can be placed on the limb while the operator is working, to confirm intraluminal position of a catheter or wire, rather than having to exchange the wire for a catheter and then perform angiography. Ideally, the ultrasound technologist would have already mapped the entire limb from groin to pedal level, becoming intimately familiar with each patient's anatomy and pathology. This allows the operator to move quickly along with the ultrasound technologist, who has an advanced understanding of the patient's arterial anatomy, including patent or occluded vessels, and will know the best window for ultrasound imaging.

In conclusion, intraoperative ultrasound is an inexpensive advanced tool, with no radiation or additional disposable equipment costs. Ultrasound gives the operator valuable information that fluoroscopy may lack. Intraoperative and pedal duplex ultrasound should be a fundamental technique for advanced CLTI interventions to aid in operative success.

References

1. Management of venous leg ulcers: Clinical practice guidelines of the Society for Vascular Surgery® and the American Venous Forum O'Donnell, Thomas F. et al. J Vasc Surg. 60(2):3S–59S.
2. Xu D, Li J, Zou L, Xu Y, Hu D, Pagoto SL, Ma Y. Sensitivity and specificity of the ankle-brachial index to diagnose peripheral artery disease: a structured review. Vasc Med. 2010;15(5):361–9. https://doi.org/10.1177/1358863X10378376.
3. Strandness DE Jr, Schultz RD, Sumner DS, Rushmer RF. Ultrasonic flow detection. A useful technic in the evaluation of peripheral vascular disease. Am J Surg. 1967;113:311–20.
4. Wütschert R, Bounameaux H. Predicting healing of arterial leg ulcers by means of segmental systolic pressure measurements. Vasa. 1998;27:224–8.
5. Hafner J, et al. Leg ulcers in peripheral arterial disease (arterial leg ulcers): impaired wound healing above the threshold of chronic critical limb ischemia. J Am Acad Dermatol. 2000;43:1001–8.
6. Darling RC, Raines JK, Brener BJ, Austen WG. Quantitative segmental pulse volume recorder: a clinical tool. Surgery. 1972;72:873–7.
7. Macdonald N. Pulse volume plethysmography. J Vasc Tech. 1994;18:241–8.
8. Lau JF, Weinberg MD, Olin JW. Peripheral artery disease. Part 1: clinical evaluation and noninvasive diagnosis. Nat Rev Cardiol. 2011;8(7):405–18.
9. Cesar C, Javier E, Anaya-Ayala H, et al. Abstract 273: Measurement of transcutaneous oxygen pressure in patients with post-thrombotic syndrome and possible clinical applications. Arterioscler Thromb Vasc Biol. 2019;39:A273.
10. Yang C, Weng H, Chen L, Yang H, Luo G, Mai L, Jin G, Yan L. Transcutaneous oxygen pressure measurement in diabetic foot ulcers: mean values and cutpoint for wound healing. J Wound Ostomy Continence Nurs. 2013;40(6):585–9. https://doi.org/10.1097/WON.0b013e3182a9a7bf.
11. Lo T, Sample R, Moore P, Gold P. Prediction of Wound Healing Outcome using skin perfusion pressure and transcutaneous oximetry: a single-center experience in 100 patients. Wounds. 2009;21(11):310–6.
12. Eiberg JP, Grønvall Rasmussen JB, Hansen MA, Schroeder TV. Duplex ultrasound scanning of peripheral arterial disease of the lower limb. Eur J Vasc Endovasc Surg. 2010;40(4):507–12.
13. Moneta GL, et al. Accuracy of lower extremity arterial duplex mapping. J Vasc Surg. 1992;15:275–83.
14. Ligush J Jr, Reavis SW, Preisser JS, Hansen KJ. Duplex ultrasound scanning defines operative strategies for patients with limb-threatening ischemia. J Vasc Surg. 1998;28:482–90.
15. Schernthaner R, et al. Multidetector CT angiography in the assessment of peripheral arterial occlusive disease: accuracy in detecting the severity, number, and length of stenoses. Eur Radiol. 2008;18:665–71.
16. Von Ziegler F, Costa MA. The role of CT and MRI in the assessment of peripheral vascular disease. Curr Cardiol Rep. 2007;9:412–9.
17. Collins R, et al. Duplex ultrasonography, magnetic resonance angiography, and computed tomography angiography for diagnosis and assessment of symp-

tomatic, lower limb peripheral arterial disease: systematic review. BMJ. 2007;334:1257.

18. Weinreb J, Rodby R, Yee J, et al. Use of Intravenous gadolinium-based contrast media in patients with kidney disease: consensus statements from the American College of Radiology and the National Kidney Foundation. Radiology. 2021;298(1):28–35.

19. Silickas J, et al. Use of computed tomography and magnetic resonance imaging in central venous disease. Methodist DeBakey Cardiovasc J. 2018;14(3):188–95. https://doi.org/10.14797/mdcj-14-3-188.

20. Sibley RC. et al. Noninvasive physiologic vascular studies: a guide to diagnosing peripheral arterial disease. RadioGraphics. 2017;37(1):346–57. https://doi.org/10.1148/rg.2017160044.

21. Sonter J, Ho A, Chuter VH. The predictive capacity of toe blood pressure and the toe-brachial index for foot wound healing and amputation: a systematic review and meta-analysis. Wound Pract Res. 2014;22(4):208–17.

22. Ato D. Pitfalls in the ankle-brachial index and brachial-ankle pulse wave velocity. Vasc Health Risk Manag. 2018;14:41–62. https://doi.org/10.2147/VHRM.S159437. Published 2018 Apr 3

23. Murphy DJ, Aghayev A, Steigner ML. Vascular CT and MRI: a practical guide to imaging protocols. Insights Imaging [Internet]. 2018;9(2):215–36. Available from: https://insightsimaging.springeropen.com/articles/10.1007/s13244-018-0597-2

24. Cavallo AU, Koktzoglou I, Edelman RR, Gilkeson R, Mihai G, Shin T, et al. Noncontrast magnetic resonance angiography for the diagnosis of peripheral vascular disease. Circ Cardiovasc Imaging. 2019;12(5):1–15.

25. Ghaye B, Szapiro D, Willems V, Dondelinger RF. Pitfalls in CT venography of lower limbs and abdominal veins. Am J Roentgenol. 2002;178(6):1465–71.

26. Tehan PE, Barwick AL, Sebastian M, Chuter VH. Diagnostic accuracy of resting systolic toe pressure for diagnosis of peripheral arterial disease in people with and without diabetes: a cross-sectional retrospective case-control study. J Foot Ankle Res. 2017;10:58.

27. Sommerset, et al. An innovative arterial duplex examination: a guide to evaluate flow in the foot using pedal acceleration time. JVU. 2019;169;11–17.

28. Sommerset, et al. Plantar acceleration time: a novel technique to evaluate Flow to the foot. AVS; 2019.

29. Sommerset, et al. Pedal flow hemodynamics in patients with CLTI. JVU; 2019.

30. Teso, et al. Pedal acceleration time: a novel predictor of limb salvage. AVS; 2021.

Beginning and Managing Underlying Comorbidities

4

Zaeem Billah, Zachary Chadnick, Kartik Kansagra,
Ali Kimyaghalam, Sreekumar Madassery,
Austin Shinagawa, Kuldeep Singh,
and Geogy Vatakencherry

4.1 Peripheral Arterial Disease Medications

Austin Shinagawa, Zaeem Billah,
Kartik Kansagra and Geogy Vatakencherry

4.1.1 Introduction

Peripheral artery disease (PAD) often occurs concurrently with other manifestations of global atherosclerosis, predominantly coronary artery, and cerebrovascular disease. Patients with PAD are at a very high risk of morbidity and mortality due to cardiovascular (CV) events such as myocardial infarction (MI), stroke, or sudden cardiac death.

Several studies have highlighted the burden of atherosclerotic disease in the PAD population, including the PARTNER trial, REACH registry, and EUCLID trial [1–3].

- According to the REACH registry, 3.7% of patients with a single bed of arterial disease had a 1-year composite outcome of MI, stroke, or CV death, with an even higher incidence of 6% in patients with polyvascular disease.
- Thus, it is imperative that modern vascular specialists treating PAD understand and optimize the medical management of atherosclerotic disease in their patients.

Medical management in the PAD population is aimed at reducing the risk of both major adverse cardiovascular events (MACE) and major adverse limb events (MALE) [4].

- MACE are typically defined as MI, stroke, and CV death, whereas MALE encompass significant interval events in PAD course progression, such as the need for peripheral revascularization or amputation/limb loss.
- Modification of cardiovascular risk factors (i.e., smoking, hypertension, dyslipidemia, and diabetes) through lifestyle and pharmaceutical intervention is the foundation of PAD medical management.

Z. Billah · K. Kansagra · A. Shinagawa
G. Vatakencherry
Department of Interventional Radiology, Kaiser
Permanente Los Angeles Medical Center,
Los Angeles, CA, USA

Z. Chadnick · A. Kimyaghalam
Department of Surgery, Staten Island University
Hospital – Northwell Health, New York, NY, USA
e-mail: Alik@auamed.net

S. Madassery (✉)
Department of Vascular and Interventional Radiology,
Rush University Medical Center, Chicago, IL, USA

K. Singh
Department of Surgery, Division of Vascular Surgery,
Staten Island University Hospital – Northwell Health,
New York, NY, USA
e-mail: Ksingh7@northwell.edu

4.1.1.1 Lifestyle Modification and Risk Reduction

The vascular specialist must assume the role of a "lifestyle coach" for their patient. Lifestyle modifications such as tobacco cessation, diet optimization, and exercise modification are crucial elements of PAD management, as these interventions alone have the potential to significantly alter a patient's disease course and functional status.

Tobacco Cessation

Smoking is an important modifiable risk factor for the development and progression of PAD.

- Epidemiological data based on the ARIC (Atherosclerosis Risk in Communities) study showed that patients who smoked for $\geq$25 pack years (versus non-smokers) were 4 times more likely to develop PAD and 1.5–2 times more likely of having CAD or stroke [5].
- Additional data found that even exposure to secondhand smoke correlates directly with the development of atherosclerotic disease [6].
- Smoking cessation is demonstrated to lower the risk of critical limb ischemia (CLI), amputation, and death, as well as slow the decline in ankle-brachial index over time.

Multiple modalities have been shown to be efficacious for achieving smoking cessation in individuals with tobacco use disorders. The EAGLES study was a randomized controlled trial (RCT) assessing the use of Varenicline, Bupropion, and Nicotine Patch in smokers with and without psychiatric disorders [7].

- It showed that Varenicline was more effective than placebo, nicotine patch, and Bupropion in helping patients who were smoking achieve abstinence. In addition, both a nicotine patch and Bupropion were more effective than a placebo alone.
- **Based on this data, Varenicline should be considered as the first-line option for smoking cessation.** This can be supplemented with more rapid-onset nicotine gum or lozenge. Smoking cessation counseling is

an adjunct to the above evidence-based therapies.

Diet Modification

Epidemiological studies have demonstrated that a healthy diet is associated with a lower incidence of PAD [8].

- Vascular specialists should encourage patients to consume a healthy diet rich in vegetables, fruits, nuts, whole grains, lean protein, and fiber, while limiting sugar and sweeteners, trans- or saturated fats, refined grains, and red meat.
- Dietary modification is especially important to address in patients with diabetes. Even so, it is crucial to consider how a patient's diet is affected by their socioeconomic status and availability of healthy food options, referring them to the appropriate resources if needed.

Parodi et al. prospectively studied the effect of aggressive hydration on 132 patients with severe claudication or rest pain whose symptoms did not improve despite maximal medical therapy comprised of risk factor reduction, supervised exercise protocols, and treatment with Cilostazol [9].

- This study showed that hydration with over 2 liters of fluid intake daily and protein supplementation (0.6 g/kg of protein daily with goal albumin above 4 g/dL) was associated with an increase in distance to claudication and even improvement in ankle-brachial index.
- However, aggressive hydration, such as in this protocol, should be avoided in patients with heart failure, dialysis dependence, and/or end-stage liver disease.

Exercise Therapy

Exercise therapy is well-studied in PAD, particularly in patients who suffer from claudication. Although the exact mechanism of improved function following exercise therapy is uncertain, there is a clear benefit of exercise therapy as evidenced by multiple trials.

The CLEVER study was a multicenter RCT that randomized 111 patients with aortoiliac PAD to optimal medical care alone, optimal medical care plus supervised exercise, or optimal medical care plus stent revascularization [10].

- This study found that there was a statistically significant increase in peak walking time for both the supervised exercise and stent revascularization groups over optimal medical therapy alone.

However, supervised exercise therapy may not be accessible or feasible for much of the PAD population. One alternative that addresses some of the barriers of supervised exercise therapy is home-based exercise therapy (HBET).

- Multiple studies, including the GOALS and MOSAIC trials, have found significant clinical value in HBET [11, 12].
- One such regimen that vascular specialists can prescribe to their patients is that of high-intensity exercise, as supported by the findings of the LITE trial [13]. This RCT compared the outcomes of low- versus high-intensity walking exercise in 305 patients, who were instructed to either walk at a comfortable pace or a pace inducing moderate-to-severe ischemic leg symptoms, respectively.
  - The trial showed that high-intensity HBET was significantly more effective for increasing 6-minute walk distance than low-intensity HBET; furthermore, the low-intensity HBET group failed to demonstrate a benefit over the nonexercise control group.

One prescription the authors recommend is exercising for 30 min at least three times a week by walking to near-maximal claudication discomfort (7/10 pain intensity), then resting (until pain subsides to a 3/10), and then resuming walking.

- Patients should be encouraged to maintain a log of their daily steps, time spent walking, and total distance walked.

- The vascular specialist can then reference this log at follow-up visits and encourage or coach the patient on their exercise habits accordingly.

4.1.1.2 Medical Optimization

Involvement in pharmacotherapy for PAD patients gives vascular specialists tremendous opportunity to dramatically alter the natural history of their patient's lives and limbs. While often managed by the patient's primary care physician, each vascular specialist should provide their expertise and guidance on optimizing the management of these conditions in the setting of PAD. Unfortunately, there is still a great deal of underutilization of life and limb-saving medical treatments in the PAD population. This section will review which therapeutic options have the strongest proven benefit in PAD, specifically lipid-lowering therapies, antihypertensives, glycemic control, and antithrombotics.

Lipid-Lowering Therapies

Lipid-lowering therapies (LLT) can reduce the deleterious effects of dyslipidemia on cardiovascular disease by rectifying imbalances in cholesterol levels, stabilizing atherosclerotic plaques, and even decreasing systemic inflammation.

- Several studies have found that a reduction in low-density lipoprotein cholesterol (LDL-c) is associated with reduced MACE and MALE [14].
- This led society guidelines to strongly recommend LLT for all patients with PAD [15, 16]. Despite this, dyslipidemia in PAD is often inadequately treated, and so vascular specialists should ensure that all patients with PAD are prescribed the appropriate LLT when possible.
- The LLT with the strongest demonstrated benefit in PAD patients are statins, ezetimibe, and proprotein convertase subtilisin/kexin type 9 (PCSK9) inhibitors.

Also, statins have also been found to improve pain-free walking distance [17]. These benefits are enhanced in patients who are suffering from CLI [18].

Table 4.1 Statin intensities as classified by the 2018 American College of Cardiology/American Heart Association Task Force cholesterol guidelines

Statin intensity	High	Moderate	Low
Average LDL-c Reduction	≥50%	30–49%	<30%
Rosuvastatin	20–40 mg	5–10 mg	
Atorvastatin	40–80 mg	10–20 mg	
Simvastatin		20–40 mg	10 mg
Pravastatin		40–80 mg	10–20 mg
Lovastatin		40–80 mg	20 mg
Fluvastatin XL		80 mg	
Fluvastatin		40 mg BID	20–40 mg
Pitavastatin		1–4 mg	

LDL-c: Low-density lipoprotein cholesterol; *XL*: Extended-release; *BID*: Twice a day

- Higher-intensity statins (Table 4.1) confer a stronger benefit than lower-intensity statins, although statin strength is sometimes limited by patient age and patient tolerance mainly due to statin-associated myopathy [19].

Overall, since it is possible that 40% of the PAD population are not receiving any form of LLT, our primary recommendation is to ensure that **all patients with PAD are on a maximally tolerated dose of statin to reduce the risk of MACE and MALE**.

- If the goal LDL-c reduction of ≥50% or LDL-c<55/70 mg/dL is not achieved with statin therapy alone, adjunctive therapy with Ezetimibe and/or PCSK9 inhibitors (Repatha, injectable drug given every 2 weeks) should be considered on an individual basis.

Antihypertensives

Hypertension is highly prevalent in the PAD population (over 80% in one registry); however, it is unfortunately less often treated in patients with PAD than those with other manifestations of cardiovascular disease [20, 21]. Inadequately treated hypertension should be identified and managed by the vascular specialist, as undertreated elevations in blood pressure are strongly associated with an increased risk of MACE [22].

Antihypertensive regimens are highly variable and are generally selected to address specific comorbidities.

- While no single antihypertensive strategy is proven to be superior, **angiotensin-converting enzyme inhibitors (ACEi) have the strongest evidence for reducing MACE in the PAD population**, as demonstrated in the HOPE trial [23–25].
- ARBs are also demonstrated to be effective for MACE reduction and are a reasonable alternative to ACEi [26, 27].
- It should also be mentioned that, although a point of historic controversy, there is a lack of evidence that β-blockers increase the risk of MALE or adversely affect walking capacity in PAD [28]. Therefore, the use of β-blockers for other indications, such as prior myocardial infarction or heart failure should not be restricted in the PAD population.

The landmark RCT SPRINT was performed to compare the outcomes of "intensive" (<120 mmHg) versus "standard" (<140 mmHg) blood pressure control in patients with increased cardiovascular risk and without diabetes [29].

- This study found a lower rate of MACE in the patients with the more aggressive systolic blood pressure goal of <120 mmHg, although the proportion of study participants with PAD was relatively low.
- As there is a lack of high-quality evidence defining the most appropriate blood pressure goals for the PAD population, the most recent 2017 ACC/AHA Task Force hypertension guidelines advise that patients with PAD be treated similarly to patients without PAD. Specifically, **these guidelines recommend a target blood pressure goal of <130/85 mmHg in the presence of atherosclerotic cardiovascular disease** [22].

Glucose-Lowering Therapies

Diabetes is a well-established risk factor for the development of PAD [30]. Patients with diabetes have a propensity for peripheral neuropathy with loss of protective sensation and thus developing non-healing wounds vulnerable to infection. Diabetes is known to elevate the risk of microvascular complications including retinopathy, neuropathy, and nephropathy; fortunately, the incidence of these complications can be reduced with proper glycemic control.

- **The target glycated hemoglobin level for patients with PAD is <7.0%.** More aggressive glucose lowering to aglycated hemoglobin <6.0/6.5% increases the risk of hypoglycemic episodes [31, 32].

Patients with Type 2 diabetes and obesity should be encouraged to lose weight by achieving a caloric deficit through dietary modification, exercise, and behavioral interventions [33].

- Weight loss of ≥10% of initial body weight is associated with a lower incidence of MACE, although an initial goal of ≥2–5% weight loss may be a more feasible goal for many patients [34].
- First-line therapy for diabetes generally also includes metformin, a safe and inexpensive medication that may be associated with a reduction in MACE [35, 36]. Renal function should always be considered in a patient prior to initiation/continuing metformin.

Two newer classes of glucose-lowering therapies, sodium-glucose transporter 2 (SGLT2) inhibitors and glucagon-like protein (GLP)-1 receptor agonists, have strong evidence for MACE reduction in patients with concomitant PAD and diabetes.

- Numerous RCTs have demonstrated this reduction in MACE with the use of SGLT2 inhibitors, specifically empagliflozin, canagliflozin, and dapagliflozin [37–40].
- SGLT2 inhibitors are also consistently associated with a reduction in heart failure hospitalizations as well as slowing the progression of renal disease [41, 42].
- Importantly, while earlier studies such as CANVAS showed canagliflozin to be associated with a significant increase in minor amputations, the later CREDENCE trial found no increased risk of MALE with canagliflozin use [38, 39]. Given the results from CANVAS, patients with active wounds should be closely observed if on canagliflozin.

- Similar cardioprotective effects were seen with multiple GLP-1 receptor agonists, specifically liraglutide, semaglutide, and dulaglutide, as demonstrated by the LEADER, SUSTAIN-6, and REWIND trials, respectively [43–45].
- In summary, **SGLT2 inhibitors and GLP-1 receptor agonists are demonstrated to have substantial benefits in the diabetic population. The American Diabetes Association guidelines recommend using these medications for all patients with concomitant PAD and diabetes, independent of glycated hemoglobin level or metformin use** [46]. However, the current cost and coverage of these medications present significant challenges for this proposed universal application.

Close coordination with primary care physicians and endocrinologists is essential to achieve optimal outcomes in these patients.

4.1.1.3 Antithrombotic Therapy

Thrombosis is suspected to significantly contribute to the progression of PAD and occurrence of MALE. There is pathologic evidence that thrombi, particularly in the infrapopliteal arteries, are a major component of luminal stenosis and occlusion [4]. Recent literature is further defining the role of antithrombotic therapy in the PAD population for MACE and MALE reduction (Table 4.2).

Antiplatelets are mainly recommended for the prevention of MACE in patients with PAD [15, 16].

- The main antiplatelet therapies used for this purpose are Aspirin and P2Y12 inhibitors (i.e., clopidogrel and ticagrelor).
- Aspirin is primarily used in patients with symptomatic PAD as its efficacy in patients with asymptomatic, marginally low ankle-brachial index (ABI) is unclear [47–49]. However, even the effectiveness of aspirin for MACE reduction in symptomatic PAD is controversial [50, 51].
- In addition, the CAPRIE trial, comparing clopidogrel and aspirin monotherapy, found clopidogrel to be associated with fewer occurrences of MACE than aspirin [52].
- The EUCLID trial found that ticagrelor confers no additional benefit in MACE reduction as compared to clopidogrel [1].

Table 4.2 Contraindications and Side Effects for Commonly Used Medications in PAD. Common side effects are classified as >1% occurrence, uncommon classified as <1% occurrence rate

Drug	Contraindications	Side effects
ACE inhibitors	**Absolute:** Pregnancy, breastfeeding, previous angioedema from ACEi, bilateral renal artery stenosis, hypersensitivity **Relative:** Impaired renal function, aortic valve stenosis, hypovolemia/dehydration, hemodialysis	**Common:** Dry cough, fatigue, dizziness, headache, fatigue, weakness, hypotension, hyperkalemia **Uncommon:** Decreased taste, upset stomach, rash, angioedema, jaundice
Angiotensin Receptor Blockers	**Absolute:** Pregnancy, breastfeeding, bilateral renal artery stenosis, hypersensitivity, use with aliskiren **Relative:** Hypersensitivity, severe liver disease, hypovolemia	**Common:** URI, back pain, sinusitis, diarrhea, cough, headache, dizziness, edema **Uncommon:** Hyperkalemia, liver failure, kidney failure, angioedema
Statins	**Absolute:** Active severe hepatic disease, pregnancy, breastfeeding, use with Gemfibrozil **Relative:** Use with other drugs which cause myopathy, CYP3A4 inhibitors	**Common:** Myopathy, transaminase elevation, **Uncommon:** New-onset diabetes, rhabdomyolysis, hepatotoxicity
GLP-1 agonists	**Absolute:** Pregnancy, hypersensitivity, GFR <30, gastroparesis, inflammatory bowel disease, MEN2A/2B, personal or family hx of medullary thyroid cancer **Relative:** GFR 30–50, pancreatitis	**Common:** Nausea, vomiting, diarrhea, dizziness, tachycardia, headaches, dyspepsia, minor hypoglycemia, injection site reaction **Uncommon:** Pancreatitis, hypersensitivity, acute renal failure, thrombocytopenia
SGLT2 inhibitors	**Absolute:** GFR <30, second or third trimester of pregnancy, ESRD/Dialysis, hypersensitivity, type 1 diabetes, or history of DKA **Relative:** Hypovolemia, osteopenia	**Common:** UTI, mycotic GU infections, URI, dyslipidemia, nausea, constipation, dysuria **Uncommon:** Hypotension, Ketoacidosis, acute kidney injury, bone fractures
Aspirin	**Absolute:** Active peptic ulcer, hypersensitivity, bleeding disorder, recent GI or intracranial bleed, severe liver disease, thrombocytopenia **Relative:** Age <21, concurrent use of anticoagulant, NSAID use	**Common:** Upset stomach, nausea, heartburn, drowsiness, mild headache **Uncommon:** Hypersensitivity, Reye syndrome, intracerebral hemorrhage, GI bleed, thrombocytopenia
P2Y12 inhibitors	**Absolute:** Hypersensitivity, active bleeding **Relative:** High bleeding risk, thrombocytopenia, neuraxial anesthesia	**Common:** Bleeding, bruising, fever, muscle pain rash/pruritus **Uncommon:** Thrombotic thrombocytopenic purpura, life-threatening bleeding
Anti-Xa inhibitors	**Absolute:** Active bleeding, hypersensitivity, valvular heart disease, **Relative:** High bleeding risk, neuraxial anesthesia, Pregnancy, severe hepatic impairment	**Common:** Bleeding, Abdominal pain, fatigue, dizziness, mild rash **Uncommon:** Life-threatening bleeding, anaphylaxis, hepatic dysfunction
Cilostazol	**Absolute:** Heart failure, ischemic heart disease, active bleeding, hypersensitivity **Relative:** Severe hepatic impairment	**Common:** Headache, diarrhea, palpitations **Uncommon:** Bleeding

- **Therefore, clopidogrel monotherapy is the antiplatelet regimen with the strongest evidence for MACE reduction.**

Dual antiplatelet therapy (DAPT) with both aspirin and a P2Y12 inhibitor is another proposed antithrombotic regimen.

- The CHARISMA trial failed to show a MACE reduction with clopidogrel-based DAPT but did find increased bleeding risk [53].
- Subsequent trials suggested a possible reduction in MACE and MALE with ticagrelor-based DAPT, but consistently at the cost of increased major bleeding risk [54, 55].
- The more novel thrombin-receptor antagonist vorapaxar was found to reduce MACE and potentially MALE in the PAD population but increased the risk of bleeding in patients with prior cerebrovascular events [56, 57].
- **Presently, there is no clear benefit of DAPT or vorapaxar for prevention of MACE and both are associated with increased bleeding risk.**

Anticoagulation is another potential strategy for primary prevention in patients with

PAD. The COMPASS trial evaluated low-dose Rivaroxaban plus Aspirin versus Aspirin alone in high-risk patients with either coronary artery disease or PAD.

- The trial found a significant decrease in MACE and all-cause mortality in the Rivaroxaban plus Aspirin group, despite an increased occurrence of major bleeding [58].
- A sub-analysis of the PAD population in this study also found a ~45% reduction in MALE, including a decreased risk of major amputation [59].
- Reduction in MACE and MALE with rivaroxaban added to aspirin was also found post-revascularization in the VOYAGER PAD trial, regardless of clopidogrel use, although an increased bleeding risk was also seen [60].
- **Given these risks and benefits, the patients who would likely have the most benefit from low-dose rivaroxaban (2.5 mg b.i.d.), plus low-dose Aspirin are those with a heavy burden of polyvascular atherosclerotic disease and concurrent low bleeding risk**.

4.1.1.4 Symptomatic Treatment

Cilostazol
Patients with claudication refractory to exercise therapy have limited therapeutic options available. Cilostazol is the medication with the strongest evidence for claudication.

- It is associated with increased pain-free and maximal walking distances (approximately 26 and 40 meters, respectively) compared to placebo [61].
- The STOP-IC trial showed decreased restenosis following angioplasty for femoropopliteal lesions with cilostazol use [62].
- However, there is insufficient evidence regarding its efficacy for MACE and MALE reduction. **It is important to be aware that cilostazol is contraindicated in patients with heart failure** [63].

Pentoxifylline
Pentoxifylline fails to show consistent improvement in walking time in placebo-controlled studies and is not considered to be an effective treatment for claudication [15].

4.1.1.5 Compression Therapy
It is important to consider that many patients with PAD may also suffer from chronic venous insufficiency. Although first-line management of venous ulcers typically includes compression therapy, the vascular specialist must be judicious about using this therapy in their patients with PAD.

- Compression therapy could reduce arterial perfusion by compressing both cutaneous microvasculature, increasing the risk of ischemic complications, as well as outflow vessels, possibly interfering with future revascularization attempts.
- Therefore, it should generally be avoided in patients with venous ulcers who also have advanced PAD [64, 65]. The vascular specialist should also consider arterial revascularization to optimize wound healing prior to initiating compression therapy in their patients with mixed arterial and venous disease.

4.2   Conclusion

The PAD population is at a significantly increased risk of major adverse cardiovascular and limb-related events. Vascular specialists must be facile with the medical management of PAD and coordinate closely in a multidisciplinary fashion to provide the most effective care to their patients. This includes both counseling their patients to pursue lifestyle changes (i.e., smoking cessation, dietary modification, and exercise therapy) as well as ensuring their patients are on appropriate pharmaceutical therapies for PAD (i.e., antithrombotic therapy and cilostazol) and its comorbidities (i.e., dyslipidemia, hypertension, and diabetes). Through actively participating in the comprehensive care of their patients, modern vascular specialists can dramatically improve their patients' lives magnitudes beyond that achieved by procedural intervention alone (Fig. 4.1).

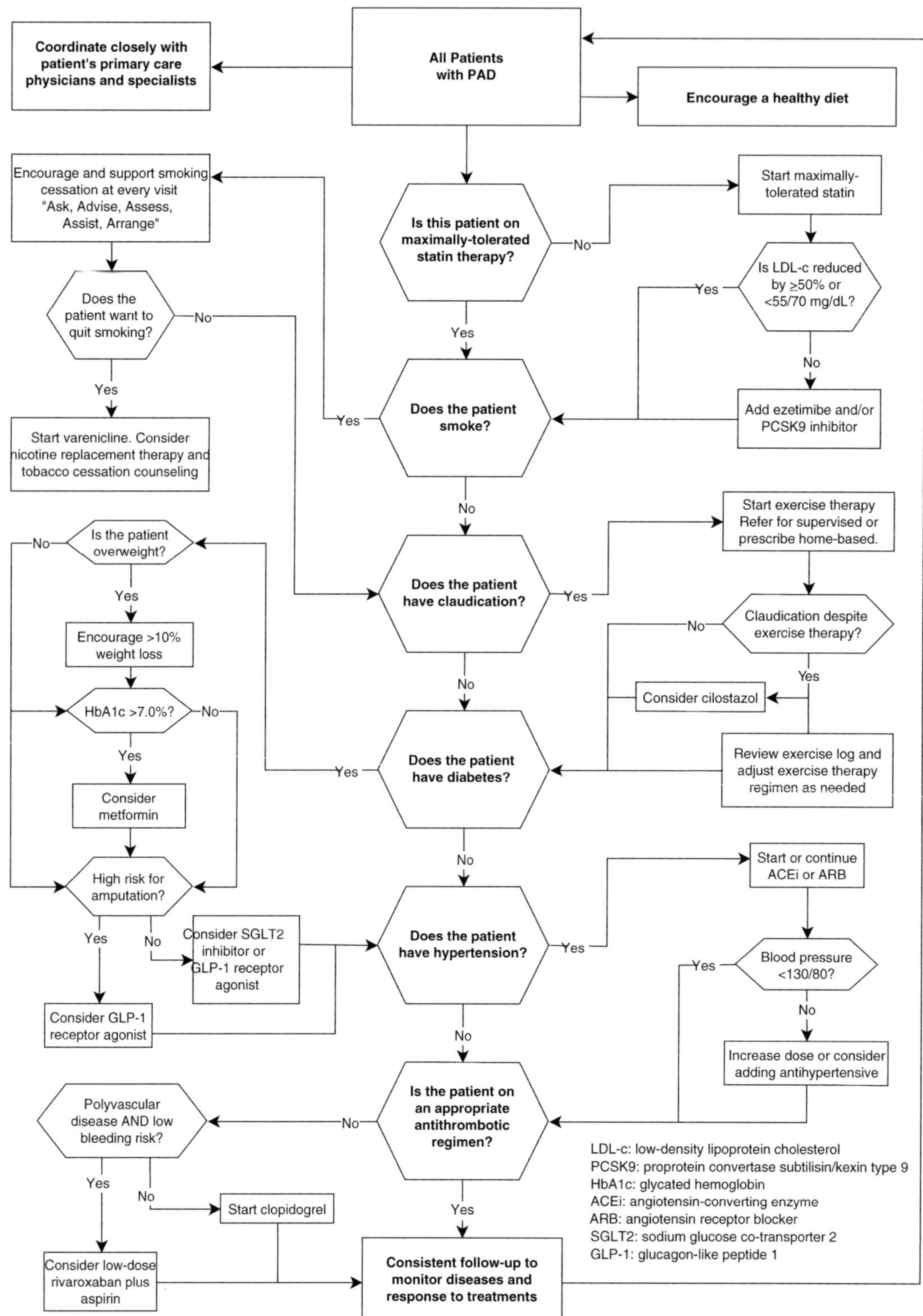

Fig. 4.1 Medical management of peripheral arterial disease flowsheet

4.2.1 Primary Recommendations for Medical Management of Pad

1. Vascular specialists must optimize the care of their patients with PAD by assisting with the medical management of cardiovascular risk factors through close coordination with these patients' primary care providers and other specialists.
2. All patients who smoke should be consistently encouraged to quit smoking and assisted in their efforts. The first-line pharmaceutical therapy for smoking cessation is Varenicline, which may be supplemented with nicotine replacement therapy and tobacco use counseling.
3. All patients should be encouraged to consume a healthy diet and aggressive hydration can be considered for patients without contraindications.
4. Patients with claudication should participate in a supervised or home-based exercise program. One example home-based prescription is walking to near-maximal claudication discomfort (7/10), resting until pain nearly subsides (3/10), and then resume walking for at least 30 minutes three times a week. Patients should also be encouraged to keep a log of their activity and the vascular specialist should coach them on their exercise habits accordingly.
5. All patients with PAD should be receiving maximally tolerated statin therapy with a goal LDL-c reduction of $\geq 50\%$ or LDL-c $< 55/70$ mg/dL. If this goal is not achieved with statin therapy alone, adjunctive therapy with ezetimibe and/or a PCSK9 inhibitor should be considered on an individual basis.
6. ACEi and ARBs should be considered as first-line therapies for hypertension in the PAD population. Blood pressure should be treated to a target of $<130/85$.
7. Patients with concomitant diabetes and PAD should be treated to a goal glycated hemoglobin of $<7.0\%$ with lifestyle and pharmaceutical intervention. SGLT2 inhibitors and/or GLP-1 receptor agonists should be considered in patients with PAD, although cost and availability might limit their current use.
8. All patients with symptomatic PAD should be considered for an antithrombotic regimen. Clopidogrel is the first-line antiplatelet therapy. Low-dose rivaroxaban added to aspirin should be considered in patients with polyvascular disease and low bleeding risk.
9. Cilostazol is helpful for increasing pain-free and maximal walking distances in patients with claudication, although it is contraindicated in heart failure. Pentoxifylline is not an effective treatment for claudication.
10. Compression therapy should be used judiciously in patients with mixed arterial and venous disease and avoided in patients with advanced PAD.

4.3 Lymphedema Management

Zachary Chadnick, Ali Kimyaghalam, and Kuldeep Singh

The lymphatic or lymphoid system is a large network of lymphatic vessels, lymph nodes, and lymphatic organs playing multiple roles in the human body related to circulation, digestion, and immune functions [66, 67]. Lymphedema occurs due to an obstruction of the lymphatic system leading to an accumulation of lymphatic fluid in the affected extremity. When the fluid load exceeds the transport capacity of the system, the fluid accumulates in the tissue leading to a proliferation of adipocytes and deposition of collagen fibers [66–68].

Lymphedema can be categorized in one of two ways. It can be classified based on the etiology of symptoms (primary or secondary) or based on the severity of symptoms (Stage I–Stage III).

Primary lymphedema occurs due to a congenital or inherited condition leading to pathologic development of lymphatic vessels and often presents in childhood but may present later. It is subdivided based on the age of onset [68].

- *Congenital lymphedema* occurs between birth and 2 years of age.
- *Lymphedema praecox* arises during puberty or pregnancy, usually before the age of 35 years.
- *Lymphedema tarda* presents after the age of 35 years.

Secondary lymphedema is much more common and occurs as the result of external factors such as a medical condition or treatment leading to disruption of the lymphatic system. Worldwide filariasis is the most common cause of lymphedema and arises due to obstruction of the lymphatic system by the parasitic worm *(Wuchereria bancrofti).*

There are several grading systems in place to categorize symptom severity including the Campisi Staging System, the American Physical Therapy Association, and the National Cancer Institute's Common Terminology Criteria for Adverse Events system, however, **the most common and well-accepted system is based on the International Society of Lymphology (ISL) 2020 guidelines**. It is a 3-stage system based on firmness of the tissue as well as response of the limb swelling to elevation. Of note, due to the presence of multiple lymphatic territories in a single limb, there may be more than one stage exhibited in different portions at any given time [68].

- Stage I is defined by an early accumulation of protein-rich fluid that subsides with limb elevation.
- Stage II involves changes in solid structures and limb elevation alone rarely reduces tissue swelling. Pitting is present in late stage I and early Stage II. Of note, in the latter portion of Stage II, the limb may not pit as excess subcutaneous fat and fibrosis develop.
- Stage III is the end stage of lymphedema characterized by hard woody skin and incorporates lymphostatic elephantiasis (Fig. 4.2). Furthermore, the presence of trophic skin changes such as acanthosis, alterations in skin character and thickness, further deposition of fat and fibrosis, and warty overgrowths are usually present in this

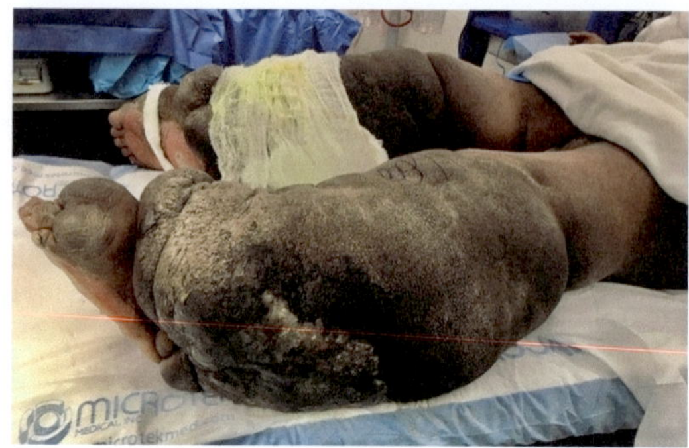

Fig. 4.2 Massive swelling of the lower leg due to chronic untreated lymphedema. Fibrosis of the skin occurs due to fluid stasis and recurrent infections leading to warty appearance and hardening of tissue

stage. Stage III lymphedema may be physically debilitating and require surgical treatment to aid in mobility and improve quality of life (Fig. 4.2).

4.3.1 Treatment Options

Lymphedema is a condition that is chronic in nature with management and treatment focusing on symptom control. There is no well-established curative treatment to fully relieve the obstruction and restore the normal flow of lymphatic channels. There is limited data supporting the various treatments recommended by the ISL for lymphedema [68, 69].

Treatment of early-stage lymphedema is primarily focused on conservative multimodal therapy with a focus on prevention of disease progression, controlling patient comfort, and reducing limb volume. **A limited number of surgical interventions exist for early stage of lymphedema including lymph node transfer and soft tissue reduction surgery, all with limited success [68]. The majority of therapy consists of various forms of compression and decongestive therapy including compression stockings, pneumatic compression devices, and physical therapy including manual lymphatic drainage and decongestive massages.** Recommendations also include avoidance of injury, constricting garments, maintenance of ideal body weight, and hygiene. Lastly, monitoring of the affected extremity using serial measurements of limb circumference, sensation, color, and skin condition is important as early intervention and prevention of progression are often easier than reversal of changes [68, 69].

The conservative measures mentioned above are the mainstay of treatment for symptom control and disease progression. Diet and exercise to maintain healthy body weight, and limb mobility

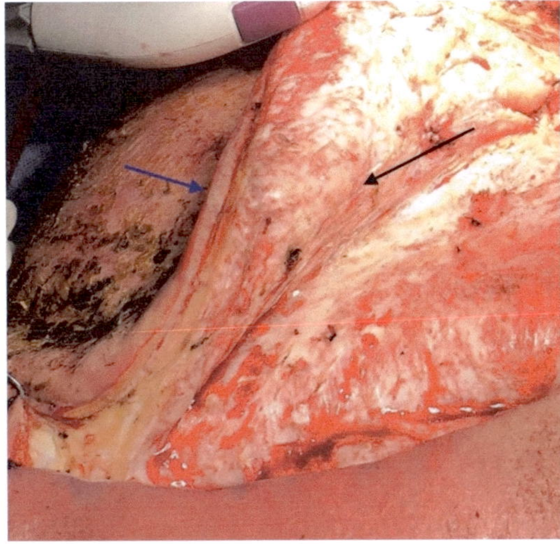

Fig. 4.3 Skin thickening (blue arrow) and fibrofatty changes (black arrow) that occur in the subdermal fat preclude less invasive options such as liposuction and physiologic surgery including lymph node transfer

are used with various levels of efficacy and limited data. **As stage and symptom severity progress the evidence suggests a stricter regimen of compression stockings and manual decompression**. In stage III lymphedema additional measures often include surgical interventions aimed at improving quality of life. There is a limited role for any pharmacological therapy and diuretics should be avoided [68, 70]. Surgical management is typically reserved for localized primary malformations, recurrent symptoms including cellulitis in the affected extremity and failed medical/conservative management.

Surgical management is categorized into physiologic techniques and reductive techniques, however, many surgeons use a combined approach [3]. Physiologic surgery consists of lymph node transplantation or lymphatic bypass. They are typically used in the early stage of lymphedema prior to deposition of excessive tissue in the extremities and severe fibrosis and skin thickening (Fig. 4.3). **The goal of reductive techniques is the removal of excessive fibrofatty tissue in a given extremity to aid in mobility and comfort of the patient.** Further management includes less invasive techniques such as liposuction, to more invasive procedures such as radical debulking of superficial tissues (Fig. 4.4). These are typically reserved for patients who have failed conservative measures and have reached stage III [68–70].

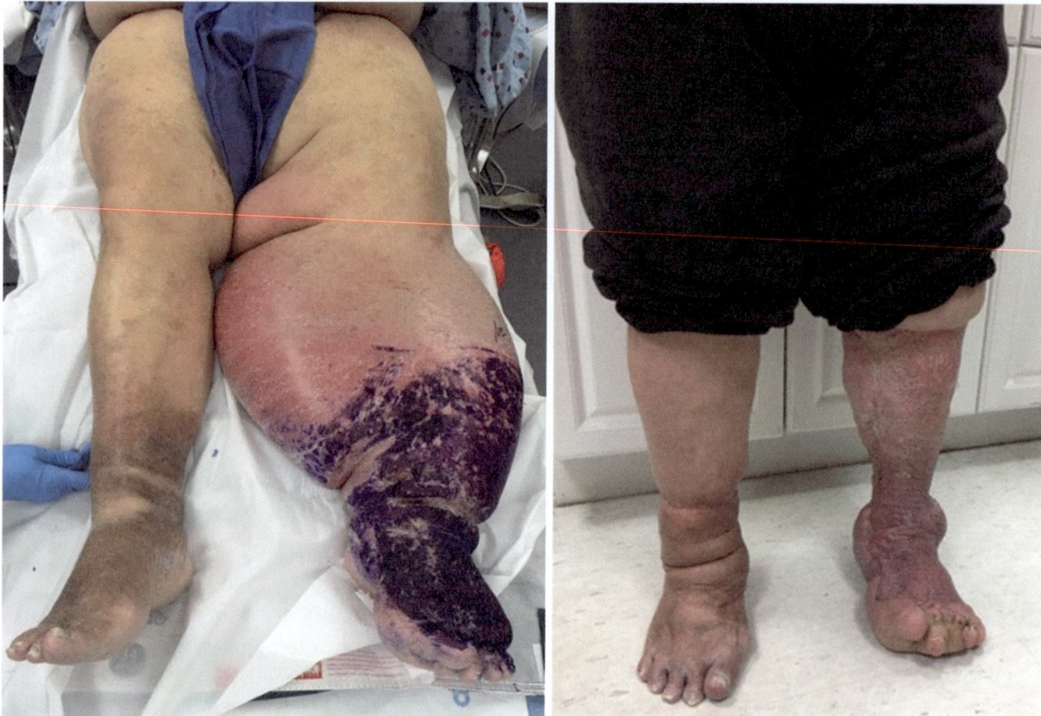

Fig. 4.4 The accumulation of the fluid caused a severe increase in weight in the legs and hence leading to debilitating back pain in this patient limiting ambulation. After radical debulking the back pain resolved and he was able to ambulate normally

References

1. Hiatt WR, Fowkes FGR, Heizer G, et al. Ticagrelor versus clopidogrel in symptomatic peripheral artery disease. N Engl J Med. 2017;376(1):32–40. https://doi.org/10.1056/NEJMoa1611688.
2. Ohman EM, Bhatt DL, Steg PG, et al. The reduction of atherothrombosis for continued health (REACH) Registry: an international, prospective, observational investigation in subjects at risk for atherothrombotic events-study design. Am Heart J. 2006;151(4):786. e1–10. https://doi.org/10.1016/j.ahj.2005.11.004.
3. Fanaroff AC, Manandhar P, Holmes DR, et al. Peripheral artery disease and transcatheter aortic valve replacement outcomes. Circ Cardiovasc Interv. 2017;10(10):e005456. https://doi.org/10.1161/CIRCINTERVENTIONS.117.005456.
4. Bonaca MP, Hamburg NM, Creager MA. Contemporary medical management of peripheral artery disease. Circ Res. 2021;128(12): 1868–84. https://doi.org/10.1161/CIRCRESAHA.121.318258.
5. Ding N, Sang Y, Chen J, et al. Cigarette smoking, smoking cessation, and long-term risk of 3 major atherosclerotic diseases. J Am Coll Cardiol. 2019;74(4):498–507. https://doi.org/10.1016/j.jacc.2019.05.049.
6. Lu L, Mackay DF, Pell JP. Secondhand smoke exposure and risk of incident peripheral arterial disease and mortality: a Scotland-wide retrospective cohort study of 4045 non-smokers with cotinine measurement. BMC Public Health. 2018;18:348. https://doi.org/10.1186/s12889-018-5227-x.
7. Anthenelli RM, Benowitz NL, West R, et al. Neuropsychiatric safety and efficacy of varenicline, bupropion, and nicotine patch in smokers with and without psychiatric disorders (EAGLES): a double-blind, randomised, placebo-controlled clinical trial. Lancet. 2016;387(10037):2507–20. https://doi.org/10.1016/S0140-6736(16)30272-0.
8. Primary Prevention of Cardiovascular Disease with a Mediterranean Diet Supplemented with Extra-Virgin Olive Oil or Nuts | NEJM. https://www.nejm.org/doi/full/10.1056/nejmoa1800389. Accessed 29 April 2022.
9. Hydration may reverse most symptoms of lower extremity intermittent claudication or rest pain – PubMed. https://pubmed.ncbi.nlm.nih.gov/32972591/. Accessed 29 April 2022.
10. Murphy TP, Cutlip DE, Regensteiner JG, et al. Supervised exercise, stent revascularization, or medical therapy for claudication due to aortoiliac peripheral artery disease: The CLEVER Study. J Am Coll Cardiol. 2015;65(10):999–1009. https://doi.org/10.1016/j.jacc.2014.12.043.

11. McDermott MM, Guralnik JM, Criqui MH, et al. Home-based walking exercise in peripheral artery disease: 12-month follow-up of the goals randomized trial. J Am Heart Assoc Cardiovasc Cerebrovasc Dis. 2014;3(3):e000711. https://doi.org/10.1161/JAHA.113.000711.

12. Bearne LM, Volkmer B, Peacock J, et al. Effect of a home-based, walking exercise behavior change intervention vs usual care on walking in adults with peripheral artery disease: the MOSAIC Randomized Clinical Trial. JAMA. 2022;327(14):1344–55. https://doi.org/10.1001/jama.2022.3391.

13. Effect of Low-Intensity vs High-Intensity Home-Based Walking Exercise on Walk Distance in Patients with Peripheral Artery Disease: the LITE Randomized Clinical Trial | Cardiology | JAMA | JAMA Network. https://jamanetwork.com/journals/jama/fullarticle/2778112. Accessed 29 April 2022.

14. Hess CN, Cannon CP, Beckman JA, et al. Effectiveness of blood lipid management in patients with peripheral artery disease. J Am Coll Cardiol. 2021;77(24):3016–27. https://doi.org/10.1016/j.jacc.2021.04.060.

15. Gerhard-Herman MD, Gornik HL, Barrett C, et al. 2016 AHA/ACC guideline on the management of patients with lower extremity peripheral artery disease: executive summary: a report of the American College of Cardiology/American Heart Association task force on clinical practice guidelines. Circulation. 2017;135(12):e686–725. https://doi.org/10.1161/CIR.0000000000000470.

16. Aboyans V, Ricco JB, Bartelink MLEL, et al. 2017 ESC Guidelines on the Diagnosis and Treatment of Peripheral Arterial Diseases, in collaboration with the European Society for Vascular Surgery (ESVS): Document covering atherosclerotic disease of extra-cranial carotid and vertebral, mesenteric, renal, upper and lower extremity arteries Endorsed by: the European Stroke Organization (ESO) The Task Force for the Diagnosis and Treatment of Peripheral Arterial Diseases of the European Society of Cardiology (ESC) and of the European Society for Vascular Surgery (ESVS). Eur Heart J. 2018;39(9):763–816. https://doi.org/10.1093/eurheartj/ehx095.

17. Mohler ER, Hiatt WR, Creager MA. Cholesterol reduction with atorvastatin improves walking distance in patients with peripheral arterial disease. Circulation. 2003;108(12):1481–6. https://doi.org/10.1161/01.CIR.0000090686.57897.F5.

18. Kokkinidis DG, Arfaras-Melainis A, Giannopoulos S, et al. Statin therapy for reduction of cardiovascular and limb-related events in critical limb ischemia: a systematic review and meta-analysis. Vasc Med Lond Engl. 2020;25(2):106–17. https://doi.org/10.1177/1358863X19894055.

19. Foley TR, Singh GD, Kokkinidis DG, et al. High-intensity statin therapy is associated with improved survival in patients with peripheral artery disease. J Am Heart Assoc. 2017;6(7):e005699. https://doi.org/10.1161/JAHA.117.005699.

20. Bhatt DL, Steg PG, Ohman EM, et al. International prevalence, recognition, and treatment of cardiovascular risk factors in outpatients with atherothrombosis. JAMA. 2006;295(2):180–9. https://doi.org/10.1001/jama.295.2.180.

21. Hirsch AT, Criqui MH, Treat-Jacobson D, et al. Peripheral arterial disease detection, awareness, and treatment in primary care. JAMA. 2001;286(11):1317–24. https://doi.org/10.1001/jama.286.11.1317.

22. Whelton PK, Carey RM, Aronow WS, et al. 2017 ACC/AHA/AAPA/ABC/ACPM/AGS/APhA/ASH/ASPC/NMA/PCNA Guideline for the Prevention, Detection, Evaluation, and Management of High Blood Pressure in Adults: A Report of the American College of Cardiology/American Heart Association Task Force on Clinical Practice Guidelines. Hypertension. 2018;71(6):e13–e115. https://doi.org/10.1161/HYP.0000000000000065.

23. Bavry AA, Anderson RD, Gong Y, et al. Outcomes among hypertensive patients with concomitant peripheral and coronary artery disease. Hypertension. 2010;55(1):48–53. https://doi.org/10.1161/HYPERTENSIONAHA.109.142240.

24. Piller LB, Simpson LM, Baraniuk S, et al. Characteristics and long-term follow-up of participants with peripheral arterial disease during ALLHAT. J Gen Intern Med. 2014;29(11):1475–83. https://doi.org/10.1007/s11606-014-2947-1.

25. Ostergren J, Sleight P, Dagenais G, et al. Impact of ramipril in patients with evidence of clinical or subclinical peripheral arterial disease. Eur Heart J. 2004;25(1):17–24. https://doi.org/10.1016/j.ehj.2003.10.033.

26. Telmisartan, ramipril, or both in patients at high risk for vascular events. N Engl J Med. 2008;358(15):1547–59. https://doi.org/10.1056/NEJMoa0801317.

27. Telmisartan Randomised AssessmeNt Study in ACE iNtolerant subjects with cardiovascular Disease (TRANSCEND) Investigators, Yusuf S, Teo K, et al. Effects of the angiotensin-receptor blocker telmisartan on cardiovascular events in high-risk patients intolerant to angiotensin-converting enzyme inhibitors: a randomised controlled trial. Lancet Lond Engl. 2008;372(9644):1174–83. https://doi.org/10.1016/S0140-6736(08)61242-8.

28. Paravastu SCV, Mendonca DA, Silva AD. Beta blockers for peripheral arterial disease. Cochrane Database Syst Rev. 2013;9 https://doi.org/10.1002/14651858.CD005508.pub3.

29. SPRINT Research Group, Wright JT Jr, Williamson JD, et al. A randomized trial of intensive versus standard blood-pressure control. N Engl J Med. 2015;373(22):2103–16. https://doi.org/10.1056/NEJMoa1511939.

30. American Diabetes Association. Peripheral arterial disease in people with diabetes. Diabetes Care. 2003;26(12):3333–41. https://doi.org/10.2337/diacare.26.12.3333.

31. Action to Control Cardiovascular Risk in Diabetes Study Group, Gerstein HC, Miller ME, et al. Effects

of intensive glucose lowering in type 2 diabetes. N Engl J Med. 2008;358(24):2545–59. https://doi.org/10.1056/NEJMoa0802743.

32. ADVANCE Collaborative Group, Patel A, MacMahon S, Chalmers J, Neal B, Billot L, Woodward M, Marre M, Cooper M, Glasziou P, Grobbee D, Hamet P, Harrap S, Heller S, Liu L, Mancia G, Mogensen CE, Pan C, Poulter N, Rodgers A, Williams B, Bompoint S, de Galan BE, Joshi R, Travert F. Intensive blood glucose control and vascular outcomes in patients with type 2 diabetes. N Engl J Med. 2008;358(24):2560–72. https://doi.org/10.1056/NEJMoa0802987.

33. American Diabetes Association Professional Practice Committee. 8. Obesity and weight management for the prevention and treatment of type 2 diabetes: standards of medical care in diabetes—2022. Diabetes Care. 2021;45(Supplement_1):S113–24. https://doi.org/10.2337/dc22-S008.

34. Look AHEAD Research Group, Gregg E, Jakicic J, et al. Association of the magnitude of weight loss and changes in physical fitness with long-term cardiovascular disease outcomes in overweight or obese people with type 2 diabetes: a post-hoc analysis of the Look AHEAD randomised clinical trial. Lancet Diabetes Endocrinol. 2016;4(11):913–21. https://doi.org/10.1016/S2213-8587(16)30162-0.

35. Holman RR, Paul SK, Bethel MA, Matthews DR, Neil HAW. 10-year follow-up of intensive glucose control in type 2 diabetes. N Engl J Med. 2008;359(15):1577–89. https://doi.org/10.1056/NEJMoa0806470.

36. Maruthur NM, Tseng E, Hutfless S, et al. Diabetes medications as monotherapy or metformin-based combination therapy for type 2 diabetes: a systematic review and meta-analysis. Ann Intern Med. 2016;164(11):740–51. https://doi.org/10.7326/M15-2650.

37. Zinman B, Wanner C, Lachin JM, et al. Empagliflozin, cardiovascular outcomes, and mortality in type 2 diabetes. N Engl J Med. 2015;373(22):2117–28. https://doi.org/10.1056/NEJMoa1504720.

38. Neal B, Perkovic V, Mahaffey KW, et al. Canagliflozin and cardiovascular and renal events in type 2 diabetes. N Engl J Med. 2017;377(7):644–57. https://doi.org/10.1056/NEJMoa1611925.

39. Perkovic V, Jardine MJ, Neal B, et al. Canagliflozin and renal outcomes in type 2 diabetes and nephropathy. N Engl J Med. 2019;380(24):2295–306. https://doi.org/10.1056/NEJMoa1811744.

40. Wiviott SD, Raz I, Bonaca MP, et al. Dapagliflozin and cardiovascular outcomes in type 2 diabetes. N Engl J Med. 2019;380(4):347–57. https://doi.org/10.1056/NEJMoa1812389.

41. McMurray JJV, Solomon SD, Inzucchi SE, et al. Dapagliflozin in patients with heart failure and reduced ejection fraction. N Engl J Med. 2019;381(21):1995–2008. https://doi.org/10.1056/NEJMoa1911303.

42. Heerspink HJL, Stefánsson BV, Correa-Rotter R, et al. Dapagliflozin in patients with chronic kidney disease. N Engl J Med. 2020;383(15):1436–46. https://doi.org/10.1056/NEJMoa2024816.

43. Marso SP, Daniels GH, Brown-Frandsen K, et al. Liraglutide and cardiovascular outcomes in type 2 diabetes. N Engl J Med. 2016;375(4):311–22. https://doi.org/10.1056/NEJMoa1603827.

44. Marso SP, Bain SC, Consoli A, et al. Semaglutide and cardiovascular outcomes in patients with type 2 diabetes. N Engl J Med. 2016;375(19):1834–44. https://doi.org/10.1056/NEJMoa1607141.

45. Gerstein HC, Colhoun HM, Dagenais GR, et al. Dulaglutide and cardiovascular outcomes in type 2 diabetes (REWIND): a double-blind, randomised placebo-controlled trial. Lancet. 2019;394(10193):121–30. https://doi.org/10.1016/S0140-6736(19)31149-3.

46. American Diabetes Association Professional Practice Committee. 10. Cardiovascular disease and risk management: standards of medical care in diabetes—2022. Diabetes Care. 2021;45(Supplement_1):S144–74. https://doi.org/10.2337/dc22-S010.

47. Antithrombotic Trialists' Collaboration. Collaborative meta-analysis of randomised trials of antiplatelet therapy for prevention of death, myocardial infarction, and stroke in high risk patients. BMJ. 2002;324(7329):71–86. https://doi.org/10.1136/bmj.324.7329.71.

48. Belch J, MacCuish A, Campbell I, et al. The prevention of progression of arterial disease and diabetes (POPADAD) trial: factorial randomised placebo controlled trial of aspirin and antioxidants in patients with diabetes and asymptomatic peripheral arterial disease. BMJ. 2008;337:a1840. https://doi.org/10.1136/bmj.a1840.

49. Fowkes FGR, Price JF, Stewart MCW, et al. Aspirin for prevention of cardiovascular events in a general population screened for a low ankle brachial index: a randomized controlled trial. JAMA. 2010;303(9):841–8. https://doi.org/10.1001/jama.2010.221.

50. Poredos P, Jezovnik MK. Is aspirin still the drug of choice for management of patients with peripheral arterial disease? VASA Z Gefasskrankheiten. 2013;42(2):88–95. https://doi.org/10.1024/0301-1526/a000251.

51. Brass EP, Hiatt WR. Aspirin monotherapy should not be recommended for cardioprotection in patients with symptomatic peripheral artery disease. Circulation. 2017;136(9):785–6. https://doi.org/10.1161/CIRCULATIONAHA.117.028888.

52. CAPRIE Steering Committee. A randomised, blinded, trial of clopidogrel versus aspirin in patients at risk of ischaemic events (CAPRIE). Lancet. 1996;348(9038):1329–39. https://doi.org/10.1016/S0140-6736(96)09457-3.

53. Bhatt DL, Fox KAA, Hacke W, et al. Clopidogrel and aspirin versus aspirin alone for the prevention of atherothrombotic events. N Engl J Med. 2006;354(16):1706–17. https://doi.org/10.1056/NEJMoa060989.

54. Bonaca MP, Bhatt DL, Cohen M, et al. Long-term use of ticagrelor in patients with prior myocardial infarction. N Engl J Med. 2015;372(19):1791–800. https://doi.org/10.1056/NEJMoa1500857.

55. Steg PG, Bhatt DL, Simon T, et al. Ticagrelor in patients with stable coronary disease and diabetes. N Engl J Med. 2019;381(14):1309–20. https://doi.org/10.1056/NEJMoa1908077.

56. Morrow DA, Braunwald E, Bonaca MP, et al. Vorapaxar in the secondary prevention of atherothrombotic events. N Engl J Med. 2012;366(15):1404–13. https://doi.org/10.1056/NEJMoa1200933.

57. Bonaca MP, Scirica BM, Creager MA, et al. Vorapaxar in patients with peripheral artery disease: results from TRA2{degrees}P-TIMI 50. Circulation. 2013;127(14):1522-9., 1529e1-6. https://doi.org/10.1161/CIRCULATIONAHA.112.000679.

58. Eikelboom JW, Connolly SJ, Bosch J, et al. Rivaroxaban with or without aspirin in stable cardiovascular disease. N Engl J Med. 2017;377(14):1319–30. https://doi.org/10.1056/NEJMoa1709118.

59. Kaplovitch E, Eikelboom JW, Dyal L, et al. Rivaroxaban and aspirin in patients with symptomatic lower extremity peripheral artery disease: a subanalysis of the COMPASS randomized clinical trial. JAMA Cardiol. 2021;6(1):21–9. https://doi.org/10.1001/jamacardio.2020.4390.

60. Bonaca MP, Bauersachs RM, Anand SS, et al. Rivaroxaban in peripheral artery disease after revascularization. N Engl J Med. 2020;382(21):1994–2004. https://doi.org/10.1056/NEJMoa2000052.

61. Brown T, Forster RB, Cleanthis M, Mikhailidis DP, Stansby G, Stewart M. Cilostazol for intermittent claudication. Cochrane Database Syst Rev. 2021;6 https://doi.org/10.1002/14651858.CD003748.pub5.

62. Iida O, Yokoi H, Soga Y, et al. Cilostazol Reduces Angiographic Restenosis After Endovascular Therapy for Femoropopliteal Lesions in the Sufficient Treatment of Peripheral Intervention by Cilostazol Study. Circulation. 2013;127(23):2307–15. https://doi.org/10.1161/CIRCULATIONAHA.112.000711.

63. Page RL, O'Bryant CL, Cheng D, et al. Drugs that may cause or exacerbate heart failure: a scientific statement from the American Heart Association. Circulation. 2016;134(6):e32–69. https://doi.org/10.1161/CIR.0000000000000426.

64. O'Meara S, Cullum N, Nelson EA, Dumville JC. Compression for venous leg ulcers. Cochrane Database Syst Rev. 2012;2012(11):CD000265. https://doi.org/10.1002/14651858.CD000265.pub3.

65. Stücker M, Danneil O, Dörler M, Hoffmann M, Kröger E, Reich-Schupke S. Safety of a compression stocking for patients with chronic venous insufficiency (CVI) and peripheral artery disease (PAD). Dtsch Dermatol Ges. 2020;18(3):207–13. https://doi.org/10.1111/ddg.14042.

66. Yang Y, Oliver G. Development of the mammalian lymphatic vasculature. J Clin Invest. 2014;124(3):888–97.

67. Randolph GJ, Ivanov S, Zinselmeyer BH, Scallan JP. The lymphatic system: integral roles in immunity. Annu Rev Immunol. 2017;35:31–52.

68. Executive Committee of the International Society of Lymphology. The diagnosis and treatment of peripheral lymphedema: 2020 Consensus Document of the International Society of Lymphology. Lymphology. 2020;53(1):3–19.

69. Ramachandran S, Chew KY, Tan BK, Kuo YR. Current operative management and therapeutic algorithm of lymphedema in the lower extremities. Asian J Surg. 2021 Jan;44(1):46–53.

70. Granzow JW. Lymphedema surgery: the current state of the art. Clin Exp Metastasis. 2018;35(5–6):553–8.

Infectious Disease Evaluation and Management

5

Nipun Atri, Nawar Hudefi, Sreekumar Madassery, and Joseph L. Mills Sr

5.1 When Should I Call Infectious Disease?

Nipun Atri

Published studies have shown that involvement of infectious diseases physicians has a positive impact on limb preservation including reducing the risk of major amputations for patients with limb ischemia and diabetic foot infections [1, 2].

An infectious disease consultation can be valuable in the following scenarios:

- **Wounds complicated by osteomyelitis**—To help determine appropriate duration and route of antimicrobial therapy.
- **Wet gangrene**—When existing dry gangrenous tissue develops severe pain, swelling, and moist appearance. This is a surgical emergency, but empiric antibiotic selection may need ID expertise.
- **Gas gangrene**—Infections caused by exotoxin-producing bacteria that progress over a noticeably brief period, and cause pain out of proportion to physical exam findings. This is also a surgical emergency, but an ID consult can help with the addition of antimicrobials with toxin suppression effects.

Additionally, involving ID in early-stage ulcers can avoid the unnecessary use of antibiotics in colonized uninfected wounds.

5.2 Is there Osteomyelitis?

Nipun Atri

Patients with limb ischemia and wounds to their extremities can have infection of the underlying bone, or osteomyelitis. Osteomyelitis can be acute (duration of a few days or weeks) or chronic (months or years). Some hallmarks of chronic osteomyelitis are presence of pieces of necrotic bone due to bone ischemia and presence of a sinus tract.

Osteomyelitis associated with limb ischemia often tends to be non-hematogenous in origin. It is often due to contiguous spread of infection from adjacent infected tissue which can be mono or polymicrobial.

N. Atri
Department of Medicine, Division of Infectious Diseases, Rush University Medical Center, Chicago, IL, USA
e-mail: Nipun_Atri@rush.edu

N. Hudefi · J. L. Mills Sr
Department of Surgery, Division of Vascular Surgery and Endovascular Therapy, Baylor College of Medicine, Houston, TX, USA
e-mail: Nawar.Hudefi@bcm.edu; Joseph.Mills@bcm.edu

S. Madassery (✉)
Department of Vascular and Interventional Radiology, Rush University Medical Center, Chicago, IL, USA

© The Author(s), under exclusive license to Springer Nature Switzerland AG 2023
S. Madassery, A. Patel (eds.), *Limb Preservation for the Vascular Specialist*,
https://doi.org/10.1007/978-3-031-36480-8_5

Osteomyelitis should be suspected if one or more of the following circumstances are present [3, 4]:

- New or worsening musculoskeletal pain in patients with poorly healing soft tissue wounds adjacent to bony structures.
- Signs of cellulitis or local soft tissue infection over existing wounds overlying bony structures.
- Ulcer duration longer than 2 weeks.
- Diabetic foot ulcers with size >2 cm^2 and/ or ability to probe to bone.
- Visibly exposed bone, particularly when evaluating the non-healing wound.
- Erythrocyte sedimentation rate (ESR) >70 mm/h.

5.2.1 What Imaging Do I Order for Osteomyelitis?

There are multiple imaging modalities, each with their own strengths and weaknesses, which play a role in diagnosis of osteomyelitis [5]. The optimal imaging modality depends upon the specific clinical circumstances and should be tailored accordingly.

The following approach is suggested based on duration of history and exam findings:

- ≥2 weeks: Start with plain X-rays
- <2 weeks: Magnetic resonance imaging (MRI)

Plain radiographs can show characteristic findings of osteomyelitis (cortical erosion, periosteal reaction, mixed lucency, sclerosis, and sequestra) but can be normal early in the disease process.

If clinical suspicion of osteomyelitis remains high despite normal appearance or without definitive characteristic features on X-rays, a more advanced imaging study (such as MRI) should be pursued.

MRI is the imaging modality with the highest sensitivity and negative predictive value for osteomyelitis. It may demonstrate abnormal bone marrow edema as early as 1–5 days following onset of infection.

5.2.1.1 Is MRI with Gadolinium Contrast Enhancement Required?

Gadolinium contrast is not required to diagnose acute osteomyelitis.

However, addition of gadolinium contrast does provide valuable information when chronic osteomyelitis is suspected. It enhances visualization of sinus tracts, fistulas, necrotic tissues and helps distinguish between abscess and phlegmon.

5.2.1.2 Other Imaging Modalities

Computed tomography (CT) is more sensitive than plain radiographs (but less so than MRI) for detection of osteomyelitis. Addition of intravenous contrast improves the detection of soft tissue abnormalities such as sinus tracts. Metallic hardware can limit CT's diagnostic yield due to artifact.

Nuclear tests such as PET/CT or three-phase bone scan are alternatives when metal hardware precludes MRI or CT, or if MRI is contraindicated. PET/CT has similar diagnostic accuracy as MRI but is cost prohibitive to be used routinely. Three-phase bone scan has high sensitivity but lower specificity for diagnosing osteomyelitis because normal bone turnover or non-infectious inflammation of bone can be confused with osteomyelitis [5].

5.3 When Do I Start Antimicrobials?

Nipun Atri

Clinicians taking care of patients with limb ischemia and wounds should attempt to establish whether there are signs and symptoms of an acute infection or not before starting antimicrobial therapy. Findings can be localized (increased pain, swelling, redness, discharge) or systemic (fever, tachypnea, tachycardia, hypotension).

Antimicrobial therapy should be promptly started for the following [6]:

- Cellulitis and abscess formation—Skin erythema (that does not improve with limb elevation), edema, warmth, purulence, or heavy drainage from wounds.
- Wet gangrene—Tissue liquefaction, warmth, erythema, and swelling present at site of previous dry gangrene.
- Gas gangrene—Muscle swelling, severe pain, thin gray "dishwater" discharge, malodor, crepitus.

The latter two processes are limb and life-threatening emergencies. If patients are noted to have them in an ambulatory setting, they should be emergently sent to the emergency room for aggressive multidisciplinary care. Besides antimicrobial therapy, such patients need surgical drainage and/or debridement.

Antimicrobial therapy is usually not immediately required for:

- Dry gangrene.
- Osteomyelitis is when no surrounding skin and soft tissue infection is present.

5.4 Demystifying Wound Cultures

Nipun Atri

Obtaining wound cultures (aerobic/anaerobic/ fungal/acid-fast bacillus) provides vital information needed for performing culture-directed therapy. However, a superficial culture taken from a chronic open wound will result in

organisms that may not be pathogenic. This often leads to unnecessary overuse of antimicrobials and contributes to additional problems, such as development of multidrug-resistant bacteria and drug-induced adverse effects like *Clostridioides difficile* infection. When infection is suspected, deep wound cultures should be taken during debridement [7, 8].

Some of the microorganisms that are often recovered from wound cultures but may not be pathogenic include:

- Coagulase-negative Staphylococci.
- *Enterococcus* species.
- *Candida* species.

Cellulitis and mild infection of ulcers is primarily caused by Streptococci (non-purulent cellulitis) and *Staphylococcus aureus* (purulent cellulitis and abscess forming).

- Chronic ulcers can additionally be infected by Enterobacterales such as *Escherichia coli*.
- Macerated wounds may contain *Pseudomonas aeruginosa*.
- Wounds associated with gangrene can have polymicrobial infections with all previously mentioned pathogens, as well as anaerobes and occasionally fungi. This knowledge should be used in prescribing an antimicrobial regimen. Local antibiograms should also be consulted in deciding the need for MRSA coverage and empiric therapy for Enterobacterales and *Pseudomonas*.

Our empiric antibiotic selection for treatment of infections is listed in Table 5.1. However, local antibiograms should always be consulted in deciding the need for MRSA coverage and empiric therapy for Enterobacterales and *Pseudomonas*. In addition, treatment should be tailored once culture and susceptibility data are available (culture-directed therapy).

Table 5.1 Empiric antibiotic selection for treatment of infection

Diagnosis	Specifics	First line	Severe penicillin allergy/second line	Duration
Cellulitis	Outpatient, Non-purulent	Cephalexin or Cefadroxil	Trimethoprim-Sulfamethoxazole or Doxycycline	5 days
	Outpatient, purulent	Trimethoprim-Sulfamethoxazole or Doxycycline	Linezolid	5 days
	Inpatient, non-purulent	Cefazolin	Vancomycin	5 days
	Inpatient, purulent	Cefazolin If history of MRSA—add Vancomycin	Consider ID consult	5 days
Abscess	Outpatient	Trimethoprim-Sulfamethoxazole	Doxycycline	5–7 days
	Inpatient	Cefazolin If history of MRSA—add Vancomycin	Consider ID consult	5–7 days
Diabetic foot infection	Mild (Ulceration with purulent discharge but minimal cellulitis, no fever	Amoxicillin/clavulanate If concern for MRSA—add Trimethoprim-Sulfamethoxazole or Doxycycline	Trimethoprim-Sulfamethoxazole or Clindamycin	5–14 days
	Moderate to severe (larger ulcer with widespread cellulitis or involving deeper structures)	Piperacillin/tazobactam or Cefepime + Metronidazole If history of MRSA—add Vancomycin	Vancomycin + Levofloxacin + Metronidazole	14–21 days
Necrotizing soft tissue infection	Inpatient (always needs surgical consultation)	Piperacillin/tazobactam + Vancomycin + Clindamycin	Vancomycin + Levofloxacin + Clindamycin	Depends on clinical improvement

5.5 When is Infection Control the Top Priority?

Nawar Hudefi and Joseph L. Mills Sr

All CLTI patients, particularly those with diabetic foot ulcer (DFU), should be initially stratified based on the Society of Vascular Surgery (SVS) Wound, Ischemia, and foot Infection (WIfI) classification system, which unlike previous classifications (Rutherford and Fontaine), which focused primarily on ischemia, includes the presence and severity of infection as a key factor in elevating limb amputation risk. This is because patients with chronic limb-threatening ischemia (CLTI), particularly those with diabetes, may present with an infected diabetic foot ulcer (DFU), a scenario associated with a markedly increased risk of early major limb amputation (Fig. 5.1).

Patients presenting with limb- and/or life-threatening infections require prompt administration of broad-spectrum IV antibiotics, rapid fluid resuscitation, and expeditious operative "damage control" debridement and drainage in the operating room to obtain source control. There are additional cohorts of CLTI patients that do not present with life-threatening infections, who also may benefit from infection control prior to revascularization. The WIfI system provides prognostic value pertaining to 1 year amputation risk and the anticipated benefit of revascularization. CLTI patients should be restaged periodically, particularly after infection control foot operations and change in perfusion status after revascularization.

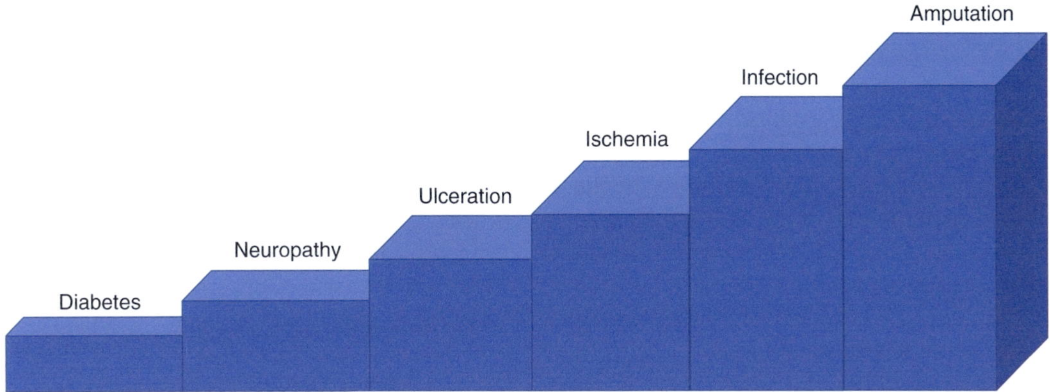

Fig. 5.1 The "stairway to amputation" as described by Rogers et al.

5.5.1 Prioritizing Source Control

5.5.1.1 Infection in DFU and PAD

Perfusion is only one of the determinants of successful limb salvage. The presence of infection profoundly increases the risk of amputation, particularly in the setting of PAD. In fact, most unsalvageable limbs are due to wound extent or the severity of infection. There is a direct correlation between the risk of amputation and increasing infection severity as infection is often the major event that prompts patients to seek out medical attention [9]. One large prospective study observed that the combination of infection and PAD tripled the risk of non-healing wounds in people with diabetes [10]. Another study of 217 diabetic patients presenting with diabetic foot ulcers found that 85% of amputations were either related to infection progression or the lack of infection resolution [11]. The increased metabolic activity and resultant small vessel thrombosis caused by infection increases perfusion demand. The ensuing non-healing wound can unmask PAD that was previously unrecognized.

5.5.1.2 Debridement Before Revascularization

The timing of infection control in relation to revascularization is a frequently encountered clinical issue. A combination of surgery and antibiotics is essential in most if not all advanced foot infections, with the goals of surgical intervention being twofold: infection (source) control and limb salvage. **By controlling the infection, draining of the purulence, and excising all necrotic and non-viable tissue, the surgeon can create a healthy wound bed primed for revascularization and wound healing.**

Therefore, it is important to initially distinguish between infections deemed to be life threatening and those that are not [12]. **Life-threatening infections result in systemic signs of toxicity such as tachycardia, tachypnea, hypotension, elevated white blood count, and fever.** These patients are typically easy to identify and very often require an expeditious trip to the operating room for emergent source control. In these cases, emergent source control may include amputation of the infected limb to prioritize saving a life over a limb (WIfI clinical stage 5).

As previously alluded to, foot infections are part of a spectrum, and therefore should not all be treated in the same manner.

- A mild infection, defined by local swelling, erythema around the ulcer, local tenderness, and superficial purulence can often be treated in an outpatient setting with antibiotics and minor drainage; revascularization can then proceed as planned by the vascular surgeon.

- However, once the local infection extends beyond the skin and subcutaneous tissue, it becomes a moderate infection and debridement may be warranted [12].
- Abscesses should be drained, the extent of the wound evaluated, and antibiotic treatment commenced.
- An infected wound or ulcer with skin undermining creates a reservoir for bacterial growth; therefore, it is necessary to debride the overlying tissue and the devitalized tissue to not only evaluate the depth and extent of the infection but also to stimulate and prepare the wound bed.
- Although there is no clear timeline on when revascularization should be pursued after debridement, most vascular specialists would agree that once appropriate infection control is obtained revascularization should be performed, if indicated, as expeditiously as possible.
- Patients who present with small non-infected ulcers or dry gangrene should be revascularized first, followed by minor digital amputations and local debridement afterward.

Some foot infections are subtle and indolent. Failure to recognize an underlying foot infection can lead to unsuccessful limb salvage attempts despite patent angioplasties or arterial bypass grafts [13]. One study looked at 454 infrainguinal bypasses in patients with CLTI and found that the presence of foot infection was a predictor of major amputation and prolonged hospital stay [14]. The data demonstrated a limb salvage rate in the non-infected group at 1 year, 3 years, and 5 years to be 88%, 79%, and 65%, respectively, compared to 78%, 61%, and 51% in the foot infection group. **This study concluded that despite revascularization, the presence of preoperative foot infection is a significant predictor of major limb amputation** [14]. Treating infection is not only life over limb, but it is often the best first step for limb salvage.

5.5.2 Lower Extremity Threatened Limb Classification System

5.5.2.1 Utility of the WIfI Threatened Limb Classification

Historically, the presence of infection in CLTI patients was ignored by most classification systems. While it is agreed that perfusion and infection are each determinant of outcomes, the extent of the wound also plays a role in predicting amputation risk. In 2014, the Society of Vascular Surgery (SVS) published the Lower Extremity Threatened Limb Classification system with the capability of characterizing the presence and severity of the wound, foot infection, and ischemia [15].

A severity grade of 0–3 (none, mild, moderate, severe) was assigned to each of the three classification components: wound, ischemia, and foot infection (WIfI) of the index limb. **Based on each of the three grades, patients are stratified into a threatened limb clinical stage that predicts the risk of amputation at 1 year and the benefit of revascularization** [15].

The premise of WIfI is that as limb disease burden progresses from clinical stage 1 (very low risk) to stage 4 (high risk), the risk of amputation increases [16]. It is recommended that any patient with suspected CLTI should be accurately staged using WIfI.

- The wound grade depends on the severity of the wound and what level of amputation is predicted to be necessary for limb salvage.
- The ischemia score is derived from hemodynamic tests (ABIs, toe pressure, transcutaneous oxygen pressure), with toe pressures preferred in people with diabetes.
- The infection grade is based upon the Infectious Disease Society of America Classification system which can be derived using clinical data [15].
- The WIfI classification system is meant to define the limb disease burden at presentation, analogous to how the tumor, node, and metastasis (TNM) system is used for cancer staging.

5.5.2.2 Prognostic Value of WIfI

While **WIfI was not designed to dictate treatment methods, it allows physicians to prioritize care, focus sequential steps in care, and to predict limb salvage outcomes.** A recent systemic review and meta-analysis evaluated the current evidence on the prognostic value of WIfI in clinical practice through the evaluation of 12 studies comprising 2669 patients with CLTI [17]. They found that the estimated risk of major amputation at 1 year was 0% for WIfI stage 1, 8% for WIfI stage 2, 11% for WIfI stage 3, and 38% for WIfI stage 4. Following a similar trend, limb salvage at 1 year for WIfI stage 1 is 95%, WIfI stage 2 at 92%, WIfI stage 3 at 91%, and WIfI stage 4 at 61%. **These data confirm that the likelihood of a major amputation increases with a higher WIfI stage while the limb salvage rate correspondingly decreases with higher WIfI stage** [17]. It has also been demonstrated that as WIfI stage increases, wound healing time is longer and reintervention rates, hospital costs, lengths of stay, and readmission rates all increase [18].

The predicted benefit of revascularization can be derived by WIfI, in a fashion similar to the prediction of amputation risk [16]. A multicenter, retrospective study reviewed 1654 CLTI patients undergoing revascularization with the aim of identifying which subgroups within the WIfI classification system benefit most from revascularization [18]. The WIfI stages were clustered into quartiles from greatest to no benefit of revascularization, Q1–Q4, respectively. The data revealed the following 1-year lower extremity amputation rates: Q1 4.4%, Q2 14.8%, Q3 28.1%, and Q4 51.2%. **This study concluded that the WIfI stage does indeed predict which CLTI patients will have the greatest and least benefit from revascularization**. The authors went on to conduct a multivariable analysis to show which of the three WIfI components most strongly predict lower extremity amputation after revascularization and found it to be the wound severity grade [18].

5.5.2.3 Importance of Restaging

The WIfI classification is not intended to be a static assessment. As a patient's course evolves with resolving infection or improved blood flow after revascularization, the limb should be restaged. A single center, retrospective study evaluated 180 limb revascularizations and found that major amputation was associated with the preoperative wound grade but the post-intervention WIfI grades at 1 and 6 months correlated strongly with amputation-free survival [19].

As recommended by the Global Vascular Guidelines, the threatened limb should be restaged after perfusion is addressed, infection is stabilized, or if the wound fails to improve despite appropriate treatment [9]. Periodic restaging can help guide subsequent decision-making regarding the need for reintervention and provide a more reliable estimate of clinical outcomes to both the treating clinician and the patient. This process is analogous to restaging a cancer patient with the TNM system after completion of a course of chemotherapy.

5.5.3 Case Example

A 69-year-old man with longstanding diabetes was admitted with an elevated WBC of 18,000 and a temperature of 102 °F. On physical examination, the lateral aspect of his right foot was red and tender. He was admitted to a hospitalist team and started on broad-spectrum intravenous antibiotics. A vascular specialist was first consulted on hospital day four, by which time the leukocytosis had risen to 27,000 and the patient had developed acute kidney injury (AKI). There was now wet gangrene with gross purulence expressible from the lateral aspect of the foot. The WIfI limb classification was determined to be wound grade 2, ischemia grade 3 (toe pressure <30 mm HG) and foot infection stage 3 (WIfI 2,3,3), WIfI Clinical stage 4, correlating to a high risk of amputation. WIfI staging can be done with a freely available app at

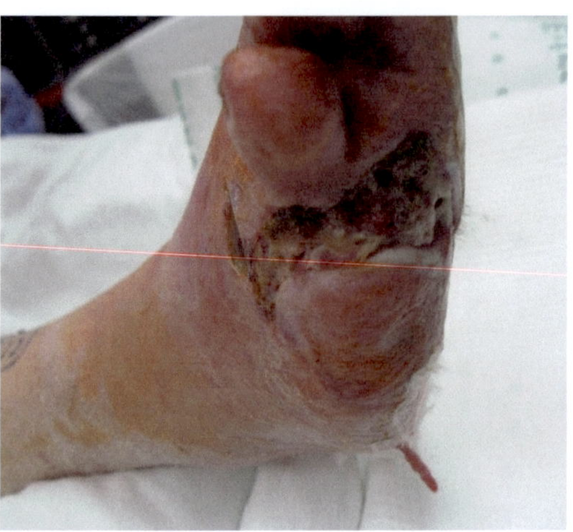

Fig. 5.2 Right foot wound status post-surgical debridement and open fifth ray amputation. Coverage of the wound was only pursued after the infection was cleared and the patient had undergone successful revascularization

the bedside (https://apps.apple.com/us/app/svs-ipg/id1014644425). Given these findings, what is the next best step in this patient's management?

5.5.3.1 Treatment

The patient has obvious signs of systemic toxicity and therefore, draining the foot infection took priority over revascularization. A right fifth ray amputation and lateral forefoot debridement were performed. Four weeks later, renal function had normalized and the infection had cleared, but there was only moderate granulation tissue (Fig. 5.2). What is the next best step in the patient's management? Now that the infection had been controlled, revascularization was clearly the next priority.

Diagnostic angiography with endovascular revascularization was performed with brisk indirect flow restored via the tibio-peroneal trunk and a robust peroneal artery (Fig. 5.3). Indocyanine

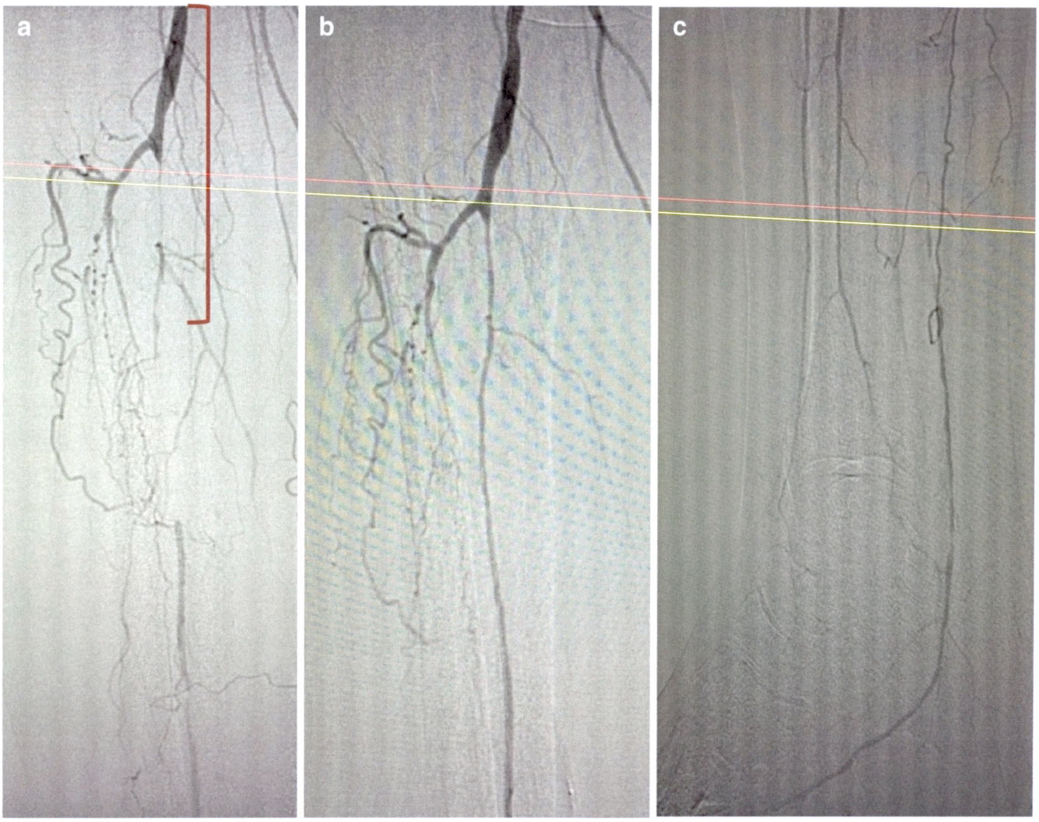

Fig. 5.3 The peroneal artery is the main run-off to the foot (**a**) Angiography revealed an occluded TP trunk and peroneal artery that were crossed and successfully treated. (**b**) Angiogram after atherectomy and balloon angioplasty of the TP trunk and peroneal artery. (**c**) Inline flow to the peroneal artery was restored with indirect perfusion to the foot via robust collaterals to the posterior tibial artery was sufficient to heel the foot (post-procedure = systolic TP 56 mm Hg); no further revascularization was needed

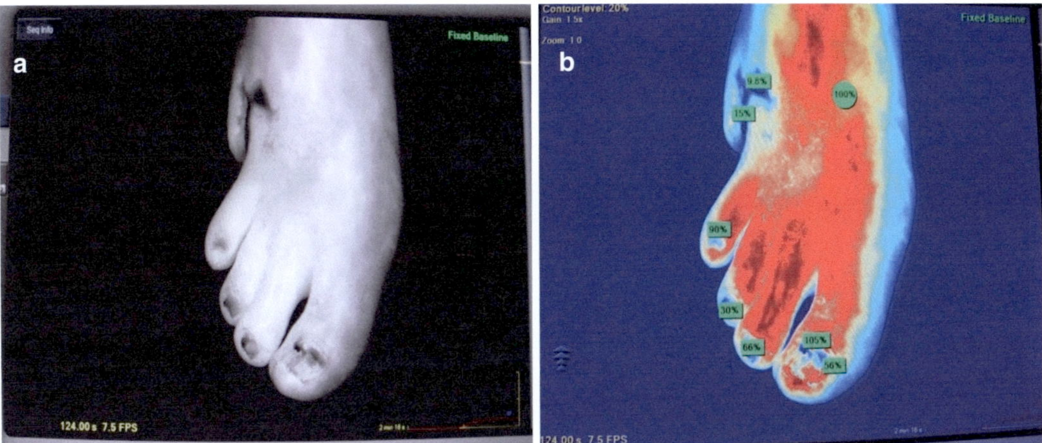

Fig. 5.4 (**a**) Indocyanine green angiography (ICGA) demonstrates quantitative information about regional foot perfusion. (**b**) An ICGA heat map is shown post-intervention

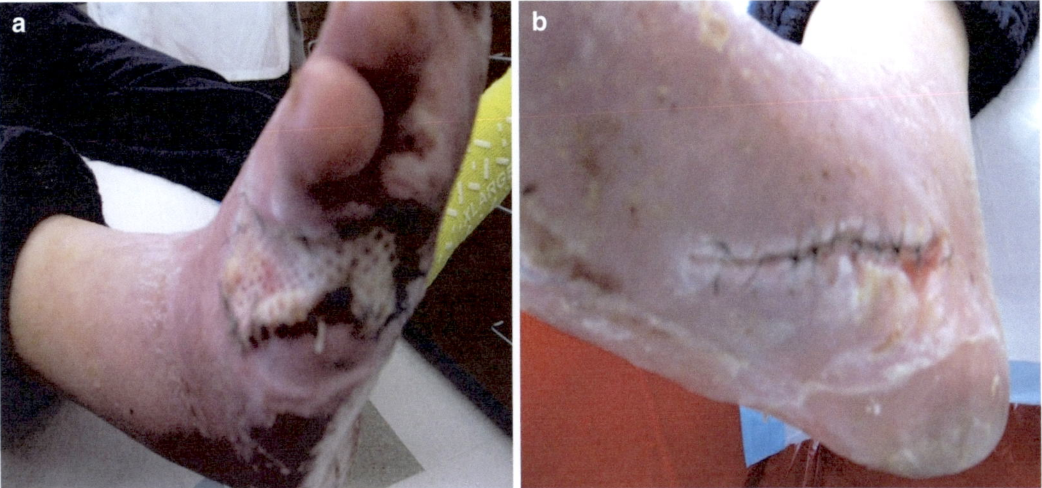

Fig. 5.5 (**a, b**) Right foot after revascularization, debridement, wound closure, and STSG; the toe systolic pressure improved from 0 mmHg to 56 mmHg. Surveillance duplex revealed a patent angioplasty. WIfI Restaging: grade 1 Ischemia and grade 0 foot infection

green angiography (ICGA) demonstrated excellent perfusion to the wound (Fig. 5.4). The patient was followed in outpatient clinic and subsequently split thickness skin grafting and wound closure was performed. Close serial outpatient follow-up was carried out to ensure proper wound care/healing, offloading footwear, and optimal medical management was achieved (Figs. 5.5 and 5.6). The patient's wound healed, major amputation was avoided, and limb salvage was achieved. The patient remains fully independent and ambulatory without recurrent foot wounds 5 years after this orderly sequence of sequential, staged management: (1) infection control; (2) revascularization; (3) final wound debridement and skin graft placement.

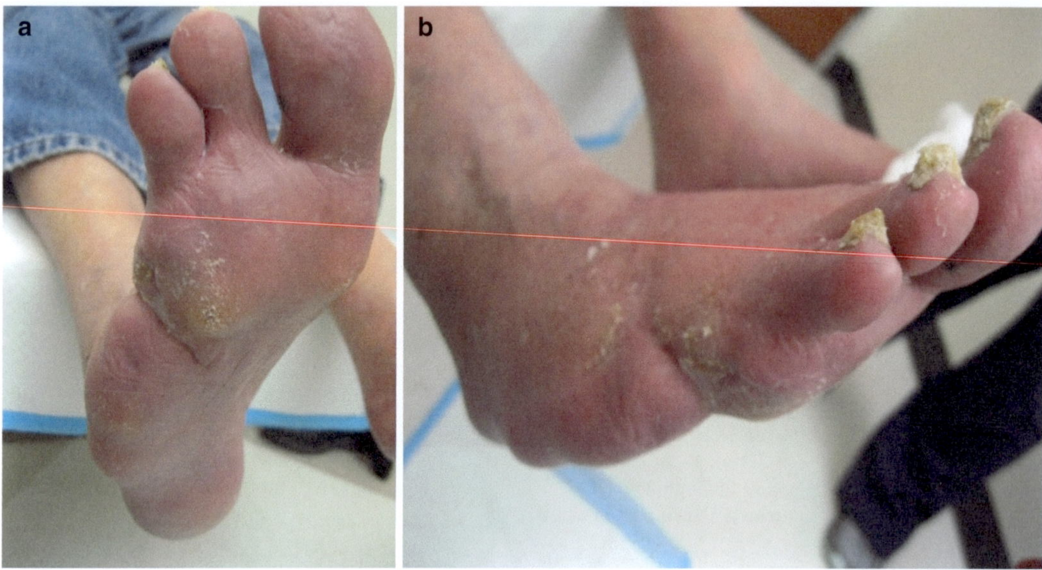

Fig. 5.6 (**a**, **b**) Wound is healed and the patient remains ambulatory 5 years post-intervention; the systolic toe pressure was 46 mmHg at the most recent follow-up assessment

5.6 Conclusion

Overall, the risk of amputation directly correlates with the presence and severity of infection, one of the key components of WIfI threatened limb staging. In the setting of PAD, infection triples the likelihood of non-healing wounds in people with diabetes [19]. Such patients are particularly vulnerable to infection and subsequent risk of amputation. **In general, non-infected ulcers and areas of dry gangrene should not be debrided prior to revascularization.** However, the situation is much different in patients presenting with a component of infection; infection must be recognized, staged, aggressively treated, and rapidly controlled. Depending on the severity of infection, emergent source control prioritizes life over limb and can also be the best first stage for saving the limb. It is recommended the threatened limb should be staged using WIfI prior to and after infection control. This system provides the most accurate prediction of limb outcomes regarding limb salvage and risk of amputation.

References

1. Brennan MB, Allen GO, Ferguson PD, McBride JA, Crnich CJ, Smith MA. The association between geographic density of infectious disease physicians and limb preservation in patients with diabetic foot ulcers. Open Forum Infect Dis. 2017;4(1):ofx015. https://doi.org/10.1093/ofid/ofx015.
2. Izumi Y. Countermeasures against infection in critical limb ischemia treatments. Ann Vasc Dis. 2018;11(3):277–80. https://doi.org/10.3400/avd.ra.18-00073.
3. Grayson ML, Gibbons GW, Balogh K, Levin E, Karchmer AW. Probing to bone in infected pedal ulcers. A clinical sign of underlying osteomyelitis in diabetic patients. JAMA. 1995;273(9):721–3.
4. Butalia S, Palda VA, Sargeant RJ, Detsky AS, Mourad O. Does this patient with diabetes have osteomyelitis of the lower extremity? JAMA. 2008 Feb 20;299(7):806–13. https://doi.org/10.1001/jama.299.7.806.
5. Dinh MT, Abad CL, Safdar N. Diagnostic accuracy of the physical examination and imaging tests for osteomyelitis underlying diabetic foot ulcers: meta-analysis. Clin Infect Dis. 2008;47(4):519–27. https://doi.org/10.1086/590011.
6. Clerici G, Faglia E. Saving the limb in diabetic patients with ischemic foot lesions complicated by acute infec-

tion. Int J Low Extrem Wounds. 2014;13(4):273–93. https://doi.org/10.1177/1534734614549416. Epub 2014 Sep 25

7. Expert Panel on Musculoskeletal Imaging, Beaman FD, von Herrmann PF, Kransdorf MJ, Adler RS, Amini B, Appel M, Arnold E, Bernard SA, Greenspan BS, Lee KS, Tuite MJ, Walker EA, Ward RJ, Wessell DE, Weissman BN. ACR Appropriateness Criteria® Suspected Osteomyelitis, Septic Arthritis, or Soft Tissue Infection (Excluding Spine and Diabetic Foot). J Am Coll Radiol. 2017;14(5S):S326–37. https://doi.org/10.1016/j.jacr.2017.02.008.

8. Bennett J, Dolin R, Blaser M. Cellulitis and superficial infections. In: Mandell, Douglas, and Bennett's principles and practice of infectious diseases. 9th ed. Amsterdam: Elsevier Health Sciences; 2020.

9. Conte MS, Bradbury AW, Kolh P, White JV, Dick F, Fitridge R, et al. Global vascular guidelines on the management of chronic limb-threatening ischemia. J Vasc Surg. 2019;69(6 Suppl):3S–125S.e40.

10. Mathioudakis N, Hicks CW, Canner JK, Sherman RL, Hines KF, Lum YW, et al. The Society for Vascular Surgery Wound, Ischemia, and foot Infection (WIfI) classification system predicts wound healing but not major amputation in patients with diabetic foot ulcers treated in a multidisciplinary setting. J Vasc Surg. 2017;65(6):1698–1705.e1.

11. van Baal JG. Surgical treatment of the infected diabetic foot. Clin Infect Dis. 2004;39(Supplement_2):S123–8.

12. Lepäntalo M, Biancari F, Tukiainen E. Never amputate without consultation of a vascular surgeon. Diabetes Metab Res Rev. 2000;16(Suppl 1):S27–32.

13. Mayor JM, Valentin W, Sharath S, Barshes NR, Chung J, Kougias P, et al. The impact of foot infection on infrainguinal bypass outcomes in patients with chronic limb-threatening ischemia. J Vasc Surg. 2018;68(6):1841–7.

14. Mills JL, Conte MS, Armstrong DG, Pomposelli FB, Schanzer A, Sidawy AN, et al. The society for vascular surgery lower extremity threatened limb classification system: risk stratification based on wound, ischemia, and foot infection (WIfI). J Vasc Surg. 2014;59(1):220–234.e2.

15. Zhan LX, Branco BC, Armstrong DG, Mills JL. The Society for Vascular Surgery lower extremity threatened limb classification system based on Wound, Ischemia, and foot Infection (WIfI) correlates with risk of major amputation and time to wound healing. J Vasc Surg. 2015;61(4):939–44.

16. Van Reijen NS, Ponchant K, Ubbink DT, Koelemay MJW. Editor's choice – the prognostic value of the WIfI classification in patients with chronic limb threatening ischaemia: a systematic review and meta-analysis. Eur J Vasc Endovasc Surg. 2019;58(3):362–71.

17. Mayor JM, Mills JL. The correlation of the society for vascular surgery wound, ischemia, and foot infection threatened limb classification with amputation risk and major clinical outcomes. Indian J Vasc Endovasc Surg. 2018;5(2):4.

18. Mayor J, Chung J, Zhang Q, Montero-Baker M, Schanzer A, Conte MS, et al. Using the Society for Vascular Surgery Wound, Ischemia, and foot Infection classification to identify patients most likely to benefit from revascularization. Journal of Vascular Surgery. 2019;70(3):776–785.e1.

19. Leithead C, Novak Z, Spangler E, Passman MA, Witcher A, Patterson MA, et al. Importance of postprocedural Wound, Ischemia, and foot Infection (WIfI) restaging in predicting limb salvage. J Vasc Surg. 2018;67(2):498–505.

Arterial Revascularization

Ibrahim Ali, Bulent Arslan, Robert Beasley,
Carlos Bechara, Pauline Berens, Venita Chandra,
Omar Chohan, Claudia Cote, Farnaz Dadrass,
Sabeen Dhand, Anahita Dua, Fakhir Elmasri,
Bryan Fischer, Ahmad Omar Hallak, Daniel K. Han,
Carmen Heaney, Kevin Herman, Uman Jaffer,
Samuel Jessula, Ahmed Kayssi, Nicole Keefe,
Neal Khurana, Maureen Kohi, Ricki A. Korff,
Prakash Krishnan, Abhishek Kumar, Chad Laurich,
Robert A. Lookstein, Sreekumar Madassery,
Alison Maringo, Jesse Martin, S. Jay Mathews,
Reuben Perez McCon, Ankit Mehta, Jim G. Melton,
Jorge Miranda, Abigail Mize,
Miguel Montero Baker, Jihad A. Mustapha,
Mohamed Nagi, Zola N'Dandu, Murat Osman,
Blake P. Parsons, Raghuram Posham,
Aishwarya Raja, Rehan Riaz, Michele Richard,
John H. Rundback, Fadi A. Saab, Gloria Salazar,
Brian J. Schiro, Eric Secemsky, Jill Sommerset,
David M. Tabriz, Jordan Taylor, Anish Thomas,
Srini Tummala, Venkat Tummala, Omar M. Uddin,
Jos Van Den Berg, Micah Watts,
Bret N. Wiechmann, and August Ysa

I. Ali · U. Jaffer · P. Krishnan
Department of Interventional Cardiology, Mount
Sinai Hospital, New York, NY, USA

B. Arslan · S. Madassery (✉) · M. Osman · R. Riaz
D. M. Tabriz · O. M. Uddin
Department of Vascular and Interventional Radiology,
Rush University Medical Center, Chicago, IL, USA
e-mail: Bulent_Arslan@rush.edu;
Murat_osman@rush.edu; rehan_m_riaz@rush.edu;
David_M_Tabriz@rush.edu;
Omar_M_Uddin@rush.edu

R. Beasley
Palm Vascular Centers, Fort Lauderdale, FL, USA

C. Bechara
Department of Surgery, Division of Vascular Surgery,
Loyola University Medical Center, Hines, IL, USA
e-mail: Carlos.Bechara@lumc.edu

P. Berens · V. Chandra
Department of Surgery, Division of Vascular and
Endovascular Surgery, Stanford Medicine,
Palo Alto, CA, USA
e-mail: pberens@stanford.edu;
vchandra@stanford.edu

O. Chohan
Great Lakes Medical Imaging,
Williamsville, NY, USA

© The Author(s), under exclusive license to Springer Nature Switzerland AG 2023
S. Madassery, A. Patel (eds.), *Limb Preservation for the Vascular Specialist*,
https://doi.org/10.1007/978-3-031-36480-8_6

C. Cote
Division of Cardiac Surgery, Department of Surgery,
Dalhousie University, Halifax, NS, Canada
e-mail: Claudia.l.cote@dal.ca

F. Dadrass · R. A. Korff · R. A. Lookstein · R. Posham
Department of Diagnostic, Molecular, and
Interventional Radiology, Icahn School of Medicine
at Mount Sinai, New York, NY, USA
e-mail: farnaz.dadrass@mountsinai.org;
robert.lookstein@mountsinai.org;
raghuram.posham@mountsinai.org

S. Dhand
Los Angeles Imaging and Interventional Consultants,
Los Angeles, CA, USA

A. Dua
Division of Vascular and Endovascular Surgery,
Massachusetts General Hospital, Harvard Medical
School, Boston, MA, USA
e-mail: Adua1@mgh.harvard.edu

F. Elmasri · V. Tummala
Lakeland Vascular Institute, Lakeland, FL, USA
e-mail: lmasri@lakelandvascular.com

B. Fischer
HCA Healthcare Tristar Division, The Surgical Clinic
PLLC, Nashville, TN, USA

A. O. Hallak
Department of Internal Medicine, Ochsner Health
System, New Orleans, LA, USA

D. K. Han
Department of Surgery, Icahn School of Medicine at
Mount Sinai, New York, NY, USA
e-mail: Daniel.han@mountsinai.org

C. Heaney · A. Mize · J. A. Mustapha · F. A. Saab
Advanced Cardiac and Vascular Centers,
New York, NY, USA
e-mail: cheaney@acvcenters.com;
amize@acvcenters:com; jmustapha@acvcenters.com;
fsaab@acvcenters.com

K. Herman · J. H. Rundback
Advanced Interventional & Vascular Services LLP,
New York, NY, USA
e-mail: jrundback@aivsllp.com

S. Jessula
Massachusetts General Hospital, Harvard Medical
School, Boston, MA, USA
e-mail: sjessula@mgh.harvard.edu

A. Kayssi
Department of Vascular Surgery, Sunnybrook Health
Sciences Centre, Toronto, ON, USA
e-mail: Ahmed.Kayssi@sunnybrook.ca

N. Keefe · M. Kohi · G. Salazar · J. Taylor
Department of Radiology, Division of Interventional
Radiology, University of North Carolina at Chapel
Hill, Chapel Hill, NC, USA
e-mail: Maureen_kohi@med.unc.edu;
gloria_salazar@med.unc.edu;
jordan.taylor@unchealth.unc.edu

N. Khurana · C. Laurich
Vascular& Interventional Specialists of Siouxland,
Dakota, SD, USA
e-mail: nkhurana@visofsiouxland.com;
claurich@visofsiouxland.com

A. Kumar
Department of Radiology, Division of Vascular and
Interventional Radiology, Rutgers New Jersey
Medical School, Newark, NJ, USA
e-mail: kumarab@njms.rutgers.edu

A. Maringo · M. Nagi · M. Richard
Department of Surgery, Division of Vascular Surgery,
Rush University Medical Center, Chicago, IL, USA
e-mail: Alison_E_Maringo@rush.edu;
Mohamed_M_Nagi@rush.edu;
Michele_Richard@rush.edu

J. Martin
Department of Radiology, Division of Interventional
Radiology, Maine Medical Center, Portland, ME, USA

S. J. Mathews
Department of Interventional Cardiology, Bradenton
Cardiology Center, Manatee Memorial Hospital,
Bradenton, FL, USA

R. P. McCon
Ochsner Health System, New Orleans, LA, USA

A. Mehta · S. Tummala
Department of Interventional Radiology, University
of Miami Health System, UM Miller School of
Medicine, Miami, FL, USA

J. G. Melton · B. P. Parsons
CardioVascular Health Clinic, Miami, FL, USA
e-mail: jmelton@cvhealthclinic.com

J. Miranda
Department of Surgery, Division of Vascular Surgery
and Endovascular Therapy, Baylor College of
Medicine, Houston, TX, USA
e-mail: Jorge.Miranda@bcm.edu

M. M. Baker
HOPE Vascular and Podiatry Institute, Houston, TX, USA
e-mail: mmontero@vascularhope.com

Z. N'Dandu
Department of Cardiology, Ochsner Health System,
New Orleans, LA, USA

A. Raja
Department of Medicine, New York-Presbyterian/
Columbia University Irving Medical Center,
New York, NY, USA
e-mail: Air9020@nyp.org

B. J. Schiro
Miami Cardiac and Vascular Institute,
Miami, FL, USA

E. Secemsky
Beth Israel Deaconess Medical Center, Harvard
Medical School, Boston, MA, USA
e-mail: esecemsk@bidmc.harvard.edu

J. Sommerset
Advanced Vascular Centers, Boston, MA, USA

A. Thomas

Mercy Clinic Heart and Vascular LLC,
St. Louis, MO, USA

J. Van Den Berg
Department of Interventional Radiology, Centro
Vascolare Ticino, Ospedale Regionale di Lugano,
Sede Civico, Lugano, Switzerland
e-mail: josua.vandenberg@eoc.ch

M. Watts
Atlantic Medical Imaging, Pleasantville, NJ, USA

B. N. Wiechmann
Vascular & Interventional Physicians,
Pleasantville, NJ, USA

A. Ysa
Department of Vascular and Endovascular Surgery,
Hospital Universitario Cruces, Bizkaia, Spain
e-mail: august.ysa@osakidetza.net

6.1 Aortoiliac Revascularization

Venkat Tummala

Aortoiliac inflow is critical for wound healing in chronic limb-threatening ischemia (CLTI) patients. Preprocedural imaging, when available, can be valuable for treatment planning of endovascular, hybrid, or open surgical interventions (Fig. 6.1) in patients with aortoiliac disease (AOID). Knowing the status of adjacent mesenteric vessels, hypogastric artery, common femoral artery, and lower extremity runoff is paramount and can have significant implications on procedural outcomes. In the setting of iliac occlusive disease, associated aortic aneurysmal disease (4–10%) poses challenges when considering endovascular vs open surgical approach [1–3]. Knowledge of unexpected pathology on CTA/MRA beforehand can be helpful to modify the treatment approach accordingly.

Endovascular approach is tailored to the location and extent of stenotic/occlusive disease and might require ipsilateral (single access), bilateral (both femoral accesses), or may require additional accesses in difficult lesions (brachial/radial access).

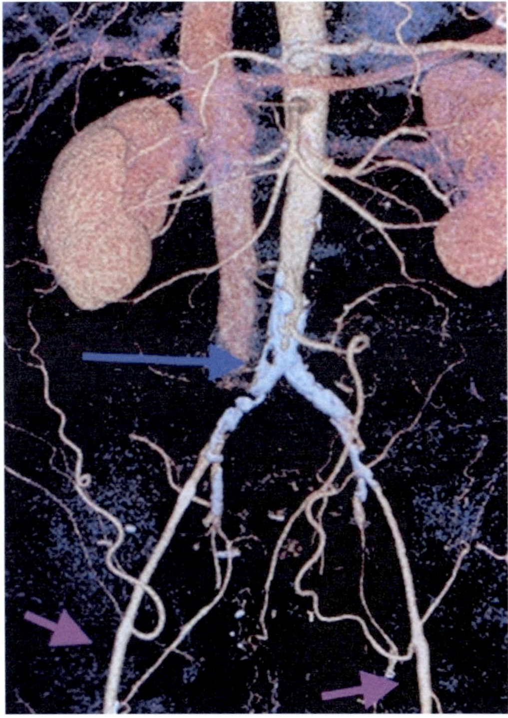

Fig. 6.1 Preprocedural CTA showing infrarenal aortoiliac occlusion (blue arrow) sparing the CFA bilaterally (purple arrows). After discussion of surgical and endovascular options, patient chose an endovascular option. However, if CFA were to be involved, hybrid option would be pursued

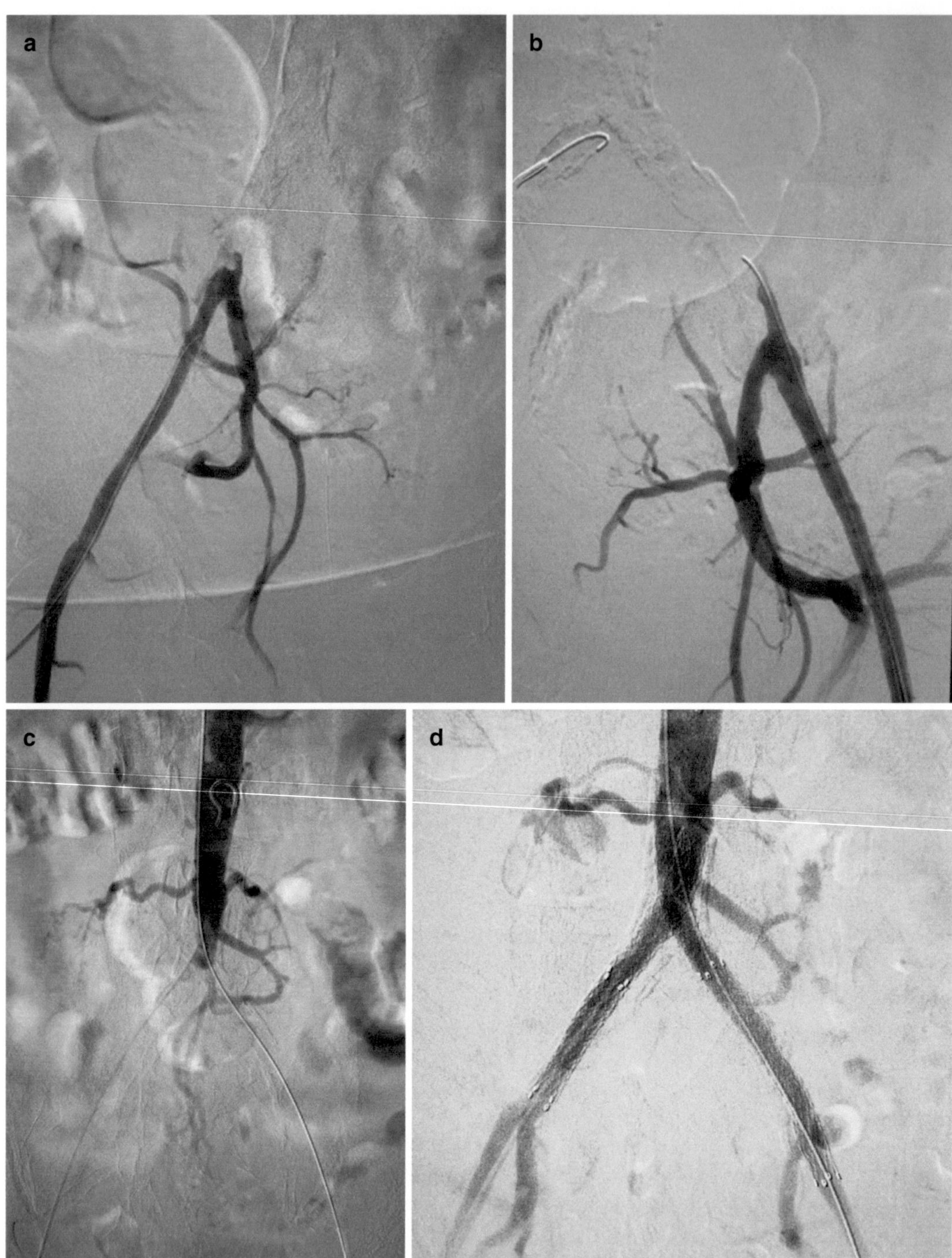

Fig. 6.2 (**a**) R CFA angiogram shows R CIA occlusion. (**b**) L CFA angiogram shows L CIA occlusion. (**c**) Occlusion of the distal abdominal aorta. (**d**) Aortoiliac reconstruction using the Kissing stent grafts at the aortoiliac bifurcation and bare metal stent extension across the hypogastric artery in an outpatient setting

The tool kit involves conventional angiographic catheters and guidewires needed for peripheral angiography. Aortoiliac interventions can be performed in a variety of practice settings including hospital and ambulatory surgery centers (Fig. 6.2).

- Ultrasound guidance during vascular access can help with first-pass success, especially with diminished femoral pulses in these patients [4].
- Initial vascular arterial access involves a 5 to 6 Fr sheath followed by upsizing to the appropriate sheath size required for stent/stent graft delivery.
- Pre-close techniques can be employed prior to the introduction of large bore delivery systems but may need to be deferred until the lesion is crossed and angioplasty is performed in patients with occlusive external iliac disease.
- IVUS can be valuable in many aspects, including but not limited to, evaluation of the extent of disease, nature of occlusion, stent sizing, and post-stent evaluation [5].
- Re-entry devices can aid in scenarios with subintimal crossing and help regain luminal entry [6]. In the setting of extensive calcific stenotic disease in the aortoiliac segments, shock wave lithotripsy can aid with delivery of large bore devices [7].
- Angiographic imaging can be tailored based on preprocedural imaging findings, when available. Oblique projections (contralateral oblique for CIA bifurcation and ipsilateral oblique for CFA bifurcation) can help in identification and characterization of ostial disease.
- Combination of antegrade and retrograde injections performed separately or simultaneously can help to map out the extent of the lesion. Delayed imaging performed after the initial bolus is useful in evaluation of reconstituted arteries that would otherwise appear occluded on initial angiography.
- Lesion crossing is typically achieved with 035″ guidewire and support catheters from a retrograde femoral access, antegrade up and over-approach, or upper extremity access. Occasionally, 018/014″ chronic total occlusion (CTO) wires can be used for a bail out (Fig. 6.3).

Many commercially available stent options exist including covered, bare metal, balloon-expandable, and self-expanding stent platforms. Stenting with percutaneous transluminal angio-plasty (PTA) has gained widespread adoption over PTA alone due to higher technical success rates and reduced risk of long-term failure [8].

- The 5-year results of the COBEST trial demonstrated that the covered stent has an enduring patency advantage over the bare metal stent in both the short term and long term.
- In addition, covered stents showed acceptable patency rates for the treatment of more severe TASC C and D lesions, and patients who received a covered stent required fewer revascularization procedures [9, 10].
  - Covered balloon-expandable stents are a viable treatment option for patients with complex aortoiliac lesions due to their higher rates of technical success and favorable patient across all devices at 12 months [11].
- Unibody bifurcated endografts such as Powerlink/AFX (Endologix, Irvine, CA) had been shown to be feasible and effective with excellent midterm patency in TASC D patients that are poor candidates for aortobifemoral bypass. The unibody configuration preserves the anatomic aortic bifurcation and allows for future up and over treatment options in CLTI patients with infrainguinal occlusive disease [12] (Fig. 6.4).

6.1.1 Hypogastric Considerations

Key considerations in aortoiliac stenting include preserving hypogastric flow and inferior mesenteric artery (IMA) when applicable.

- If the celiac and superior mesenteric artery (SMA) are compromised, covering the IMA could lead to disastrous mesenteric ischemia.
- Hypogastric artery occlusion can lead to pelvic ischemia and can severely impair quality of life due to buttock claudication and possible new-onset erectile dysfunction in males [13, 14].
- When CIA disease spans into the external Iliac artery, bare metal stenting can be performed to preserve the hypogastric artery [15] (Fig. 6.5).

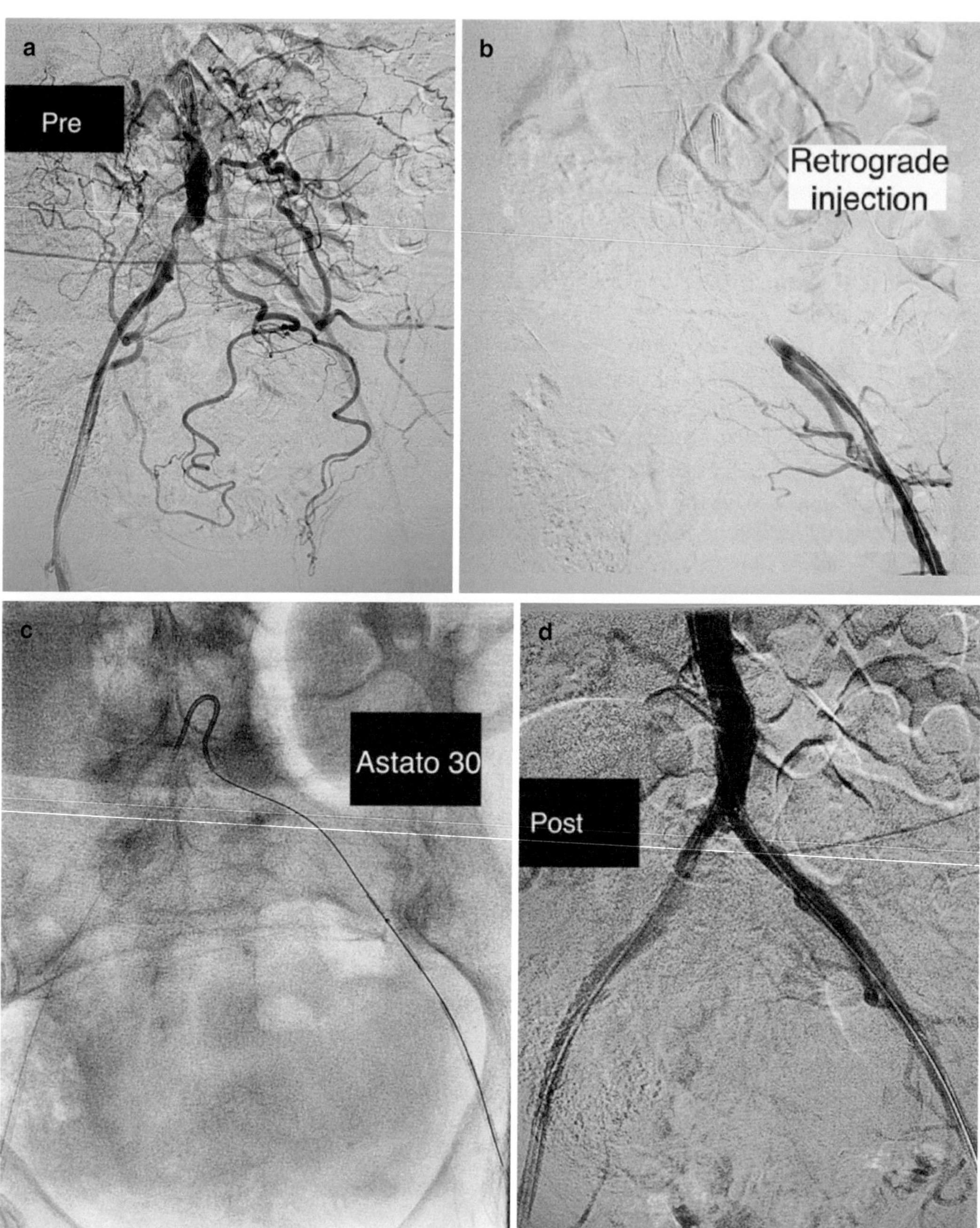

Fig. 6.3 (**a**) Aortogram via R CFA access showing high-grade R CIA tight stenosis and L CIA occlusion. Length of L CIA occlusion and proximity to L hypogastric origin not clear on this view. (**b**) Retrograde L CFA injection identifies the distal extent of LCIA occlusion and its relationship to L hypogastric origin. (**c**) Successful L CIA CTO crossing using both antegrade and retrograde approach with 018″ wire. (**d**) Successful reconstruction of bilateral CIA using kissing balloon-expandable kissing stents. Overlapping bare metal stent extended into L EIA for flow-limiting dissection

Focal aortic flow-limiting stenosis/occlusion can be treated with stent graft and PTA while avoiding major visceral branches. Stent size and type can be chosen based on the anatomical location of the lesion, lesion type, aortic diameter, access vessel size, etc. (Figs. 6.6 and 6.7).

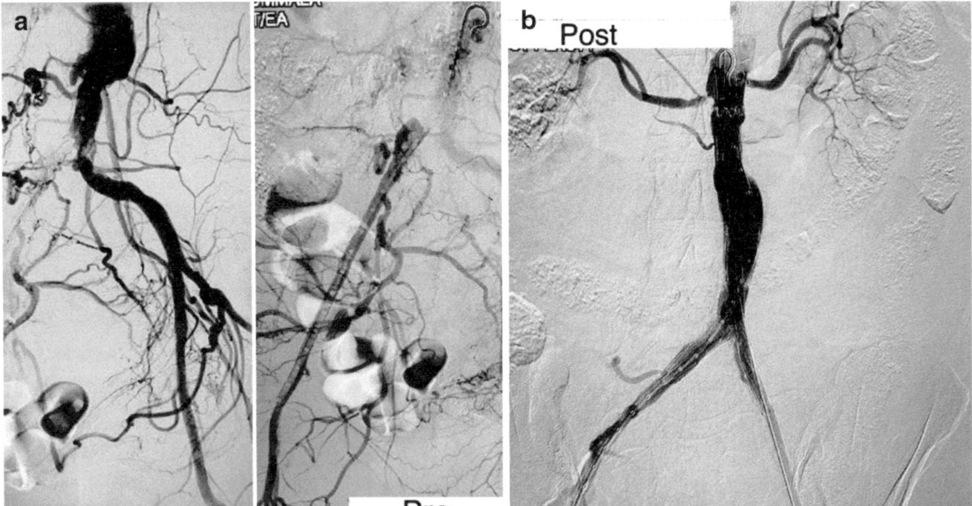

Fig. 6.4 (**a**) Elderly patient with aortic aneurysmal and right Iliac occlusive disease treated with AFX unibody bifurcated endograft using a percutaneous approach. Heavy calcific burden noted at aortoiliac confluence and intravascular lithotripsy used to facilitate endograft delivery. (**b**) Completion angiogram shows successful aortoiliac reconstruction while excluding associated aortic aneurysm

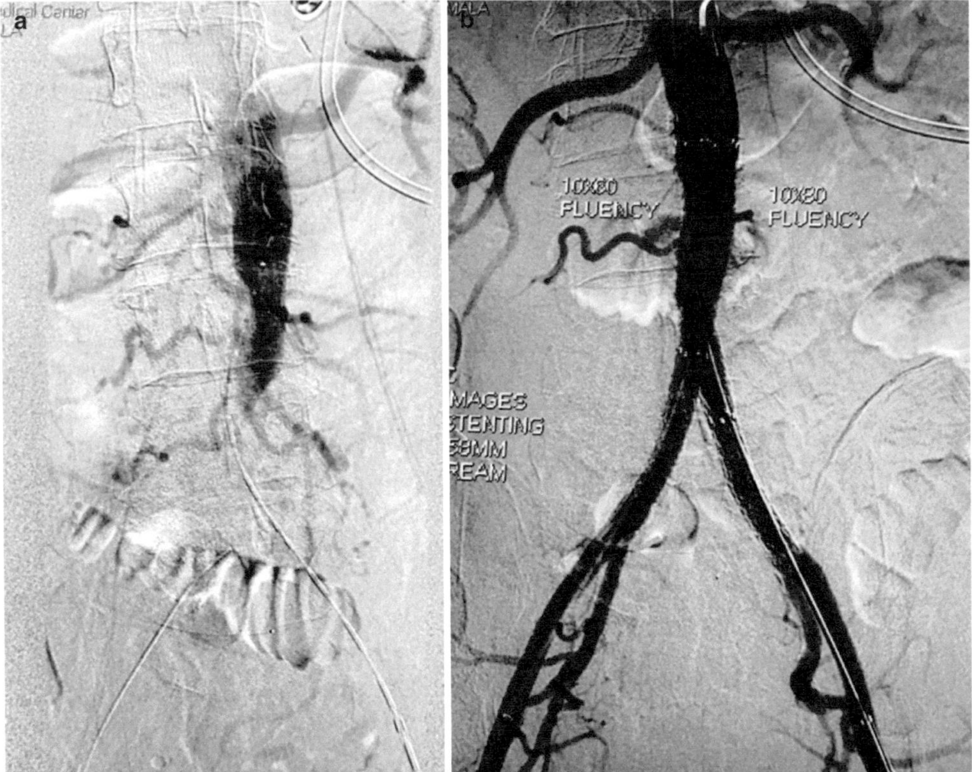

Fig. 6.5 (**a**) Abdominal aortogram from femoral approach shows infrarenal distal aortoiliac occlusion. Retrograde injection (not shown) revealed patent hypogastric arteries bilaterally, with disease limited to distal CIA bilaterally. (**b**) Completion angiogram shows successful aortoiliac reconstruction using double-barreled self-expanding covered stents in aorta and balloon-expandable covered stents in the CIA bilaterally. Hypogastric arteries bilaterally were preserved

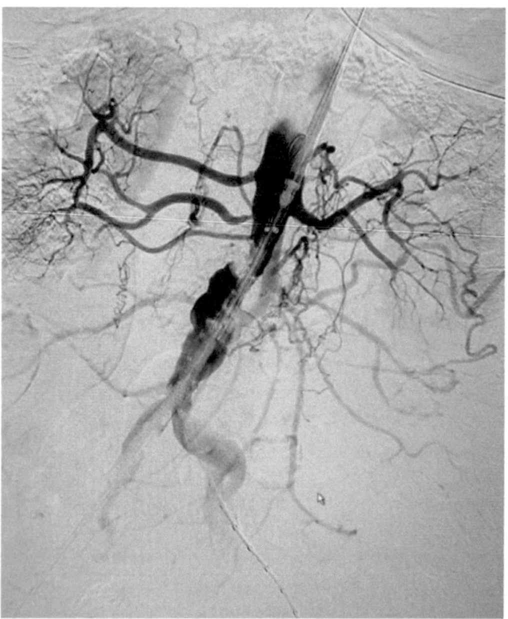

Fig. 6.6 Elderly patient with severe focal infrarenal aortic calcific stenosis, poor open surgical candidate

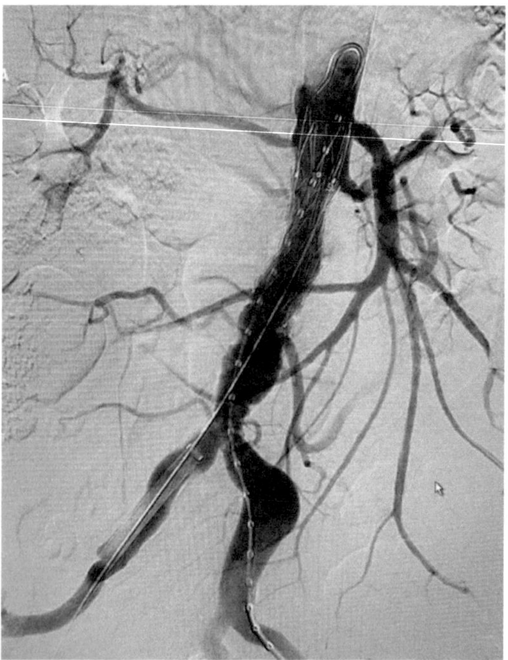

Fig. 6.7 Treated with Endurant II Aortic cuff (Medtronic, Minneapolis, USA). The accessory R renal had to be compromised due to lesion extending to the ostium. Main renals and IMA were preserved

6.1.2 CERAB and C-CERAB

In cases of more extensive disease involving the infrarenal aortoiliac confluence, covered endovascular reconstruction of aortic bifurcation (CERAB) and Chimney CERAB (C-CERAB) has gained popularity.

- CERAB was introduced in 2013 to improve endovascular and clinical outcomes aimed at minimizing the turbulence and stasis seen with kissing stents, by employing a more anatomical and physiological reconstruction [16, 17].
    - Freedom from target lesion revascularization (TLR) at 12 months was found to be 100% [18]. Three-year outcomes employing CERAB showed a 97% limb salvage rate [19].
- In this technique, a balloon-expandable stent graft is first deployed in the aorta followed by flaring of the proximal edge to match the patent adjacent aorta. Then, two appropriately sized kissing balloon-expandable stents are placed into the aortic stent graft creating a raised new aortic bifurcation (Fig. 6.7). VBX (W.L. Gore & Associates, Arizona, USA), LifeStream (BD & Co, Arizona, USA), and other commercially available balloon-expandable stent grafts can be employed in CERAB [11, 20]. Chimney CERAB has been shown to be technically feasible and can be an alternative to open surgery for complex aortoiliac disease [21].
- C-CERAB is employed for juxta renal/visceral disease with placement of additional stent graft to preserve the juxtaposed renal/visceral artery.

An additional consideration in lesions where the aortic and iliac disease is non-contiguous is that spaced targeted stenting of the lesions can be accomplished without raising the aortic bifurcation (Fig. 6.8).

In AIOD associated with CFA disease, a hybrid approach can be undertaken with femoral endarterectomy and aortoiliac endovascular reconstruction performed in the same setting (Fig. 6.9).

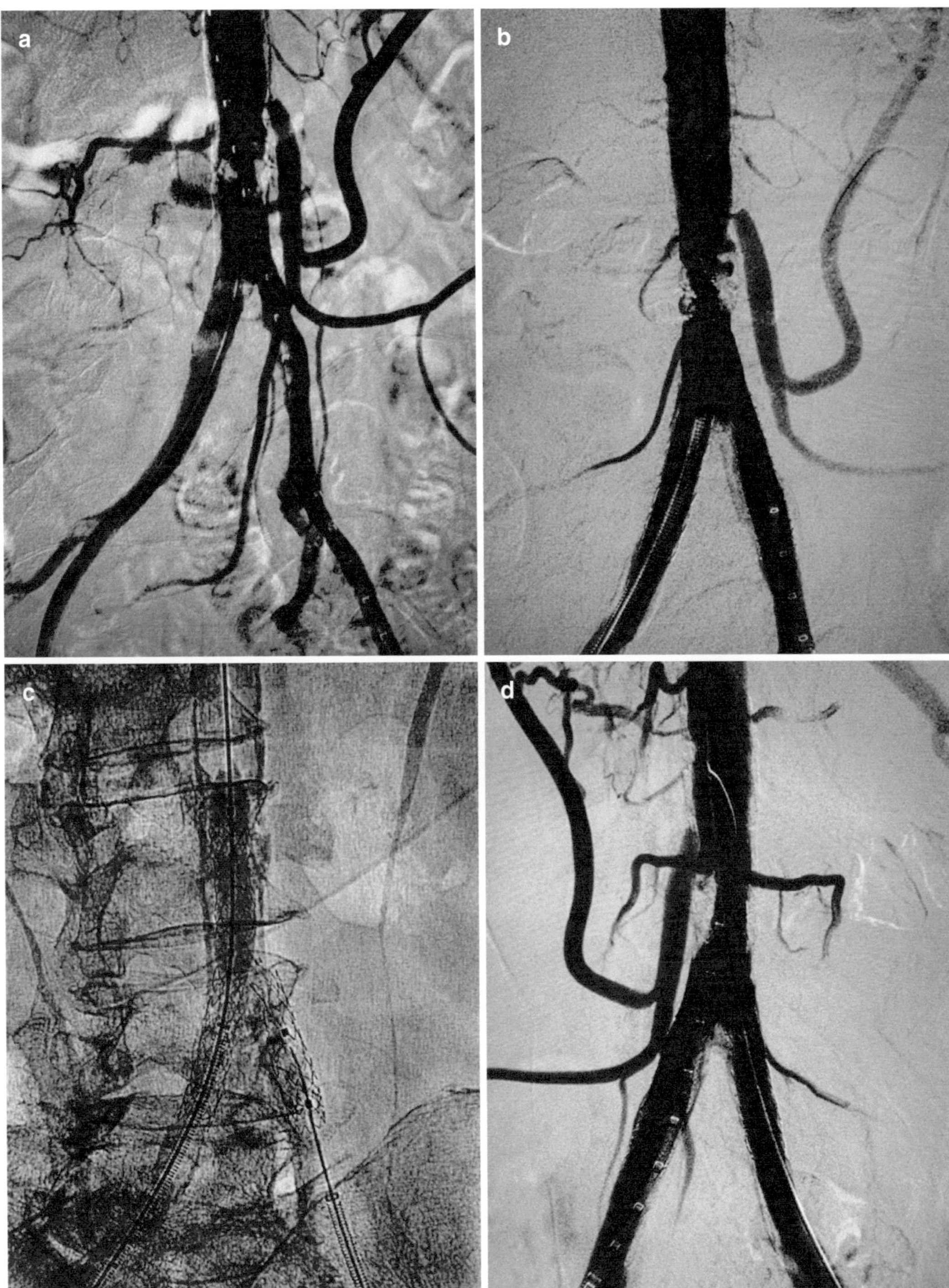

Fig. 6.8 (a) Angiogram showing focal high-grade calcific infrarenal aortic stenosis caudal to IMA takeoff. Bilateral popcorn calcific CIA stenosis noted sparing the distal most aorta. This was treated by separate spaced aortic and bilateral CIA balloon-expandable covered stents, without raising the bifurcation. IMA was preserved. (b) Kissing CIA stents placed without raising aortic bifurcation. (c) Followed by aortic balloon-expandable covered stent placement avoiding IMA coverage. (d) Completion angiogram showing successful aortoiliac reconstruction without raising the bifurcation. IMA preserved

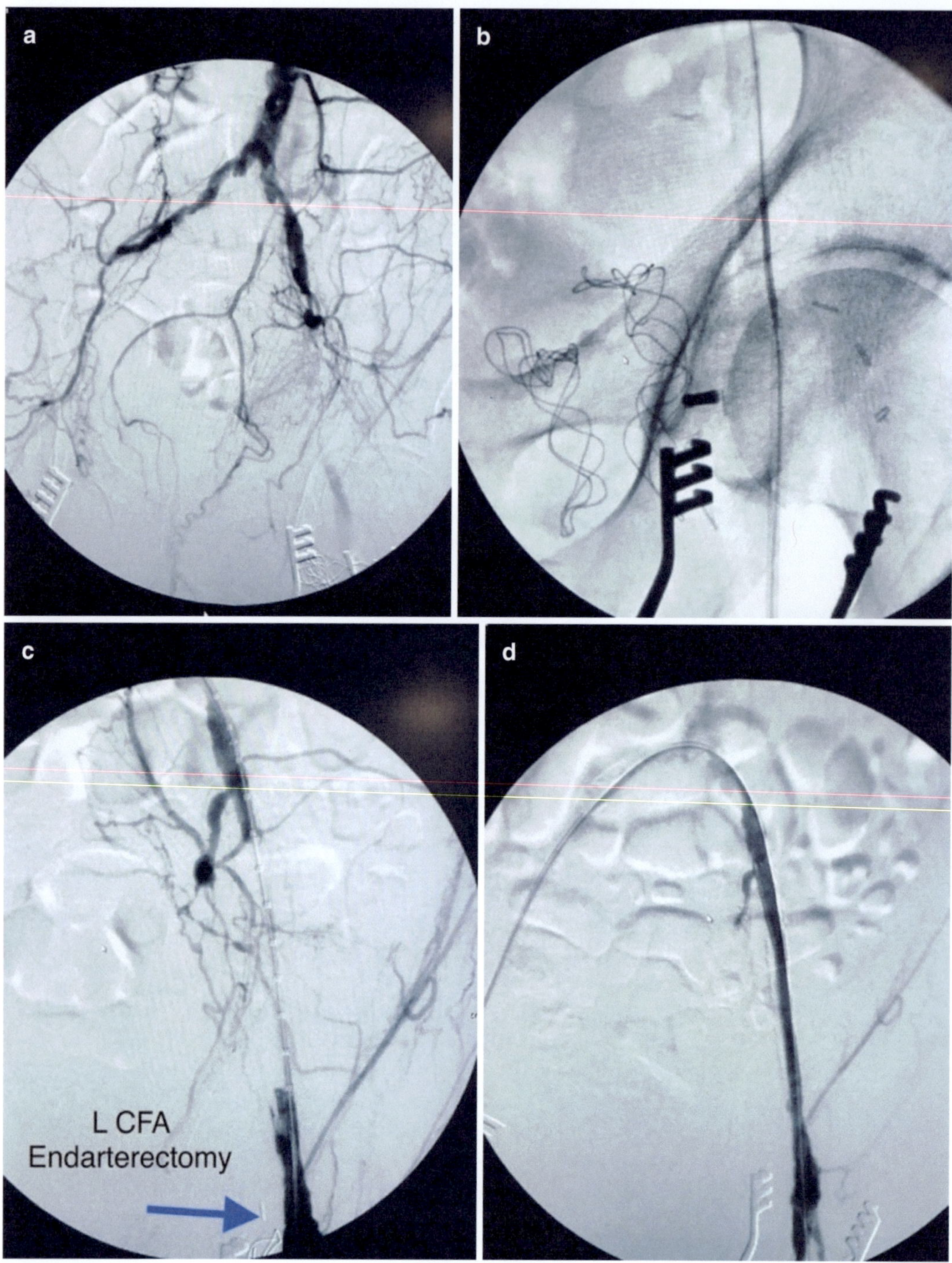

Fig. 6.9 (**a**) CLTI patient with bilateral external iliac occlusive disease and CFA involvement. Treated using hybrid approach with femoral endarterectomy and fixing iliac inflow endovascularly. (**b**) Fluoroscopy image showing successful external Iliac artery crossing using ante- grade and retrograde approach with wire flossed and externalized. (**c**) Left CFA endarterectomy done followed by pelvic angiogram showing the extent of L EIA occlusion. (**d**) Successful stenting of L EIA avoiding extension across the inguinal ligament

6.1.2.1 Conclusion

Successful aortoiliac revascularization in AIOD is vital for achieving limb salvage. Familiarity with various endovascular techniques and proper execution can translate to improved clinical outcomes. Advances in endovascular technologies and improved proficiency continue to provide alternatives to open surgery in TASC C and D lesions, especially in poor open surgical candidates.

6.1.3   When to Consider Aortobifemoral and Femoro-Femoral Bypass?

Daniel K. Han

6.1.3.1 Aortobifemoral Bypass

Endovascular interventions for aortoiliac occlusive disease (AIOD) have good patency rates, and as such, the number for aortobifemoral bypasses (ABFs) that are being performed today has substantially decreased, as they are a more invasive procedure with higher rates of perioperative morbidity and mortality.

- For patients with limited areas of disease (short-segment iliac or aortic disease), angioplasty with stenting can lead to high technical success and long-term patency.
- Especially when considering that patients with isolated AIOD often present with claudication, an ABF that requires an open laparotomy/retroperitoneal incision can be considered overly aggressive.

For patients with critical limb ischemia or significant life-limiting claudication, an ABF has excellent long-term patency and can provide a very durable result. In well-selected patients, ABF can have a mortality rate as low as 2% and a 10-year patency rate of around 75%.

Consideration for ABF should include the following:

- Anatomic Considerations
  - Extent of Disease.
    ABF should be limited to those patients with extensive AIOD. While TASC II guidelines have made suggestions for what "extensive" means, in today's practice, several lesions that are considered TASC C and D can still be effectively treated using endovascular options. Lesions that are challenging for endovascular intervention include the following:
    - Small caliber iliac arteries.
    - Extensive calcification of the iliac arteries.
    - Long-segment CTO of the external iliac, common iliac, and distal aorta.
    - Prior failed endovascular intervention.
    - Patients with ulcerated plaques at high risk for distal embolization.
  - Inflow.
    ABF is typically considered for patients who have a clampable portion of the infrarenal aorta.
    If the common iliac artery and internal iliac arteries are patent, the surgeon may consider performing an end-to-side anastomosis to maintain antegrade flow into the pelvic circulation.
    If the common iliac arteries or the internal iliac arteries are occluded, an end-to-end anastomosis allows for better sitting of the bypass graft in the retroperitoneum.
  - Outflow.
    The common femoral artery is the most common target for an ABF.
    While disease in the distal superficial femoral and popliteal arteries may be

acceptable, the profunda is important for the long-term patency of the ABF.

- As such, many surgeons will perform an extended profundaplasty at the time of the distal anastomosis to ensure adequate outflow.
- The ability to reconstruct a diseased profunda artery at the time of revascularization is another benefit of ABF over endovascular interventions.
  - Patient Factors.
    Medical comorbidities limiting general anesthesia.
    Age and life expectancy.
    Prior abdominal surgery: The loss of normal surgical planes from prior surgery can lead to longer operative times and increased complication rates.
    Body habitus: In addition to providing technical challenges from body habitus, obese patients have significantly increased wound complication rates. Given that most ABFs are performed using a bifurcated prosthetic conduit, an infection of the prosthetic graft can be catastrophic.
    Patient preference: A thorough discussion of risks and benefits of all revascularization approaches should be had prior to selecting ABF as the treatment of choice.

Take Home: ABF may be the preferred revascularization option in good risk younger patients with extensive AIOD.

6.1.3.2 Femoro-Femoral Bypass

A fem-fem bypass is not as durable as an ABF and reported that 5-year patency rates range around 60–70%. With the increasing experience and success of endovascular revascularization for AIOD, the number of fem–fem bypasses performed for PAD has decreased in recent times. In fact, the most common indication for a fem–fem bypass today may be in the setting of an endovascular aortic aneurysm repair with an aorto-uni-iliac device.

However, the common femoral arteries are readily accessible with a surgical cutdown, and a fem–fem bypass can be performed with general, regional, or even local anesthesia. As such, a fem–fem bypass is an important option in the armamentarium of a vascular surgeon for extra-anatomic iliac artery reconstruction across many different pathologies.

Similar to the discussion above for ABF, the decision to perform a fem–fem bypass for peripheral arterial disease must take into account the following considerations:

- Anatomic Considerations.
  - A fem–fem bypass is considered for patients with **unilateral** iliac artery occlusive disease. Similar lesions may provide a challenge for endovascular intervention:
    Small caliber iliac arteries.
    Extensive calcification of the iliac arteries.
    Long-segment CTO of the external iliac and/or common iliac arteries.
    Prior failed endovascular intervention.
    Patients with ulcerated plaques at high risk of distal embolization.
- Inflow and Outflow.
  - The success of fem–fem bypass depends on the presence of a patent aorta and single iliac artery to serve as the inflow vessel for both lower extremities and free of hemodynamically significant lesions.
  - Similarly, the donor common femoral artery needs to be free of disease. In cases of significant CFA disease, a concomitant endarterectomy can be performed. The same holds true for the recipient CFA.
    Similar to an ABF, the profunda artery is important for patency of a fem–fem bypass. In cases of significant profunda origin disease, an extended profundaplasty can be performed at the time of the fem–fem bypass.
    The impact of distal SFA disease on the patency of a fem–fem bypass is unclear in the setting of a patent profunda artery.

The final thing to consider is that a fem–fem bypass can limit access options for future lower extremity interventions. While the bypass graft can be accessed directly, repeat access of a prosthetic bypass can lead to pseudoaneurysms or graft infection, which can lead to suboptimal outcomes and significant morbidity in a patient.

6.2 When to Choose Alternate Access

6.2.1 Pedal Approach

Blake P. Parsons and Jim G. Melton

6.2.1.1 Why Choose Pedal Access for Peripheral Arterial Intervention?

There are many benefits when performing peripheral intervention from a primary pedal approach. Benefits include the following:

1. Decreased risk of bleeding/access complications.
   (a) Common femoral artery access, especially in high BMI patients, can increase the risk of bleeding complications. Tibial artery access significantly lowers access bleeding/vascular risk. Tibial artery access can safely be performed with less than 0.5% risk of major vascular injury, similar to radial artery access.
2. Decrease in radiation exposure to you and the patient.
   (a) Tibial artery access limits the need for increased fluoroscopy time and dose over the pelvis as associated with traditional up and over access from a contralateral common femoral artery approach. This can contribute to a significant reduction in radiation dose to the patient and physician. This also equates to a significant reduction in procedure time.
3. Decrease in contrast utilization and increase ability to cross difficult atherosclerotic lesions.

   (a) There is increased ability to gain access through difficult atherosclerotic lesions secondary to increased pushability and access of the soft cap of atherosclerotic plaque. This decreases the need for mapping angiography. Utilization of intravascular ultrasound can also significantly decrease the need for angiography. Cases can routinely be performed with less than 40 cc of contrast.

Clinical Evaluation

There is no significant change in the clinical evaluation of peripheral arterial disease patients when comparing pedal approach for access versus traditional common femoral artery access. Evaluation is still focused on a good clinical examination that is supplemented with noninvasive vascular testing that was described in previous chapters.

- However, evaluation of the tibial arteries can be difficult with noninvasive testing especially if performed by technicians who are not comfortable with its evaluation and patients with medial calcinosis.
- Clinical evaluation with palpation of the abdominal aorta and bilateral common femoral arteries, supplemented with handheld Doppler interrogation of the popliteal artery, proximal and distal anterior tibial artery, proximal and distal dorsalis pedis artery, distal peroneal artery, and distal posterior tibial arteries (Fig. 6.10) are crucial in determining arterial options for access and likely distribution of patient's disease.
- Doppler arterial examination enables not only determination of access point patency but helps determine the likelihood of a proximal lesion given the audible sound of monophasic, biphasic, or triphasic signal. All aspects of the physical examination and clinical evaluation will determine whether a primary pedal approach is appropriate.

Access

The use of ultrasound is key to successful access into the tibial arteries. Ultrasound is carefully uti-

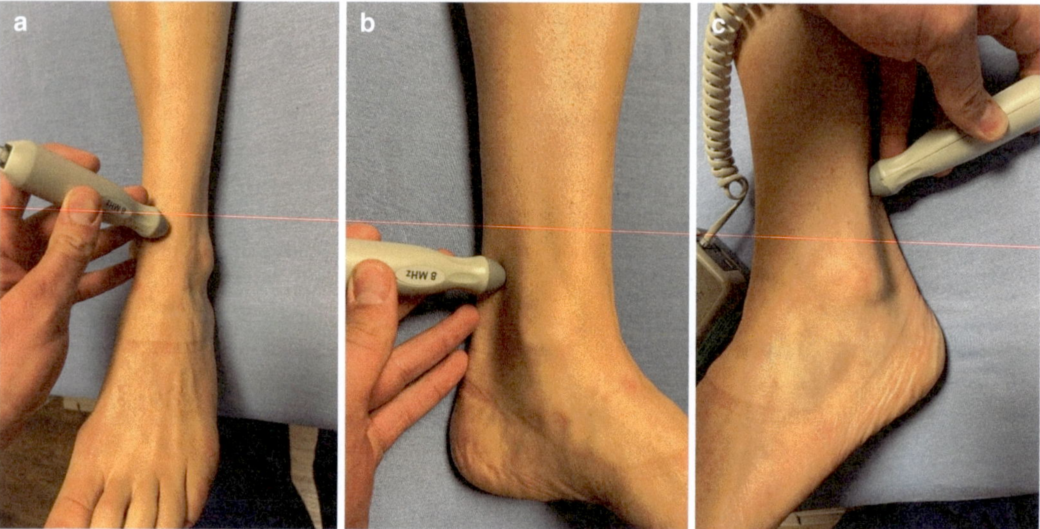

Fig. 6.10 Typical location for hand help Doppler interrogation of (**a**) anterior tibial artery. (**b**) Posterior tibial artery. (**c**) Peroneal artery

lized to evaluate patency of both the anterior tibial and posterior tibial arteries.

- Upon first becoming comfortable with pedal access, it is preferred to attempt on patients with patent two- or three-vessel runoff.
- Determining access of the tibial artery should consider the angiosome of the underlying pathology and vessel size and degree of atherosclerosis.
- Access can be performed into an occluded tibial artery with attempt to recanalize, therefore decreasing the possibility of vascular injury and/or injury to single patent tibial artery.
- Upon becoming more comfortable with tibial artery approach, access can be gained on patients with single-vessel tibial artery runoff for the potential of increased successful revascularization.

Evaluation of the tibial artery should be performed within 4–6 cm of the ankle joint (Fig. 6.11). Accessing the tibial arteries more proximally will be limited secondary to tibial artery depth/visualization.

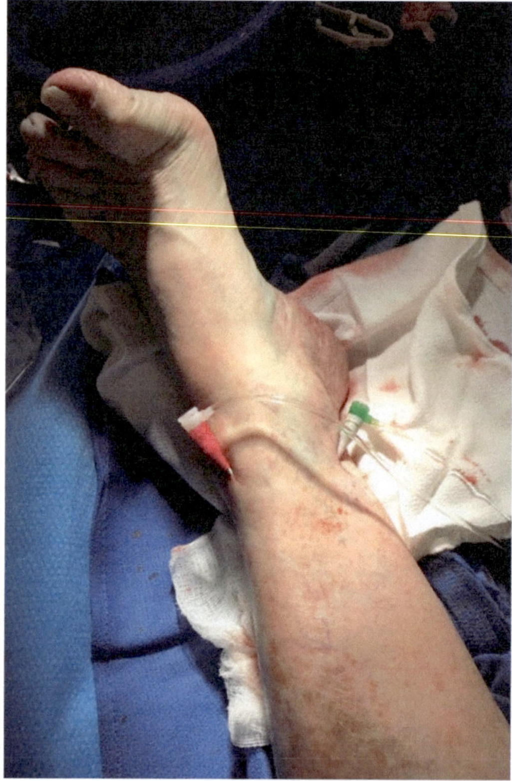

Fig. 6.11 Access into the left anterior tibial artery with 5/4 Fr slender sheath and posterior tibial artery with 6/5 Fr sheath

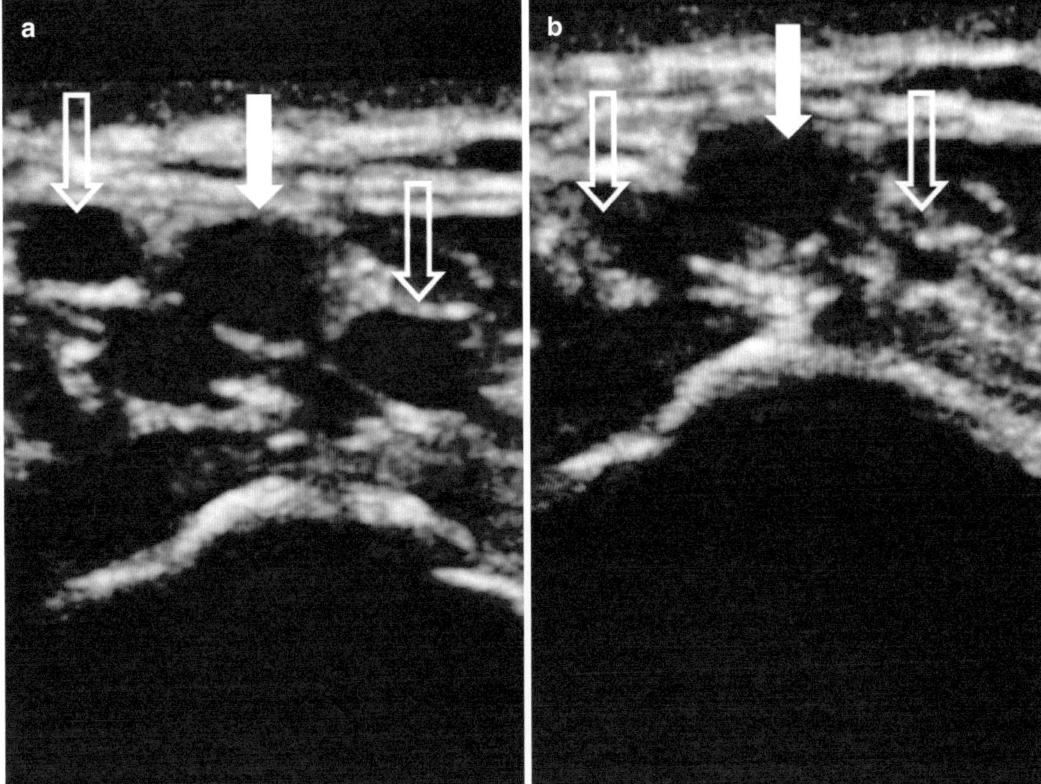

Fig. 6.12 (a) Ultrasound evaluation of tibial artery (solid white arrow) with paired tibial veins (open white arrows). (b) Ultrasound evaluation of tibial artery with mild compression demonstrating compression of tibial veins (open white arrows) with patency of tibial artery (solid white arrow)

- There is also increased risk of bleeding with access in a more proximal location. Ultrasound evaluation demonstrates a tibial artery with a pair of tibial veins (Fig. 6.12).
- There is increased success in access and decreased risk of injury with tibial arteries 2 mm or larger.
- The overlying skin is anesthetized with 1% lidocaine, and ultrasound-guided access is made with direct ultrasound visualization of the needle tip intraluminal. Access using a 4 cm 21-gauge micropuncture needle is preferred. A 0.018″ access wire should then successfully be advanced intraluminally under ultrasound and fluoroscopy. Angiography can then be performed through vascular sheath or transitional dilator.
- If there is concern for small vessel disease, the inner dilator of a 3 Fr introducer sheath can be advanced intra-arterially with subsequent arterial runoff performed for visualization of arterial runoff below the ankle and evaluation of the pedal loop (Fig. 6.13).

Slender sheaths are preferred for tibial artery access. Typical sheaths utilized are thinned-walled 4/5 Fr and 5/6 Fr.

- 6/7 Fr sheaths can be placed when needed for patients with minimal calcification and vessel diameter greater than 3.5 mm.
- Braided sheaths are preferred given some issues with kinking at the access site.
- A cocktail is administered consisting of heparin and nitroglycerin.
  - Typical cocktail administered includes 3000 units heparin and 200 mcg nitroglycerin through the indwelling sheath.

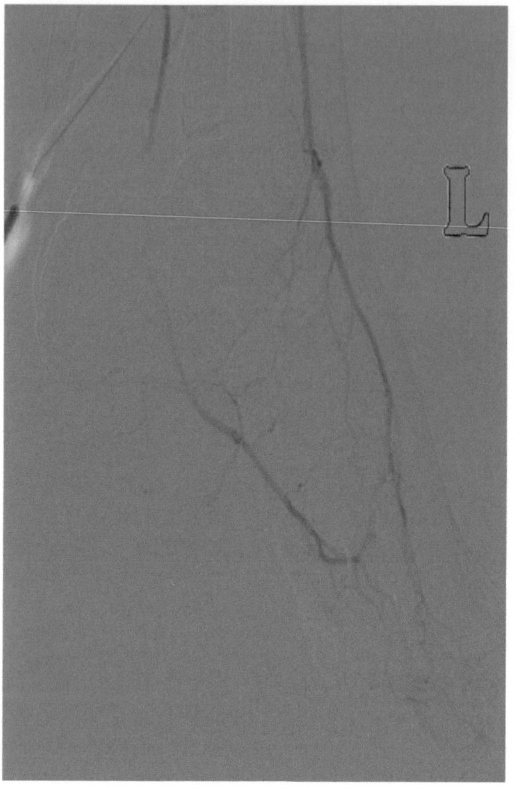

Fig. 6.13 Digital subtraction angiography of left foot performed through posterior tibial artery access and placement of the inner dilator of 3F access sheath

 – Heparin is then dosed through peripheral IV on a weight-based scale per the performing physician.

6.2.1.2 Primary Pedal Intervention

Upon review of patient's physical examination and retrograde angiogram, physician should have a good idea of the disease location.

- If intervention will likely be warranted in the aortoiliac distribution or femoral–popliteal distribution, a 5/6 Fr thin-walled sheath should be utilized.
- If patient's disease is small vessel and involving primarily a tibial artery distribution, intervention can be performed through a 4/5 Fr thin-walled sheath. Upon evaluation from a retrograde angiogram from your tibial artery access, guidewires and crossing catheters are advanced centrally. Typical working wires are similar to wires utilized in a standard antegrade fashion.

A primary pedal approach can routinely be utilized for interventions of the iliac arteries, superficial femoral artery/popliteal artery, and tibial arteries. By using a primary pedal approach, multilevel arterial inventions can be performed in a single intervention.

- Once retrograde angiography and evaluation of the tibial arteries have been performed, a 0.014″ or 0.018″ guidewire is typically advanced centrally.
- If chronic total occlusion is demonstrated along the femoral–popliteal or iliac artery distribution, standard crossing techniques can be utilized as from an antegrade approach.
- A 0.035″ catheter can be advanced into the distal abdominal aorta to allow pelvic angiography. The catheter can then be retracted into the iliac arteries with angiography of the intended leg and visualization of peripheral arterial disease.
- The use of intravascular ultrasound is highly recommended for evaluation of plaque morphology, subintimal versus intraluminal location, dissection, and precise intervention to disease segments only.
  - By utilizing intravascular ultrasound, this will significantly decrease your total contrast utilization and radiation exposure to you and the patient.

Re-entry devices such as Pioneer (Philips) and Outback (Medtronic) can be used from a retrograde approach. All atherectomy devices that accommodate a 6 Fr vascular sheath can be utilized. These include rotational, orbital, directional, and laser and lithotripsy options. If stent placement is warranted within the femoral–popliteal territory, all intra-arterial stents that accommodate a 6 Fr vascular sheath can be utilized.

- By coming from a retropedal approach, precise SFA stent placement at the femoral bifurcation can be easily accomplished, minimizing risk of compromise to the profunda femoris artery.

- Stents will need to be placed from proximal to distal fashion so that there is no risk of passing a secondary stent through an initial stent causing stent migration and/or inability to advance the secondary stent centrally.
- If iliac artery intervention is warranted it should be performed initially, prior to intervention in the femoral/popliteal or tibial arterial territory. Iliac artery intervention can be safely performed from a tibial artery access.

However, all precautions and preparation should be taken if urgent femoral artery access is needed and/or cover stent placement is warranted for underlying vascular injury.

- The largest balloon-expandable stent that can be deployed through a 6 Fr sheath is a 9 mm x 28 mm Herculink (Abbott). However, 8 mm balloon-expandable stents are routinely utilized and can be overdistended to 9 mm when warranted.
- If iliac arteries are larger in size warranting larger stent sizes, then common femoral artery access may be warranted in a staged fashion.
- External iliac artery disease can be easily treated with self-expanding nitinol stents up to 12 mm through a 6 Fr vascular sheath. Angioplasty balloons on 0.018 platforms such as Sterling (Boston Scientific) will allow you utilize up to 10 mm diameter balloon through a 6 Fr sheath.
- Angioplasty balloons on 0.035 platforms will allow treatment up to 12 mm through a 6 Fr vascular sheath. However, removal of larger balloons can be tight through tibial arteries and 5/6 Fr thin-walled sheaths.

Interventions on the tibial arteries and the pedal loop can be performed from a retropedal approach.

- An up and over-approach can be utilized from the anterior tibial artery into the peroneal artery or posterior tibial artery and posterior tibial artery access into the anterior tibial artery.
- A modified 4 Fr SOS Omni Select catheter or 90-degree Berenstein (Fig. 6.14) can be used to easily cannulate the intended tibial artery.
- 0.018″ and 0.014″ microwires are preferred for below-knee tibial artery intervention.
- 90 cm crossing catheters such as Rubicon (Boston Scientific) or Quick-Cross (Philips) can be used to provide ample support and gain access through dense calcification within the distal tibial arteries and into the forefoot/pedal loop.
- Atherectomy devices, such as Rotablator (Boston Scientific), Excimer Laser (Phillips), 1.5 mm Phoenix (Philips), and Orbital Diamondback (CSI) can be used in the tibial arteries from up and over-approach. Angioplasty is performed from 0.014″ and 0.018″ balloon platforms, and 90 cm length balloon shafts are preferred for ease of use. Tibial artery stent placement can be performed if warranted with a variety of coronary and dedicated peripheral arterial stents.

Postoperative Care

If there is concern for arterial spasm, nitroglycerin can be administered prior to removal of the tibial artery sheath.

- The vascular sheath should be removed with relative light to moderate traction. Hemostasis can be achieved using manual pressure and or banding.
- While pressure is being applied to the access site, periodic interrogation with handheld arterial Doppler is recommended on the distal tibial arteries in comparison with preoperative evaluation.
- Manual pressure is typically performed for 15–20 min. One of the postoperative benefits of tibial artery access is that the patient can immediately sit up in postoperative recovery and eat and drink once appropriately recovered from sedation.
- After hemostasis has been achieved, the patient will be evaluated for 20 min followed by the patient being positioned on the edge of

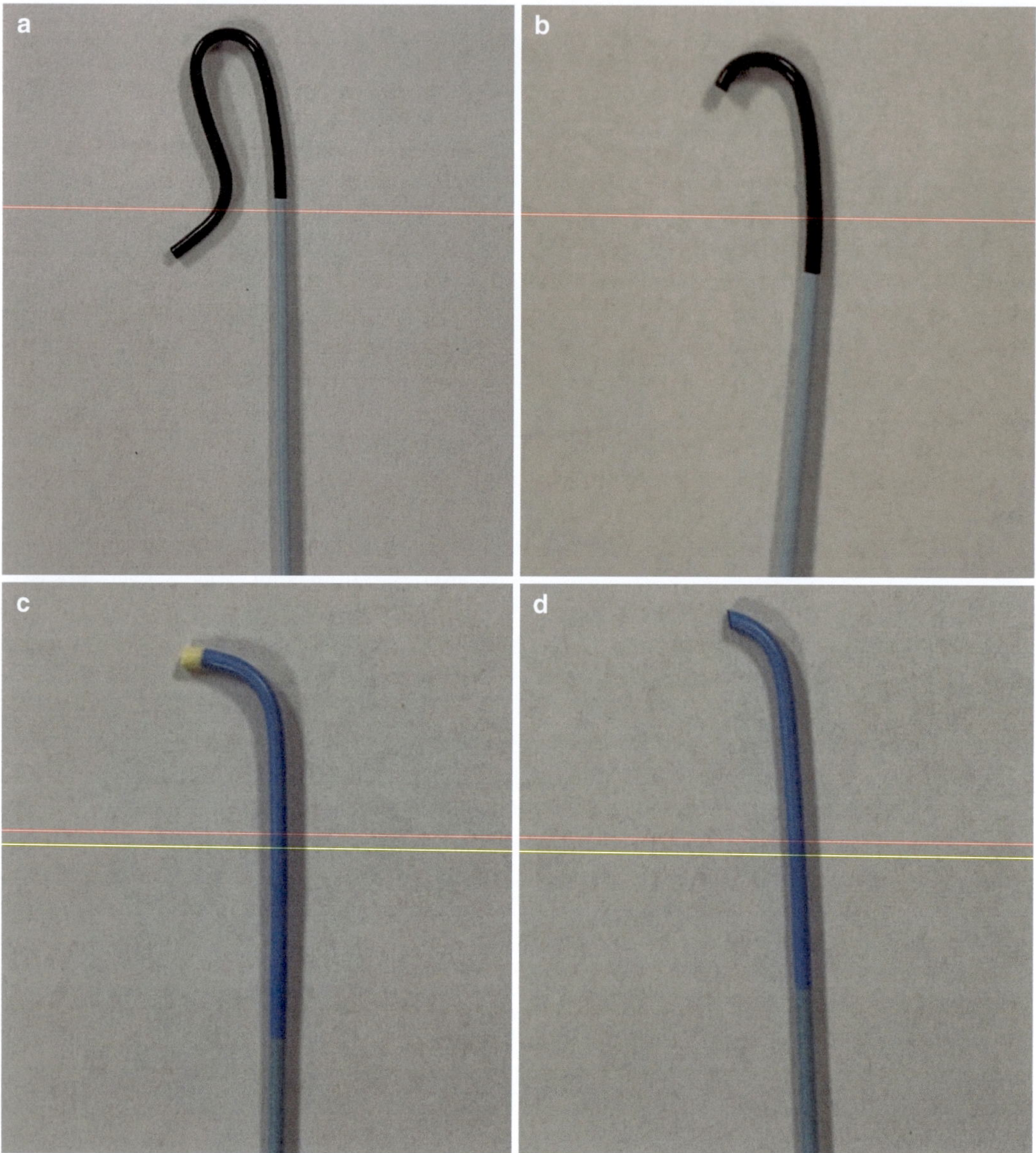

Fig. 6.14 (**a**) 4 Fr SOS Omni Select catheter. (**b**) Modified 4 Fr SOS Omni Select catheter with cut made at descending portion. (**c**) 4 Fr 90° Berenstein catheter (**d**) Modified 4 Fr 90° Berenstein catheter with cut made 1–2 mm from distal tip

the bed with leg in a dependent position for another 20 min. If there is no concern for bleeding/hematoma, the patient is then walked to ensure adequate hemostasis prior to discharge.

Postoperative care with antiplatelet therapy and clinical evaluation is unchanged from routine common femoral artery access procedures. During follow-up clinical visitation, the tibial arteries, specifically the access artery, should be evaluated with handheld arterial Doppler distal to site of access to ensure patency. Arterial duplex ultrasound can also be performed if needed.

Postoperative Complications

Inability to remove a tibial artery access sheath secondary to arterial spasm is extremely rare. However, administration of nitroglycerin and/or verapamil through the tibial artery sheath and topical nitroglycerin can be performed with light continuous manual traction.

- If access into a single tibial artery runoff was performed, there may be issues with vasospasm/small periarterial hematoma and decreased perfusion to the foot.
- Typically, this will resolve without any intervention over the next 10–15 min as vasospasm resolves.
- If there is continued concern, topical nitroglycerin paste can be placed over the access artery and placing the lower leg and foot in a warm blanket.
- If ischemia persists and there is concern for further damage, repeat angiography from an antegrade approach and potential angioplasty across the access site may be warranted.

Approximately 30% of patients will have some mild postoperative soreness within the area of access, which will typically resolve over the next 3–4 days.

- Postoperative pain is most commonly secondary to small hematoma formation along the neurovascular bundle. The risk of major vascular injury is less than 1%.

6.2.1.3 Use of Extra-Vascular Ultrasound (EVUS) for Pedal Access and Guiding Therapy

Abigail Mize, Jihad A. Mustapha, and Fadi A. Saab

The use of ultrasound has historically been used for diagnostic evaluation of arterial disease in the lower extremities, in addition to a multitude of other diseases throughout the body. Implementation of the modality for interventional procedures to directly visualize vascular structures provides additional safety and information to promote better outcomes for patients with cardiac and vascular disease. To standardize the approach of treating chronic total occlusions (CTO), we will describe multiple techniques for the utilization of ultrasound within the interventional suite, referred to as extra-vascular ultrasound (EVUS). EVUS is used for safe access of tibial arteries, crossing CTOs, treating lesions, and placing devices within vessels. These techniques require good understanding of how the vessels and devices appear under ultrasound. This section focuses on the use of EVUS to define CTO parameters and how to utilize EVUS to aid in crossing these lesions.

Introduction

The use of ultrasound for interventional procedures was a natural evolution of the current technology and has been established as a time-honored tool that decreases rates of complication and increases accuracy [22–26].

- Patients with CLI can require an average of 1.9–2.4 procedures each to achieve complete revascularization [27]. All these factors expose patients to higher rates of complications that may offset the benefit achieved from revascularization.
- Utilization of ultrasound to obtain femoral access for revascularization procedures has been shown to decrease the rate of complications and improve accuracy [26]. Due to disease complexity and comorbidities surrounding CLI patients, the next step in ultrasound utilization is to incorporate it into treatment strategy.
- The term extra-vascular ultrasound (EVUS) refers to the use of transcutaneous ultrasound imaging to visualize vascular structures and equipment during the interventional procedure. The modality provides live feedback for the operator to plan and adjust their treatment plan.

This chapter will provide the vascular interventionalist with essential information required to incorporate EVUS into their practice. Terms described here are new and reflect the novelty of the concept. The authors believe the utilization of

EVUS in revascularization of patients with CLI and PVD will be essential as our patient population becomes older and more complex.

Ultrasonic Features of Arteries

To understand how to use EVUS to deliver therapy, the operator must develop a clear understanding of how these vessels appear under ultrasound. Traditionally, interventionalists depend on angiography to define the vascular lumen. This has pushed a lot of operators to describe imaging obtained via angiography as "luminograms," meaning the contrast defines the inner borders of the lumen. Depending on the location of the structure of interest, different probes with different frequencies are utilized to obtain the best image resolution possible.

- Larger vessels with greater than 3 cm depth, such as common femoral, superficial femoral, and popliteal arteries, are imaged with a standard vascular linear ultrasound probe, with frequencies ranging from 9 to 12 MHz.
- Smaller superficial arteries, such distal tibial and pedal arteries, are imaged with a higher resolution vascular ultrasound probe, sometimes referred to as a "hockey stick" probe, with frequencies ranging from 15 to 20 MHz. Varying frequencies of the ultrasound probes depend on system manufacturer.

Ultrasound images are displayed on the screen based on how quickly sound waves reflect off structures and return to the probe. Soft or fluid-filled structures display as dark or black on the screen with more dense or calcified structures displayed as bright white [28]. This concept directly correlates to the visualization of the artery wall layers on EVUS.

- The intimal layer of the artery is comprised of the endothelial lining of the inner lumen and appears as a thin bright white line on EVUS.
- The medial layer is made up of smooth muscle cells with heavy blood saturation, creating a dark echolucent appearance.
- The collagenous adventitia appears as a mixed echogenic outer later just beyond the dark adventitia.
- Lower extremity arteries can have plaque formation across the three vascular layers, and EVUS can be used to clearly define plaque position to influence treatment decision-making and device placement (Fig. 6.15).

EVUS for Pedal Access

When utilizing EVUS for tibial artery access, the vessels can be identified in a short-axis (transverse) view. The distal posterior tibial artery is best identified just posterior to the medial malleolus and the anterior tibial artery is best identified in the top of the ankle. Choosing the best access point depends on the location of treatment required.

- Tibial access should be obtained in the distal third of the calf, approximately 3–4 finger

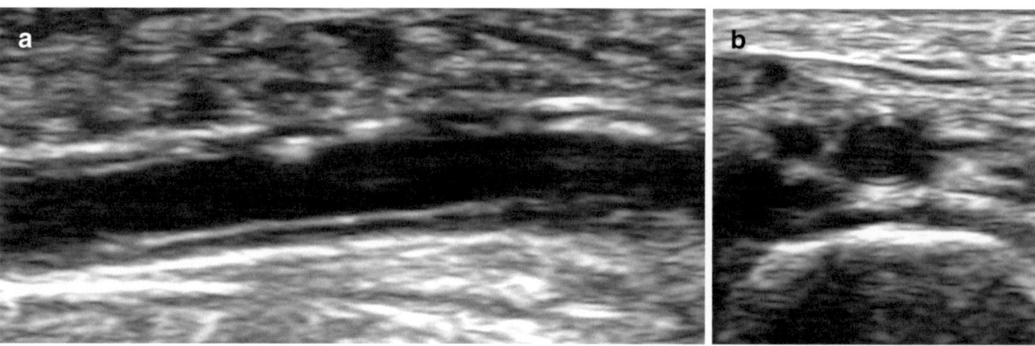

Fig. 6.15 (**a, b**) Long- and short-axis extra-vascular ultrasound (EVUS) image of a tibial artery with definition of all three arterial walls

widths above the ankle joint to prevent puncture of the muscle compartments.

- The tibial arteries in patients with CLI tend to be calcified along with low intravascular pressure from more proximal disease, which may pose as a technical challenge.
- In the setting of multilevel occlusive disease, the distal artery wall may be more pliable than normal due to low filling pressures and puncturing the artery wall with the needle may require the operator to change the angle of entry. In addition, because of the lack of stiffness of the arterial wall the vessel may escape the needle trajectory.
- The operator may also face difficulty with the amount of pressure required to successfully puncture given the low filling pressure and lack of artery wall stiffness. The vessel may collapse under such pressure, and eventually, the needle will puncture the posterior wall. This represents a true Seldinger technique. The operator will have to withdraw the needle very slowly while gently advancing the wire to aid in releasing posterior wall from the needle and allowing the access wire to easily advance within the true lumen. Figure 6.16 shows a longitudinal view of needle access into the distal PT.

Imaging protocols for diagnostic ultrasound assessment of tibial arteries vary by institution. In a CLI center, technologists perform an extensive evaluation, or mapping, of the three tibial arteries. In addition, particular attention is paid to areas of disease, vessel integrity, and proximal and distal CTO location. Evaluating collateral flow and communication between tibial arteries is of particular importance for the operator in planning the revascularization approach.

- As tibiopedal access becomes an essential part of treating CLI patients, the use of arterial mapping can define patients that have adequate targets for tibial access.
- A phenomenon described as the white stop sign refers to complete loss of vessel lumen preventing successful access. In these patients, the distal tibial artery is completely opacified with calcified plaque along the length of a segment of the vessel.
- EVUS can distinguish this feature from short areas of occlusion, a situation in which the operator can choose another location within the same vessel to access, usually above or below the occlusion to obtain successful access.

Table 6.1 shows a list of common US landmarks the operator can depend on to identify position within the vascular tree

EVUS is also able to identify prominent branches of the tibial arteries. The proximal anterior tibial (AT) artery gives way to the anterior tibial and posterior tibial recurrent branches. Identifying this landmark is important because in many instances the AT occlusion occurs in the proximal segment. The posterior recurrent branch tends to compensate for the AT if occluded. This branch is commonly mistaken for the AT.

- This collateral tends to be tortuous and becomes very small toward the ankle. It is important to recognize this vessel, especially with retrograde tibial access, in order to prevent the wire from naturally sub-selecting this branch.

Another important landmark for tibial access is the anterior and posterior communication branches of the peroneal artery. While each patient is different, EVUS with color Doppler can identify the communicating vessels, usually

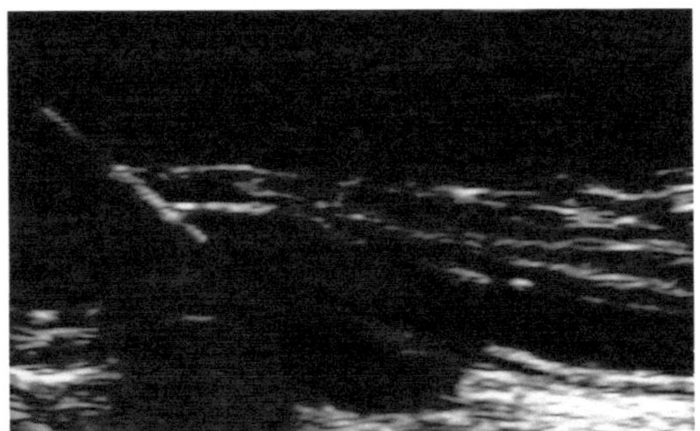

Fig. 6.16 An access needle is visualized on EVUS while obtaining retrograde pedal access

Table 6.1 Tips for EVUS Guided Procedures

Detailed Anatomical Map for Procedure Planning •Multiple modalities including duplex ultrasound, CTA, and MRA may be used. •Selective angiography has a better correlation with arterial duplex imaging and in patients with PVD [30]. •Assessing adequate conduits for access approach.
EVUS Characteristics of Arteries •Layers of the arterial wall define the intima, media, and adventitia to provide safest and most effective therapy. •Plaque location and type to ensure safe access and appropriate therapy. •Calcium content within the vessel may impact imaging. *Severe calcification will create acoustic shadowing rendering US imaging obsolete. Calcium can be as dense as bone tissue and does not allow the sound waves to penetrate beyond the anterior wall of a vessel. In these cases, EVUS may not be effective.*
EVUS Anatomical Landmarks •Identification of the head of the femur for groin access. •Identification of collateral branches and bifurcations. •Identification of the muscle compartments within the calf for tibial access.
Characteristics of Endovascular Devices •Echogenic tip needle. •Bright double lumen of a catheter or sheath. •Bright single line of a wire. •Moving/rotating of atherectomy device. •Stent strut identification.
Chronic Total Occlusion Mapping •The proximal CTO cap morphology, architecture, shape. •The distal CTO cap morphology, shape. •Collaterals at the proximal CTO cap.

around or just above the ankle. Ideally, if the operator can visualize the takeoff of these vessels, access can then be achieved above their termination allowing blood flow beyond the access point to the foot.

Ultrasonic Features of Endovascular Therapeutic Devices

Needles and Wires

Needles are made of stainless steel and may have indentation along the distal length of the needle for better ultrasound visualization, referred to as an "echogenic tip" needle. It is essential to visualize the needle as the skin is punctured, and the needle is advanced toward the artery. Wires are made up of multiple different types of material to ensure lubricity and mobility of the wire to prevent sticking to anatomical structures or devices. The metal of the wire is easily identified with ultrasound and is visualized as a bright white line. Because of the movement of the wire and the density of the material, reverberation artifact is often seen. Identifying the true position of the wire will eliminate any complications from this artifact.

- CTO crossing with EVUS is an advanced technique that allows the operator to directly visualize the wire cross into the CTO, avoiding the subintimal space, and ensures that the wire maintains a true luminal position for the length of the CTO to provide the best treatment possible.

Catheters and Sheaths

Identifying sheath location during intervention is pertinent, especially for treatment in close proximity to the tip of the sheath. The sheath is visualized as two bright white parallel lines due to the density of the sheath wall under EVUS. Catheters look very similar under EVUS, however tend to be much smaller in size. Visualization of catheters depends on material utilized to build the device. Typically, larger catheters (0.035″ and 0.018″) are easier to visualize due to their size. Some catheters are double braided increasing the echogenicity of the catheter.

- Catheters with a bend tip offer a particular advantage as the operator rotates the device, and this is well observed with EVUS. This in turn will allow the operator to engage areas within the vessel such as the CTO cap or guide the wire away from side branches to avoid complications during treatment.

Balloons

Angioplasty balloon catheters are made up of multiple layers. Depending on the balloon type (rapid exchanged or over the wire), the shaft of the balloon appears as a lumen with a wire through it. As the balloon is advanced, the thickening of the catheter indicates that the bladder portion of the balloon has come into view. Once balloon position is confirmed under EVUS and fluoroscopy, EVUS-guided inflation of the balloon allows for direct visualization of the arterial wall interrogation.

- Balloons that are underinflated or undersized will demonstrate a dark echogenic gap between the balloon wall and the arterial wall.
- Properly sized inflated balloons will demonstrate no gap with complete balloon opposition to the arterial wall, and in some cases, a step down is visualized at the proximal and distal end of the balloon to account for vessel recoil.
- Sometimes, the lesion will not immediately comply with balloon inflation. Slow inflation with EVUS guidance allows live monitoring of vessel wall compliance to ensure adequate and safe balloon inflation while avoiding fluoroscopy.

Atherectomy and CTO Crossing Devices

The appearance of atherectomy devices varies depending on the mechanical component. For Diamondback orbital atherectomy (CSI), the metal crown is covered with a synthetic diamond coating to modify the surface of the plaque, allowing for more effective adjunctive therapy. EVUS allows for visualization of the crown interrogation of plaque. Laser atherectomy creates an ablation bubble ahead at the tip of the catheter and creates micro-cavitation within the artery to disintegrate plaque. The micro-cavitation bubble created when the catheter is activated can be visualized with EVUS.

Stents

Stents deployed in the infrainguinal region are most often self-expanding, while stents deployed in the tibial arteries tend to be balloon expandable. Regardless of the type of stent, all stents are well visualized under EVUS due to the thin metal struts that are highly echogenic. Identifying the location of the stent struts allows the operator to successfully interrogate an occluded stent while avoiding crossing behind the stent. Operators can visualize wires, catheters, and balloons traversing the stent, preventing equipment from getting stuck behind a stent strut, or creating a false lumen between the stent and the arterial wall. EVUS-guided sizing and deployment of a stent can also be performed with precision. For example, EVUS-guided stent deployment performed from a retrograde tibial approach in the ostium of the SFA allows the operator to avoid stenting across and jailing the profunda femoral artery (Fig. 6.17).

Ultrasonic Features of Chronic Total Occlusion (CTO)

CTOs are some of the most complex arterial pathologies to treat and are composed of a proximal cap and distal CTO cap, often with mixed plaque types along the length of the occluded segment. Depending on the length and age of the occlusion, the CTO segment may have a hibernating lumen in between the proximal and distal caps. In extreme cases, the whole vessel between the proximal and distal cap is occluded.

EVUS can be used to assess the type and location of the CTO cap. Mapping the morphology of

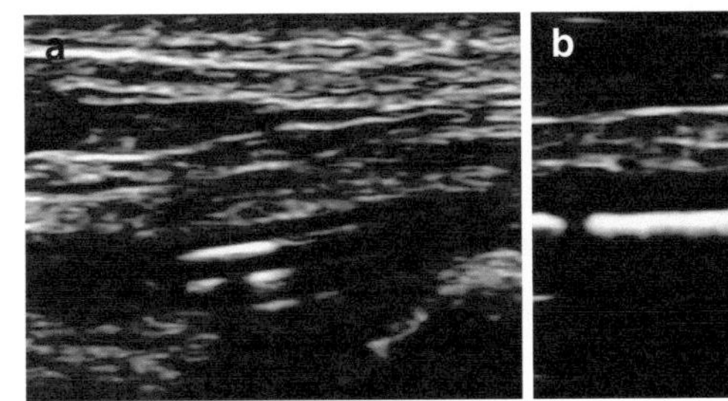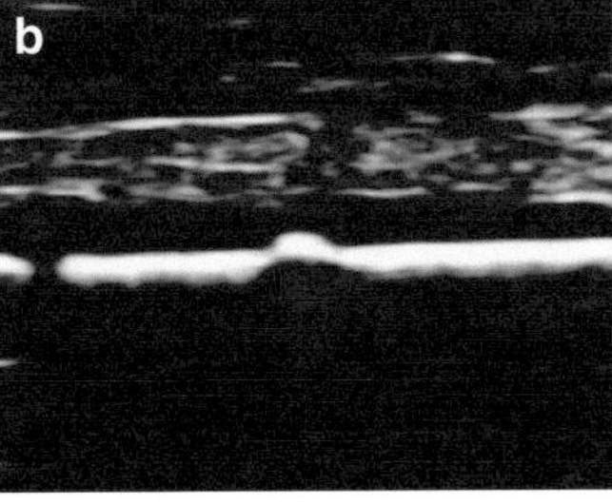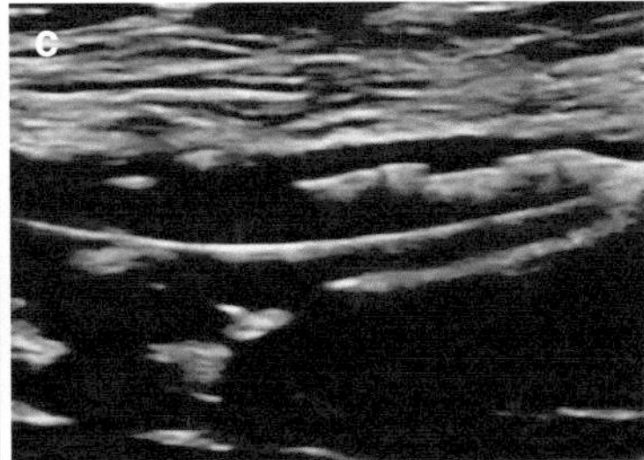

Fig. 6.17 (a) A support catheter is seen traversing an occluded tibial artery, (b) an orbital atherectomy crown visualized while treating a tibial artery, and (c) a stent is deployed utilizing EVUS guidance to avoid jailing the profunda femoral artery

the CTO caps will allow better assessment of access approach and treatment options. While the composition and calcium content may differ from one CTO cap to another, one common quality observed among most CTO caps is the shape.

- The chronic total occlusion crossing approach based on the plaque cap morphology (CTOP) analysis evaluated patients with CTOs involving the SFA/poplitcal and tibial rcgions [29].
- Shape of the CTO cap was categorized into two shapes: concave and convex. The shape is determined based on the shape of the cap from an antegrade direction. For example, Fig. 6.18 shows a concave-shaped CTO cap. This CTO cap is imaged via EVUS and angiography.
- The cap description also allows the operator to predict which CTO cap will allow for true lumen wire crossing of the vessel and which will direct the wire into the subintimal space.

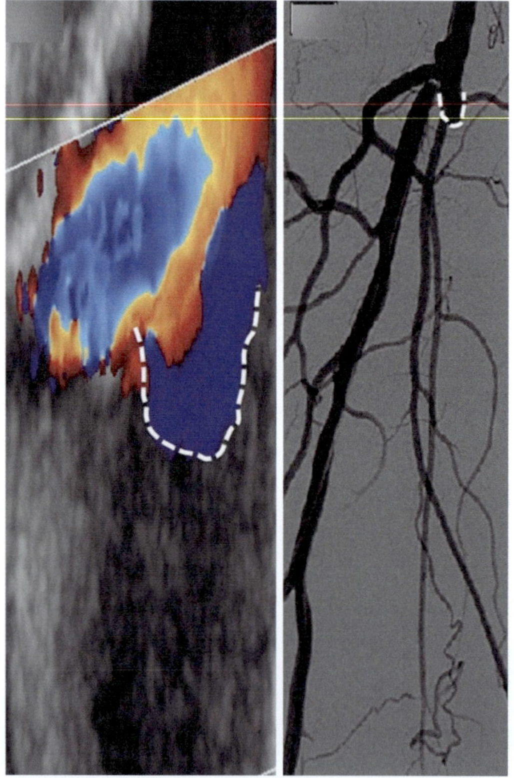

Fig. 6.18 A concave CTO cap is assessed with EVUS and angiography

- A convex CTO cap will include flat-shaped caps, oblique caps, or oblique caps leading to a collateral. All of these are features suggestive of a cap that is difficult to penetrate. Based on a simple dichotomous distinction between the caps and the fact there are usually proximal and distal caps, there would be four possible combinations in patients with CTOs.
- Utilizing EVUS to assess for CTOP cap morphology will allow the operator to choose whether or not to implement retrograde pedal access to mediate CTO crossing.

Conclusion
EVUS utilization for endovascular intervention in CLI is a viable option for patients with complex disease including multilevel and multivessel CTOs. Patients with CLI can benefit from the utilization of EVUS as it may significantly lower the use of contrast and radiation exposure, especially during access and CTO crossing. EVUS is an effective tool in obtaining pedal access and can guide the treatment of complex tibial disease. The utilization of EVUS in CLI interventions should be an essential tool for operators tackling advanced PVD and CLI.

6.2.2 Femoro-Popliteal Access and Closure

S. Jay Mathews

6.2.2.1 Introduction
While radial and pedal access may be preferable and relatively safe alternative accesses, sometimes they are not feasible nor effective for certain pathologies. Popliteal, antegrade superficial femoral artery (SFA), and retrograde superficial femoral artery (SFA) access offer additional interventional options for challenging anatomies. However, careful considerations must be made to optimize the ergonomics of the procedure while ensuring patient safety during and after the case.

6.2.2.2 Popliteal Access
Popliteal access allows for retrograde crossing of difficult superficial femoral artery (SFA) occlu-

sions, especially when the cap morphology is not amenable to antegrade crossing. In the modern era, direct pedal access is usually preferable to popliteal access, offering similar retrograde crossing capabilities with easy vessel closure via extra-vascular compression [31].

- In terms of alternative access, popliteal access is considered one of the least desirable points of entry due to difficulty in compression.
- As a result, postoperative pseudoaneurysms, hematomas, and bleeding are more common [32].
- In the setting of poor tibial vessel caliber or tibial occlusion, and where modified Schmidt access (direct access into an occluded vessel segment) is not successful, direct popliteal access may be preferable as long as the vessel is not diseased.

Access is most commonly performed with the patient in the prone position after which the patient is flipped supine [32].

- If this is a planned procedure, the preparation process can be simplified as the patient can have a limited draping performed for sheath access after which a complete draping done in the supine position.
- Ideal use a longer sheath (25–45 cm) to facilitate easy access once supine. Performance of the entire procedure can also be done in the prone position, but obese patients or those with airway management issues may not tolerate long-duration interventions without anesthesia support.
- Alternative methods of access include placing the patient in the lateral decubitus position, but this is ergonomically less ideal for access. The "frog-leg" position has been described for popliteal access with external rotation and gentle knee flexion, either from posterior puncture or anteromedial access [32, 33].
- Given the proximity of the tibial, peroneal, and more proximal sciatic nerves, access should not be performed without extra-vascular ultrasound (EVUS). Moreover, the popliteal vein also may lay on top of the artery,

which can lead to inadvertent arteriovenous fistula formation with through-and-through access.

Ideally, access should be kept as small as possible potentially utilizing 2.9 to 4/5 Fr thin-walled sheaths or sheathless approaches (i.e., Bareback). Avoidance of the popliteal artery as the solo access will allow for balloon compression of the entry site at the end of the procedure from an alternate femoral access above. Data are limited with larger sheaths as these may be prone to more vascular complications. Vascular closure devices (VCDs) have been used with some success [34].

- Given the mobility of the vessel, extra-vascular closure devices may be less reliable leading to hematoma or pseudoaneurysm formation [35].
- Active VCDs (intravascular hemostatic plugs, active fixation/clips, and suture-mediated closure) may be potentially effective but at the risk of acute vessel closure, dissection, or other vascular complications [36].

6.2.2.3 Antegrade SFA Access

Antegrade femoral approaches are utilized over contralateral femoral access when contralateral access is unfavorable. This can be due to bifurcation issues (e.g., acute iliac angulation, extreme iliac tortuosity, bifurcated endografts, or iliac stents), inadequate shaft length for below-the-knee (BTK) interventions, or inadequate support for difficult crossing [37]. Antegrade SFA access may be preferable to antegrade common femoral access [38, 39].

- In patients with even mild amounts of truncal obesity, the angle at the inguinal crease will be unfavorable resulting in more perpendicular access into the common femoral artery [40].
- Angulation of entry may also drive the access wire into the profunda rather than down the SFA. The proximal superficial femoral artery is fairly superficial under the skin and may allow a more favorable shallow entry angle avoiding kinking of the sheath.

- Ultrasound-guided access of the proximal superficial femoral artery is reliable [41].
- Closure of the SFA can be challenging as manual hemostasis below the femoral head is impaired by lack of adequate compression.
- VCD closure of the access site can be performed similar to a retrograde common femoral approach, except in an opposite fashion. More distal antegrade access increases risk of closure-related complications, but active vascular closure devices may help secure the access more reliably.
- In this pictured example, after antegrade ultrasound-guided SFA access (Fig. 6.19a) and completion of the procedure, the Celt ACD vascular closure device is utilized given its low-profile and easy fluoroscopic visualization (Fig. 6.19b).

Ergonomics are more challenging with an antegrade approach. If positioning the patient on the table in standard fashion, after micropuncture access of the SFA, the access can be switched to a 45 cm braided sheath, which can be curved either ipsi- or contra-laterally and secured with adhesive dressing.

- The contralateral thigh may be preferable as the angulation will be less extreme, which will be less likely to adversely impact stent deployment systems or delivery of other equipment (Fig. 6.20a).
- Alternatively, the patient can be positioned with the feet at the head of the table (Fig. 6.20b). This will allow for more natural access angle, but should be utilized with an anesthesia halo to avoid covering the patient's face with the drape. The fluoroscopic image

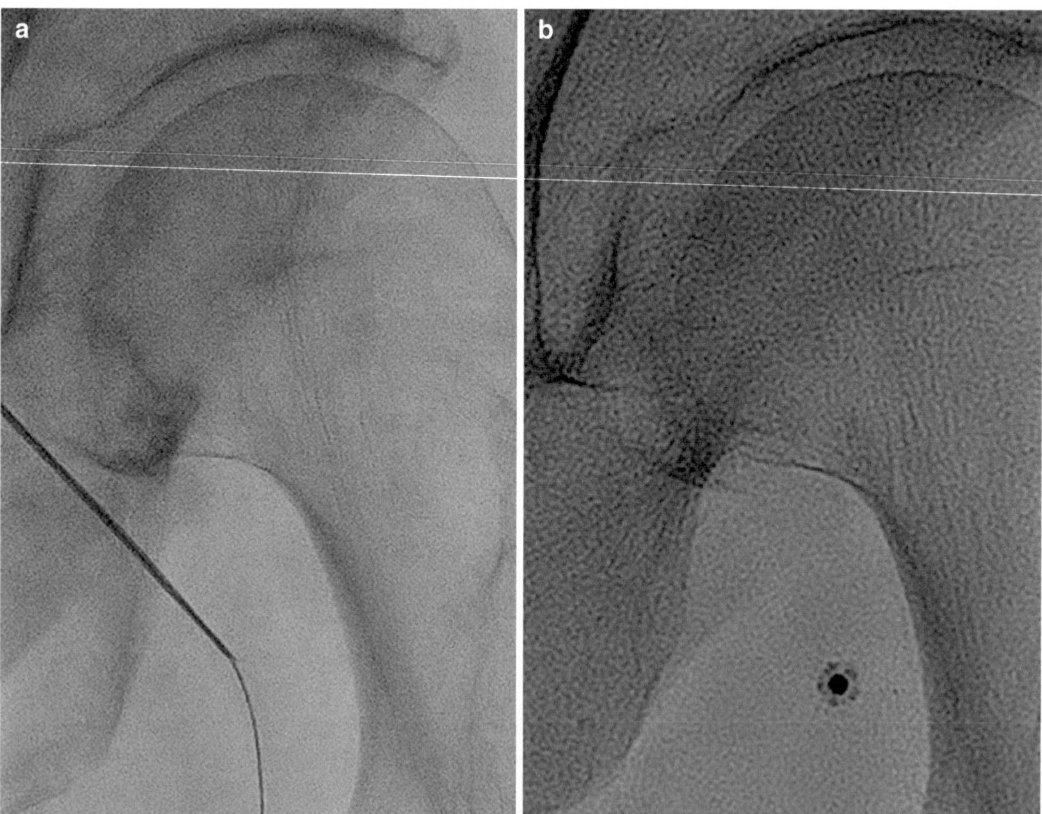

Fig. 6.19 (**a**) Antegrade SFA access. (**b**) SFA Celt ACD occlusion

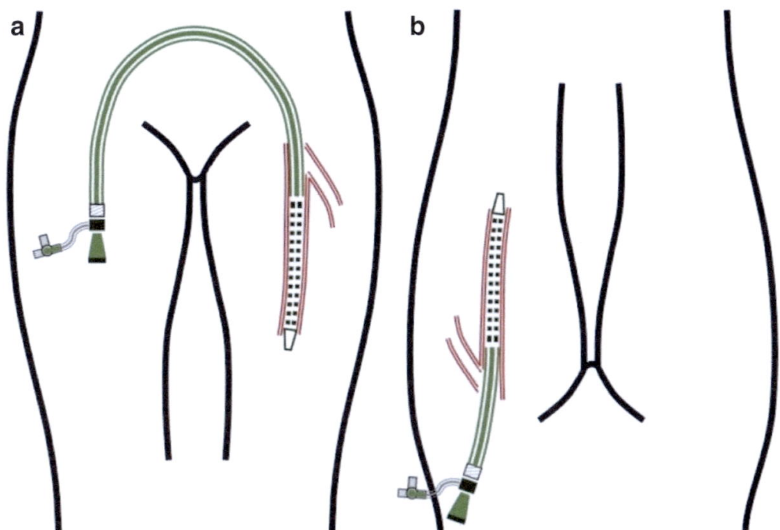

Fig. 6.20 (**a**) Antegrade SFA access with a 45 cm long sheath with operator standing on contra the contralateral side. (**b**) Antegrade SFA access, with a short (13–30 cm) sheath, patient inverted and operator on ipsilateral side

can be also flipped digitally to the correct orientation.

6.2.2.4 Retrograde SFA Access

Proximal retrograde SFA access has been well described as an alternative to common femoral access in patients with high profunda bifurcations or unfavorable common femoral anatomy. Large vessel access for structural heart procedures and endovascular aortic repair has successfully utilized this technique [42].

- Distal retrograde SFA access is more challenging but sometimes necessary when antegrade crossing of an SFA occlusion is not possible or successful, especially with extreme calcium or stent fractures leading to unfavorable subintimal crossing.
- Retrograde access below the adductor canal has been well described and can be safely performed [43]. EVUS should be utilized when possible but may be challenging as visualization through the musculature may be poor, especially in obese patients. Fluoroscopic guided access may be necessary utilizing road mapping from a proximal injection site.

Occasionally, a modified Schmidt technique can be used within an occluded stent [44].

- This can be performed with a micropuncture needle through the strut interstices, with advancement of an 0.018″ stiff wire (ideally nitinol based to avoid kinking) torqued into a drill-like appearance through several rotations.
- This wire is continuously spun clockwise and counterclockwise with steady force. A micropuncture sheath or sheathless technique can be used with a 0.018″ crossing catheter after which the wire can be directed or snared into the proximal access.
- Sheathless approaches for balloon crossing and even stenting is also possible from the retrograde SFA access [45].
- Of note, closure of the SFA puncture is usually easily performed with balloon tamponade from a proximal access, but occasionally with extreme calcium, a persistent channel may form requiring adjunctive use of a covered self-expanding stent.

6.2.2.5 Case Example

An 81-year-old man with diabetes, dyslipidemia, and chronic tobacco abuse presented with a Rutherford 5 left hallux wound. Antegrade crossing of a severely calcified SFA was not possible (Fig. 6.21). The tibial vessels could not easily be identified on EVUS due to occlusion and poor caliber. Direct SFA access below the adductor

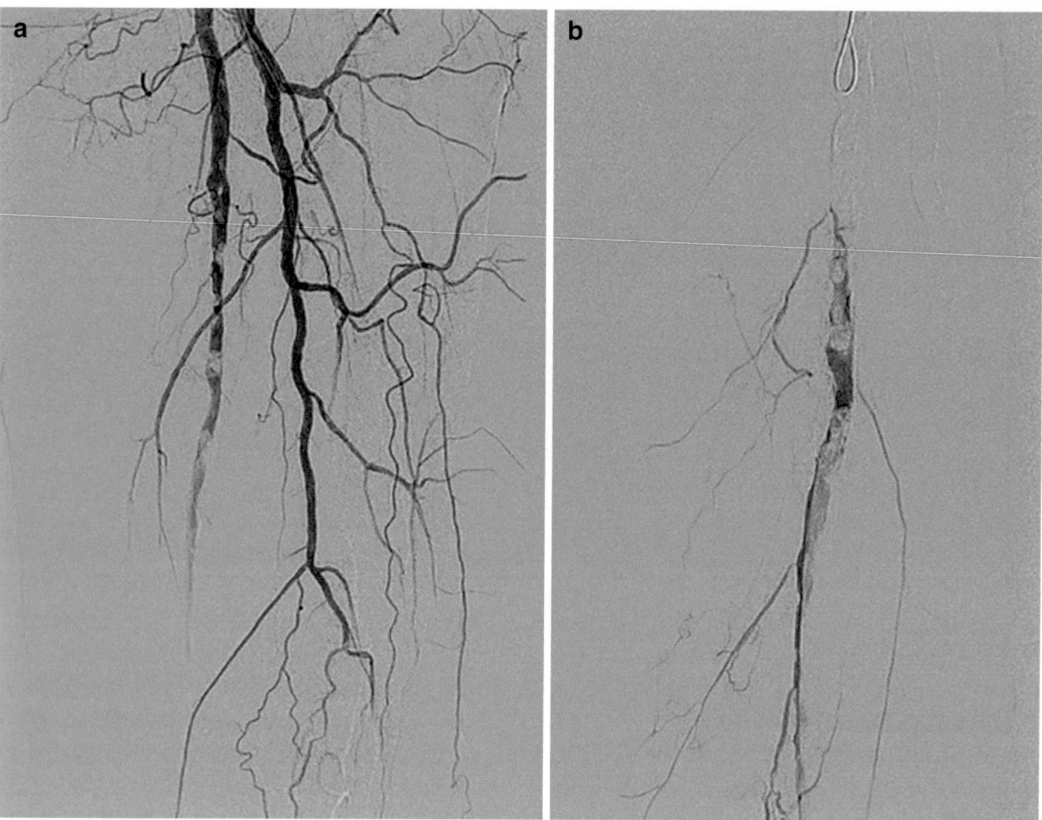

Fig. 6.21 Diagnostic angiogram showing heavily calcified arteries, with distal SFA CTO and mid-popliteal artery reconstitution (**a**) and inability of antegrade wire crossing (**b**)

canal was performed with ultrasound guidance (Fig. 6.22). A micropuncture sheath was left in place with wire crossing retrograde. After antegrade atherectomy, drug-coated balloon angioplasty, and prolonged percutaneous transluminal angioplasty (PTA) were performed. A persistent leak was seen once the micropuncture sheath was removed (Fig. 6.23a). Ultimately, a focal Viabahn (W.L. Gore & Associates, Inc.) covered stent was necessary to seal the leak (Fig. 6.23b).

6.2.3 Arm Access for Peripheral Arterial Disease

Ricki A. Korff, Raghuram Posham, and Robert A. Lookstein

Transradial access (TRA) is an essential component of the endovascular peripheral arterial disease (PAD) treatment toolbox. A radial approach is typically selected in cases where it is difficult or unsafe to access the common femoral artery, in patients with previous abdominal endografts or bifurcation stenting, or if anticoagulation is unable to be stopped [46]. With the currently available tools, plain balloon angioplasty, bare metal stenting, and atherectomy are the only treatment options for treating infrainguinal PAD via radial access, and covered stent graft are yet to be available. New longer devices that are small enough to fit through a 6 Fr sheath have expanded the scope of PAD interventions that can be performed via TRA. In the past, axillary and brachial accesses were used for interventions requiring larger sheath sizes where femoral access was contraindicated. Now that technological advancements have facilitated radial artery access up to 6 Fr in most patients and even 7 Fr in some patients, axillary and brachial accesses are

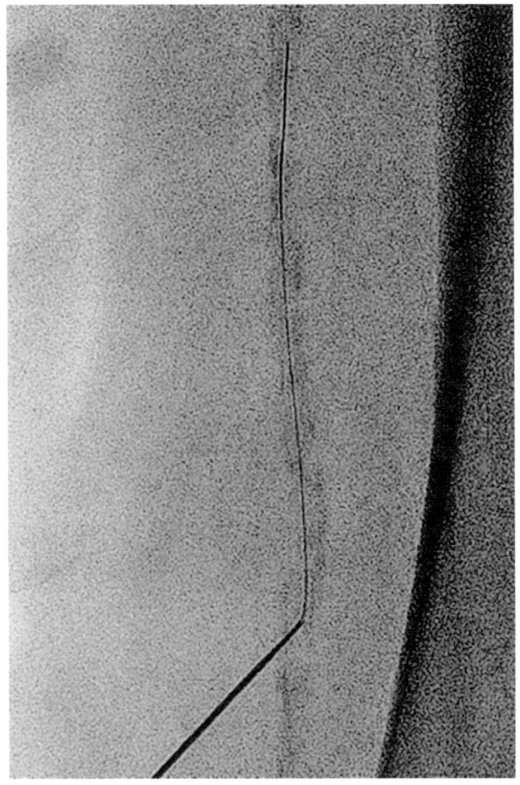

Fig. 6.22 Distal retrograde SFA access after failed antegrade access and no suitable tibial access

rarely used. While with good ultrasound-guided access and other techniques, the common femoral use is still standard for many operators without significant complications; however, alternative access and tools are of interest to many and growing.

6.2.3.1 Device Selection for Radial Access

Prior to performing a peripheral arterial intervention via transradial access, preprocedural planning and knowledge of available devices are essential.

- In a typical transradial PAD case, radial access is obtained, a 6 Fr radial sheath is placed, and a radial cocktail is administered.
- A guidewire and catheter such as the 110 cm OPTITORQUE Sarah Radial Catheter (5 Fr, Terumo) are used to navigate the infrarenal abdominal aorta.

- The system is then exchanged for a stiff support wire such as a 260 cm angled GLIDEWIRE (0.035″, Terumo) and an angled catheter such as an angled GLIDECATH (4 Fr, 120/150 cm, Terumo).

Common and external iliac artery lesions:

- Crossed with a support catheter (i.e., 3.2 Fr × 150-cm Quick-Cross Select catheter, Philips) over a support wire. If stenting is indicated, the stiff support wire is then exchanged for a super stiff 0.035″ 260 cm Amplatz wire in preparation for stent deployment.
- The largest diameter stent that can be deployed via TRA is a 12 mm diameter × 60 mm length self-expanding stent, which is available on a 6 Fr × 120 cm platform (Boston Scientific Epic Stent). This allows for stenting of the majority of external iliac arteries and common iliac arteries in select patients.
- There are currently no drug-coated balloons indicated for treatment of the iliac arteries.
- Numerous percutaneous transluminal angioplasty (PTA, POBA) balloons are available on 6 Fr platforms reaching up to 12 mm in diameter, with working lengths capable of treating iliac artery lesions, compatible with both 0.035″ and 0.018″ wire systems (Fig. 6.24).
- For treatment of external iliac artery lesions, the 10 mm diameter self-expanding WALLSTENT is available on a 6 Fr × 135 cm platform (Boston Scientific).

For treatment of common femoral and superficial femoral artery (SFA) lesions:

- The short introducer sheath and diagnostic catheter are exchanged for a long stiff introducer sheath and support guiding catheter. Examples of long stiff sheaths include R2P Destination Slender Sheath (6 Fr, 119/149 cm, Terumo), Pinnacle Destination Guiding Sheath (6 Fr, 45 cm, Terumo) with a 100 cm GLIDECATH (5 Fr, Terumo), R2P SLENGUIDE Catheter (7 Fr OD, 6 Fr ID, 120/150 cm, Terumo), Sheathless Eaucath (6.5–7.5 Fr OD, 4–5 Fr ID, 100 cm, Asahi),

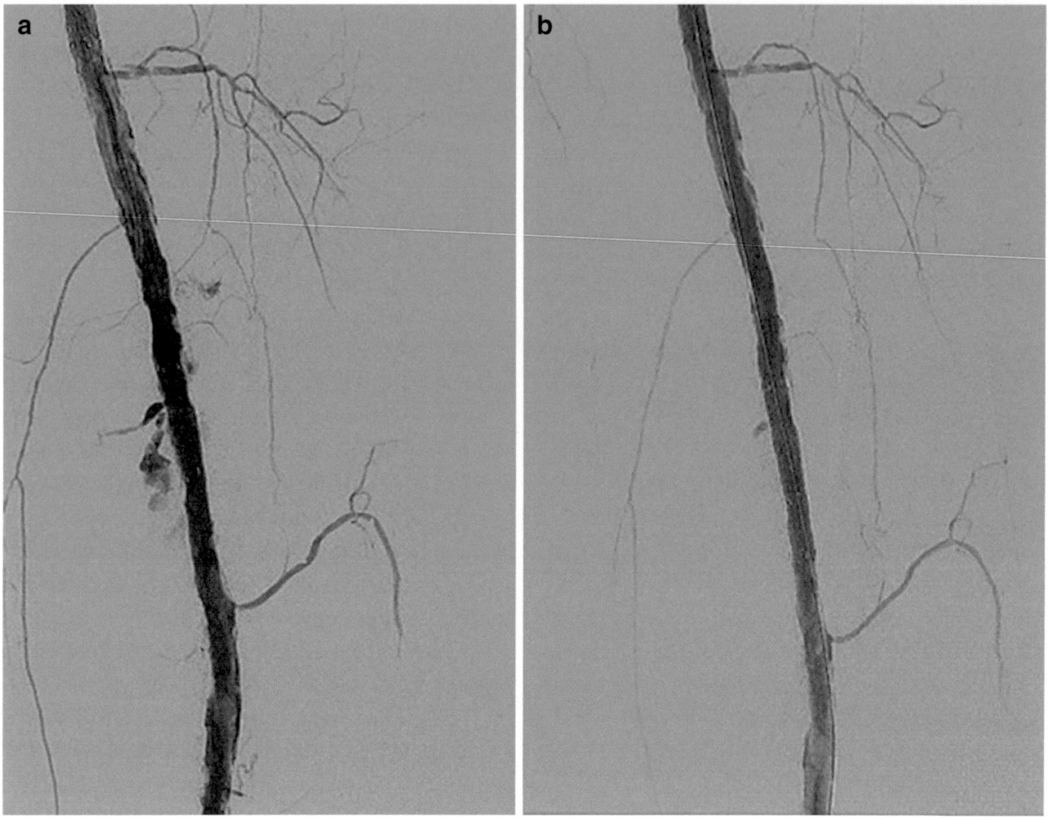

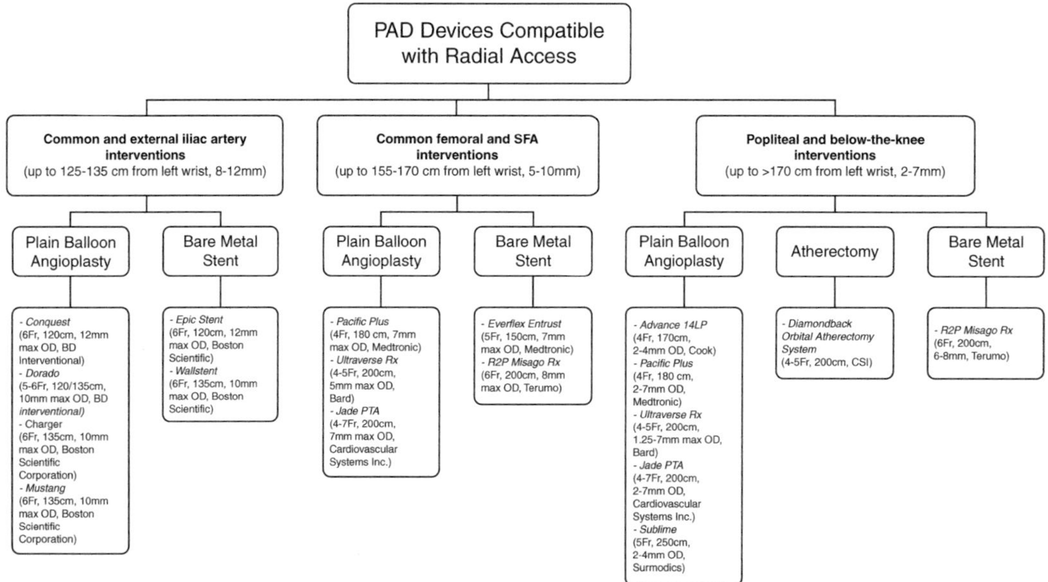

Fig. 6.23 Persistent SFA access site bleeding after prolonged angioplasty (**a**). Followed by resolution of SFA access site bleeding after covered stenting (**b**)

Fig. 6.24 Peripheral arterial disease devices compatible with radial access. *PAD* peripheral arterial disease, *SFA* superficial femoral artery, *OD* outer diameter

and the Flexor Shuttle Sheath (5 Fr, 110 cm, Cook).

- Next, a crossing support catheter (e.g., 3.2 Fr × 150 cm Spectranetics Quick-Cross Select catheter) is advanced to the proximal SFA.
- The GLIDEWIRE is then exchanged for a stiff microwire, such as the 0.018″ × 300 cm Boston Scientific V-18 Control steerable guidewire.
- Once the lesion is crossed, the Quick-Cross Catheter is removed in preparation for intervention.
- Device options for angioplasty and stenting of common femoral and SFA lesions are outlined in Fig. 6.24.

For popliteal artery and below-the-knee lesions:

- Occlusions are crossed with a longer crossing catheter such as the 5 Fr 200 cm Vipercath XC support catheter and crossing wire. *Of note, greater than 200 cm of the wire must be outside of the patient to safely advance a 200 cm support catheter.*
- Longer crossing wires include 475 cm ViperWire Advance 0.14″, 400 cm Medtronic Nitrex 0.035″, 350-450 cm Terumo GLIDEWIRE 0.035″, and 335-475 cm Cardiovascular Systems 0.014″.
- Device options for angioplasty, stenting, and atherectomy of popliteal and below-the-knee lesions are listed in Fig. 6.24. A detailed list of the tools available for use in TRA PAD cases and a description of the procedural steps for treating a variety of infrainguinal PAD lesions via TRA are available in the literature [47, 48].

6.2.3.2 Limitation and Bailouts for Upper Extremity Access

Although a transradial approach is a great option for patients on anticoagulation or with groins that are unsafe or difficult to access, not all patients are candidates.

- In patients with a radial artery smaller than 2 mm, there is an increased risk of radial artery occlusion after TRA.

- In addition, the use of larger-sized sheaths increases the risk of radial artery complications such as radial artery occlusion and spasm [49].
- A 6 Fr sheath at a minimum is typically necessary for PAD cases to ensure adequate catheter and stent platform compatibility, so TRA is typically avoided in patients with a small radial artery.
- In patients with an incomplete superficial palmar arch and a Barbeau D waveform, radial access has traditionally been avoided. However, this has become more controversial as new data emerge suggesting that an incomplete superficial palmar arch is not associated with increased risk of upper extremity dysfunction after transradial access [50]. Regardless, it is important to discuss these risks, complications, and alternative options.

In patients with known aortic arch atherosclerosis or calcification, there is a theoretical risk of stroke from atherosclerotic emboli during endovascular manipulation within the aorta, and a femoral approach is considered safer. In practice, these risks may be overstated [51, 52]. In addition, in patients with a radial loop (tortuosity of the radial artery), it may be difficult to navigate tools to the lower extremities.

- Radial access should also be avoided in patients with advanced chronic kidney disease or end-stage renal disease to preserve the radial artery for future hemodialysis access.

With the available tools, we are currently able to treat lower extremity peripheral arterial disease below the inguinal ligament with plain balloon angioplasty, atherectomy, and bare metal stenting via radial artery access. New longer devices that are small enough to fit through a 6 Fr sheath have expanded the scope of PAD interventions that can be performed via TRA. For example, the 200 cm shaft length R2P MISAGO stents that are now available in the USA allow us to treat arterial lesions and dissections in popliteal arteries as small as 6 mm.

- Although drug-coated balloons (DCB) are frequently used to treat femoropopliteal lesions, currently available DCBs are only available with a shaft length up to 130 cm and are unable to be used with a transradial approach.
- Similarly, while drug-eluting stents (DESs) play an important role in the treatment of infrapopliteal PAD, DESs with shafts long enough to treat these lesions via left radial access are not available.

The full range of endovascular PAD tools is not yet available in lengths compatible with a transradial approach.

- Re-entry devices with shafts long enough to reach the infrapopliteal vessels from the arm are not currently available.
- In addition, covered stents are currently only available in catheter lengths up to 135 cm and on a 6-F platform, so bailout options from the wrist are limited if infrainguinal vessel perforation is encountered. In this case, prolonged balloon tamponade and preparation of the groin for additional femoral artery access would be required.

6.2.3.3 My Sheath Is Stuck, Now What?

One drawback of radial artery access is that the small diameter of the radial artery makes it prone to spasm when larger sheaths are used. Radial sheath entrapment is a rare but serious complication of radial artery access. Increased risk factors include small radial artery diameter, larger sheaths, more catheter exchanges, longer procedure times, and patient anxiety.

- First-line treatment typically includes intra-arterial vasodilators such as nitroglycerin and verapamil, although administration may be limited by hypotension or bradycardia.
- Additional options include increasing sedation, warming the patient's forearm, waiting and retrying, local injection of nitroglycerin around the radial artery, and deep sedation or general anesthesia.
- An additional novel option includes the flow-mediated vasodilation technique. In this method, a blood pressure cuff is used to occlude the brachial artery for 5 min, and then, the cuff is briskly released, leading to a smooth muscle relaxation and vasodilatory response in the radial artery and allowing for radial sheath removal [53, 54].
- Regional brachial plexus block has also been described as a rescue measure [55].
- Several case reports describe the use of lubricants initially designed to reduce friction between atherectomy devices and guidewires including ViperSlide and Rotaglide. Intra-arterial administration of these lubricants has been shown to facilitate radial sheath removal when sheath entrapment is encountered that is refractory to traditional vasodilators and increased sedation [56–58].
- There have also been case reports of radial sheath entrapment treatment with papaverine, an opium-derived alkaloid that leads to vasodilation [59].
- In severe radial sheath cases refractory to these measures, particularly in cases where longer destination sheaths are used for PAD cases, surgical removal may be required [60] (Fig. 6.25).

Radial Sheath Entrapment Treatment

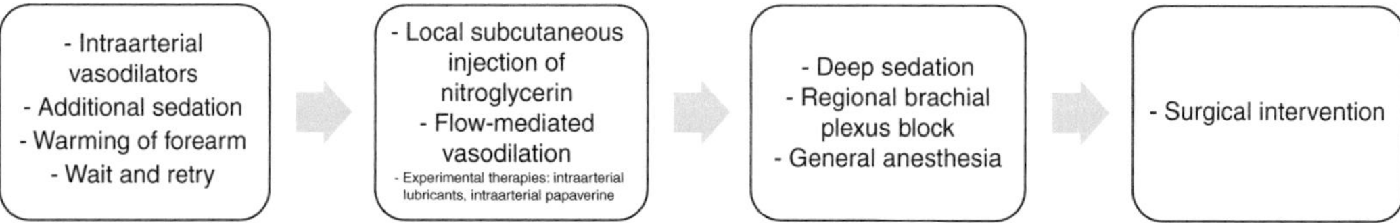

Fig. 6.25 Radial sheath entrapment treatment options

6.2.3.4 Axillary and Brachial Access and Closure

In certain PAD cases in which a larger sheath size is required and femoral access is infeasible, axillary or brachial access may be considered. Larger bore access via the proximal arm allows for treatment with covered stents (e.g., Viabahn Covered Stent, 5–13 mm, 7–12 Fr × 120 cm platform, Gore) and drug-coated balloons (e.g., Ranger Balloon, 7 mm, 6 Fr × 150 cm platform, Boston Scientific) that are not available on platforms designed for radial access.

To access the axillary artery, a vascular surgeon will typically perform a surgical cutdown. More recently, axillary access via a percutaneous approach has been proposed to avoid the need for surgical axillary artery exposure.

- The axillary artery is accessed in the distal first or proximal second segment where it is compressible against the second rib [61]. The first segment of the axillary artery lies superficial to the anterior and posterior divisions of the brachial plexus and generally has the fewest arterial branches, making this the safest access location [62].
- For closure of percutaneous axillary artery access, closure devices may be used off-label, although there is increased risk of access site complication. In the literature, Perclose is the most common device used to close percutaneous axillary arterial access, with ANGIO-SEAL and Mynx also described.
- The most frequent complications include hematoma, pseudoaneurysm, and brachial plexus injury, which is often transient [63].

Due to the risk of vascular complication and injury to the brachial plexus with brachial and axillary artery access, these sites of access are typically not considered first line. With appropriate patient selection and procedural planning, a large percentage of cases in which femoral access is contraindicated can be performed safely from the wrist.

6.3   CO$_2$ Tips and Tricks

Rehan Riaz

Carbon dioxide (CO$_2$) is an odorless, widely available, and nontoxic gas that is rapidly cleared from tissues in the human body and thus a safe alternative contrast agent in the vascular system, especially in patients with an iodinated contrast allergy or renal failure. Combined with digital subtraction angiography (DSA), CO$_2$ angiography can be applied in complex endovascular procedures such as portal vein interventions, renal artery stenosis, and abdominal aortic aneurysm repair. However, widespread use in lower extremity arterial disease is not as prevalent due to many factors, mostly due to lack of experience and to an overstated fear of complications. A more thorough understanding of the unique characteristics of CO$_2$ and diligent attention to technique, with minor alterations to angiographic practices outlined in this chapter, minimizes this threat and allows its safe and successful utilization. With minor variations in angiographic technique, imaging with CO$_2$ can be equivalent to conventional iodinated contrast media (Fig. 6.26).

Iodinated contrast media have evolved over the years, but the inherent risks of contrast-induced nephropathy (CIN) and allergic reaction to contrast have persisted. Although recent observational studies question the prevalence and severity of CIN following contrast exposure, a decline in renal function has been shown to occur 48–72 h after contrast administration in some patients [64].

- Conditions prevalent in patients with lower extremity arterial disease, such as preexisting renal disease, diabetes mellitus, smoking, hypertension, advanced age, and concurrent cardiovascular disease, have been shown to increase this risk [65].
- Periprocedural hydration is the only effective countermeasure at this time, with the use of N-acetylcysteine and/or sodium bicarbonate producing unproven and mixed results [66].

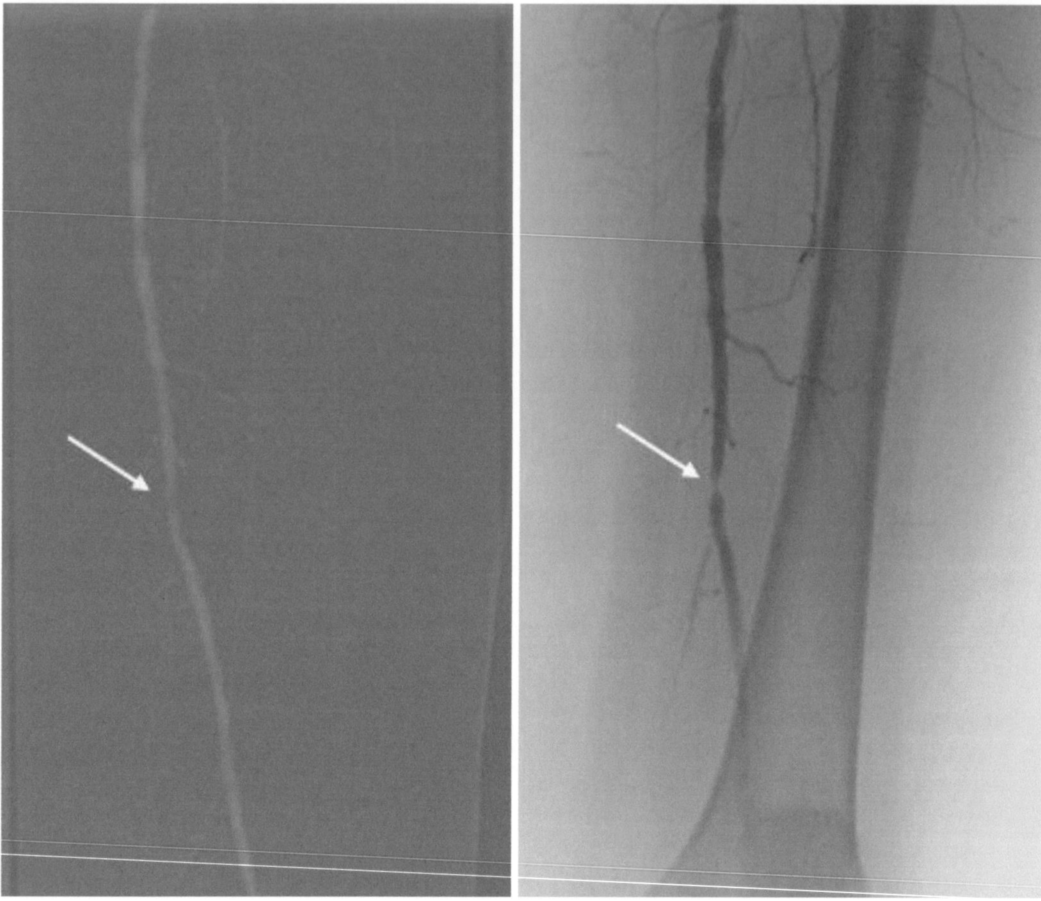

Fig. 6.26 CO_2 angiogram (left) demonstrating a severe stenosis in the distal SFA (arrow). This has an identical appearance to images obtained with iodinated contrast (right)

The risk of contrast allergy reactions range from pruritus and a mild rash to anaphylaxis. Premedication protocols are widely used to lower the severity of these symptoms. Nonetheless, breakthrough reactions occur and, in some patients, complete avoidance of contrast is needed [67].

- Carbon dioxide (CO_2) is the only safe contrast agent available in patients with renal failure and hypersensitive allergic reactions to iodinated contrast media.

6.3.1 Advantages

Carbon dioxide is a nontoxic gas that is widely available and is cheaper than other contrast media. As a natural by-product of the human body, it cannot cause a hypersensitive or allergic reaction and there is no evidence of renal or hepatic toxicity.

There are several attributes that make CO_2 an ideal contrast agent, specifically a high solubility and buoyancy with a low miscibility and viscosity.

- As a result, it can be injected into the arteries below the diaphragm.
- For veins, it can be injected throughout the body without concerns for a clinically significant gas embolism, unless patient has a cardiac defect such as a patent foramen ovale.
- When CO_2 mixes with the water in blood, a majority of it is converted into carbonic acid and bicarbonate. In the lungs, this bicarbonate is effectively converted back into CO_2 and expelled from the alveolar capillaries, with

first-pass lung clearance of approximately 60 mL completely dissolving in 30–60 s [68].

- This high solubility means repeat large bolus injections can be given with essentially no limit to the total amount of CO_2 used, as long as 1–2 min is allowed in between injections to allow for complete clearance.
- In patients with multiple CO_2 injections and underlying pulmonary hypertension or emphysema, it is prudent to increase the time interval between large injections to 3–5 min [69].

CO_2 is lighter than blood, allowing it to float while preferentially opacifying the anterior aspect of the blood vessel. While this has significant implications in large vessels such as the aorta/aortic aneurysms and the IVC, in vessel sizes less than 10 mm seen in the lower extremity this is negligible as the CO_2 gas bubble displaces the blood in more than 80% of the lumen [68].

- Elevation of the legs by 15 degrees or Trendelenburg positioning can further optimize infrapopliteal arterial visualization.

- The buoyancy and fluid displacement also allow better visualization of collateral pathways.
- Unlike iodinated contrast media that mixes and dilutes with blood resulting in poor visualization or washout, the use of CO_2 allows the delineation of reconstituted segments distal to complete occlusions and antegrade, retrograde, and contralateral vascular filling due to reflux from the point of administration.
- Due to its low viscosity, large volumes of contrast (up to 30 mL) can be injected through a 3 Fr microcatheter, standard end-hole catheters, and even around the guidewire in a catheter using a Touhy Borst connector or through the sidearm of a sheath with a stent delivery or angioplasty system in place (Fig. 6.27) [70].
- Intraprocedurally, flushing with 5 cc of CO_2 every 3 min can prevent clot development in the catheter and sheath as this completely displaces any blood that may be stagnating within.

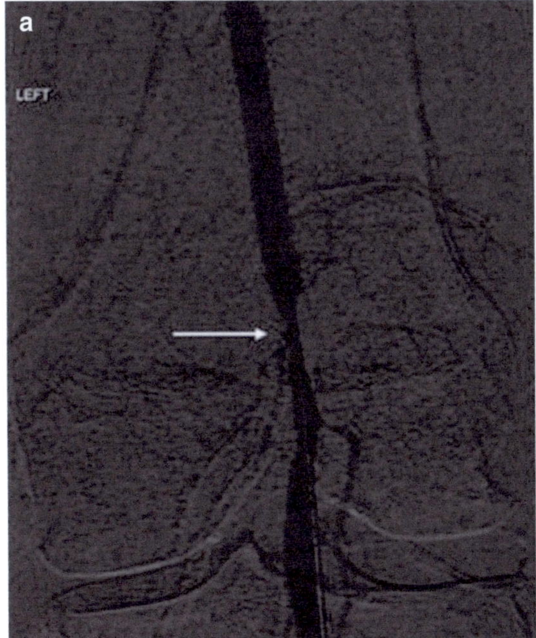

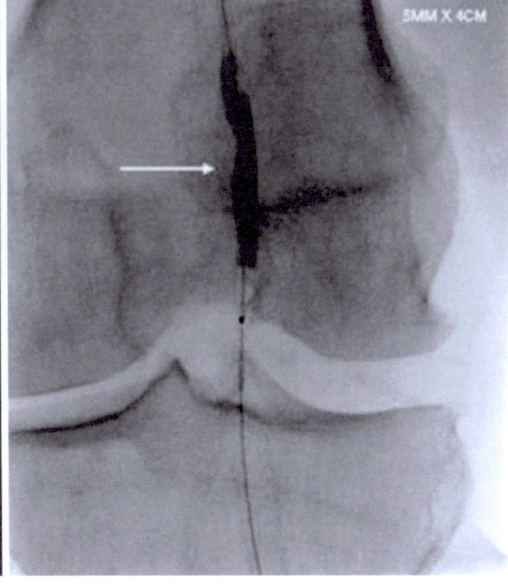

Fig. 6.27 Angiograms can be performed with stent delivery or angioplasty balloon systems in place due to the low viscosity of the gas. (**a**) CO_2 angiogram performed through the sheath (5 Fr) with the balloon in place, demonstrating stenosis in the popliteal artery (arrow) and confirming balloon position. This would not be possible with iodinated contrast or would require a much larger sheath to allow concurrent administration. (**b**) Image obtained during angioplasty

6.3.2 Disadvantages

However, CO_2 is a colorless and odorless gas, making it impossible to visually detect air contamination. CO_2 is compressible and can result in explosive delivery with pressure build-up, requiring a specialized delivery system to avoid these pitfalls.

- CO_2 should not be used in the arterial system above the diaphragm due to the potential for neurotoxicity and myocardial ischemia, or in the abdominal aorta with the patient in prone position as this can cause spinal artery embolism [71].
- Brachial artery injections using CO_2 should be avoided given the risk of reflux into the thoracic aorta and subsequently into the cerebral vasculature.
- Patients with an intracardiac septal defect or pulmonary arteriovenous malformation are also at risk of a paradoxical gas embolism.
- Since CO_2 is a negative contrast agent, any motion by the patient or from bowel gas significantly degrades the image.
- Although the nonmixing of CO_2 is usually a beneficial characteristic, this also makes the gas susceptible to bolus fragmentation at bifurcation points or other areas of high turbulence, resulting in a false-positive stenotic appearance (Fig. 6.28). Patient condition permitting a small amount of iodinated contrast may still be needed to detect true stenosis or resolve equivocal findings.

6.3.3 General Principles of CO_2 Angiography

6.3.3.1 Patient Monitoring
- All patients should be monitored with electrocardiogram and pulse oximetry, and if possible capnography.
- Heavy sedation should be avoided during angiography as respiratory depression and hypotension, which may be the only signs of air contamination, can be mistaken for oversedation.
- If there is air contamination in the system, systemic blood pressure will begin to fall within 20 s of CO_2 delivery, and if it drops by more than 10 mmHg, the delivery system must be inspected for any source of contamination. Although pulse oximetry reflects the status of lung perfusion and oxygen delivery to the tissues, it is not an early warning sign for an air embolism. Oxygen saturation levels can easily remain above 90% despite systemic hypotension from air embolism or excessive CO_2 administration.
- The blood pressure should be checked immediately and 1 min after each CO_2 injection. Furthermore, imaging of the distal lower extremity is greatly affected by motion. In an overly sedated patient, the transient leg discomfort that occurs with CO_2 injection can result in excessive motion artifact if the patient cannot consciously hold still.

6.3.3.2 Carbon Dioxide Delivery
99.99% medical-grade CO_2 must be used with a 0.2 µm filter to remove any contaminants, and the catheter must never be directly connected to the CO_2 source.

1. Plastic bag reservoir method in which a large CO2 tank is kept at the facility and used to fill a sterile bag with stopcocks and one-way valves.
2. CO_2mmander/AngiAssist: The CO_2mmander is the only FDA-approved portable medical CO_2 delivery system. The most commonly used and easiest to adapt (Fig. 6.29).
3. Automatic CO_2 injectors: Similar to the ubiquitous iodinated contrast power injectors, an automated CO_2 injector offers the benefit of precise control of CO_2 volume and pressure while limiting radiation exposure. While first-generation models were too bulky and expensive, newer iterations (Angiodroid, INSPECT 3005R) are used in Europe with promising initial experiences [72].

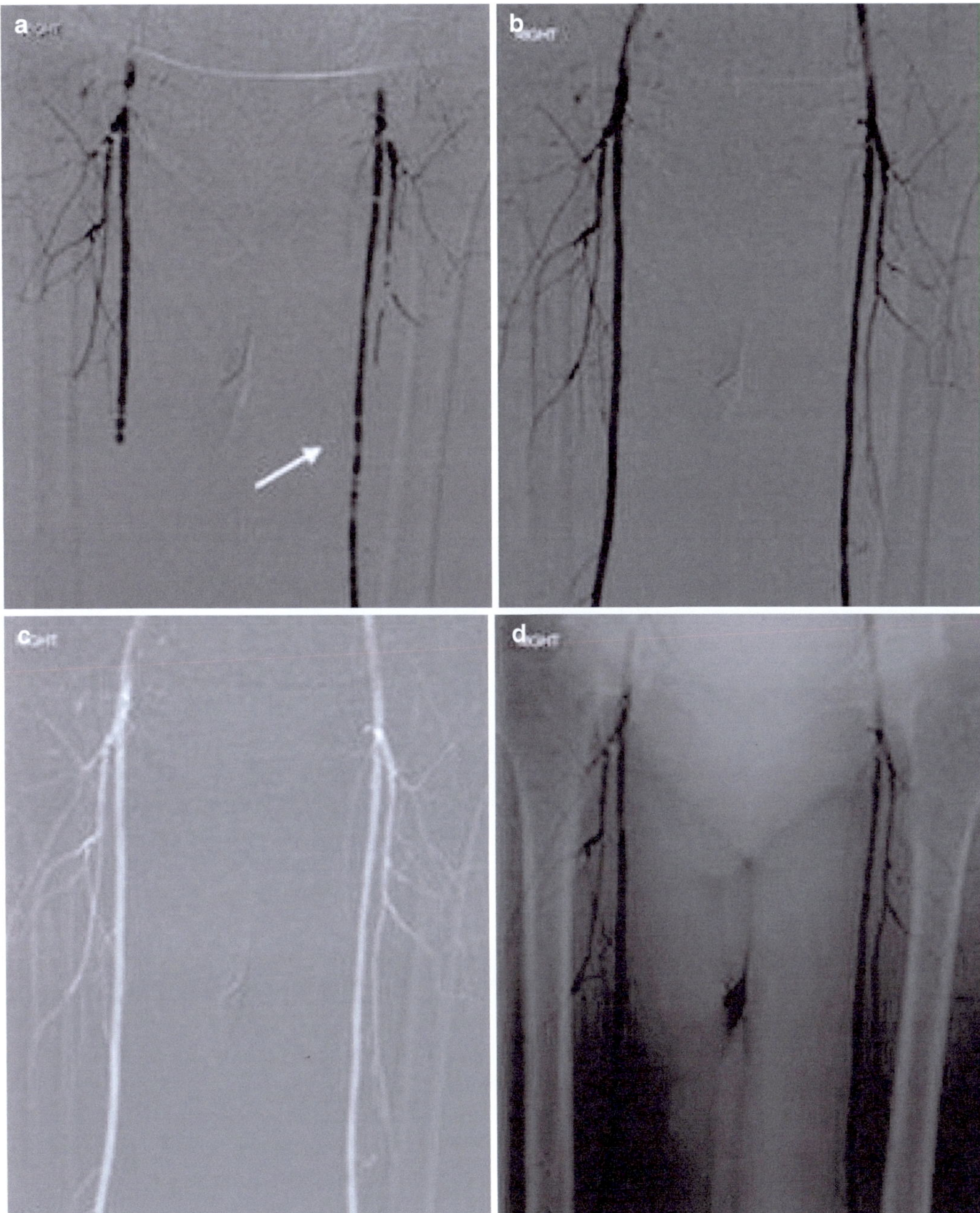

Fig. 6.28 Digital stacking. This is essential due to the breakup of the CO_2 bolus that occurs when the gas travels well beyond the injection. In this example, bilateral run-offs were performed with the catheter in the abdominal aorta. The fragmentation into smaller bubbles results in incomplete luminal opacification (**a**). Stacking provides an accurate representation of the entire lumen by integrat-ing individual segments seen on individual frames (**b**). CO_2 images are commonly inverted during postprocessing (**c**) as clinicians are more familiar with seeing positive contrast images (**d**). Higher frame rates, digital masking, and prevention of patient motion are critical to allow for successful stacking

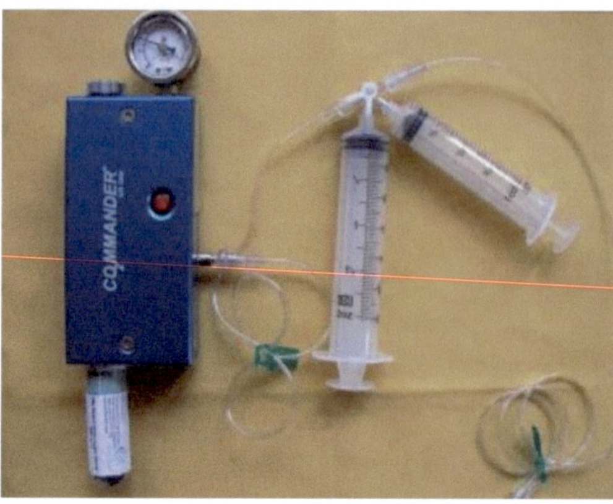

Fig. 6.29 Carbon dioxide delivery system. The CO_2mmander/AngiAssist system is a self-contained apparatus that allows switching from repeated reservoir filling to administration due to a proprietary K-valve stopcock without risking air contamination

6.3.3.3 Imaging Parameters

In most modern fluoroscopy hardware packages, there is a CO_2-specific protocol that must be utilized to fully take advantage of the benefits and avoid the pitfalls of imaging with CO_2 mentioned above. There are minor differences in technique between imaging systems, and because of the unique properties of CO_2, the diagnostic findings when comparing CO_2 imaging to iodinated contrast angiography have been shown to be nearly equivalent (Fig. 6.30) [73]. In fact, as a negative contrast agent, CO_2 allows a better evaluation of preexisting stents and the degree of stent patency in the setting of dense plaque, or when there is a concern for stent compression/fracture or poor wall apposition.

6.3.3.4 Technique for Standard Aortogram and Lower Extremity Runoff

After retrograde access in the contralateral femoral artery using the standard Seldinger technique and placement of a sheath, a 4 or 5 Fr end-hole catheter is positioned just above the aortic bifurcation.

- If evaluation of the aorta is needed, the catheter may be advanced to the level of the renal arteries instead. A somewhat forceful injection of 30–60 cc of CO_2 is needed. It is essential to first flush the catheter with 3–5 cc of CO_2 to clear the blood in the catheter, which decreases gas compression and potential explosive delivery.
- If an aortic aneurysm is present, most of the CO_2 will be trapped in the anterior portion of the aneurysm due to the buoyancy of the gas. This trapped gas can be dissipated by gently rolling the patient from side to side.
- AP and oblique projection angiograms of the pelvis are obtained from the level of the bifurcation, with volumes of 15–30 cc being sufficient to visualize the common and external iliac arteries. 1 mg of glucagon can be administered intravenously to minimize bowel gas motion. The internal iliac arteries are usually not well seen because of their dependent path.

The catheter is then advanced into the contralateral external iliac artery, and additional injections (15–30 cc) are performed to evaluate the femoral and popliteal arteries. The catheter can then be advanced into the superficial femoral artery to evaluate the infrapopliteal vessels, with 15–20 cc of CO_2 being sufficient. If the catheter cannot be advanced into the iliac or femoral vessels due to atherosclerotic disease, a microcatheter can be advanced coaxially into the popliteal artery and gentle injections of 5–10 cc are performed.

Distal CO_2 injection usually results in reflux and visualization of the more proximal vessels as well (Fig. 6.31). If the vessels are suboptimally visualized with these doses, the volume of CO_2 injected can always be increased. Concurrently, intra-arterial injection of nitroglycerin (100–300 µg) and elevation of the foot by 15–30° improve visualization by vasodilation and preferential infragenicular flow of CO_2, respectively. Small amounts of diluted iodinated contrast can be employed to better visualize the distal runoff and pedal vessels.

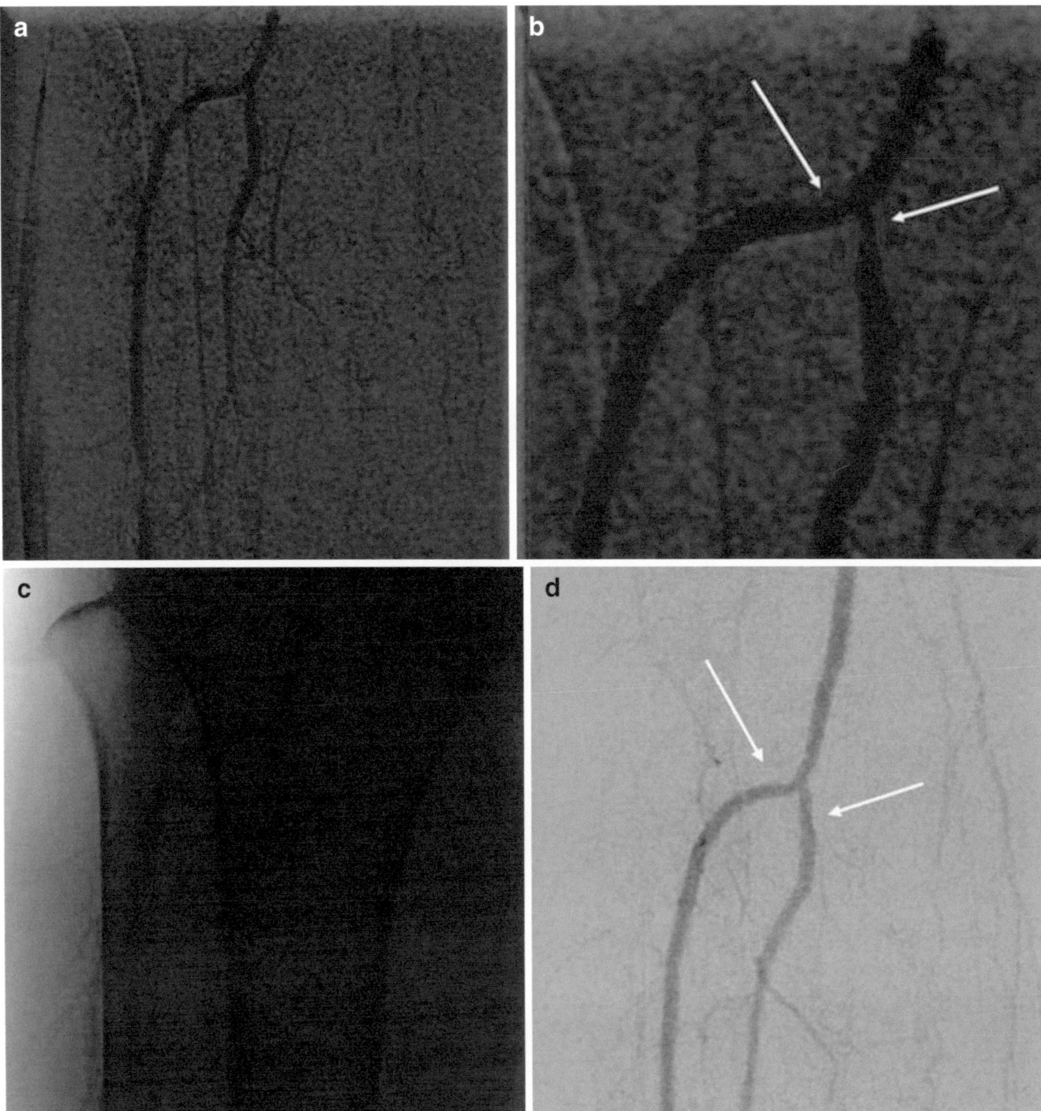

Fig. 6.30 Angiogram of the infrapopliteal vessels of the right lower extremity demonstrating pseudostenosis due to turbulent flow at bifurcation points. CO_2 angiogram (**a**) shows apparent stenosis (arrows) at the origin of the ante-rior tibial artery and tibioperoneal trunk, better seen on magnified view (**b**) of this area. Native (**c**) and digital sub-traction angiography (**d**) images using iodinated contrast show there is no true stenosis

Patient cooperation is vital at this stage, as even minor motion of the extremity eliminates the masking protocol and renders the acquired images nondiagnostic. A discussion prior to the proce-dure with the patient highlighting the importance of remaining still, light sedation, practice runs with coaching during the injection, and even using a leg immobilizer can all improve image quality.

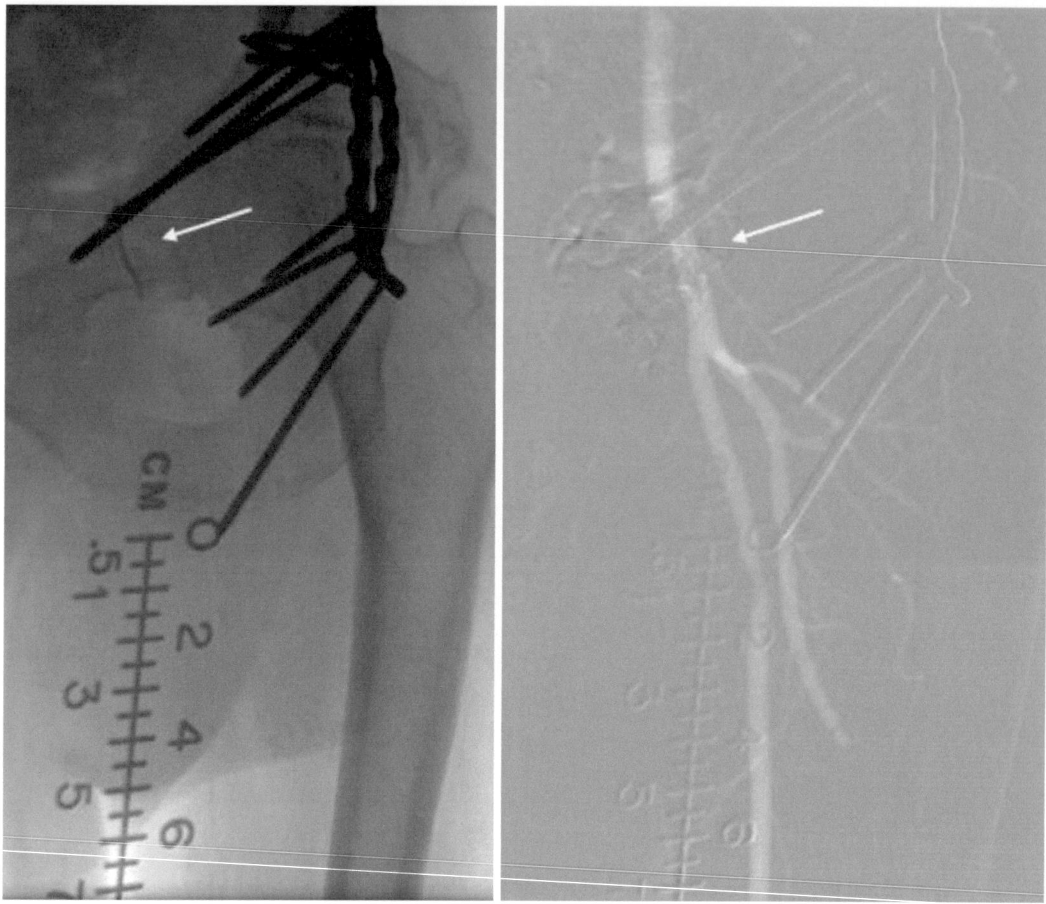

Fig. 6.31 Reflux properties of CO_2. Although the catheter tip is located in the common femoral artery (arrow), the more proximal common femoral and external iliac arteries are well visualized

Key points to optimize peripheral arterial imaging:

- Selective distal catheterization with microcatheter.
- Elevate the area of interest (15–30°).
- Vasodilate with nitroglycerin (100–300 µg).
- Postprocessing with masking and stacking software with high frame rate of acquisition.
- High-contrast X-ray technique with high mA and low kV.
- Patient cooperation.

6.3.4 Complications/Adverse Effects

Almost all of these are minor, temporary adverse effects. When they do occur, they are usually related to the following:

- Operator error as a result of air contamination.
- Excessive dose delivered without adequate time for clearance.
- Inadvertent injection in an undesired location.

- If there is explosive delivery of CO_2 into the peripheral vessels, pain and discomfort may occur, but this lasts for approximately 1–2 min. Additional non-serious adverse effects include nausea and abdominal pain during aortography, which resolves in 2–3 min upon resorption of the gas.
- Serious adverse effects include air contamination, vapor lock, thrombotic atheroembolism, spinal cord ischemia, and neurotoxicity.
- Accidental administration of air in the aorta (or iliac vessels due to reflux) can cause bowel ischemia and infarction.
- Vapor lock can occur due to tapped CO2 mixing with nitrogen and oxygen, and so, nitrous oxide (N_2) general anesthesia should be avoided when CO_2 use is planned. This should be suspected with worsening, persistent abdominal pain occurring during angiography, especially in the setting of superior mesenteric artery occlusive disease.
- A thrombotic embolism occurs with explosive CO_2 delivery resulting in the showering of atheromatous plaque. In smaller vessels, this may result in peripheral embolic lesions. When this occurs in the aorta, this can also lead to bowel ischemia and pancreatitis, irreversible kidney damage, or spinal cord ischemia. Transient spinal cord ischemia has been reported, with patients endorsing temporary paresthesias that resolve as the CO_2 dissolves. If symptoms persist, spinal fluid drainage may be required.

6.3.4.1 Conclusion

Carbon dioxide is a safe, valuable, and versatile alternative to traditional contrast in evaluating and treatment of peripheral arterial disease in the lower extremity. CO_2 should be considered first line in all infradiaphragmatic arterial imaging in patients with renal insufficiency or known contrast allergy. Knowledge of the limitations of CO_2 angiography and an obsessive

level of care is needed to avoid the adverse effects associated with air contamination and vapor lock, with absolute avoidance of use in the thoracic aorta and cerebral vessels. Fortunately, most of the techniques for the safe administration of CO_2 are easily learned and applied and most interventionalists will quickly become competent.

6.4 Dealing with Heavy Calcium

6.4.1 Tricks for Rock Hard Superficial Femoral Artery and Popliteal Complete Total Occlusions

Jos Van Den Berg

While in the past minimally invasive treatment was mainly restricted to relatively simple lesions, nowadays heavily calcified, long total occlusions of the superficial femoral artery (SFA) can be treated by endovascular means. This chapter will provide an overview of the problems that may arise during access, crossing, and final treatment of such calcified long occlusions. Solutions to overcome these problems will be discussed, and a brief overview of the various treatment strategies will be given.

6.4.1.1 Access

In most cases, access is obtained at the level of the common femoral artery (CFA), either for a retrograde crossover approach or an ipsilateral antegrade approach. When ultrasound-guided access is used for access, calcifications of the anterior wall may render confirmation of the intraluminal position of the needle tip difficult, due to the presence of acoustic shadowing (Fig. 6.32). As an alternative fluoroscopy guidance may be used, and in these cases, the presence of extensive calcification may help in identifying the CFA and the femoral bifurcation. Both techniques can be used to facilitate the

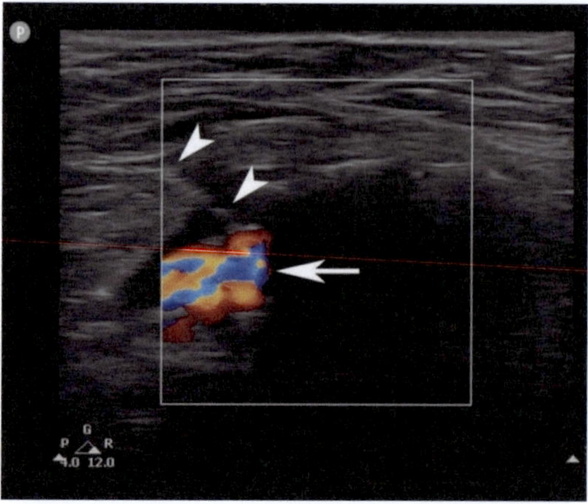

Fig. 6.32 Duplex ultrasound image demonstrating acoustic shadowing of heavily calcified anterior wall of the common femoral artery; only part of the needle (arrowheads) can be seen, "shadow" obscuring needle tip; note abrupt ending of Doppler signal caused by calcification (arrow)

choice of an optimal puncture site, while avoiding puncture of an anterior wall calcification.

Access/puncture of the anterior vessel wall may be difficult due to extensive calcifications (hard, bone-like) causing the needle to slip off to the lateral or medial side of the target vessel. In addition to the problems posed by the acoustic shadowing for access, it may be difficult to further monitor the course of the needle under ultrasound (the needle will move out of plane). Fluoroscopy can be used to "chase" the artery that is slipping away, in such a way that the needle will "follow" the "escaping" artery until it enters. Even when using this technique, it may be difficult to enter the artery with a standard 18G arterial access needle, and in this scenario, a so-called coaxial needle system can be used. This coaxial system consists of the 18G needle (that remains with its bevel against or slightly into the vessel wall, providing additional support) with a 21G puncture needle inside that can be "drilled" into the arterial wall by rotating the 21G needle back and forth inside the 18G needle (Fig. 6.33a, b).

Once needle access has been obtained and a standard access wire has been placed intraluminally, and it may be difficult to advance the introducer sheath. The smaller the sheath, the less problems that will be encountered in advancing the introducer (a 4F sheath has almost the same outer diameter as an 18G needle). In case the calcium is expected to create a non-surmountable barrier for the sheath, it is recommended to use a short (75–90 cm) extra-stiff guidewire (e.g., Lunderquist 0.035″) from the start. This guidewire will provide a lot of support and will allow access of the sheath, even in the most severe calcifications. Alternatively, an 0.018″ guidewire-based sheath (micropuncture set) may be used, although the guidewire of this system oftentimes does not provide the required support, especially in obese patients.

All the techniques described here can also be used for retrograde distal access to the distal SFA and popliteal artery (Fig. 6.33c, d).

6.4.1.2 Crossing

The first approach is to use a 4 or 5F diagnostic catheter or a support catheter with a standard 0.035″ hydrophilic guidewire.

- In cases of high-grade heavily calcified stenoses, it is advisable to use supportive 0.018″ guidewires with a (shapeable) nitinol tip to allow for navigation through the (oftentimes) meandering, extremely narrow lumen (Fig. 6.34a–c).
- Sometimes downgrading to 0.014″ guidewires may be necessary in order to be able to cross extremely narrow segments. The additional use of support (micro)catheters may enhance the probability of successful crossing.

The same intraluminal strategy may also be followed in cases of heavily calcified chronic total occlusions, but in these cases, it is more likely that the guidewire will follow a subintimal course. Due to the increased resistance encountered in heavily calcified arteries, it may be necessary to use a stiff hydrophilic guidewire in order to be able to advance the crossing catheter. In case advancement of the 4F or 5F catheter is not feasible, it is recommended to exchange the (stiff) guidewire for a supportive microcatheter, creating a so-called coaxial catheter system (Fig. 6.35a). The 4- or 5F catheter needs to have a 0.038″ lumen in order to accommodate the

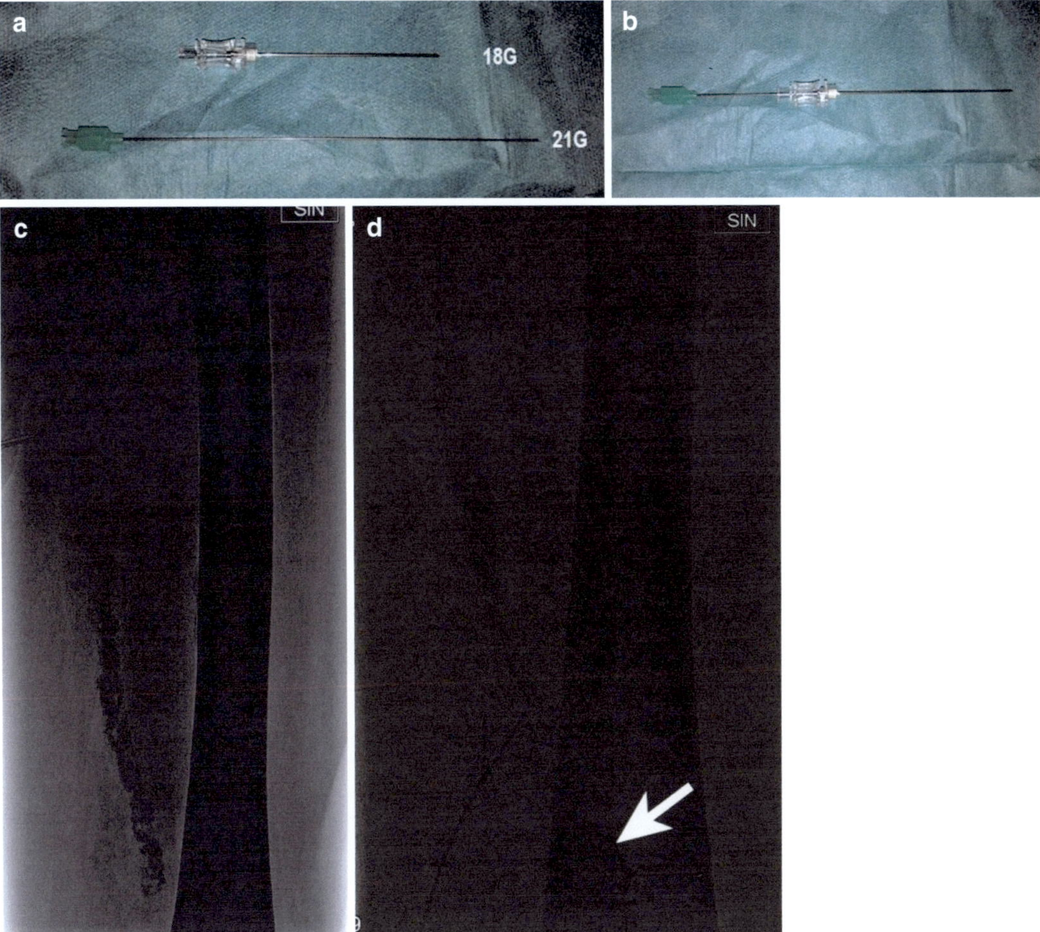

Fig. 6.33 (a) Photograph of 18G standard access needle and 21G needle for coaxial access. (b) Photograph of the two needles assembled. The 21G needle needs to be at least 5 cm longer than the 18G needle. (c) Fluoroscopic image of the left upper leg demonstrating extensive calci-fication in patient with SFA occlusion. (d) Fluoroscopic image of retrograde puncture with 21G needle after failed antegrade crossing (distal perforation with contrast extravasation; arrow); the needle can be seen curving by the force applied, with needle tip not entering the vessel

microcatheter. A continuous saline flush through a Y-connector that is mounted on the main catheter may be applied to reduce the probability of thrombus formation in the space between the two catheters and will reduce friction when advancing the microcatheter. For SFA crossing, the use of a microcatheter that is compatible with an 0.018″ guidewire is recommended (Fig. 6.35b–f).

In case of "spontaneous" re-entry failure, one can resort to re-entry devices, consisting of a catheter with a curved needle that can be pushed outside of the catheter in order to perforate the intima and re-enter into the intraluminal space.

Advancement of these devices can be cumbersome, especially in highly calcified arteries, and predilation of the catheter track with a 2–3 mm diameter balloon may be necessary.

- As a (less costly) alternative, a distal retrograde puncture can be performed and the (intraluminal or subintimal) retrograde and (subintimal) antegrade pathways of the catheters/guidewires may be connected using various techniques.

- In case both retrograde and antegrade pathways are subintimal, the "rendez-vous" can be

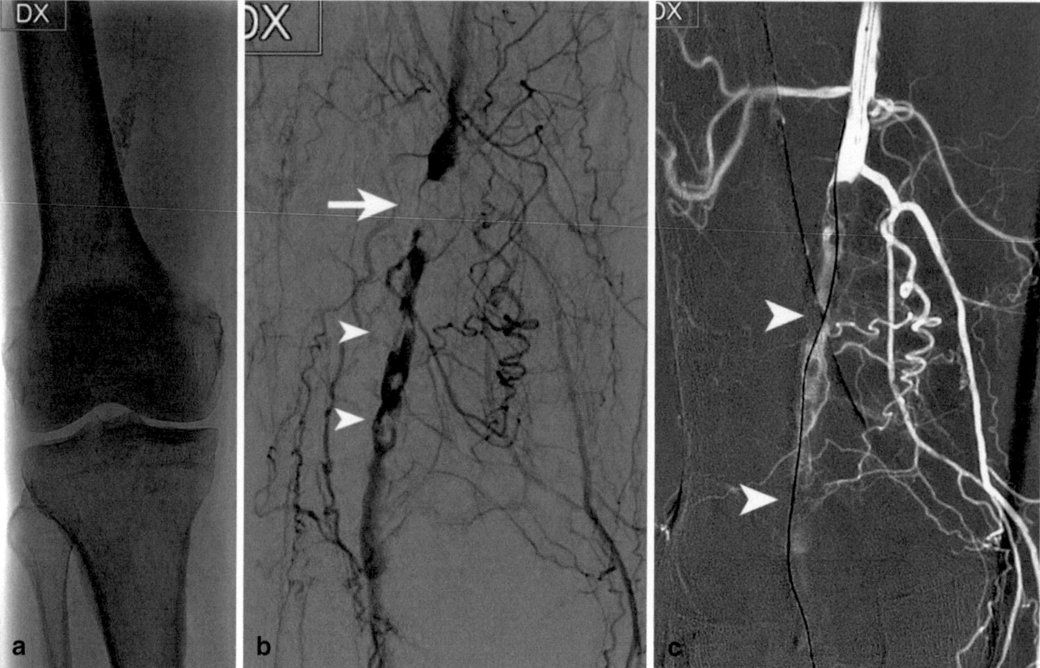

Fig. 6.34 (**a**) Fluoroscopic image of the right upper leg demonstrating extensive calcification in the distal SFA and popliteal artery. (**b**) DSA image demonstrating high-grade stenosis of the distal SFA (arrow) and multiple eccentric stenoses of the popliteal artery (arrowheads). (**c**) Roadmap image demonstrating successful intraluminal passage of 0.018″ guidewire (arrowheads)

accomplished relatively easy with the use of a curved tip catheter from one side that "snares" the (curved) guidewire tip that is coming from the other end (Fig. 6.36a, b).

- In case the distal guidewire has maintained an intraluminal position, the intimal layer that is interposed between the intraluminal and subintimal pathway needs to be "ruptured" with a PTA balloon, which can either come from distal (CART technique) or proximal (reverse CART; Fig. 6.36c–h) [74]. The balloon should be of a diameter that is identical or slightly bigger than the reference vessel diameter, since an undersized balloon will not allow for breaking of the intimal layer [75, 76]. Once the connection between the two pathways has been established, "snaring" can be performed as described above.

For very focal, short highly calcified lesions an alternative technique may be used that consists of the use of the back end of an 0.018″ guidewire together with a 4-5F diagnostic catheter that is centered at the proximal edge of the occlusion. In case a stable, centered position cannot be achieved with a diagnostic catheter, centering can be facilitated by using a PTA catheter that is inflated just proximal from the occlusion. Multiple obliques should be used to confirm directionality. This technique should be used with extreme caution and should never be used in tortuous vessel segments (Fig. 6.37a–c).

6.4.1.3 Treatment

Calcification is an independent predictor of patency and late lumen loss in drug-coated balloon angioplasty [77, 78]. Stent scaffold may also have difficulty in fully expanding, which often cannot be improved once deployed. More aggressive vessel preparation is oftentimes necessary to deal with calcified lesions. Atherectomy devices (rotational, orbital, and to a lesser extent directional atherectomy) can be used to reduce the plaque burden [79–81]. Other devices aim for

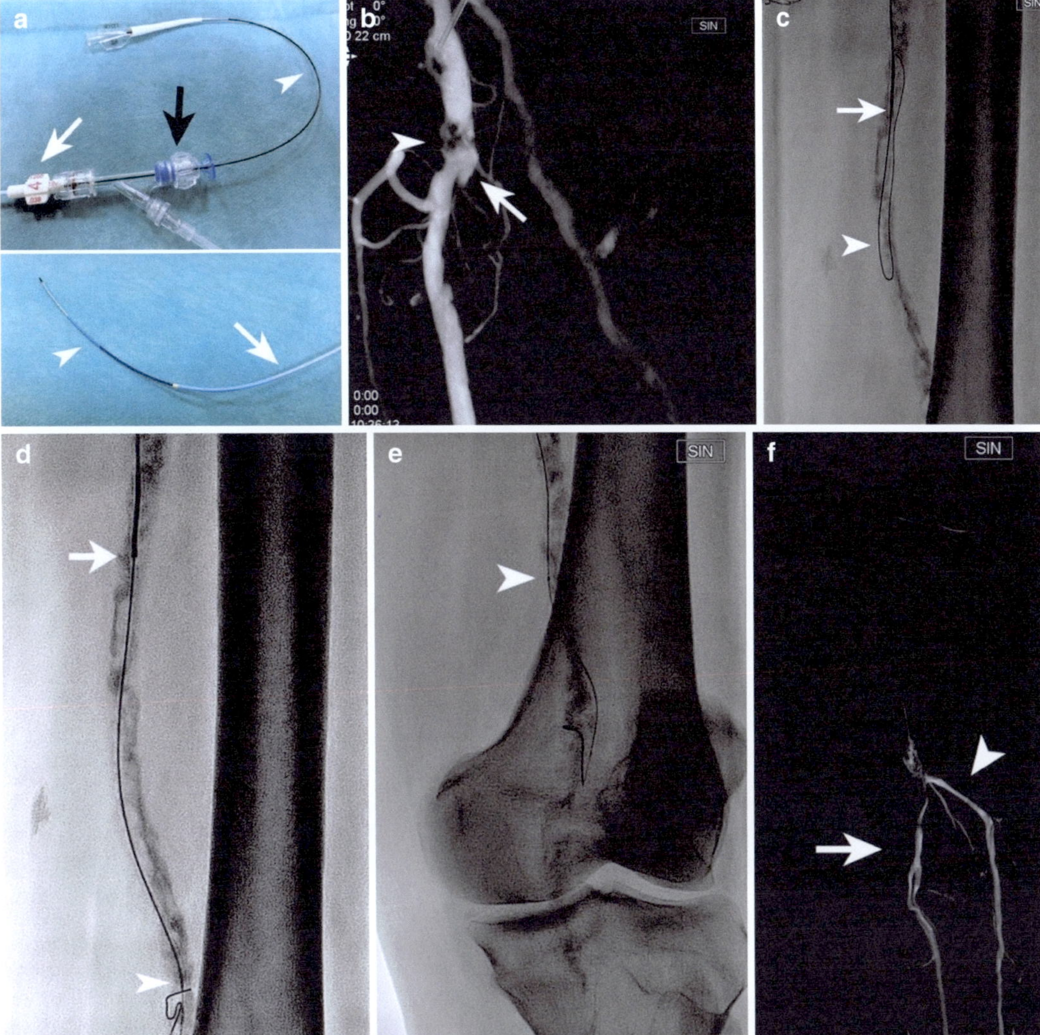

Fig. 6.35 (a) Photograph of coaxial catheter system with Y-connector (black arrow), diagnostic catheter (white arrow), and microcatheter (arrowhead). (b) Roadmap image of left common femoral artery with high-grade stenosis (arrowhead) and occlusion of the SFA with short proximal stump (arrow); patient with total occlusion until distal P3 segment (not shown). (c) Fluoroscopic image after subintimal recanalization of the SFA occlusion with 4F diagnostic catheter (arrow) and stiff GLIDEWIRE (arrowhead); advancing beyond this point was not possible. (d) Fluoroscopic image with coaxial catheter system in place; diagnostic catheter (arrow) and distal position of microcatheter (arrowhead) and 0.018″ guidewire; (e) Fluoroscopic image after further subintimal recanalization with microcatheter (arrowhead indicates tip). (f) Roadmap image obtained using microcatheter after spontaneous re-entry of guidewire intraluminally, demonstrating patency of (stenotic) tibioperoneal trunk (arrow) and anterior tibial artery (arrowhead)

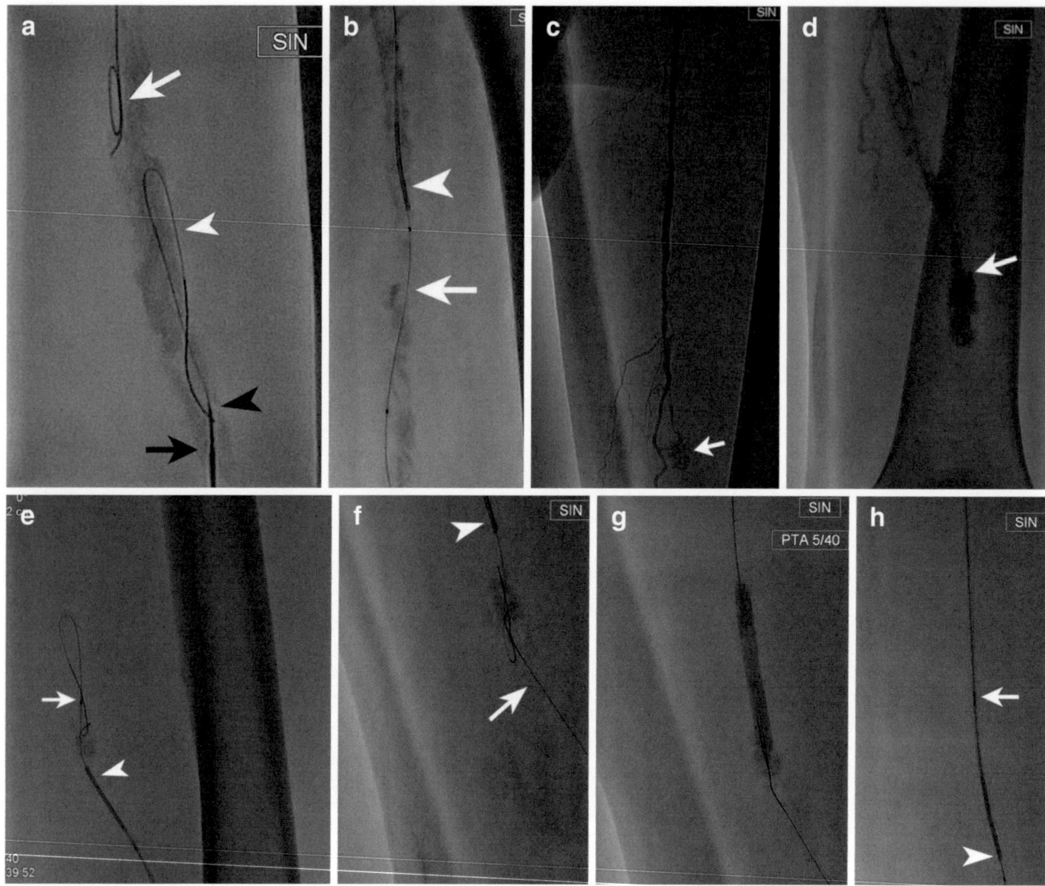

Fig. 6.36 (**a**) Fluoroscopic image showing subintimal passage of antegrade (white arrow) and retrograde guidewire (arrowhead); note coaxial needle system in place (18G needle black arrow, 21G needle black arrowhead). (**b**) Fluoroscopic image after "snaring" of guidewire and microcatheter (arrow) by diagnostic catheter (arrowhead) . (**c**) Unsubtracted angiographic image showing occlusion of the SFA with short-segment calcification (focal, homogeneous; arrow). (**d**) Fluoroscopic image: subintimal recanalization attempt led to extra-vascular course of guidewire with contrast extravasation (arrow). (**e**) Fluoroscopic image of second attempt with primary distal approach; coaxial catheter system was used (microcathe- ter indicated by arrow, diagnostic catheter by arrowhead); re-entry was not possible. (**f**) Fluoroscopic image after antegrade access showing antegrade diagnostic catheter (arrowhead) and retrograde guidewire (arrow); it was not possible to establish a connection between the two subintimal pathways. (**g**) Fluoroscopic image of "reverse CART" with proximal balloon of sufficient diameter to "crack" the intima; note presence of distal wire and position of balloon proximal from calcification. (**h**) Fluoroscopic image after "snaring" of microcatheter (from distal, arrow); arrowhead indicates tip of antegrade catheter

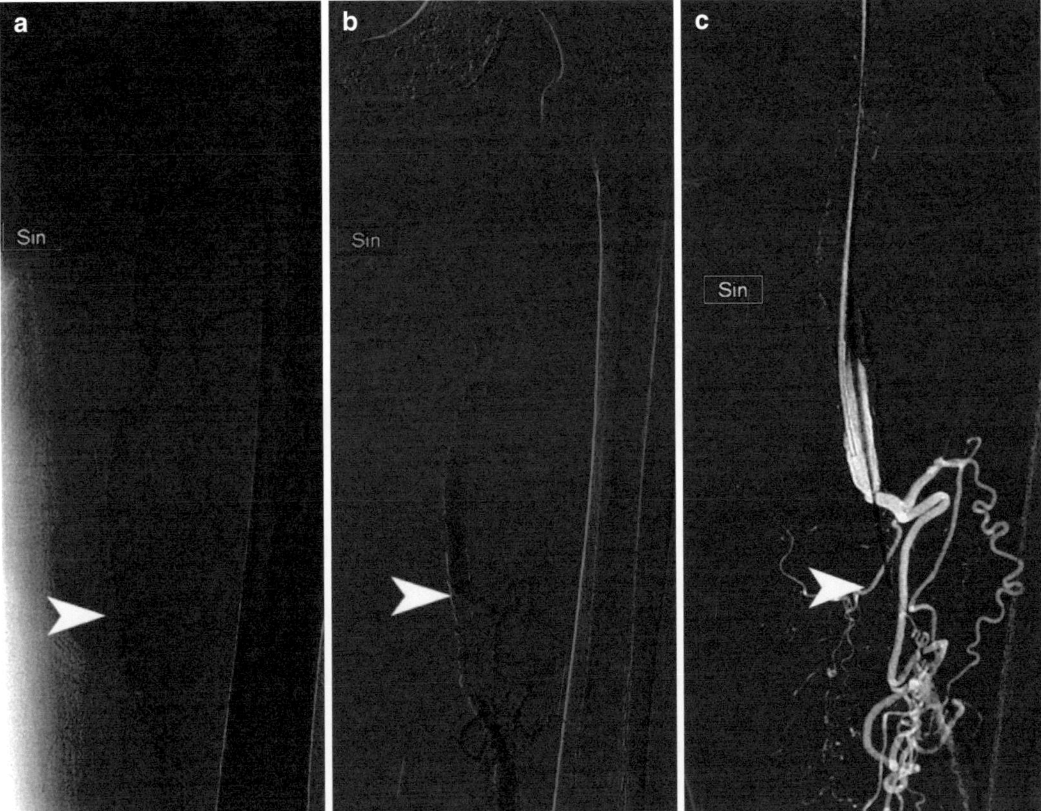

Fig. 6.37 (**a**) Fluoroscopic image of left upper leg, with extensive calcification; arrowhead indicates start of the occlusion. (**b**) DSA of occlusion with absence of "stump" and outflow into large collateral (arrowhead). (**c**) Roadmap image showing back end of wire (arrowhead) pushed through proximal cap after centering of diagnostic catheter

plaque modification (intravascular lithotripsy (IVL), rotational atherectomy, and laser).

- Reducing plaque burden and/or plaque modification will decrease the likelihood of bailout stenting, and in case stenting is needed, it will be easier to achieve proper stent expansion.
- Vessel preparation probably will increase the uptake of drug in case drug-coated balloons are used.
- One of the disadvantages of atherectomy devices is the potential risk of distal embolization, and therefore, distal filter protection devices are recommended with most. The risk of embolization is lower when using IVL [82, 83].
- There are no RCT data that favor the use of one device over another, while comparison of studies with different devices is hampered by the fact that no uniform classification of the degree of calcification is used across the various studies. It is therefore not possible to illustrate exactly which device is best suited for vessel preparation and final treatment.

6.4.2 When Should I Consider Intravascular Lithotripsy?

Bryan Fischer and Sreekumar Madassery

The introduction of intravascular lithotripsy has provided a viable solution for calcified occlusive arterial disease, which is the most difficult of arterial plaque types to manage from an endovascular or even surgical approach. Plain balloon angioplasty (POBA) has limited success in disruption and caliber increase when dealing with heavy calcium. Historically, options for patients with small calcified iliac vessels undergoing endovascular aneurysm repair were either limited to surgical conduit via open retroperitoneal iliac exposure or aggressive endovascular maneuvers like "Pave and Crack" (covered stent placement to avoid rupture, followed by very high-pressure balloon angioplasty and then bare metal stenting). This approach has been adopted in the heavily calcified femoropopliteal segments as well. Since then, the ability to consider minimally invasive options has increased with the application of IVL technology, which decreases the risk of vessel injury or rupture during device/sheath passage and can reduce the need for scaffold use such as the pave and crack approach [84].

- The most commonly used IVL is the Shockwave lithotripsy balloon catheter (Shockwave Medical).
- IVL uses a balloon-based catheter containing multiple lithotripsy emitters, which when activated by a generator system, fire within the fluid-filled balloon to create sonic pressure waves in sequential patterns for a prescribed number of pulses and time, with refractory periods in between.
- These waves cause disruption of calcium within the media and intimal walls of arteries, resulting in increased vessel compliance. This approach is similar to procedures performed for kidney stones.
- There are several available balloon sizes currently including the M5, M5+, and S4 (Shockwave Medical) catheters, which range in size from 2.5 mm to 8 mm in diameter. These are in varying lengths and sheath compatibility (5–7 Fr).
- With POBA, the consequences of high atmospheric pressure from this option unfortunately resulted in higher dissection rates, limited patency, and increased vessel rupture risk. Failure to identify high-risk vessels prior to dilation can result in inferior results and places the patient at higher risk for vessel occlusion or rupture.

- Whether involving the iliac, SFA/pop, or tibial vessels, the patients most likely to benefit from selective IVL treatment are those with increasing density and circumferential calcified disease of the vessel wall.
- In the iliac vessels, its use allows for easier passage of larger devices and thus expands patient access such as in TAVR procedures, without increasing risk of rupture or vessel occlusion secondary to dissection.

There has been a growing body of data to validate the use of IVL within PAD patients. The Disrupt PAD III trial was a randomized trial with 306 lesions randomized to IVL plus drug-coated balloon (DCB) versus POBA plus DCB, with 83% severe calcium and approximately 13 cm lesion length. This resulted in primary patency of 80.8% vs 70.9% at 1 year and 74.4% vs 57.7% at 2 years, favoring IVL plus DCB. There was also 77% reduction of type C or greater dissections, no complications, and 75% reduction in bailout stenting favoring IVL with DCB [85]. Recently, the Disrupt BTK 1 study, which was a prospective safety study for infrapopliteal arteries in 20 patients followed to 30 days, shows 100% freedom from TLR in these patients which were 100% severely calcified and 75% that were Rutherford V [83]. While these data are small, a randomized infrapopliteal large study is currently enrolling [88].

The SFA/popliteal vascular bed presents additional challenges to treatment due to lesion length and the kinetics of this infrainguinal segment. Heavy calcium in the vessel wall adds an additional obstacle for even the most advanced interventionalist.

- The benefit of IVL in the carefully selected patient is best seen with intravascular ultrasound imaging after adequate delivery of energy to the vessel wall.
- Furthermore, aggressive post-dilation or scaffolding is seldom needed when IVL is used prior to definitive treatment.
- Of note, debulking/vessel modification with atherectomy prior to IVL in the SFA/pop is an accepted practice; however, there are many

who prefer not to use atherectomy prior to balloon lithotripsy, with the benefit being a near zero risk of distal embolization with lithotripsy alone.

There are nuances to use of IVL which should be understood:

- The balloon is only inflated to a sub-nominal pressure, until it effaces the area of calcific stenosis, usually around 1 mm Hg. The balloon pressure is increased incrementally after each cycle of IVL at the target site, until a maximum of 4 mm Hg is reached with the indeflator device.
- As the sonic waves are created, operators will notice a slow decreased in pressure, which indicates that the compliance of the arterial wall is increasing, and continued inflation is performed.
- By using low-pressure angioplasty/lithotripsy, there is less significant dissections and avoidance of perforation, which is common in conventional angioplasty of calcified stenoses.
- It is not uncommon to see EKG changes during lithotripsy, which are artifactual and warning your procedural nurses or anesthesia will alleviate unnecessary stress.
- With heavy calcified severe stenosis, sometimes predilation of the target area may be required to pass the IVL balloon.
- For very stenotic lesions, centering the middle emitter at the tightest area is ideal as typically multiple lithotripsy waves are created in the center compared to the periphery.
- IVL likely has the least chances of embolization as it is intended for circumferential calcium and disrupts the calcium without grinding, cutting, or other methods. However, if there is eccentric, chunky, or coral reef calcium, pushing any device across these lesions can result in embolization even without activating the device.

The increasing use of IVL has been instrumental in changing the algorithmic approach for calcified vessels. In patients with at least 180^0 or circumferential calcium, best evaluated on IVUS,

then IVL may be the ideal tool to prep the vessel for maximum definitive treatment. Regardless of preference, intravascular lithotripsy represents a significant breakthrough for patients who historically had few viable options for the treatment of heavily calcified disease, reduces significant dissections or perforations, and likely provides enhanced drug delivery and scaffold expansion.

6.4.2.1 Case: Courtesy of Sreekumar Madassery, MD

This is a case study of 70-yo male with DM2, HTN. ESRD who has a right dorsal foot suspected diabetic ulcer (Fig. 6.38). Despite wound care, there has been stalling of any wound healing. After obtaining noninvasive imaging with noncompressible tibial vessels, decision was made to perform diagnostic lower extremity angiogram. Angiogram demonstrated heavy calcific burden with significant stenosis of the anterior tibial artery, P3 segment of the popliteal artery, and focal CTO of the peroneal artery origin. Utilizing antegrade access, the anterior tibial artery was able to be traversed and IVL was performed of the proximal anterior tibial artery. Attempts to cross the TPT trunk into the peroneal in the antegrade direction were unsuccessful. The patent proximal peroneal artery was directly accessed under fluoroscopic guidance, and an 014 wire was used to revascularize the CTO with bareback catheter support. Once the wire was externalized after rendezvous, IVL of the P3 popliteal artery and peroneal artery was performed (Fig. 6.39a–d). After IVL, the anterior tibial and peroneal artery were further angioplastied with scoring balloons (Fig. 6.40a–c). Patient on follow-up did show progressive wound healing with continued wound care.

6.4.3 When to Use Laser?

Micah Watts

Laser atherectomy is a safe and effective method to debulk arterial atherosclerotic plaque to improve results of subsequent angioplasty. Additionally, its ablative mechanochemical characteristics make it useful in treating mixed plaque

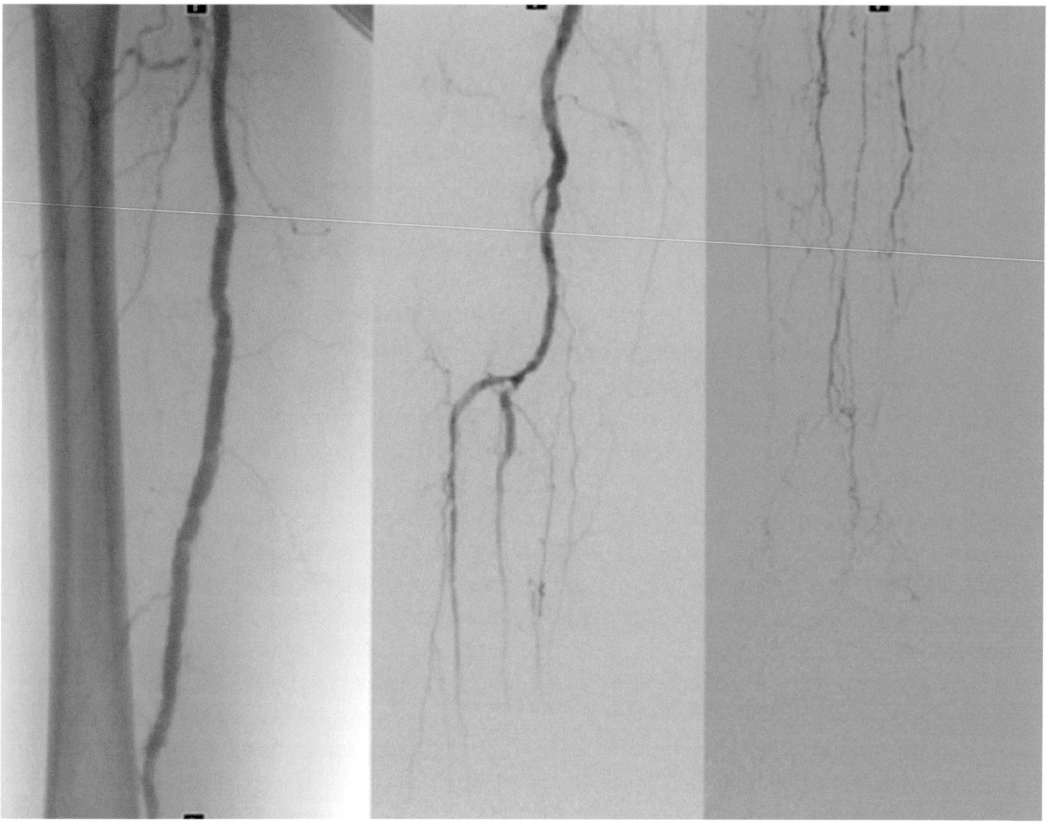

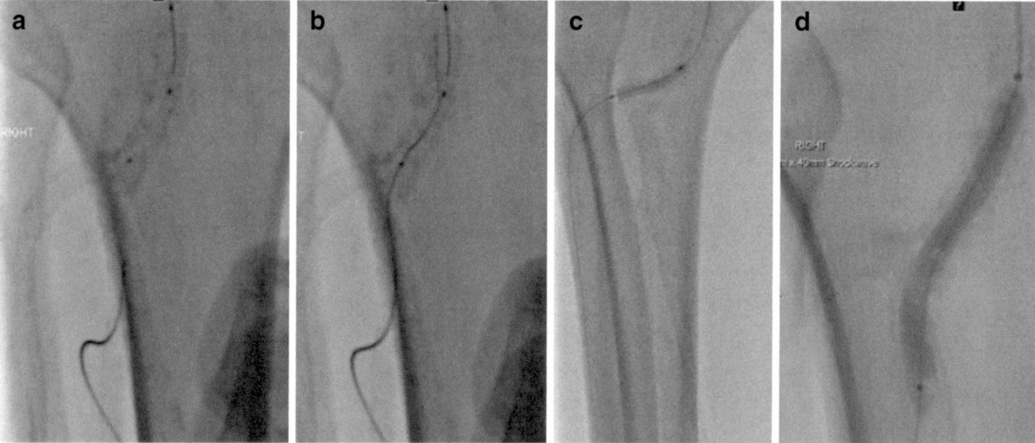

Fig. 6.38 Diagnostic angiogram of a 70-yo pt. with DM2, ESRD, and a non-healing right dorsal foot diabetic ulcer

Fig. 6.39 Heavy calcific burden can be seen in the images **a–d**. After antegrade access, direct peroneal retrograde access (**a**) followed by rendezvous in the P3 segment (**b**). IVL was performed of the proximal anterior tibial (**c**), TP trunk, and the P3 segment (**d**)

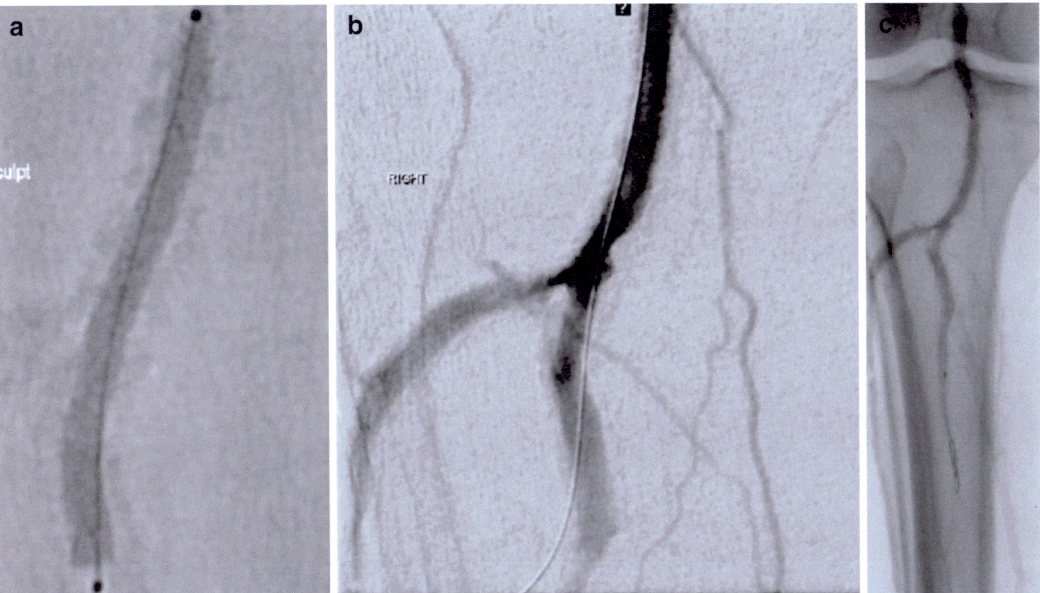

Fig. 6.40 After IVL pretreatment, angioplasty of the peroneal CTO and P3 segment was performed (**a**). Completion angiograms (**b, c**) show markedly improved caliber of the treated segments, with no dissection or perforation, with avoidance of scaffold placement

morphologies and thrombus. Data for laser atherectomy, including in-stent restenosis (ISR), are convincing, but are limited in the setting of calcified vessels. Algorithms for heavily calcified above and below-the-knee arteries are proposed.

6.4.3.1 Laser History and Background

The mainstay of endovascular peripheral arterial revascularization remains balloon angioplasty. Unfortunately, the patency rates of POBA (plain old balloon angioplasty) are often short lived with potentially unacceptable restenosis rates. Restenosis after PTA can be as high as 60% at one year depending on the location, length, and characteristics of the original lesion [87].

Current consensus dictates that arterial wall injury from barotrauma during balloon angioplasty is the main cause of restenosis. High balloon pressures exerted unevenly across the arterial wall, and atherosclerotic plaque causes overstretching, plaque rupture, and wall trauma that results in growth factor production eventually leading to proliferation of endothelial and smooth muscle cells and ultimately resulting in arterial stenosis (referred to as intimal hyperplasia) [88].

Heavily calcified arterial stenoses will often require higher pressure angioplasty and potentially lead to more barotrauma on the surrounding tissues, ultimately leading to potential early restenosis, intimal dissection, or possible vessel rupture [89].

A commonly employed tool to attempt to "debulk" atherosclerotic plaque is endovascular atherectomy. The hypothesis behind debulking the plaque is that removing the plaque from the artery will allow for revascularization with either lower pressure angioplasty, or perhaps without angioplasty at all. Multiple atherectomy technologies exist including those meant to sharply excise and remove the plaque, those meant to break the plaque into very small pieces to be removed by the body's reticuloendothelial system, and laser atherectomy that targets the molecular bonds of the atheroma literally ablating the plaque and transforming it into vapor [90].

6.4.3.2 Laser Technical Details

The technical details and physics of LASER (Light Amplification by Stimulated Emission of Radiation) is beyond the scope of this discussion.

However, the basics of the lasers used for plaque ablation are important to understand.

- Lasers emit very high-intensity light at a single wavelength in either continuous or pulsed modes. Currently available clinical laser atherectomy devices are "Excimer" lasers, which are a combination of the words "excited" and "dimer."
- In the case of laser atherectomy, the excimer referred to is xenon chloride (XeCl). Current laser technologies take advantage of both the photochemical and acoustic mechanical laser–tissue interactions, both of which are nonthermal leading to the moniker "cool laser." The high-energy UV photons target and destroy molecular bonds. At the same time, short high-energy pulses lead to local shockwave formation inducing local tissue ablation.
- These lasers only function in pulsed mode, as continuous lasers tend to have an unacceptable safety profile [90].

Current laser atherectomy systems work at wavelengths of 308 nm (Philips Medical CVX-300 laser system) or 355 nm (AngioDynamics Auryon System).

- The Philips laser has been FDA approved since 1993 and has significant safety and efficacy data, including indication for in-stent restenosis from the EXCITE ISR trial [91].
- The Auryon laser claims to have a better safety profile in that the UV photons at this frequency are more selective for atherosclerotic plaque and fibrous tissue than healthy arterial endothelium, though data are limited as its FDA clearance was granted in 2020 [92]. The Auryon also claims that its short pulse length increases power for more effective ablation of calcium.
- The Philips laser comes in large sizes with a rotating mechanism to help treat a larger lumen size, while the Auryon system offers aspiration with its larger catheters and has a blunt blade to help dissect through partially ablated plaque while traversing the lesion.

- A wavelength of 355 nm used by Auryon, as opposed to 308 nm, will not interact with calcium or blood and therefore does not require a continuous saline flush.
- Only the Philips laser has customizable fluence and rate controls.

6.4.3.3 Laser Atherectomy in Calcified Arteries

Clinical evidence for laser atherectomy in calcified vessels is lacking [93]. A small observational single-center study characterized femoropopliteal lesion types in patients presenting for peripheral arterial disease treatment using intravascular ultrasound (IVUS). These lesion types included calcific, heterogeneous, homogenous, and restenotic. Each lesion was then treated with three passes of the Philips excimer laser at three different settings identified as "low, medium, and high" based on manufacturer recommended rate and fluence settings. The lesion was re-imaged with both DSA and IVUS after each pass allowing for visualization of luminal gain achieved by the laser in each lesion type. Based on the defined endpoints of change in percent stenosis and change in minimal lumen area, laser atherectomy proved to be an effective treatment for heavily calcified lesions when treated with a low and subsequent medium power setting (2.0 or 2.3 mm laser treated at 40 mJ/mm^2 and 60 Hz followed by 60 mJ/mm^2 at 40 Hz). Treating the lesion with a third pass at the "high" setting did not gain additional benefit (Fig. 6.41) [94].

In the author's practice, laser atherectomy is found to be useful in a wide variety of femoropopliteal plaque morphologies as well as in ISR. However, it is especially effective in heavily calcified tibial stenoses.

- The laser fiber is produced in a variety of sizes with the smallest size available measuring 0.9 mm. These fibers have a very low crossing profile and track well over a 0.014″ wire. Most atherectomy devices require a proprietary wire or are very limited in wire choices that can safely pair with the device. The 0.9 mm laser fiber is safe to use with any wire. This

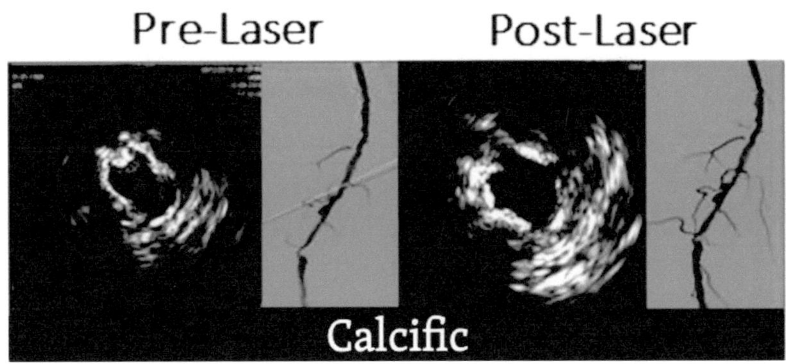

Fig. 6.41 Intravascular ultrasound image showing pre- and post-laser plaque morphology

becomes very significant in the case when a specialized wire is needed to cross a very small lumen in a heavily calcified stenosis or occlusion.

- Often, no balloon or device can track effectively over the wire to facilitate wire exchange for a specialized atherectomy wire. The 0.9 mm laser fiber is the only Philips laser fiber that can produce a rate of 80HZ. At this rate, there are significant acoustic mechanical effects, which allow for disruption of intraluminal calcium.
  - Once the laser fiber has treated the calcium sufficiently to pass through the stenosis, stepwise inflation with increasing sized balloon angioplasty can be completed (Fig. 6.42).

6.4.3.4 Tips
- Two commercially available laser systems.
  - Philips CVX-300.
    - 308 nm wavelength.
    - Randomized data to support on label use for ISR.
    - 0.9 to 2.0 mm fibers with adjustable fluence and rate, larger fibers oscillate to increase ablation area.
    - Will violently interact with contrast material and can create heat-related damage to the vessel.
  - AngioDynamics Auryon:
    - Slightly altered wavelength (355 nm) to interact more with calcium and less with healthy arterial wall.

0.9 to 2.35 mm sizes, larger sizes have aspiration.

Blunt blade on tip to help dissect through and cross-lesions while ablating.

- Laser has a modest, but measurable effect on calcium.
  - Can be very useful in calcified vessels when no other catheter or balloon will crossover the wire. Laser fibers will work over guidewires of any construction or coating.
- Acts as a workhorse atherectomy device since it will effectively treat lesions of multiple types including mixed morphology and thrombus.
- No moving parts to damage or catch on indwelling stents.
- Unlikely to provide optimal vessel preparation on severely calcified lesions.
- May benefit from an embolic protection filter when treating lesions with mixed morphology, in-stent restenosis, or when acute to subacute thrombus is present.
- The Philips laser can be used in a "step-by-step" fashion. This entails advancing the blunt tip of the laser catheter to an occlusion, firing the laser to advance into the cap, advancing the wire a short distance and following with the catheter. This can be continuously repeated with the wire contained within the catheter for short distances. This can be an excellent way to recanalize occluded ISR or traverse through fractured stents when a wire would pass through the interstices.

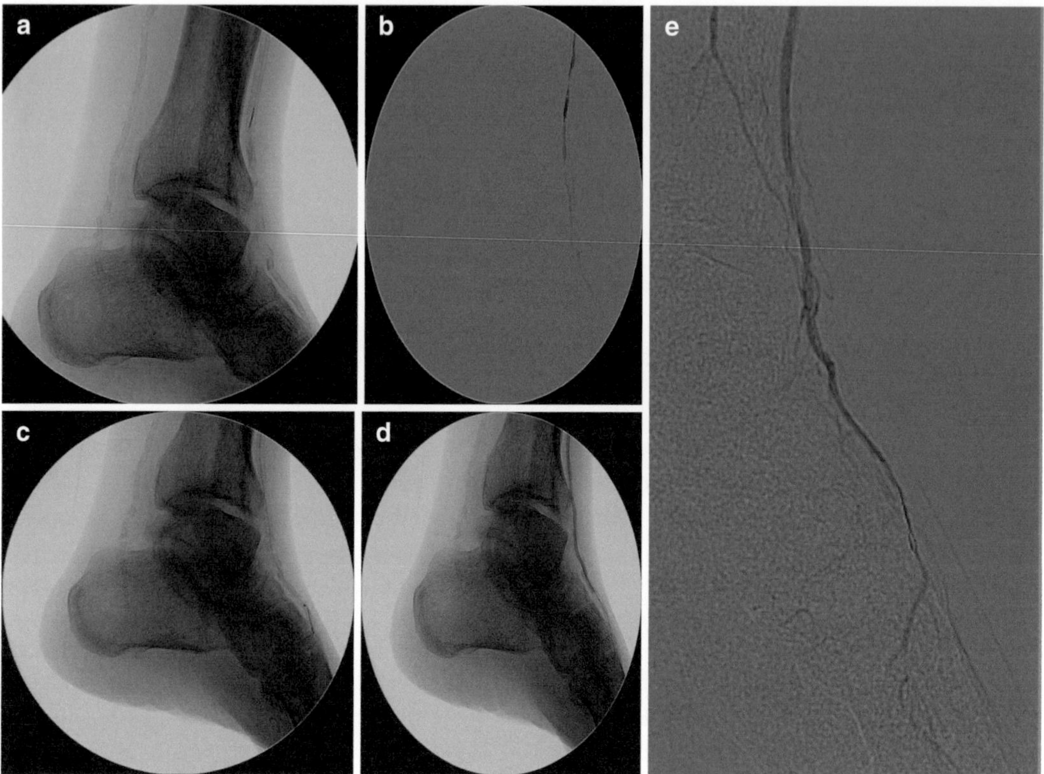

Fig. 6.42 (**a**) Native view of a heavily calcified distal anterior tibial artery and dorsalis pedis artery in a 68-year-old man with Rutherford 6 changes in his forefoot. (**b**) Subtracted image of a selective distal anterior tibial arteriogram showing essentially complete occlusion in the region of heaviest calcification just anterior to the ankle joint. (**c**) 1n 0.014″ GLIDEWIRE advantage (Terumo medical) was able to cross the heavily calcified lesion. An ultralow-profile balloon could not cross the heavily calci-fied stenosis at the level of the ankle. A 0.9 mm Philips laser catheter set to 80 mJ/mm² and 80 Hz was able to achieve enough luminal gain to pass the device into the dorsalis pedis artery. (**d**) After increasing luminal area with laser atherectomy, sequential angioplasty of the distal anterior tibial artery was completed to 1.5, 2, and 2.5 mm. (**e**) Post-angioplasty DSA demonstrates brisk inline flow to the forefoot without residual stenosis

6.5 Crossing Devices

John H. Rundback and Kevin Chaim Herman

Chronic total occlusions (CTOs) are often the principal challenge to successful endovascular therapy, with failure frequently due to long lesion length, extensive calcification, and location in the infrapopliteal region, as well as small arterial caliber and absent distal targets. Fundamentally, crossing may be achieved either using subintimal or intraluminal techniques (and often with a combination of both). Subintimal recanalization is often necessitated by the absence of a traversable vessel lumen or due to the configuration of the proximal and distal caps [95]. Cap morphology can be utilized to determine if a primary retrograde or primary antegrade wire approach will have greater initial success; caps that are concave toward the CTO segment will better direct wires intraluminally across microchannels and through the target lesion rather than through marginal collaterals adjacent to the occlusion.

While most CTOs can be crossed using traditional wire and catheter techniques, there also exist a number of dedicated CTO devices that are designed to disrupt occlusive caps and allow wire penetration into more difficult CTOs [96]. It is important for all interventionalists to have some familiarity with crossing devices for selected

Table 6.2 Common commercially available crossing devices in the USA

Company	Product	Catheter (F)	Wire (inch)	Length (cm)	Description
Avinger, Inc.	Kittycat 2	5	0.014	150	Peripheral OTW preshaped CTO crossing catheter
	Wildcat	6	0.035	110	Peripheral OTW CTO crossing catheter
Baylis Medical Company, Inc.	PowerWire	–	0.035	250	Nitinol core PTFE coated distally tapered tip delivering radiofrequency energy
BD Interventional	Crosser 14S	5	0.014	106, 146	Recanalizes CTOs through ultrasonic mechanical vibration and cavitation; available in OTW and RX configurations
	Crosser S6	5	–	106, 154	
Cordis	Frontrunner XP	3.1	–	90, 140	Actuating distal tip creates a channel through occlusions via blunt microdissection
Medtronic	Viance	2.9	0.014	150	Torque handle for fast manual spinning
Ra Medical Systems, Inc.	DABRA Laser	5	–	150	Laser recanalization closed tip catheter
Reflow Medical, Inc.	Wingman 14	2.7	0.014	65, 135, 150	Extendable radiopaque guide tip (extendable tip) and activating handle
	Wingman 18	3.8	0.018	90, 135, 150	
	Wingman 35	4.6	0.035	65, 90, 135	
Upstream Peripheral Technologies	GoBack	2.9, 4	0.0140.018	80, 120	23.8-gauge needle that can be extended from the catheter tip with a slight radial curve to allow for directional crossing

cases, particularly when an intraluminal recanalization is desired for best case management.

There are numerous commercially available devices categorized as crossing devices, including high-tip strength microcatheters with the most common and purpose-specific tools shown in Table 6.2 and Fig. 6.43. Each of these devices has unique physical properties, specifications, configurations, and advantages. In general, preference is based upon user experience and individual outcomes.

6.5.1 Trial Results

Overall, the data regarding crossing devices are somewhat limited.

- In the PFAST-CTO trial of the Viance device, 38/45 (84%) of CTO (avg length 19.5 cm, 42% moderate/severe calcification) were successfully traversed [97].

- The TruePath crossing device was utilized in 85 subjects with a mean occlusion length of 16.6 cm, with facilitation of crossing with the device or any guidewire in 80% [98]. This device is no longer in use.

- The Wing-It trial also demonstrated 90% success in a cohort of 85 patients including SFA, popliteal, and tibial arteries [99].

- The Crosser device, which also has an atherectomy indication, was also utilized in multiple vascular beds (n = 85, 83.5% SFA/popliteal) and successfully allowed distal wire placement in 83.5%.

  - Interestingly, this was a challenging cohort, with an average lesion length of only 11.7 cm, but including 55% severely calcified mostly mature (average occlusion duration 15 months) CTOs [100]. Serious

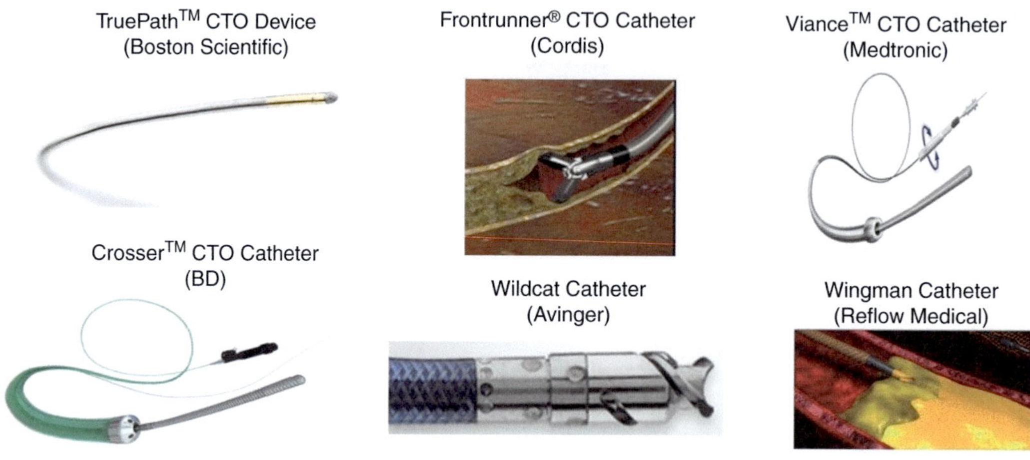

Fig. 6.43 Images of crossing devices

adverse events including device-related perforation, embolization, or flow-limiting dissection were rare (<5%) in all of these studies.

6.5.2 Clinical Utilization

While the selection of a particular crossing device is largely operator preference, some guidance can be considered.

- In our experience, the PowerWire has predominantly been used in refractory chronic central venous occlusions that fail bidirectional wire catheter crossing techniques.
- The Frontrunner, Wingman 35, Wildcat, and DABRA systems are for larger iliac through popliteal arteries and may be limited in more tortuous arteries due to the bigger caliber and more rigid construction of the catheters.
- In contrast, the Wingman 18 and 14 platforms (Fig. 6.44) and the Kittycat crossing device are more suitable for smaller popliteal and tibial occlusions, with the Kittycat being advantageous for operators who also have the compatible optical coherence technology to assure intraluminal positioning.
- The Crosser catheter is more versatile in crossing calcified arteries and older occlusions (Fig. 6.45).
- Finally, the newly introduced GoBack catheter needle extension can be activated both as a CTO device or a re-entry device providing some unique functionality.

6.5.3 Conclusion

Crossing devices represent a class of endovascular tools with a sole purpose to aid in crossing of chronic total occlusions. Although these devices have not been randomized against traditional wire catheter techniques (particularly with the use of retrograde access strategies), these devices are successful in approximately 80% of cases and have very low complication rates.

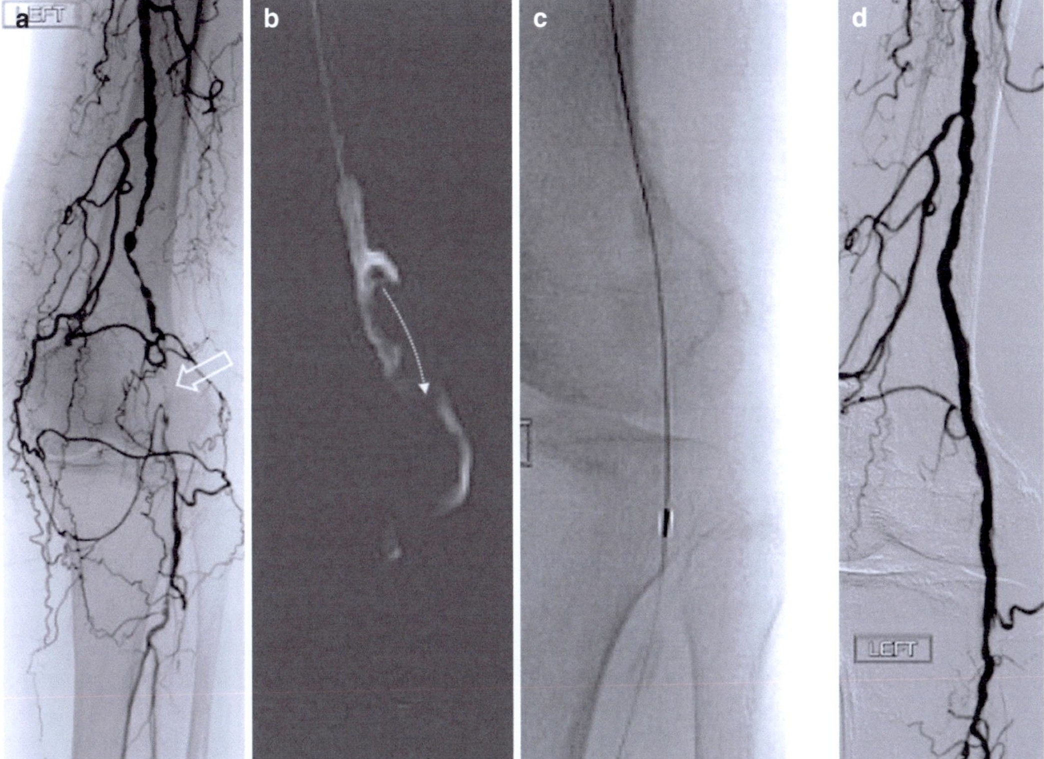

Fig. 6.44 Popliteal CTO crossing with the Wingman device. (**a**) Initial angiogram shows a severe stenosis of the popliteal artery with a short-segment occlusion (open arrow) (**b**) Magnification image of the occluded segment demonstrates a large intraluminal calcific plaque, which repeatedly resulted in subintimal wire passage; activation of the Wingman catheter allowed central lesion crossing (dotted arrow) and intraluminal wire crossing (**c**) following orbital atherectomy and angioplasty, and completion angiography (**d**) demonstrates an excellent initial result

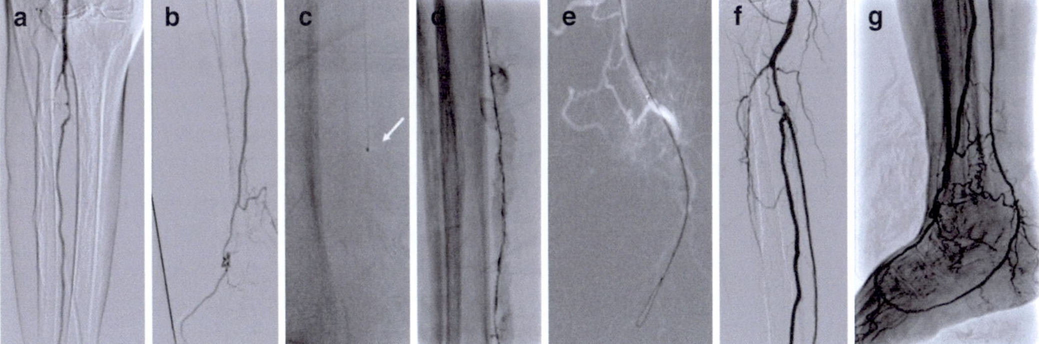

Fig. 6.45 Successful recanalization of long tibial CTO with a Crosser catheter. (**a, b**) Chronic occlusion of the posterior tibial artery in a patient with a plantar heel wound. (**c**) The Crosser 14 device and Usher catheter (arrow) were used for recanalization after failed wire crossing. (**d**) After using the Crosser 14 catheter, there is now noted to be patency of the posterior tibial artery to the ankle. (**e**) Successful knuckle wire crossing of the common plantar artery into the pedal arch after recanalization of the posterior tibial artery. (**f, g**) Final angiogram after angioplasty showing restored uninterrupted posterior tibial artery flow through the pedal arch

6.6 Managing In-Stent Restenosis

Anish Thomas

Self-expanding nitinol stents revolutionized the treatment of patients with chronic PAD. They are able to address some of the limitations of percutaneous transluminal angioplasty including flow-limiting dissections, elastic recoil, and residual stenosis. Despite the advancements in technology, up to one-half of all patients that receive bare metal standard nitinol self-expanding femoropopliteal stents will require secondary interventions due to in-stent restenosis (ISR) [101, 102].

6.6.1 Classification

A classification system for femoropopliteal ISR was proposed by Tosaka et al., in which ISR lesions are assigned based on their angiographic appearance [103, 104]. They are as follows:

- **Class I (Focal ISR): It** includes lesions less than or equal to 50 mm in length that are positioned in the stent body, stent edge, or both.
- **Class II (Diffuse ISR): It** includes lesions that are greater than 50 mm in length.
- **Class III (Totally Occluded ISR):** It includes totally occluded stents.

Lumen loss within the stent is from neointimal hyperplasia, extracellular matrix, and often in complete in-stent occlusions have some component of thrombus.

6.6.2 Crossing In-Stent Occlusions

Oftentimes, crossing in-stent complete occlusions is not challenging. In most cases, this can be accomplished antegrade with a support catheter and a hydrophilic glide wire. Using a looped wire helps to ensure that the wire remains within the architecture of the stent.

In cases where there is a flush occlusion and stent fractures, crossing antegrade may not be possible. In addition to standard retrograde tibial access, direct retrograde stent puncture of the occluded stent is easy, safe, and effective to facilitate retrograde crossing. This can be done under ultrasound or fluoroscopy.

Crossing some occlusions may be difficult with a wire and support catheter especially in extremely fibrotic occlusions with under-expanded stents. Other tools to cross these occlusions within the stent architecture exist, for example, using laser atherectomy leading with the laser catheter itself, especially using the turbo-power catheter.

6.6.3 Management

Current endovascular management strategies to treat femoropopliteal ISR include the following:

- Drug-coated balloon (DCB) angioplasty.
- Atherectomy combined with DCB.
- Stent grafts to reline the stents.
- Drug-eluting stents (DES).

PTA alone for ISR is ineffective as the nitinol cage limits positive remodeling that would otherwise occur in an unconstrained vessel. While the immediate result might appear angiographically pleasing, this is often from dehydrating the plaque, which will re-expand over a short time. The recurrence rate following PTA alone for ISR is therefore high [104]. There is no proven benefit in the use of cutting balloons over conventional balloon angioplasty in ISR [105].

However, there may be a role in vessel preparation in severely fibrotic and hyperplastic lesions with a cutting or scoring balloon prior to drug-coated balloon (DCB) angioplasty to further improve the efficacy of ISR. DCB angioplasty has shown to be superior to conventional PTA in ISR [106]. However, the efficacy significantly decreases with class II and III ISR [107]. This is not unexpected due to the limitations of balloon angioplasty for ISR, as described above.

- Debulking the neointimal tissue within the stents using atherectomy followed by PTA has been shown to be superior to PTA alone, using numerous atherectomy devices.
- Commonly used atherectomy devices for ISR that are currently FDA approved include Excimer Laser atherectomy (Philips), Jetstream ™ (Boston Scientific), Pantheris (Avinger), and Rotarex™ (BD).
- While the use of the SilverHawk directional atherectomy system has been described to have high acute procedural success in the hands of experienced operators, it is contraindicated for use because of the potential risk for cutter entrapment on the stent that can result in serious adverse events.

Similar to combining atherectomy with PTA, combining atherectomy with DCB angioplasty is appealing and has been shown to be safe and effective, with some data showing better outcomes compared to use of DCB angioplasty alone.

Treating in-stent occlusions can result in distal embolization that can compromise the runoff, causing further ischemia. If one suspects a significant amount of thrombus within the occlusion, which can be confirmed with IVUS or when a guidewire flies through the stent, catheter-directed thrombolysis or mechanical thrombectomy prior to atherectomy or DCB might be warranted. Debris can also be generated from use of atherectomy. Using distal embolic protection can help in mitigating this complication. Stent grafts or PTFE-covered stents like Viabahn have been shown to be effective in the treatment of ISR [108]. These covered stents act as a mechanical barrier for migration of smooth muscle cells and neointimal hyperplasia.

- In patients with a predominantly thrombotic occlusion, there may be significant residual thrombus despite use of thrombolytics or mechanical thrombectomy. In these cases, relining the scaffold might be necessary to prevent distal embolization.
- This should be done with caution in patients with limited runoff. It is important to size the Viabahn stent appropriately to reduce graft infolding that can increase the risk of acute or subacute stent thrombosis.
- The use of drug-eluting stents (DESs) in femoropopliteal ISR has been studied with use of the Zilver PTX DES [109] that showed promising 1- and 2-year clinical outcomes with low stent fracture rates.
- Surgical bypass remains an option for treating these patients, especially those who are low surgical risk and have good autologous conduit and those with repetitive failures of long-segment stenting.

6.7 Femoropopliteal and Femorotibial Bypass

Daniel K. Han

As with all bypasses, the following should be considered for open surgical reconstruction of the infrainguinal arterial system.

1. **Inflow**
   (a) The common femoral artery is the most commonly used inflow source for infrainguinal bypasses. In the case of a diseased common femoral artery, an endarterectomy can be performed at the time of the bypass to ensure a good inflow source can be established.
   (b) If there is proximal profunda disease, an extended arteriotomy can be made onto the profunda at the time of the endarterectomy to perform a profundaplasty.
   (c) In the case of a disease-free common femoral and superficial femoral artery, the popliteal artery can also be considered as inflow for an infrapopliteal bypass. Limited length of vein conduit may be another reason for choosing a distal superficial femoral or popliteal artery as the inflow source.
2. **Outflow**
   (a) Patency of a bypass graft is also heavily dependent on the outflow pressure. A bypass to a healthy outflow vessel that

runs to the foot and gives off several branches will allow for high flow through the bypass graft. Conversely, a bypass into a diseased outflow vessel or a vessel that leads into a desert foot can cause high outflow pressure and diminished flow in the graft.

(b) A prosthetic bypass to the tibial arteries has poor long-term patency. While there are adjunctive techniques that are described and used to improve success rates (vein patch, composite vein conduit, distal arteriovenous fistula), the long-term patency of prosthetic tibial bypasses is significantly worse than fem-pop bypasses (prosthetic and vein) and tibial vein bypasses.

- Despite this, a fem-tibial prosthetic bypass may be beneficial for patients with critical limb ischemia that may not otherwise be able to heal their wound.

(c) Vein bypasses to the infra-malleolar targets have also been described. Depending on the status of the pedal loop and intra-foot arteries, a bypass to the infra-malleolar dorsalis pedis or posterior tibial arteries can also be a beneficial option for the correct patient.

3. **Conduit**
   (a) Vein is best.
   (b) Vein is best.
   (c) Vein is best.
   (d) A vein conduit should always be the preferred option for a lower extremity bypass as the long-term patency is far superior to a prosthetic bypass. The great saphenous vein (GSV) is the preferred bypass conduit. The GSV can be harvested using one long incision or skip incisions. While not the widely adopted practice for vascular surgeons, some have also described endoscopic vein harvest, similar to use in coronary artery bypasses.
   (e) While a vein conduit is best, using a suboptimal vein as a conduit may not provide the same benefits over a prosthetic conduit.

(f) Length is often an issue when using a vein conduit, particularly for infrapopliteal bypasses. Several studies have described splicing good vein conduits together can lead to comparable patency rates as a single-length great saphenous vein (GSV). Splicing of arm veins has also been described as an acceptable option for a bypass conduit.

(g) The vein conduit can be reversed or non-reversed in orientation. Reversing the vein allows for minimal manipulation of the vein, as the valves will be in the correct direction of flow.

- Reversing the vein can sometimes lead to significant size mismatch as the peripheral saphenous vein is often substantially smaller than the more central GSV at the saphenofemoral junctions.
- To minimize size mismatch, some surgeons opt to keep the vein in non-reversed orientation. A valvulotome device is used in these cases to lyse the valves to allow for blood to circulate in the correct direction.

(h) Some surgeons prefer to perform an in situ venous bypass when using the GSV for fem-pop or fem-tibial (particularly posterior tibial artery) bypasses. In this procedure, only the proximal and distal portions of the GSV are initially exposed. A valvulotome device is used to lyse the venous valves, and then, proximal and distal anastomoses are made. Following completion of the anastomoses, major branches along the GSV that steal blood from the distal target are identified (using color duplex or angiogram). Cutdowns are made over these branches, which are then ligated.

4. **Additional Considerations**
   (a) **Clamping**
   - In addition to selecting an appropriate, disease-free inflow and outflow targets, one should consider where the surgeon will be controlling the vessel for surgical anastomoses. Significant circumferential calcification on a vessel may make clamping the vessel hazardous,

necessitating more extensive dissection (i.e., to a healthier portion of artery in the retroperitoneum for inflow).

- For tibial targets, many surgeons opt to use a tourniquet to avoid clamping the artery all together, as the small tibial vessels can be more prone to clamp injury. In the case that a tourniquet is insufficient in achieving vessel control due to extensively calcified arteries, an intraluminal Fogarty balloon can be used to limit bleeding during anastomosis. In the case that a clamp must be used, surgeons may opt to use a doubled vessel loop or a very light atraumatic clamp such as a bulldog.

(b) **Tunneling**
- The bypass graft can be tunneled anatomically from the common femoral artery using a subsartorial, transpopliteal fossa tunnel. This tunnel allows for the shortest length from the inflow source to the outflow target and can be valuable in the case of limited vein conduit.
- Anatomical crossing from the popliteal fossa to the anterior tibial artery requires tunneling through the interosseous membrane in between the tibia and fibula. This membrane can be tight, and care must be taken to develop a sufficient tunnel to ensure no pinching of your bypass graft.
- The graft can also be left extra-anatomic in the subcutaneous tissue where the GSV was harvested or in a superficial, extra-anatomic tunnel. No meaningful differences in patency have been described.

6.7.1 Patient Selection

Sreekumar Madassery

Most high-level operators will keep in mind that the data for autologous vein bypass when performed by an experienced surgeon have a very good and long patency rate in low-risk patients. This result may not be achieved in high-risk patients and in those who do not have native veins suitable for bypass. Additionally, when endovascular procedures are performed by experienced interventionalists, the option for bypass is not lost. This can be seen when endovascular-first approaches are performed often by surgeons who could perform a bypass instead. The recovery, complications, re-operations, and other issues are not to be taken lightly, and these are some of the reasons why an endovascular-first approach may often be prudent. In the authors' practice, if the patient has the following characteristics:

- Younger patients.
- Long-segment infrainguinal occlusion, particularly flush ostial SFA occlusions.
- Adequate proximal and distal targets.
- Native veins still present.
- Low operative risk.

Then, the preference would be to send for surgical consideration. Additional surgical first approach would be for patients with isolated common femoral artery disease and those with infected bypass grafts. Patients who have had multiple endovascular reinterventions of full metal jacket stented patients or simply repetitive interventions and agreeing to surgery are some other situations to consider for surgical management.

The patient and family should be offered both options with appropriate information and clear discussion of risks/benefits. Additional attributes are often important to consider when determining which approach is ideal for a patient, including those with ESRD, non-ambulatory patients, and limb status. Each patient and their situation must be evaluated globally, and the decision of appropriate management should be custom tailored to their lives, needs, and desires. The best outcomes are those when the multiple vascular specialties can work together in creating treatment plans in each institution.

There have been no exact data-driven guidelines to help operators decide if bypass is the best option for patients compared to an endovascular approach. The exponential growth of endovascular procedures being performed by all three vascular specialties (IR, VS, and IC) does not necessarily prove that endovascular management is the right approach. Until recently, no large-scale, randomized trial has ever been conducted to answer this question. The BEST-CLI study was intended to be such a trial and is specific to CLI/CLTI patients. The results of this study were just presented in November 2022 at the AHA meeting in Chicago. There is certain to be a considerable forthcoming dissection of the data that will be critically reviewed and will likely result in several publications related to it after this book is in print. However, the boiled-down summation presented was that for patients with CLI/CLTI, they fared better from a MALE and mortality standpoint when a greater saphenous vein (GSV) conduit was available for bypass, compared to endovascular intervention. When no native GSV was present, outcomes between surgical bypass and endovascular intervention were similar. There are many underlying considerations for later discussion, including the breakdown of specialties performing the procedures, the type of endovascular approaches utilized, and some of the surprising findings in the cohorts. This study was a tremendous undertaking nonetheless, in order to try and answer some of the questions we do not have a clear understanding of, other than anecdotal experience. Time will tell how the results will be properly utilized. In the meantime, continued efforts to work together with all specialties are the only way patients will end up with the best outcomes.

6.7.2 When and Why Axillofemoral Bypass?

Mohamed Nagi, Alison Maringo,
and Michele Richard

Axillofemoral bypass remains the standard revascularization procedure for aortoiliac occlusive disease in patients who are unsuitable candidates for inline revascularization with aortoiliac or aorto-femoral bypass. The reported patency of axillofemoral bypass remains >70% at 5 years [110]. Axillofemoral bypass provides a favorable revascularization option in patients who have significant surgical risk. There are no reported studies comparing patency and outcomes of axillo-PFA bypass compared to CFA.

6.7.3 Axillofemoral Bypass Technique

The first part of the axillary artery is typically used as the inflow artery for axillofemoral bypass. This is done to minimize the risk of graft disruption secondary to movement at the shoulder. An incision approximately 5 cm in length is placed one fingerbreadth below the middle third of the clavicle. The pectoralis major fascia is opened in a longitudinal fashion and the muscle fibers of the pectoralis major are split. The pectoralis minor muscle can be divided to facilitate exposure.

The axillary vein will first be encountered anterior and caudal to the axillary artery. This can be mobilized and retracted inferiorly with the aid of a vessel loop. Crossing venous branches can be ligated and divided to facilitate exposure. Careful dissection of the axillary artery is essential to avoid injury to the cords of the brachial plexus. Care should be taken to avoid injury to the lateral pectoral nerve and the cephalic vein by retraction devices [111, 112].

The common femoral arteries are exposed through short longitudinal incisions if an axillo-bifemoral configuration is planned or unilaterally for axillounifemoral cases.

An externally supported 8 mm PTFE or Dacron graft is most commonly used. In cases of particularly small native vessels, a 6 mm graft can be considered. The graft tunnel is created retrograde from the femoral incision to the axillary incision along the mid-axillary line in the subcutaneous plane. The graft should course anterior to the anterior superior iliac crest and anterior to the inguinal ligament. The tunnel should remain extra-anatomic and not enter the abdominal or thoracic cavities. A counter incision can be employed midway if the tunneling device is not long enough. The graft should be tunneled deep to the pectoralis major muscle and lie medial to the pectoralis minor muscle. Care should be taken to ensure no twists or kinks result from tunneling. If performing axillobifemoral bypass, the contralateral groin anastomosis can be performed after creating a suprapubic tunnel for the graft. A bifurcated graft or two segments of straight graft can be used [111, 112].

After tunneling, the patient can be systemically heparinized with 100 units/kg of IV heparin and clamps are then placed. The graft is stipulated at both ends and end-to-side anastomoses are performed. Graft redundancy at the axillary end is necessary to prevent excessive tension, which could result in anastomotic disruption with arm movement and abduction. The axillary arteriotomy is performed as medially as possible, given this segment of the artery is least mobile. The axillary artery is more friable compared to the femoral artery, and care should be taken to avoid dissection or vessel injury from clamp placement or suturing. The distal anastomosis is performed on the CFA (if SFA outflow is preserved) or the PFA (in cases of SFA occlusion).

Upon bypass completion, a handheld sterile Doppler probe can be used to assess flow. Flow in the donor arm should be assessed by checking the radial pulse [111, 112].

6.8 Percutaneous Femoropopliteal Bypass: Detour Approach

Fadi A. Saab, Jihad A. Mustapha, and Carmen Heaney

Peripheral arterial disease of the femoropopliteal arterial segment is the most common cause of intermittent claudication [113]. Once this disease progresses to lifestyle-limiting claudication, or to critical limb ischemia, physicians generally agree revascularization is necessary. Minimally invasive endovascular interventions are now reported to be more common than bypass surgery, as the revascularization treatment of choice for this disease [114]. Vascular bypass surgery is not as desirable from the patient perspective due to general anesthesia, prolonged hospital stays, and higher risk of post-surgical infection, hemorrhage, or nerve injury. While advances in endovascular therapy have provided additional, less invasive options for patients, there are some lesion characteristics that do not lend themselves to safe, minimally invasive solutions that provide durable patency.

6.8.1 Challenging Lesion Characteristics

Short to mid-length lesions have been proven safe and effective for revascularization in balloon angioplasty, drug-coated balloon, and stent trials. Longer lesions, those greater than 20 cm, have historically been treated with open femoropopliteal bypass surgery. Open bypass surgery offers long-term patency. However, open femoropopliteal bypass surgery is associated with a 30-day morbidity rate of 37% due to complications such as infection and hemorrhage [115]. Additionally, patients with advanced PAD and CLI are wrought with comorbidities such as advanced age, coronary artery disease, diabetes, chronic kidney disease. These long lesions are often further challenged by the presence of chronic total occlusions and diffuse calcification. These challenges lend to the unmet need of safe, durable approaches to the treatment of long-segment femoropopliteal disease. Twenty years into the endovascular revolution, patients with long-segment femoropopliteal disease still have limited treatment options.

6.8.2 The Innovative DETOUR Procedure

The PQ Bypass proprietary Detour system, which includes the Torus stent graft, Detour crossing device, and Detour snare, may be the solution to durable endovascular revascularization of long-segment femoropopliteal disease. At the time of this writing, final results of the DETOUR II investigational device exemption trial are pending. The DETOUR II is a prospective, multicenter trial evaluating the Detour system for percutaneous femoral–popliteal bypass in patients with extremely long, complex lesions in the superficial femoral artery (SFA). The study enrolled 202 patients in 36 sites in the USA and Europe and is assessing freedom from major adverse events within 30 days of the index procedure as the primary safety endpoint. The primary effectiveness is primary patency at 12 months.

The DETOUR I study enrolled 77 patients with de novo, chronic total occlusions, or in-stent restenotic femoropopliteal lesions ≥10 cm. Primary safety and efficacy endpoints were met, and patency was demonstrated to be equivalent to open bypass surgery. Primary efficacy endpoint was primary patency at six months (PSVR ≤ 2.5) with no target lesion revascularization. CE Mark was granted in February 2017 [116, 117].

Results of this trial showed that the technology is certainly feasible with low rates of complications. It also addresses the primary concern of developing deep vein thrombosis (DVT). DVT was not a common complication in the trial population.

6.8.3 Technique

The Detour procedure creates an artery-to-vein-to artery pathway originating in the superficial femoral artery (SFA) crossing into and traveling through the femoral vein, and then returning into the popliteal artery, completely bypassing the diseased part of the vessel (Fig. 6.46).

6.8.3.1 Procedure: Proximal Anastomosis

After obtaining access within the tibial vein, a snare is advanced to the proximal femoral vein, creating a target within the femoral vein. Meanwhile, after obtaining arterial access (typically in the contralateral limb), a sheath is advanced to the CFA. The bypass is typically started from the proximal SFA. A catheter with proprietary re-entry mechanism employing a needle that is advanced from the SFA to femoral vein can create the original connection between the proximal SFA and the proximal femoral vein. The snare in the proximal femoral vein acts as the trapping mechanism when the needle is advanced from the artery to the vein. The needle penetrates the venous wall into the snare. A 0.014″ wire is then passed through the needle and released from the re-entry device, from the SFA into the femoral vein. Once the needle is through the snare, the 0.014″ wire is further advanced, and the snare will trap the wire and pull it from the SFA to the femoral vein. The wire is further pulled to the popliteal vein in preparation of crossing from the popliteal vein to the popliteal arterial reconstitution.

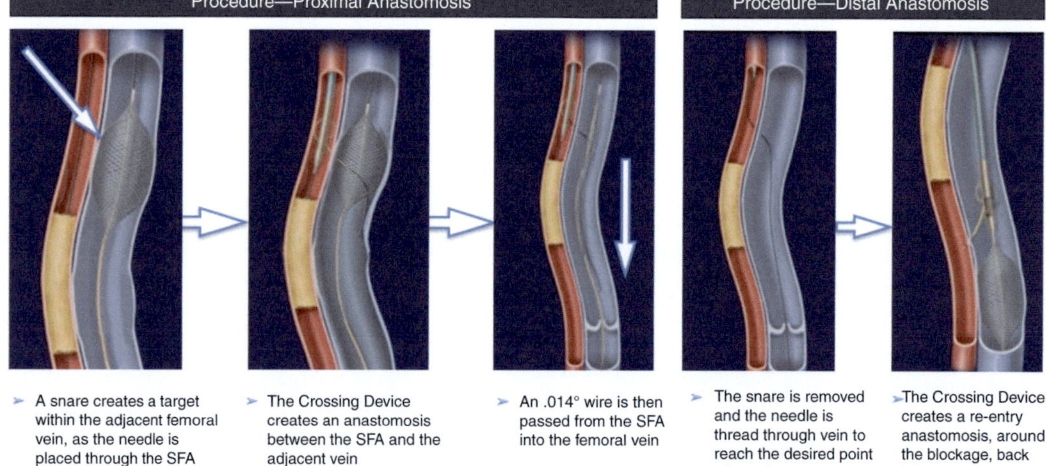

Fig. 6.46 Detour system creates an artery-to-vein-to artery pathway

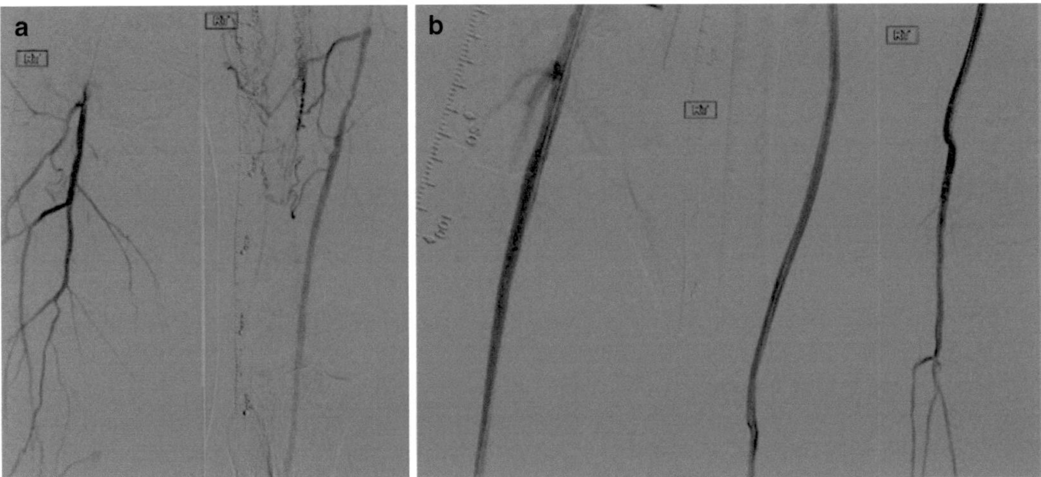

Fig. 6.47 (**a**) Angiogram pre-percutaneous femoropopliteal bypass showing long superficial femoral artery (SFA) chronic total occlusion (CTO). (**b**) Final angiographic result of successful percutaneous femoropopliteal bypass

6.8.3.2 Procedure: Distal Anastomosis

At this point, there is a wire extending from the proximal SFA through the femoral vein to the popliteal vein. The SFA/femoral vein anastomosis site gets predilated with typically a 4.0 balloon. There will be no extra-vascular extravasation. The crossing device is advanced through the proximal anastomosis site to the popliteal vein. An angiogram will show arterial reconstitution. The re-entry device has an orientation fluoroscopic marker that can help the operator orient the needle to the popliteal artery from the popliteal vein. Once the needle crosses into the artery, an 0.014″ wire is advanced. This essentially establishes a wire connection from the SFA to the femoral vein back into the reconstituted arterial site within the popliteal artery. We essentially bypassed the CTO via the above-described steps. The distal crossing site from the vein into the artery is further predilated with another 4.0 mm balloon. The operator will exchange the 0.014″ wire to an 0.035″ for further support. A proprietary self-expanding covered stent is advanced from the popliteal artery to the femoral vein and back into the proximal SFA. The proximal 2 cm of the self-expanding stent is not covered and will serve to stabilize the stent into the CFA without covering the takeoff of the profunda (Fig. 6.47a, b).

6.8.4 Conclusion

The Detour system and associated percutaneous femoropopliteal bypass technique appear to be a revolutionary step in treating patients with lifestyle-limiting claudication via minimally invasive, safe, and effective means. This technology could revolutionize the way we treat long CTOs.

6.9 Hidden Thrombus

6.9.1 Atherectomy Versus Mechanical Thrombectomy

S. Jay Mathews

6.9.1.1 Introduction

Chronic occlusions within peripheral vessels may have heterogeneous pathologies. Intravascular ultrasound (IVUS) shows that while some patients may have fibrocalcific or calcified chronic total occlusions (CTOs), many patients will also have combinations of soft plaque or a core of thrombotic material. In one series, 79% of CTOs had thrombus comprising up to 34% of the plaque volume [118].

Patients with diffuse disease or discrete distal disease may develop a column of stasis.

- This material can organize and remodel, but often may remain in a state of flux due to autologous fibrinolytic mechanisms.
- During crossing of these lesions or use of vessel preparation technologies including atherectomy devices, the potential for distal embolization and "trash foot" exists.
- Additionally, the nonocclusive stasis of flow from stenotic disease can propagate thrombus formation, which often presents as a long-segment "CTO" when in reality the long segment may be mostly thrombus.

6.9.1.2 Hidden Thrombus

The "wire test" is a simple way to predict a core of soft plaque or thrombus. IVUS often cannot distinguish between these pathologies, but both can embolize distally. Often after penetrating an initial hard cap, a lubricious wire will easily cross a native occlusion or in-stent restenotic segment.

- The classic example is an occluded Viabahn-type (W. L. Gore & Associates, Inc.) covered stent with a typical fibrotic cap/edge stenosis and a soft core. However, this can also be seen in bare metal stents and native occlusions with varying degrees of severity.

6.9.1.3 Mitigating Risk

With easy wire crossing, prophylactic aspiration thrombectomy prior to atherectomy and/or percutaneous transluminal angioplasty (PTA) may prevent distal embolization. "Laser CAT" is one technique that has been proposed where upfront thrombectomy with Indigo CAT 6/7/8 (Penumbra, Inc.) is performed prior to laser atherectomy. However, the technique is easily modified to other mechanical or aspiration thrombectomy devices and atherectomy tools. No comparative data exist yet as to which combination is most effective, however as a hole may reduce unnecessary scaffold placement, ICU stays for thrombolysis and overall hospital stay.

Typically, the cap is crossed proximally, but the wire should not penetrate the distal cap.

- The distal cap can serve then as a native embolic filter. The Indigo catheter is advanced over the wire under aspiration.
- The wire can then be removed, and aspiration can be performed backward (with or without rotation of the catheter). If desired, a smaller 0.014″ wire can be left in place if wire position is critical but maximizing aspiration lumen is important.
- Usually at this point, thrombectomy can be performed while penetrating the distal cap. Optional angiography can be performed to verify the residual plaque volume.
- After this, laser atherectomy with either of the current catheter-based laser systems, Spectranetics (Philips, Inc.), or Auryon (AngioDynamics, Inc.) is performed and can be done sized to at least two-thirds of the vessel lumen for maximal efficacy.

Thrombolytic-assisted intervention has also been proposed for patients with hibernating thrombus in CLTI. One series suggested reduced lesion length (average reduction of 150 to 30 mm) and improvement in Inter-Society Consensus for the Management of Peripheral Arterial Disease (TASC) II Classifications post-thrombolysis [119].

- Use of adjunctive thrombolytics must be weighed against systemic bleeding complications, though this could be mitigated with use of reduced-dose local thrombolysis combined with thrombectomy when appropriate.

Combination aspiration thrombectomy and atherectomy devices like Rotarex (BD, Inc.) or JET Stream (Boston Scientific, Inc.) offer promising solutions for these type of lesions [120, 121]. However, in order to be successful, both features need to be equally effective.

- One series in patients with CTOs failed to find improvement between rotational thromboatherectomy with drug-coated balloon (DCB) vs. DCB alone suggesting that this approach

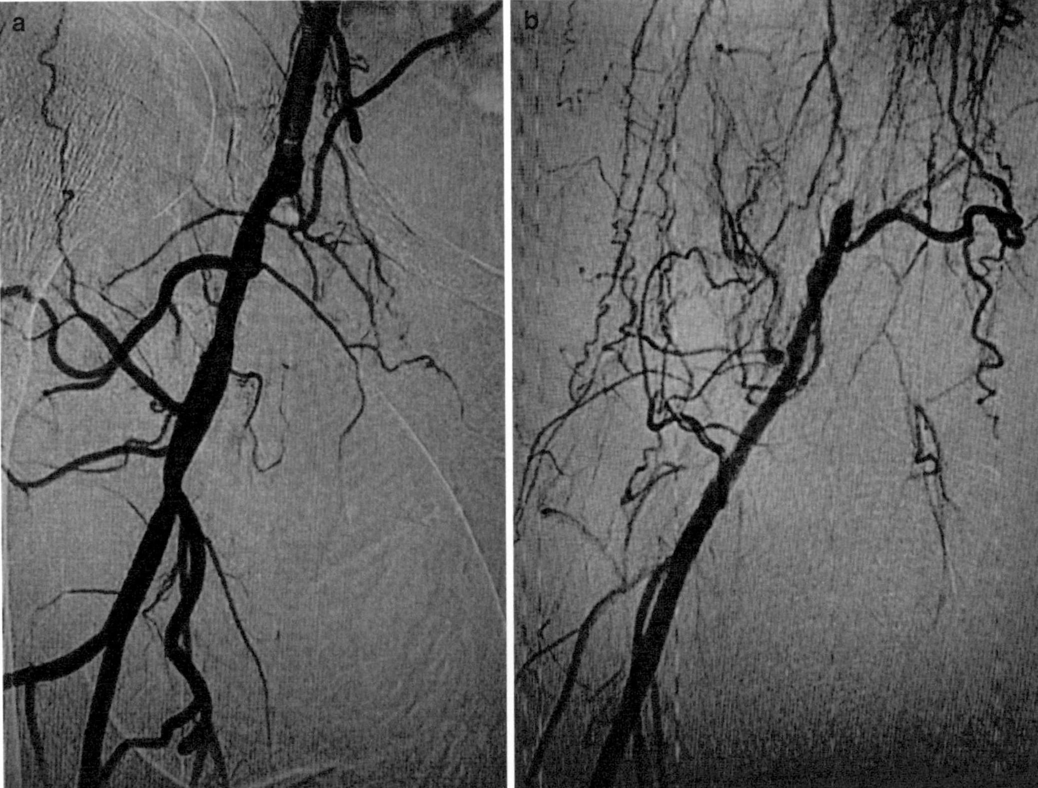

Fig. 6.48 Long-segment native and in-stent restenotic occlusion (**a** – proximal; **b** – distal)

may not be as useful in all chronic occlusions, especially those without significant embolization risk [122].

- Laser atherectomy with smaller fibers with <1 mm/s crossing speeds should ablate thrombus but may prove challenging to reliably prevent embolization with long occlusions.
- One series with both chronic and subacute thrombus found 100% improvement angiographically with laser treatment alone, but 85.7% of filters filled with macro-debris (>2 mm) [123].
- Therefore, prophylactic embolic protection may be advised with bulky soft plaque or thrombus. If thrombectomy is not used up front, there is a risk that the material in the occlusion channel may overwhelm the capacity of the filter, allowing for spillover and distal embolization.

6.9.1.4 Case Example

A 65-year-old woman with diabetes, dyslipidemia, and chronic tobacco abuse presented with Rutherford 3 claudication symptoms and long-segment native and distal in-stent restenotic total occlusion (Fig. 6.48a, b). Proximal crossing was not possible, but retrograde crossing via pedal access revealed easy wire passage through a soft distal cap. The wire was used to penetrate the proximal cap, and body floss was performed. Thrombectomy using an Indigo Lightning 7 catheter (Penumbra, Inc.) was performed from above. Post-angiography revealed that the central soft occlusive column was gone, leaving only the dense circumferential rind of plaque (Fig. 6.49a, b). Laser atherectomy was performed with a 2.0 mm Turbo-Power Laser Catheter (Philips, Inc.) with full rotation with increasing fluence and frequency. After this, focal force balloon

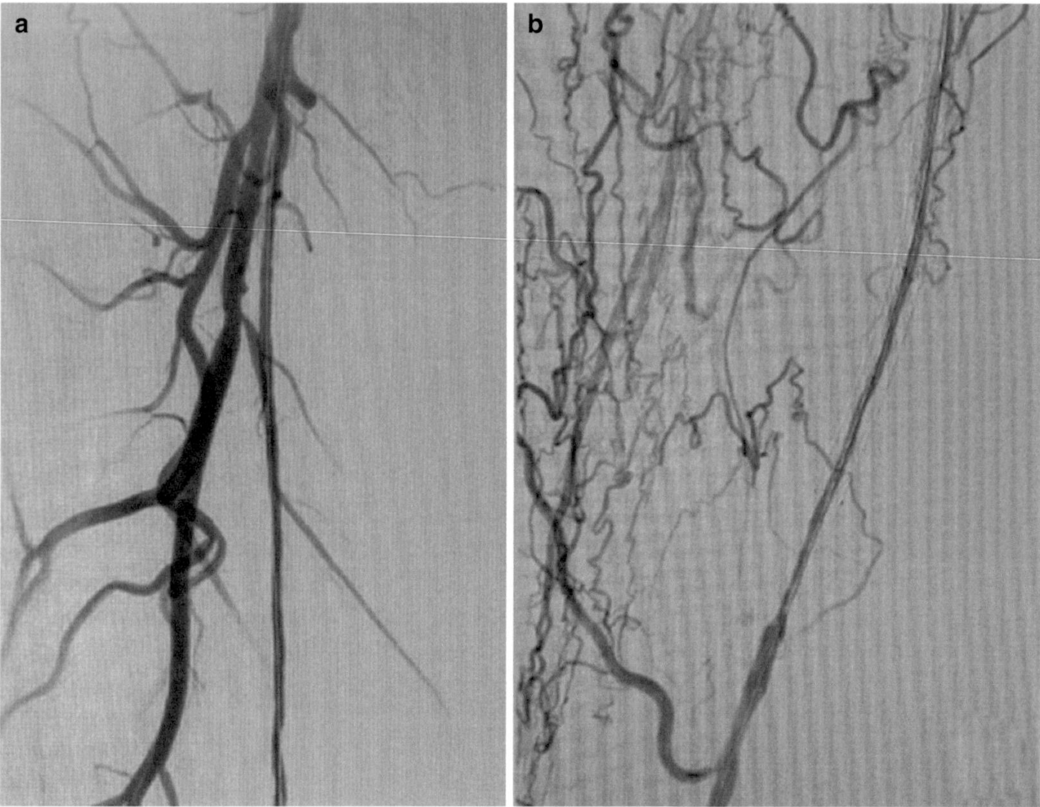

Fig. 6.49 Residual plaque burden post-Indigo mechanical thrombectomy (**a** – proximal; **b** – distal)

angioplasty was performed followed by treatment of the entire segment with drug-coated balloon angioplasty (Fig. 6.50a, b).

6.9.2 Heparin-Induced Thrombocytopenia (HIT) and Thrombolysis Management

Omar M. Uddin and David M. Tabriz

Introduction: Intravenous unfractionated heparin is one of the most often and generally used medications throughout all forms of medical facilities. Most often, this is used for DVT prevention, active anticoagulation in patients with arterial or venous thrombus, bridging from oral anticoagulants, and so on. With the preponderance of use, development of adverse reactions, such as heparin-induced thrombocytopenia (HIT or HITT) has increased.

- HIT is a life-threatening complication of heparin exposure related to antibody development against the platelet factor 4-heparin complex.
- Approximately 12 million patients in the USA have exposure to heparin and the incidence of HIT ranges from 1 to 5% in patients with prolonged heparin exposure following surgery.
- HIT is associated with venous and/or arterial thromboembolism, and complications include myocardial infarction, limb ischemia, end-organ failure, and death [124–127].

HIT Phases: Five phases of HIT are commonly described:

- Suspected HIT.
- Acute HIT.
- Subacute HIT A.
- Subacute HIT B.
- Remote HIT.

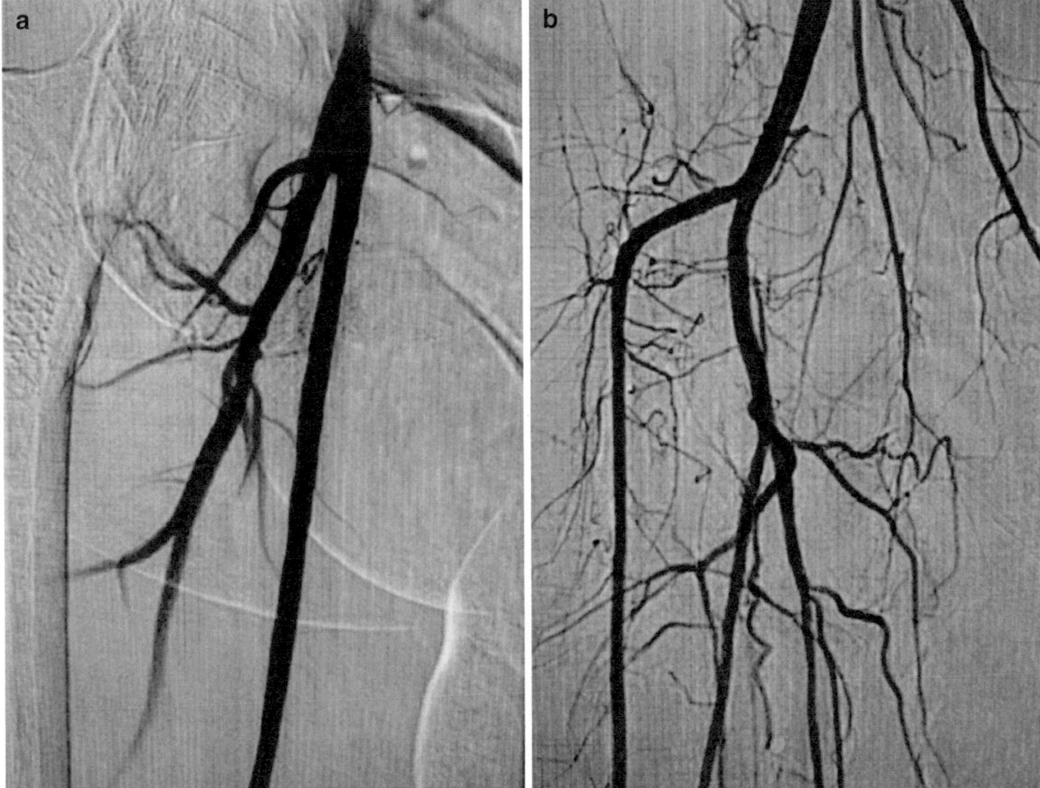

Fig. 6.50 Final angiography after laser atherectomy and drug-coated balloon angioplasty (**a** – proximal; **b** – distal)

This section concentrates on HIT management suspected intraprocedurally and not explicitly during each phase.

Pathophysiology: IgG antibodies are formed within 4–10 days of heparin exposure, directed at the heparin-platelet factor 4 complex (PF4). A conformational change in the platelet factor 4 proteins is thought to function as a neoantigen. Thus, *antibodies are heparin-dependent.*

Anti-heparin–PF4 antibodies bind to heparin–PF4 complexes on the platelet surface, their Fc region is captured by Fc receptors and/or glyco-protein Ib/IX of adjacent platelets causing a positive feedback loop of further platelet activation. This leads to greater substrate availability for heparin to bind. IgG-coated platelets are removed from the circulating blood by macrophages causing *consumptive coagulopathy.*

Thrombosis is secondary to widespread platelet activation and endothelial injury. Procoagulant microparticles are released by activated platelets and direct effect of HIT antibodies on the endothelial cell, leading to increased thrombin generation and tissue factor expression.

6.9.2.1 Diagnosis

4 Ts Score: It estimates pretest probability of HIT based on clinical features.

- **T**hrombocytopenia:
  - Platelet decreased >50% or nadir >20,000: **2 points.**
  - Platelet decreased 30–50% or nadir 10 to 19,000: **1 point.**
  - Platelet decreased <30% or nadir <10,000: **0 points.**
- **T**iming in relation to heparin exposure.
  - Onset between 5–10 days: **2 points.**
  - Fall at 5–10 days but unclear of true onset: **1 point.**
  - Platelet fall <4 days without recent heparin exposure: **0 points.**

- Thrombosis.
  - Confirmed thrombosis after heparin exposure: **2 points.**
  - Recurrent or progressive thrombosis: **1 point.**
  - None: **0 points.**
- Other causes of thrombocytopenia.
  - None apparent: **2 points.**
  - Possible: **1 point.**
  - Definite: **0 points.**
- Scoring:
  - 0–3 points: low probability (HIT risk <1%)
  - 4–5 points: intermediate probability (HIT risk 10%)
  - 6–8 points: high probability (HIT risk 50%).

For intermediate or high probability 4Ts score, obtain *immunoassay*. Treat for presumptive HIT until excluded.

If positive, obtain *functional assay* (not readily available at many institutions).

6.9.2.2 Management

For intraprocedural anticoagulation management in the suspicion or setting of HIT, suggest use of argatroban or bivalirudin.

Medication: **Argatroban**

1. Mechanism of action: direct thrombin inhibitor.
2. *Intra- or post-procedural anticoagulation:*
   (a) Bolus: none.
   (b) Continuous infusion:
   - Normal organ function: 2 ug/kg/min.
   - Liver dysfunction: 0.5–1.2 ug/kg/min.
   - Laboratory monitoring: adjust to APTT 1.5–3.0× baseline.

Medication: **Bivalirudin**

1. Mechanism of action: Direct thrombin inhibitor.
2. *Intra- or post-procedural anticoagulation:*
   (a) Bolus: None.
   (b) Continuous infusion:

- Normal organ function: 0.15 mg/kg/min.
- Renal or liver dysfunction: consider dose reduction.
- Laboratory monitoring: adjust to APTT 1.5–2.5× baseline.

6.9.2.3 Thrombolysis (Fibrinolytic) Management in Patients with HIT

Introduction: Systemic or catheter-directed fibrinolytic therapy dates to laboratory studies in 1933 noticing that strains of bacteria could dissolve fibrin clot. Streptokinase was studied in humans to attempt to dissolve hemothoraces and vascular thrombi in the 1940s and 1950s, respectively, with refinement resulting in recombinant tissue plasminogen activator (rtPA) developed in the 1980s.

Fibrinolytic therapy for peripheral arterial occlusion: Three multicenter trials in the 1990s fostered the surgical alternative approach to acute limb ischemia: the Rochester series, Surgery or Thrombolysis for the Ischemic Lower Extremity (STILE) trial, and Thrombolysis or Peripheral Arterial Surgery (TOPAS) trials. These combined with other studies resulted in endovascular catheter-directed thrombolysis (CDT) becoming the preferred initial treatment particularly when (1) limb ischemia symptoms present for less than 2 weeks, (2) no absolute contraindications to fibrinolytic therapy (see below), and (3) the predicted time to reestablish antegrade flow is short enough to preserve limb viability [128–131].

Indications for thrombolysis: Acute or subacute arterial or venous thrombosis can consider thrombolysis in conjunction with mechanical thrombectomy to address acute thrombus.

6.9.2.4 Contraindications of Thrombolysis

1. Absolute: Recent intracranial hemorrhage, intracranial neoplasm, active bleeding, recent intracranial or spinal surgery, and severe uncontrolled hypertension.
2. Relative: History of ischemic stroke and recent internal bleeding.

Medication: Alteplase (TPA)

1 Mechanism of action: Thrombolytic (converts plasminogen to plasmin to degrade fibrin and fibrinogen).

2 *Intra- or post-procedural anticoagulation:*
   (a) Bolus: operator discretion. Typically, < 5 mg.
   (b) Continuous infusion: 0.05–0.1 mg/kg/hr. via infusion catheter.
      • Laboratory monitoring: fibrinogen levels.

6.9.2.5 Thrombolysis Protocol

There is a wide variability in concurrent anticoagulation administration, interval of fibrinogen monitoring, and changing thrombolytic dose during thrombolysis [132]. An example protocol for patients with suspected HIT is provided:

Example thrombolysis with anticoagulation protocol in setting of HIT/HITT used at our institution:

• 0.5 mcg/kg/min argatroban + alteplase 0.5–1 mg/h.
• Fibrinogen monitored every 4 h.

   (a) If fibrinogen <100, decrease alteplase by 50% and recheck in 2 h.
   (b) If fibrinogen <75, decrease alteplase by 50% and administer 2 units of FFP.
   (c) If fibrinogen <50, discontinue alteplase and administer 2 units of FFP. Initiate normal saline through infusion catheter.

6.10 Tibial Calcium Management

6.10.1 Device Selection

Omar Chohan, MD

6.10.1.1 Tibial Disease

1. Big artery disease (BAD) = below knee/above ankle (Figs. 6.51 and 6.52).
   (a) Transmitting vessels – sends blood through to feet.
   (b) Disease affects tibial vessels to pedal loop.
   (c) Atherosclerotic disease.

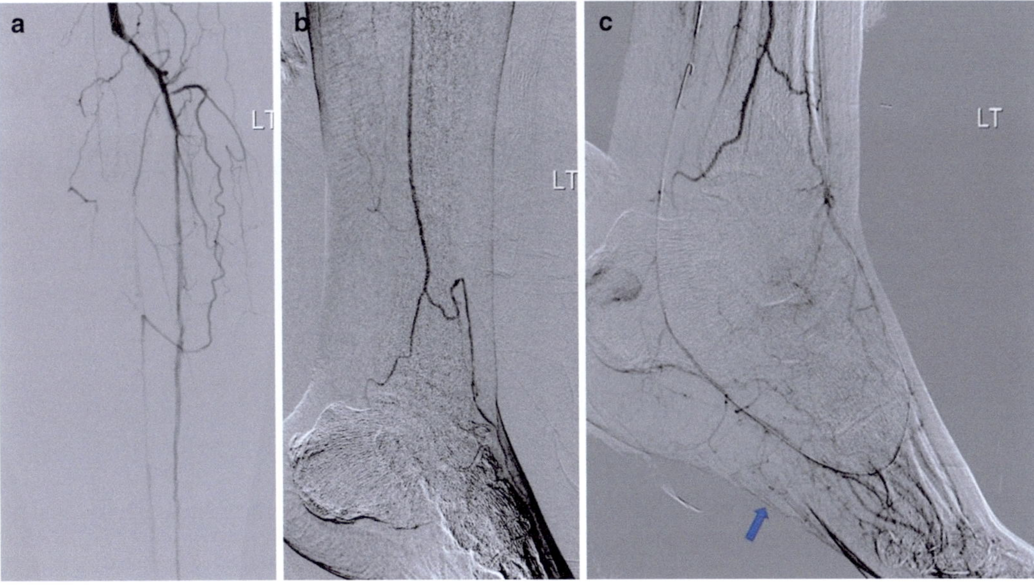

Fig. 6.51 (a–c) Left lower extremity runoff demonstrates BAD; Flush occlusion of the posterior tibial artery and distal occlusion of the anterior tibial artery. Peroneal artery reconstitutes to supply foot distally and opacifies the pedal loop, large digital arteries, and small vessels with poor distribution to tissue (blue arrow). Patient was scheduled for trans-metatarsal amputation

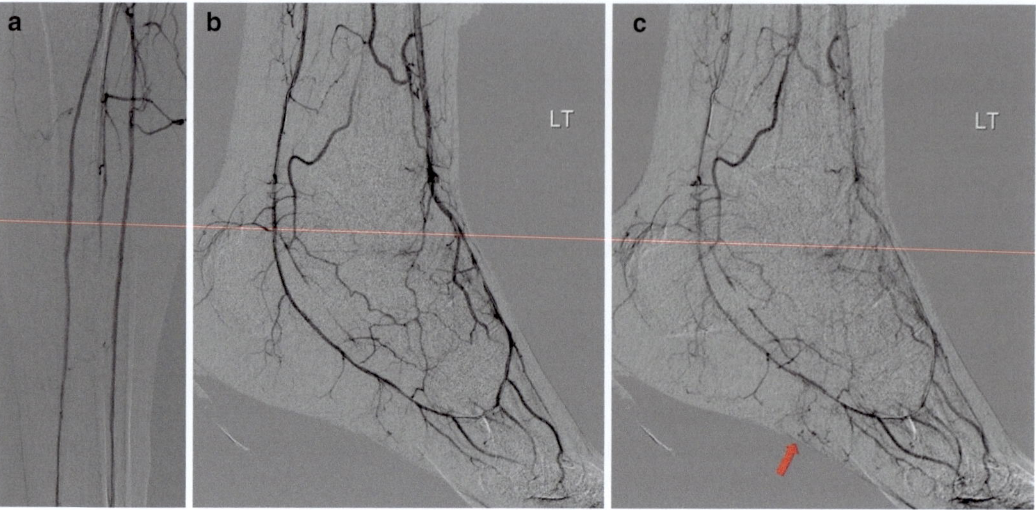

Fig. 6.52 (**a–c**) Left lower extremity runoff demonstrates BAD following orbital atherectomy and angioplasty; revascularization of anterior and posterior tibial artery provides inline flow to pedal loop, large digital arteries, and small vessels distributing flow to tissue (red arrow). No amputation was required

2. Small artery disease (SAD) = blow ankle (Fig. 6.53).
   (a) Distribution vessels – delivers blood to feet tissue.
   (b) Disease affects distal metatarsal arteries and capillary outflow.
   (c) DM; medial artery calcification (MAC). Often see tram-track calcium.
   (d) Often "no-option" CLI patients, or "desert foot."
   (e) Calcium morphology.
      • Atherosclerosis.
         – Luminal plaque; soft or calcified.
         – Can be of various lengths and sizes.
      • Medial artery calcification.
         – Intramural plaque contained within media.
         – Often diffuse and appears as "railroad tracks" on CT, X-ray, or fluoroscopy.
   (f) Approach to device selection.
      • Stenosis or occlusion length.
      • Calcium density and location.
      • Thrombus.
      • In-stent restenosis.

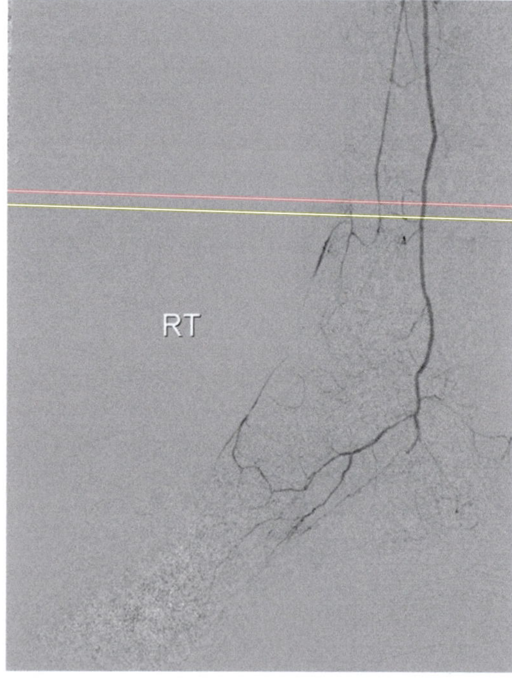

Fig. 6.53 Right lower extremity runoff demonstrates SAD. Posterior tibial artery supplies pedal loop, however, thready digital arteries and essentially nonexistent small vessels. Revascularization would not improve distribution. This patient required amputation

Table 6.3 Device types and their uses

Atherectomy	Directional	Rotational		Photoablative		Orbital	IVL
Device	Hawk	Jetstream	Rotablator	Excimer	Auryon	Diamondback	Shockwave
Focal Ca	++					+	+
Diffuse Ca	+	+	+			++	+
Thrombosis		+			+		
BTK	+		+	+	+	+	+
ISR	+			+	+		
CTO	++	+	++	+	+	++	

3. Device types (Table 6.3).
   (a) Atherectomy.
       - Orbital.
           - Diamondback.
               Eccentric crown mounted on wire rotating at high speeds.
               Can achieve luminal gain larger than crown size due to orbital rotation resulting in plaque removal and differential sanding.
               Useful in heavy calcium and long-length segments.
               Sands calcium into debris less than blood cell, however caution or avoid when using with chunky/coral reef type calcium.
       - Rotational.
           - Jetstream.
               Front cutting tip and aspiration ports.
               Useful for mixed plaque morphologies and thrombus.
               Not useful for BTK.
           - Rotablator.
               Rotating burr centrally mounted.
               Sands and removes plaques.
               Useful in heavy calcium and long-length segments.
           - Phoenix.
               Front cutting tip.
               Not useful for BTK.
       - Directional.
           - HawkOne.
               Cutting blade contained in tubular housing.
               Can be turned and directed toward plaque to exercise.

DEFINTIVE LE study – 800 patients.
   - ~90% success.
   - 3% distal embolization.
   - 12-month freedom from major amputation 95%.
   - Laser.
       - Excimer.
           High-energy monochromatic light beam vaporizes plaque.
           Can penetrate proximal fibrous cap in CTO.
           Can be used for in-stent restenosis.
           LACI trial.
           - 93% limb salvage rate at 6 months.
       - Auryon.
           Laser photoablation like Excimer.
           Has an aspiration port on larger catheter sizes which can be used in mixed plaque and thrombus.
   - Intravascular Lithotripsy (IVL).
       - Shockwave.
           Semi-compliant balloon mounted on a catheter delivering ultrasonic waves.
           Uses low pressure compared to POBA.
           Softens and remodels dense calcium improving luminal gain and recoil.
           Can be used in conjunction with traditional atherectomy or alone.

6.10.2 Non-POBA Balloons

Micah Watts

Improved intraprocedural imaging, including routine use of IVUS, has increased the awareness of arterial dissection after PTA [133]. It is believed that treatment failure including restenosis or thrombosis may result from untreated or undiagnosed dissections.

- The theorized mechanism of this is a combination of flow limitation due to luminal obstruction and exposure of the thrombogenic subintimal layers of the vessel.
- Dissections can be treated with prolonged balloon angioplasty, stenting, or an endovascular tack device. Prolonged angioplasty is not always effective.
- Stenting and Tack (Philips Inc.) placement causes either continuous outward force or inflammatory stimulus that may accelerate restenosis.
- Any method of treating a dissection will accelerate neointimal hyperplasia accelerating the rate of restenosis.
- Preventing dissections by decreasing barotrauma during angioplasty has become the goal in development of multiple endovascular devices [134].

6.10.2.1 Cutting and Scoring Balloons

Cutting balloon (Boston Scientific) angioplasty has been available in the United States since 2005 and was the first device designed to dilate fibrotic stenoses at lower atmospheric pressure. Three or four atherotomes, or small blades, are mounted onto a noncompliant angioplasty balloon. When the balloon is inflated, these blades score the plaque to allow for lower pressure angioplasty. Small studies demonstrated superiority regarding restenosis with cutting balloon vs conventional balloon in femoropopliteal angioplasty [135].

The original cutting balloons were limited to short lengths and required relatively large sheath sizes. The technology was updated, although without blades, with the release of AngioSculpt (Philips medical), which is available in tibial artery sizes from 2.0 to 4.0 mm and lengths up to 100 cm delivered via a 5F or 6F sheath. The AngioSculpt balloon is a semi-compliant balloon wrapped in a helical configuration with three rectangular flexible nitinol struts, which grip the artery to prevent slipping and concentrate the force of the angioplasty 15 to 25 times that of conventional angioplasty along the struts [136].

Multiple small studies demonstrated excellent primary patency with low rates of clinically significant dissection or bailout stenting when using AngioSculpt as a primary treatment modality [137, 138]. Other scoring balloons have been released subsequently from other medical device companies and function similarly.

6.10.2.2 Chocolate

The chocolate balloon (Medtronic) is a semi-compliant angioplasty balloon mounted inside a nitinol restraining cage. When the balloon is inflated, the constraining cage creates a series of pillows and grooves, which interact with the vessel wall. The pillows are balloon segments that extend from the cage and provide gentle focal force to the arterial wall. The appearance of the pillows constrained by a nitinol grid gives the appearance of a classic chocolate bar divided into rectangular segments. The design of the balloon is to encourage uniform inflation pressures and allow the balloon "pillows" to exert the force on the arterial wall, while the metallic cage elements brace the balloon to the wall and act as a barrier to dissection propagation. The restraining cage also helps prevent overinflation and excessive barotrauma while protecting the vessel from the torsional forces inherent in unfolding a traditional angioplasty balloon during inflation [139].

The chocolate balloon is designed to treat both above and below-the-knee arteries with diameters as low as 2.5 mm and lengths up to 120 mm via a 5 Fr sheath. It is designed to be sized 1:1 to the normal vessel lumen to result in fewer dissections and bailout stents and less neointimal hyperplasia.

- Chocolate BAR, a post-market multicenter registry focusing on safety and efficacy followed 226 patients with tibial artery chocolate balloon interventions showing excellent 12-month results in freedom from bailout stenting and freedom from target lesion revascularization (TLR) [140].

6.10.2.3 Intravascular Lithotripsy

Adapting technology from urologic extracorporeal lithotripsy, the Shockwave intravascular lithotripsy (IVL) device delivers sonic energy to the vessel wall via a balloon inflated to sub-nominal pressures. An electric generator sends small electric charges through the mixture of saline and contrast in the balloon, which vaporizes the fluid and creates a rapidly expanding and contracting pressure wave. The pressure wave passes through soft tissue and preferentially impacts hard tissue including both intimal calcium and medial calcium. The sonic pressure causes microfractures along the calcium, thus increasing vessel compliance. The more compliant vessel is then ready for definitive therapy to maximize luminal expansion. Shockwave IVL catheters are available in femoropopliteal sizes from 3.5 to 8 mm in 6 cm lengths and in tibial sizes ranging from 2.5 to 4 mm in 4 cm lengths. The balloons are available on an 0.014″ platform [141]. Femoropopliteal balloons are routinely used off-label in the iliac arteries. The DISRUPT PAD and DISRUPT PAD studies were discussed in prior sections. Early results seem very positive for IVL [82].

6.10.2.4 Serranator

The Serranator PTA serration balloon catheter (Cagent Vascular, Wayne, PA) is the latest specialty balloon to enter the market. The Serranator is a semi-compliant angioplasty balloon with three or four embedded metallic strips with serrated scoring elements designed to apply greater than one thousand times the force to the vessel wall compared to POBA.

- This focal force creates an interrupted line along the vessel surface allowing for plaque modification and controlled expansion at low pressures. Those two factors combine to create fewer dissections and less recoil with the ability to more effectively and safely treat calcified, highly fibrotic, and complex lesions.
- Serranator PTA balloons are available for above and below the knee. Below-the-knee sizes range from 2.5 to 3.5 mm and lengths range from 40 to 120 mm. These have three metallic strips. Above-the-knee sizes range from 4 to 6 mm and lengths range from 40 to 120 mm. These are equipped with four metallic strips.
- Long-term data are still lacking as Serranator is new to the market, but safety and efficacy have been proven in the PRELUDE studies. The PRELUDE ATK studies enrolled 25 patients with femoropopliteal lesions and demonstrated very low residual stenosis at very low inflation pressures, the majority of which measured less than 6 atm.
- The PRELUDE BTK study showed similar luminal gain at low pressures with minimal bailout stenting. Results in both studies included qualitative core laboratory review of IVUS or OCT, which consistently demonstrated the focal perforations from the metallic strips [142, 143].

6.10.2.5 Tips

- Very long percutaneous old balloon angioplasty (POBA) balloons (up to and exceeding 300 mm) are available for tibial angioplasty. With the rare exception of complete tibial artery occlusion, these apply forces unevenly to different portions of the vessel.
  - If using a long balloon, it can be inflated to nominal pressure and examined for remaining as it is. If waists are present, deflate the balloon and pretreat that area with a specialty balloon to decrease the pressure applied to that spot, and in turn, to the unaffected arterial wall touched by the balloon.
- Drug-coated balloon technology for the tibial arteries has been slow in development. Specialty balloons can improve the outcome of tibial angioplasty without the use of medication.
  - Though many studies have subsequently shown no definite increase in the risk of death after the use of paclitaxel bearing

devices, some may still wish to avoid drug delivery when possible.

- Debulking atherectomy can similarly decrease required angioplasty pressures, but may increase the risk of complication including downstream embolization in certain lesions.
- As data continue to show positive results with tibial stenting and as new tibial stents are being designed and released, effective low-pressure angioplasty in calcified lesions may improve stent expansion and allow for optimal results after tibial artery stenting.
- Shockwave IVL is routinely used in heavily calcified iliac arteries to aid in the delivery of large sheaths for structural heart procedures and growing use in the infrainguinal arteries down to the tibials.
  - A stent that has been deployed into heavy calcium and has poorly expanded can be treated with Shockwave IVL to attempt better expansion by fracturing the calcium that is constraining the stent.
- Predilation with a scoring balloon may perforate the intima and allow for a larger-sized POBA balloon to treat the lesion at a lower pressure.
- "No stent zones" include the P2 segment of the popliteal artery and the common femoral artery, making these excellent places to use specialty balloons to minimize the risk of dissection and necessity for bailout stenting. Stenting in these areas has been performed however lack significant data as of yet.

6.10.3 Tibial Scaffold Options

Jesse Martin and Robert Beasley
Currently, there are no FDA-approved stents for use below the knee. For many years, balloon-expandable coronary drug-eluting stents have been used as a bailout for failed tibial angioplasty with good outcomes (Figs. 6.54 and 6.55). One limitation is areas of external compression, such as below the calf level, limits use of these stents. Past trials looking at self-expanding stents for below-the-knee use have not had favorable results [144]. However, now in FDA-approved clinical trials, there are multiple dedicated below-the-knee tibial stents that are showing promise.

6.10.3.1 Indications for Below-the-Knee Stenting

1. Critical limb ischemia (Rutherford criteria 4–6).
2. Severe vessel recoil (>50% reference vessel) following balloon angioplasty.
3. Long-segment CTO occlusions unlikely to respond to angioplasty alone.
4. Lesions involving the proximal 2/3 tibial vessels (for current technology using balloon-expandable coronary drug-eluting stents).
5. Flow-limiting dissections.
6. Bailout for vessel perforation with active extravasation.

6.10.3.2 Contraindications for Below-the-Knee Stenting

There are few if any ABSOLUTE contraindications in the setting of critical limb ischemia. There are, however, RELATIVE contraindications:

1. Contraindication or intolerance to antiplatelet/anticoagulant therapy.
2. Contrast dye reaction.

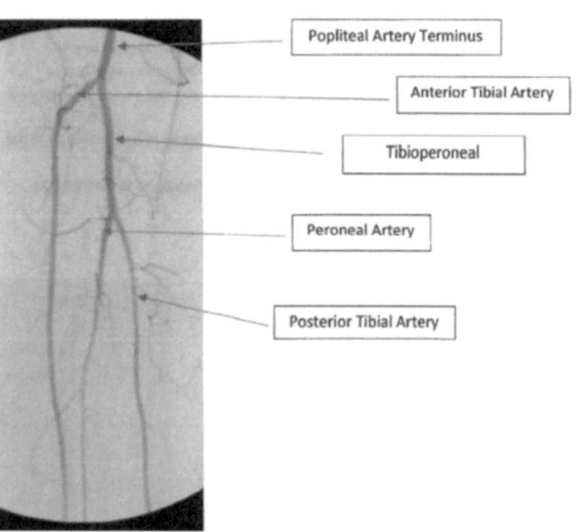

Fig. 6.54 Normal anatomy for standard tibial artery stenting procedures. Image courtesy of Robert E. Beasley, MD, Palm Vascular Centers

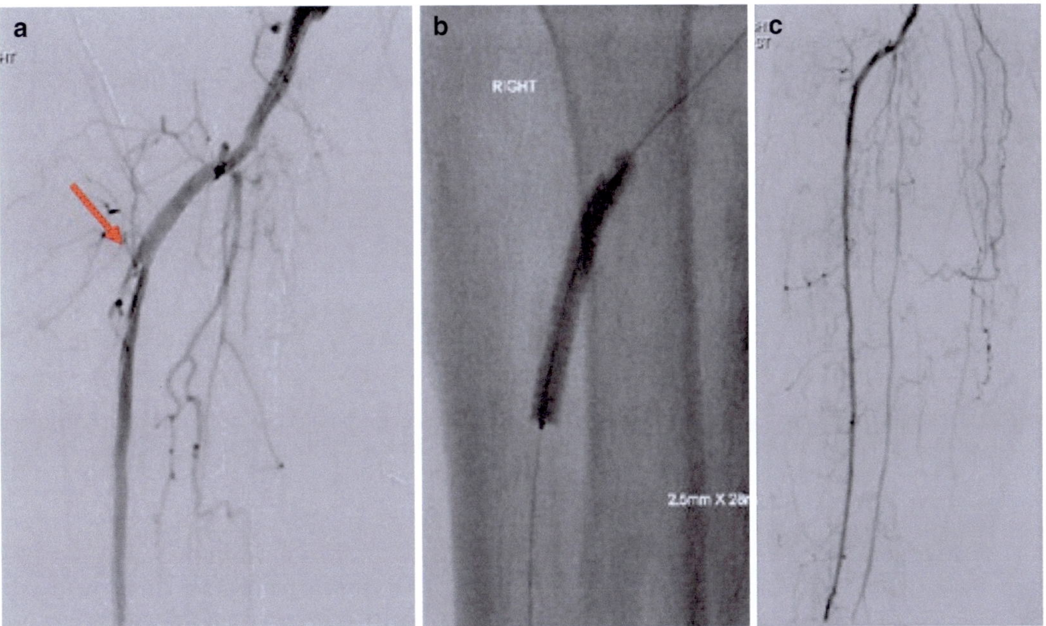

Fig. 6.55 (**a**) Post-SAFARI and angioplasty of the right anterior tibial artery resulting in significant dissection (red arrow). (**b**) Coronary drug-eluting bare metal stent placement. (**c**) Completion angiogram with resolution of dissection

6.10.3.3   Current Tibial Scaffold Options with Trial Data and Future Tibial Stent Platforms

1. In the ACHILLES Trial that took place at 17 European centers, balloon-expandable coronary drug-eluting stents were randomized to plain balloon angioplasty for treatment of tibial lesions in patients with CLI.
   (a) DES showed significantly lower restenosis rates (22.4% versus 41.9%), higher patency (75.0% versus 41.9%), and improved Rutherford classification at 12 months [145].
2. In the Yukon-BTK trial, 161 patients were randomized to receive balloon-expandable coronary drug-eluting stents versus balloon-expandable coronary bare metal stents.
   (a) The DES showed significantly higher primary patency (80.6% versus 55.6%) and improved Rutherford class [146].
3. In the XCELL registry, which evaluated the Xpert self-expanding bare metal stent (Abbott Vascular), 120 patients were enrolled in a multicenter trial.
   (a) Significant binary in-stent restenosis was seen with a rate of 68.5% at 6 months and only 49% had complete wound healing at 6 months [144].
4. Future stent possibilities at the time of this writing include three tibial stents that are currently in the FDA IDE trial.
   (a) The Microstent (Micro Medical solutions) is a tightly woven nitinol stent that is currently being studied in the STAND trial.
   (b) The Eluvia stent (Boston Scientific) is a drug-coated self-expanding nitinol stent that is currently being studied in the SAVAL trial.
      - Results of this study were released at CIRSE meeting in Barcelona 2022 showing it did not meet is primary safety and efficacy endpoints.
   (c) The ESPRIT stent (Abbott Vascular) is a drug-eluting bioresorbable scaffold that is currently being studied in the LIFE-BTK trial.

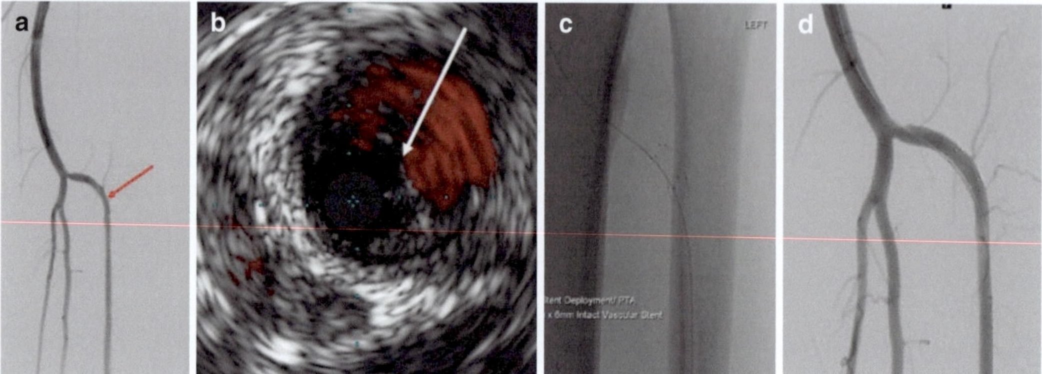

Fig. 6.56 (**a**) Post-angioplasty of the left anterior tibial artery resulted in focal subtle dissection (red arrow). (**b**) IVUS color flow image showing significant dissection flap (white arrow). (**c**) Deployment of two tack dissection repair scaffolds. (**d**) Completion angiogram with satisfactory tacking of dissection flap

TACK Dissection Repair

The TACK (Philips Inc.) endovascular dissection repair is a Self-Expanding scaffold with low outward radial force, with the only intent of tacking up the dissection flaps post-intervention, which otherwise can be a source of restenosis or thrombosis (Fig. 6.56). These small stents, with minimal metal component, come preloaded on catheters for above-the-knee and below-the-knee sizes, from 1.5 mm up to 8 mm vessel diameters. These are not intended for stenosis recoil management, which are reserved for conventional stents/scaffolds. In using this device, one can avoid using unnecessary stent material, which itself can induce more downstream or follow-up stenosis.

- The TOBA II BTK study has followed 233 patients out to 3 years with below-the-knee application and showed approximately 70% K-M Freetom from CD-TLR and ~ 94% K-M target limb salvage.
- Most operators prefer to use drug-coated balloon angioplasty before TACK placement to assist in reducing restenosis.

6.11 Distal Popliteal and Trifurcation Disease Management

Ibrahim Ali, Uman Jaffer, and Prakash Krishnan

We know that there is significant elastic recoil in the tibial vessels with balloon angioplasty alone, and oftentimes, prolonged balloon inflations are needed for better vessel patency. To date, however, our only bailout scaffold for recoil, residual stenosis, flow-limiting dissection, or perforation of the tibial vessels are stents.

Various trials evaluating below-the-knee arterial disease management are summarized below and in Table 6.4:

- Bare metal stents (BMSs), both balloon-expandable and self-expandable, have been compared with PTA and have shown no clinical benefit with regard to 1-year primary patency or TLR [147].
  - Additionally, BMSs have a high rate of restenosis [147].

Table 6.4 Results over various trials evaluating below–the- knee arterial disease management

Trial	Randomization groups	Number of patients	Primary outcome	Lesions
Yukon-Btk	Sirolimus-eluting stent vs BMS	161 CLI and Claudication Rutherford 2–5	12-month patency (80.6% vs 55.6%; $P = 0.004$)	Single de novo, <5 mm
Destiny	XIENCE everolimus-eluting stent vs BMS	140 CLI Rutherford 4–5	12-month patency (85.2% vs 54.4%; $P = 0.0001$)	Maximum of two focal lesions. Total lesion length <40 mm. Excluded bifurcations
Achilles	Sirolimus-eluting stent vs standard PTA	200 CLI Rutherford 3–5	12-month restenosis by angiography (22.4% vs 41.9%; $P = 0.019$)	Total lesion length <120 mm. Excluded bifurcations
Ideas	DESs (zotarolimus/ sirolimus/everolimus stents) vs paclitaxel drug-coated balloons (DCBs)	50 CLI Rutherford 3–6	6-month angiographic restenosis (28% vs 57.9%; $P = 0.046$)	Single lesions >70 mm
Padi	Paclitaxel-eluting stent vs PTA/BMS	137 CLI Rutherford 4–6	5-year amputation-free survival (31.8% vs 20.4%; $P = 0.041$)	Single lesion <60 mm

- In contrast, the emerging evidence for the use of drug-eluting stents (DESs) in infrapopliteal disease is promising [145, 146, 148, 149].
  - Therefore, we suggest using DES, including coronary DES, in all bifurcation lesions when, and if, a scaffold is required, with an effort to minimize the amount of stented area [150, 151].
  - It is important to keep in mind there are little to no data on the long-term patency on drug-eluting stents in bifurcation lesions below the knee. Our recommendations are based on DES performance in single lesions [151].
- A non-drug-eluting tibial stent, the MircoStent (Micromedical Inc.), which is a closed-cell nitinol self-expanding stent currently under trials, may hold future promise as well [152].
- Treatment of bifurcation lesions may evolve to include bioresorbable vascular scaffolds (BVS), as to leave no footprint. In a recent registry publication analyzing the Absorb BVS by Abbott, the BVS showed freedom from restenosis of 86.6% at 24 months. Additionally, we await the results of the LIFE-BTK randomized trial [152].

In complex bifurcation lesions of the tibial vessels, we have primarily adapted coronary bifurcation techniques to tackle these lesions.

- Primary techniques are provisional, culotte, T-stenting, mini-crush, and kissing stents. Below, we explain each [150].

6.11.1 Single Stent Technique/ Provisional (Fig. 6.57)

- Preferred, least complex.
- Typically, a side branch is not involved.
- Steps: Wire placed down main branch and stent is deployed into main vessel with side branch jailed (i.e., stent from TP trunk into peroneal artery jailing the posterior tibial). If significant dissection in a side branch, one

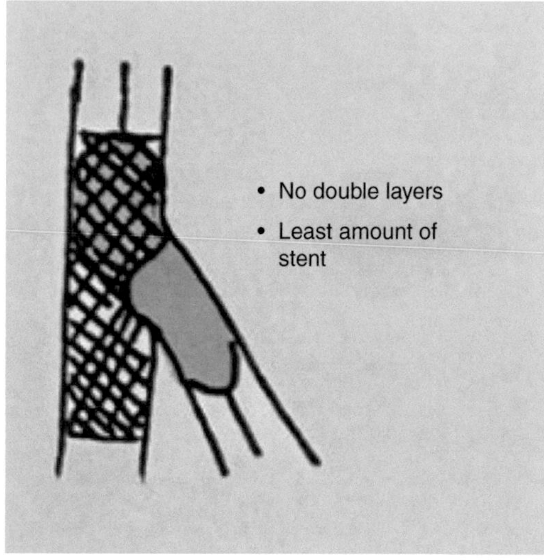

Fig. 6.57 Single stent technique

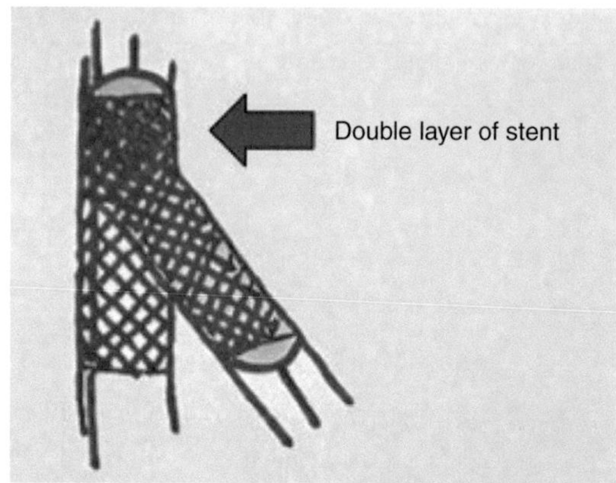

Fig. 6.58 Culotte technique

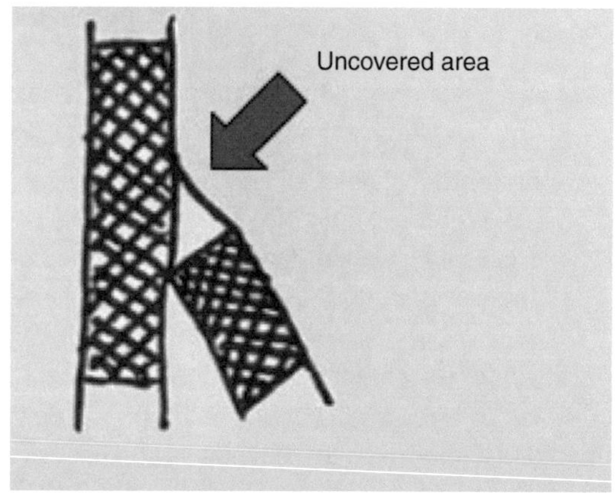

Fig. 6.59 T-stenting technique

would need to rewire side branch via stent struts from main vessel stent and balloon ostium of the side branch with final KBI (kissing balloon inflation).

6.11.2 Culotte Technique (Fig. 6.58)

- Good technique for true bifurcation lesions with similar size of two branches (main branch and side branch).
- Side branch ostium will definitely be covered; however, two layers of metal will be left in the proximal main vessel (prior to bifurcation).
- Steps: Wire main branch and side branch. Stent the more angulated branch first. Then, cross into the side branch via struts of main branch stent and dilate struts open. Deploy the second stent into side branch with proximal portion of the stent in the main vessel overlapped with first stent. Re-cross the first stent in the main branch and then perform KBI.

6.11.3 T-Stenting (Fig. 6.59)

- This is a relatively less complex bifurcation technique, which is great for lesions that do not involve the side branch ostium due to difficulty in fully covering side branch ostium.

- No overlap between main branch and side branch stents so less metal left behind proximally prior to bifurcation.
- Steps: Wire main branch and stent main branch. Next, cross the main branch stent struts into side branch with wire and deploy stent in the proximal portion of the side branch. Perform KBI to complete.

6.11.4 Mini-Crush Technique (Fig. 6.60)

- Variation of the T-stenting which addresses inherent lack of side branch ostium coverage with T-stent technique.
- Good for bifurcations with side branch ostial involvement as ostium is always covered. In addition, unlike culotte technique only a sin-

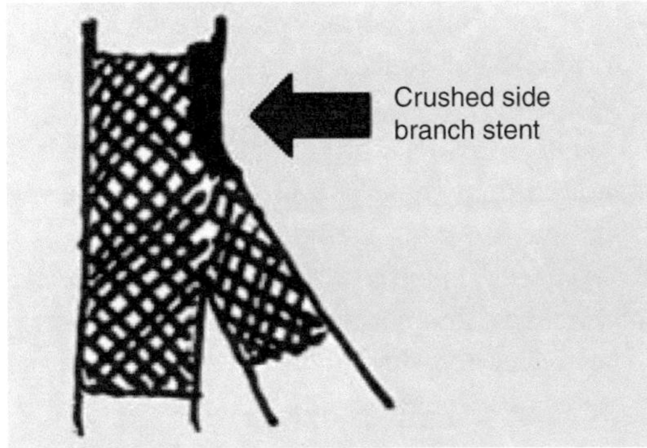

Fig. 6.60 Mini-crush technique

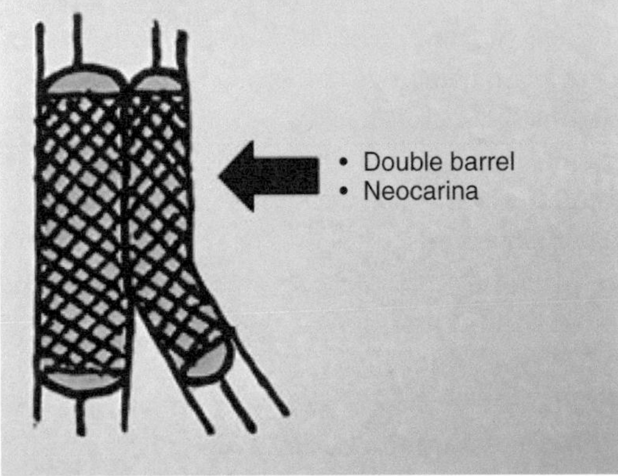

Fig. 6.61 Kissing stent technique

gle layer of stent is left behind in the main vessel proximal to the bifurcation.

- Steps: Side branch is wired, and stent is placed in the side branch with small portion of proximal portion of stent protruding into main vessel. Next, the main branch is wired, and stent is placed in the main branch of bifurcation protruding out into main vessel and deployed such that it "crushes" the proximal portion of the side branch stent against the vessel wall. Finally, the side branch is rewired and KBI is performed.

6.11.5 Kissing Stent Technique (Fig. 6.61)

- New metallic neocarina created in proximal main vessel (i.e., TP trunk) as two stents deployed simultaneously from proximal main vessel into each respective bifurcating vessel (side branch, main branch).
- Similar to technique used for aorto-iliac bifurcating lesions with kissing technique used there.
- Best for shallow angles (60° to 90°).
- Less time-consuming as no need to re-cross for KBI.
- The downside is that it is theoretically creating a smaller lumen in the proximal main vessel with neocarina.
- Steps: Wire both side branch and main branch and place appropriately sized stents in each vessel with proximal ends of both stents protruding in the proximal main vessel. Simultaneously inflate both stents.

6.12 Distal Emboli Management

S. Jay Mathews

6.12.1 Introduction

Any peripheral intervention carries the inherent risk of distal embolization (DE). Mitigation of this risk involves identifying patients at highest risk, those who will be most impacted adversely by embolization, and intraprocedural prevention strategies.

Embolic debris is seen in most peripheral arterial interventions, occurring in 70–100% of cases as seen by examination of embolic protection or by Doppler studies [153]. However, clinically significant embolic lesions requiring mechanical or pharmacomechanical treatments remain low (<3%) [153, 154]. TASC (Transatlantic Inter-Society Consensus) II D lesions, angiographic thrombus, and prior history of amputations are independent predictors of DE [154]. In addition, patients with critical limb ischemia, greater number of treatment vessels, and emergent cases seem to have higher DE [153]. The use of atherectomy devices can also lead to DE [155].

6.12.2 Prevention

In appropriate patients, distal embolic protection devices (EPD) may mitigate macroembolic debris.

- Most embolic protection filter devices feature a pore-size between 100 to 150 micrometers, potentially allowing microembolic material below that size.
- While typically not clinically significant, this material can lead to no-reflow in various vascular beds. An alternative to traditional EPD devices is use of external compression.
- The "HIRANODOME" (Interim hemostatic technique with HIgh pressure for Regional blood flow in the superficial femoral Artery, NOninvasive Distal protection Occlusion MEthod) technique utilizes an external band to compress the popliteal artery [156].
- Alternatively, the use of pneumatic compression with a blood pressure cuff inflated over the calf may also be effective [157]. With distal compression during proximal intervention, a column of static blood is created which can be removed with manual or mechanical aspiration thrombectomy. In this fashion, DE can be reduced. Distal compression carries the advantage of not requiring specialized EPD, trauma to the intima with inadvertent EPD migration, or distal "spillover" from a full EPD.

In patients at high risk for DE, prophylactic EPD may be advised. Some have proposed use of filters in patients with chronic total occlusion, in-stent restenosis, thrombotic lesions, calcific lesions >40 mm, and long-length lesions (>140 mm) [158]. Complex patients with single-vessel runoff or use of atherectomy devices may warrant EPD placement.

- While EPD does offer some protection, it is not without some risk as DE can still occur despite use (>4% in one series) [159].
- In general, in the presence of acute or subacute thrombus, thrombectomy should be performed to reduce the risk of distal embolization and avoid overwhelming the capabilities of an EPD.

6.12.3 Treatment

Treatment strategies for distal embolization depend on pathology.

- Macrovascular arterial thrombotic embolization may respond to simple aspiration (manual or powered).
- Microvascular embolization (<1 mm) may respond to infusion of thrombolytics for 6 to 24 h post-procedure.
- In the setting of extensive thrombosis, it may be necessary to perform lytic (TPA) infusion in order to separate out discrete atherosclerotic disease from thrombotic material.
- Cholesterol, atheromatous debris, and calcium fragments will not respond to lysis [160]. A combination of aspiration and thrombolysis may be effective [161]. In this situation, direct-powered aspiration devices like Indigo Lightning 7 or CAT Rx for tibial–pedal vessels (Penumbra, Inc.) may be effective [162].
- Thrombectomy devices like the Wolf (Boston Scientific, Inc.) may have greater extraction force than powered aspiration devices as it uti-

lizes a nitinol weave to ingest mixed morphology material in antegrade fashion.

- Basket embolectomy devices (e.g., Pounce [Surmodics, Inc.], Excipio SV [Contego, Inc.], etc.) may also have a role with removal of calcific debris, but risk further distal embolization as the device needs to be advanced beyond the occlusion before removal.

- Combination aspiration and extraction techniques may be effective. Atherectomy and/or PTA may restore flow with discrete lesions, but also carries the risk of further distal embolization. Some operators have proposed using small underinflated balloons (2–3 mm in size) and performing Fogarty embolectomy into an aspiration catheter.

6.12.4 Case Example

A 75-year-old woman with diabetes, chronic kidney disease, dyslipidemia, and former tobacco abuse presented with Rutherford 4 symptoms. During inflow intervention of the SFA, she developed DE with occlusion of both the anterior tibial and tibioperoneal trunk (Fig. 6.62). Mechanical powered aspiration thrombectomy utilizing the Indigo Lightning 7 catheter (Penumbra, Inc.) was first performed into the tibioperoneal trunk. Due to difficulty in crossing due to the presence of tibioperoneal disease, a balloon-assisted tracking technique was used with an underinflated 3 mm balloon (Fig. 6.63a). The catheter was advanced during balloon deflation with simultaneous aspiration. Then aspiration was performed into the anterior tibial artery (Fig. 6.63b). There was dissection seen in the tibioperoneal trunk (Fig. 6.64a). Flow restoration was demonstrated with intact three-vessel runoff after drug-eluting stent placement into the tibioperoneal trunk (Fig. 6.64b).

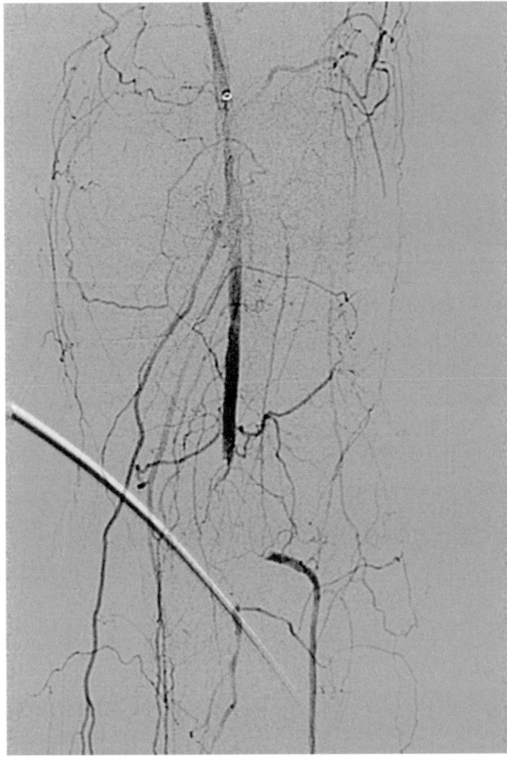

Fig. 6.62 Occlusion of the distal popliteal, tibioperoneal trunk, and proximal anterior tibial arteries due to distal embolization

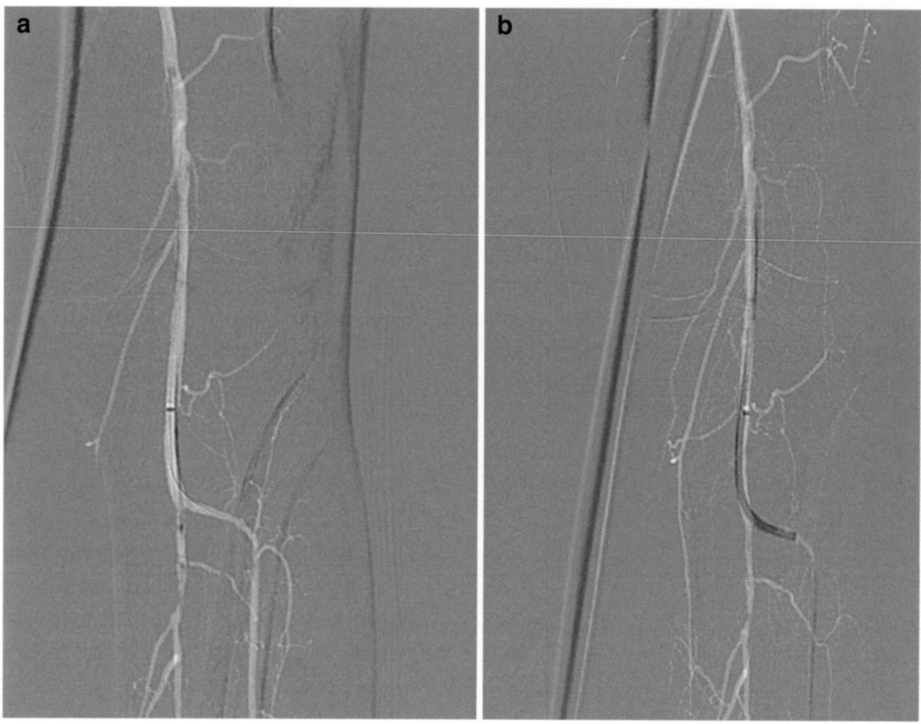

Fig. 6.63 Advancement of the Indigo Lightning 7 catheter (A – tibioperoneal trunk; B – anterior tibial artery)

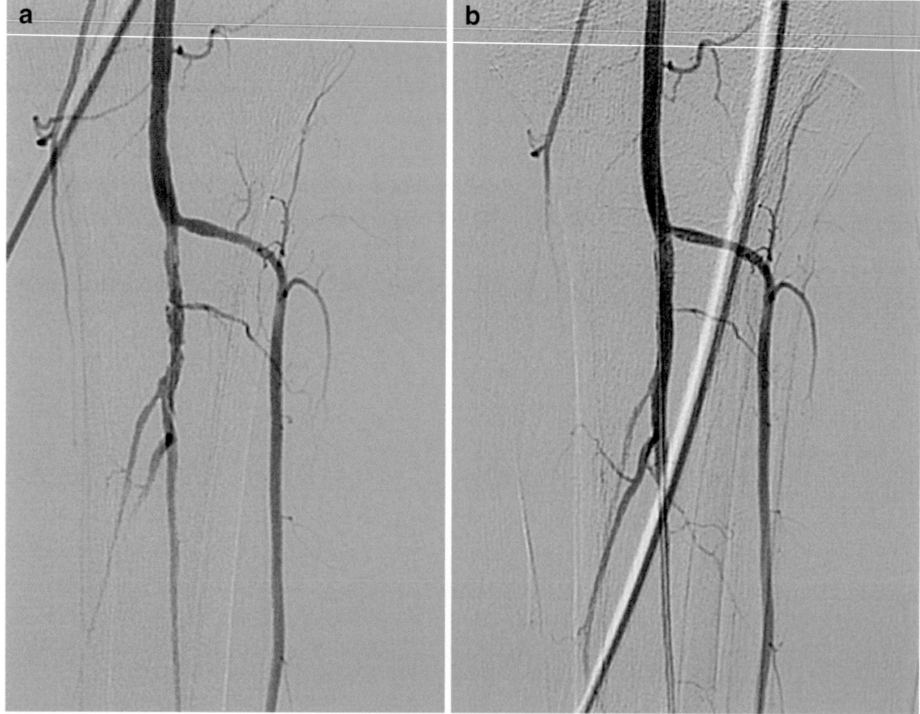

Fig. 6.64 Final angiography (**a** – post-thrombectomy; **b** – post-stenting of the tibioperoneal trunk)

6.13   Blue Toe Syndrome Management

Sabeen Dhand, MD

Blue toe syndrome is manifested by a cyanotic toe caused by ischemia from small end artery occlusion, most commonly due to atheroembolic disease. Several other conditions may also present with blue discoloration of toes and a careful history, physical exam, and noninvasive workup can aid in the diagnosis and management of this condition. Here, we will discuss the condition as well as the appropriate workup and management of syndrome.

Presentation: Sudden onset of a unilateral, painful blue toe (Fig. 6.65). Can also present with multiple toes and/or involve both feet depending on the etiology.

Causes: Several causes of blue toe syndrome exist, which all relate to a common mechanism: Obstruction of the small digital arteries supplying the toe leading to ischemia [163, 164]. A careful history from the patient can help determine the etiology of the syndrome.

1. *Embolic Disease (most common):*

   Most embolic causes are related to atherosclerotic and aneurysmal sources. Unstable, friable plaques can result in fragmentation and emboli of cholesterol debris and/or fibrinoplatelet aggregates into the tiny arteries of the digits. This results in mechanical occlu-

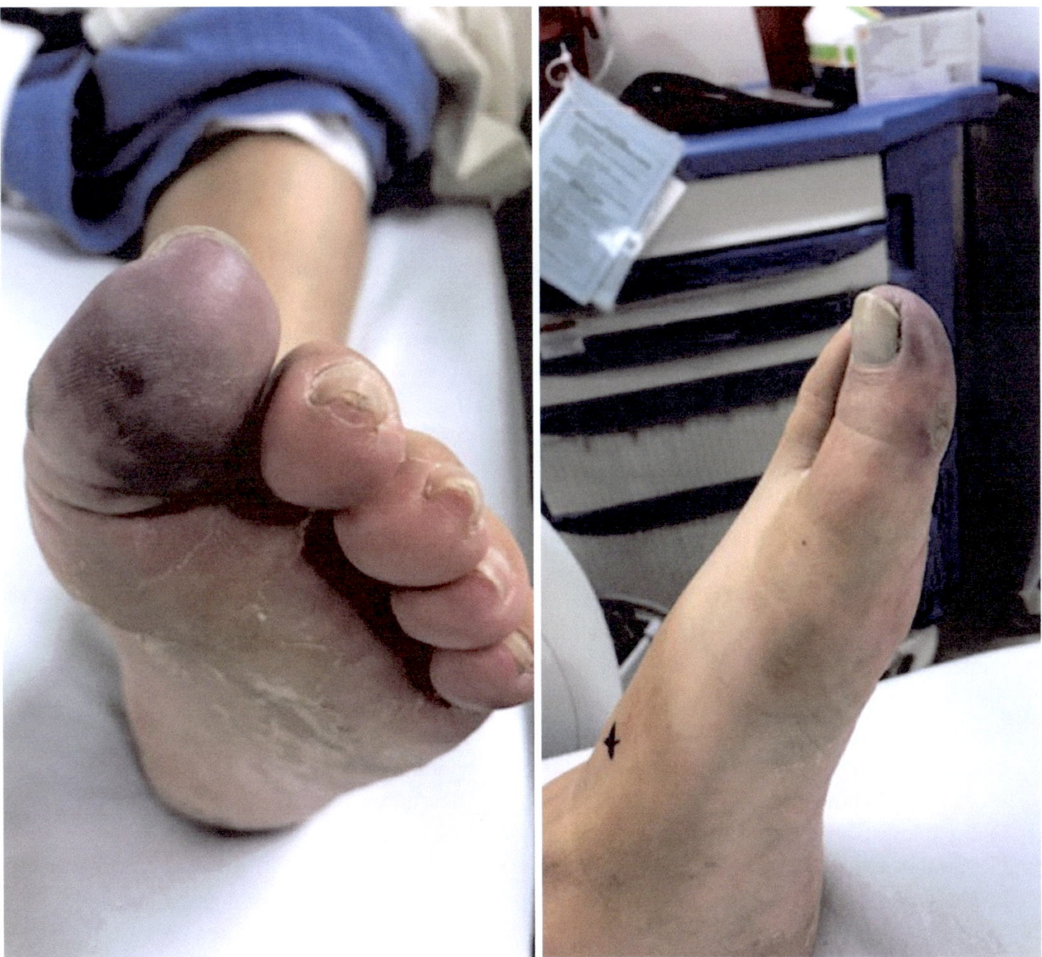

Fig. 6.65 Bluish, purplish discoloration of the first digit on the left foot

sion of the digital artery, with development of ischemia that characteristically presents with cyanosis and pain [163–166].

Most lesions are from the infrarenal abdominal aorta to the distal popliteal artery. Suprarenal lesions usually present with visceral organ ischemia (i.e., splenic or renal infarct) rather than lower extremity digital ischemia, although these may still occur [163, 164]. Similarly, intracardiac thrombus and or valvular vegetative disease can also serve as a source for emboli [163, 164, 167].

2. *Vasculitis*:

Inflammation of blood vessels results in vasospasm and/or immune complex deposition, resulting in endothelial proliferation, eventually narrowing or obstructing digital arteries. Since vasculitides are systemic, involvement is usually bilateral and symmetric. A commonly referred to disorder includes Raynaud's disease, although other examples include microscopic polyarteritis, polyarteritis nodosa, and system lupus erythematosus [163, 164].

3. *Hyperviscosity:*

Blood viscosity increases when there is increased cellularity (red blood cells, platelets, proteins, etc.). This increased thickness slows down blood flow leading to stasis and promoting thrombosis of digital arteries. Conditions include polycythemia, leukemia, cryoglobulinemia, and macroglobulinemia. Findings can often involve multiple toes, can be bilateral, or also involve larger arteries and organs [163, 164].

4. Hypercoagulability:

Numerous conditions are associated with a tendency to thrombosis due to abnormal blood vessels, platelets, or coagulation factors. Again, thrombosis leads to focal digital ischemia, frequently involving multiple digits or other vascular territories. Examples include malignancy, antiphospholipid syndrome, essential thrombocytopenia, and disseminated intravascular coagulation [163, 164].

5. Calciphylaxis:

Calcium deposits and accumulates in blood vessels and the skin, resulting in obstruction of arteries, as well as skin lesions, including ulcerations and even gangrene. This condition is rare and serious, carrying a very high mortality rate [164, 168].

6. Medications:

Anticoagulation and thrombolytics can destabilize friable plaques and promote fragmentation of cholesterol or fibrinoplatelet emboli into distal vascular beds [164, 169, 170]. Corticosteroids have also been shown to cause blue toes due to inhibited platelet activation in the setting of endothelial damage, thus exacerbating a hypercoagulable or hyperviscous state [171].

Illicit drug use is also associated with blue toes, including cocaine and amphetamines, as result of vasoocclusive disease [172].

7. Iatrogenesis:

A recent angiogram can disrupt atherosclerotic lesions, promoting fragmentation and embolization. This can be related to the wire or from intervention, such as angioplasty [163, 164].

Any podiatric surgery that manipulates the foot or toes can also damage the vascular bed within the forefoot, leading to temporary or permanent digital ischemia [164, 173].

8. Nonocclusive mimickers of blue toe syndrome: trauma (ecchymosis, venous hemorrhage), reflex sympathetic dystrophy, and acrocyanosis [164].

6.13.1 Physical Examination

- Initially petechia, then bluish or purplish discoloration, or mottling of the toes.
- Partial or entire involvement of the toe – usually well demarcated.
- Distribution: single toe, multiple toes, or bilateral.
- Ulceration or gangrene may be present.
- Sluggish capillary refill.
- Cool to touch.
- Tender to palpation or manipulation.
- Palpable pedal pulses often present.
- Proximal livedo reticularis: blue-red mottling of the foot or calf (Fig. 6.66).

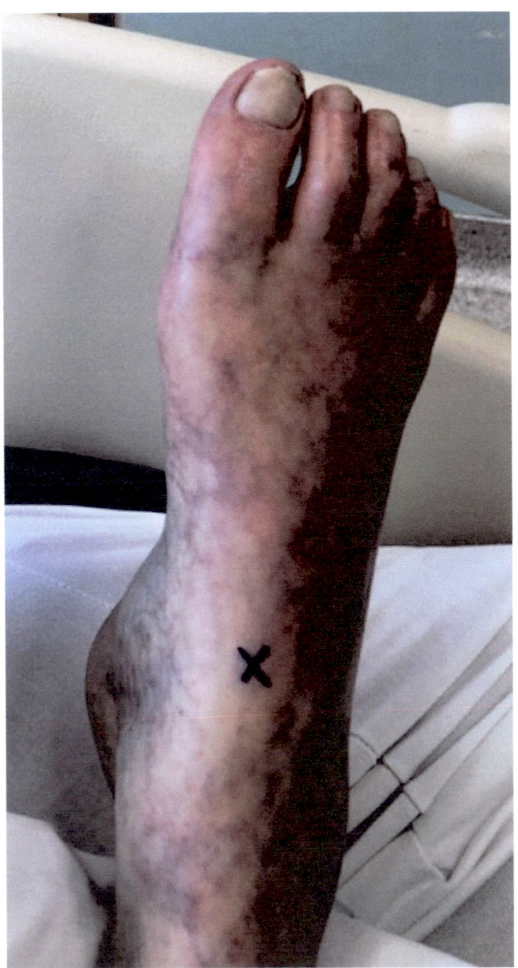

Fig. 6.66 Livedo reticularis affecting the right foot. This condition is represented as blue-red mottling of the skin in a net-like, or reticular, pattern

6.13.1.1 Evaluation

A sudden, unilateral blue painful toe should raise high suspicion for an embolic source [164]. In these cases, the identification of the offending lesion with noninvasive imaging is vital to determine management and prevent further embolization and ischemia.

Duplex ultrasonography is widely available and good at identifying disease in the femoro-popliteal segment. However, since up to 40% of the offending lesions may originate in the aorta or iliac arteries, additional evaluation with computed tomography angiogram (CTA) or magnetic resonance angiogram (MRA) is necessary [164]

(Fig. 6.67). Even if a femoropopliteal lesion is identified on duplex ultrasound, CTA, or MRA is still recommended, since these modalities better characterize the morphology and location of the lesions, which significantly aids in treatment planning and device selection (Fig. 6.68).

Therefore, when atherosclerotic disease is suspected as a cause for blue toes, workup should begin with duplex sonography of the lower extremities followed by CTA or MRA covering the entire length of the aorta and the bilateral lower extremities. Morphology characteristics that are seen on these studies include severe focal stenoses/occlusion, noncalcified ulcerated plaques, and penetrating ulcers [174, 175]. Aneurysms at any location with irregular mural thrombus are also at risk for peripheral embolization.

If a cardiac source is suspected, echocardiography (transthoracic or transesophageal) is recommended [163]. In addition, intravascular ultrasound (IVUS) during endovascular therapy can also further delineate and characterize vulnerable plaques [176].

In cases where no obvious embolic source is identified, then other systemic causes of blue toe syndrome should be investigated, if the history alone did not easily identify the cause [164].

6.13.1.2 Treatment

The goal of treatment is to control the underlying source and prevent further embolization, occlusion, and eventual tissue (digit/limb) loss. This requires medical therapy in combination with endovascular or surgical approaches (for atheroembolic causes).

Treatment starts with antiplatelet therapy and anticoagulation.

- Primary choices usually include aspirin and heparin, which can be used as a bridge to oral anticoagulation of choice.
- Other antiplatelet agents, such as clopidogrel or dipyridamole, have also been used [164, 167, 177].

Following the identification and characterization of the offending lesion, definitive treatment

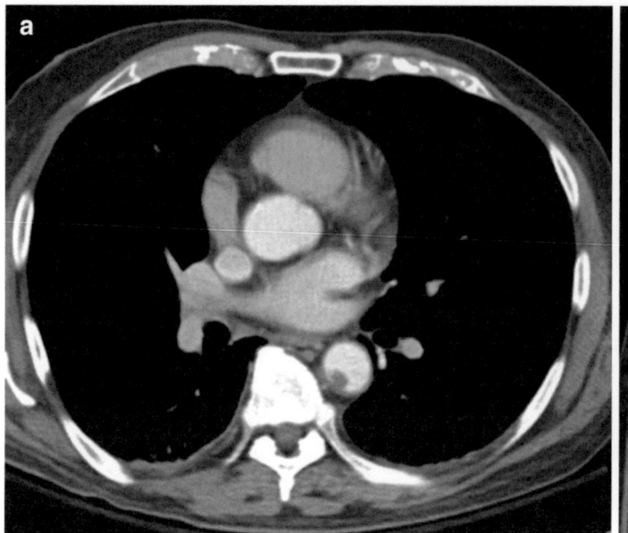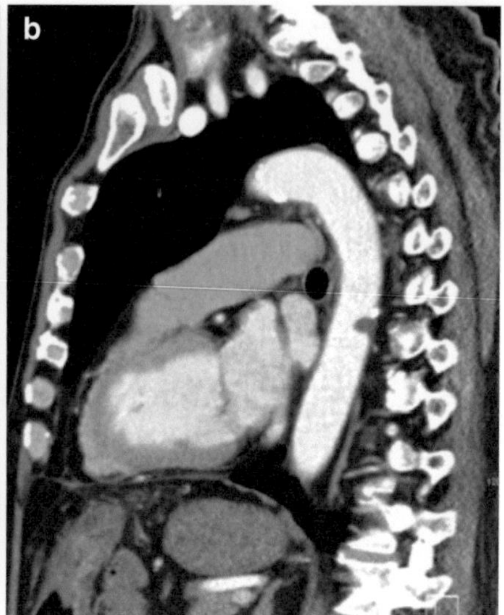

Fig. 6.67 (**a**) Axial and (**b**) sagittal views of a computed tomography angiogram of the thoracic aorta demonstrating an irregular adherent plaque in a patient presenting with renal infarcts and tissue loss involving the bilateral feet. The remainder to the patient's aorta and lower extremity arteries did not demonstrate suspicious lesions to account for the emboli

can be performed via an endovascular or surgical approach.

- Thoracic and abdominal aortic syndromes are typically treated via an endovascular approach, if possible. A stent graft is utilized, excluding the offending lesion, whether it be eccentric mural thrombus in an aneurysm, adherent aortic thrombus, or a penetrating ulcer (Fig. 6.69).
- Femoropopliteal aneurysms, however, are usually treated surgically with ligation and bypass, although endovascular options with stent grafting are also possible in appropriate candidates.

Atherosclerotic lesions with friable plaques are now most exclusively treated via an endovascular approach. In most cases, a bare metal stent or stent graft is utilized to stabilize and exclude the lesion [178]. Adjunctive therapies such as atherectomy and thrombectomy can also be utilized with caution [167, 177, 179–181]. Embolic protection devices can be used to prevent further embolization during various endovascular therapies (Fig. 6.70). Surgical options still include endarterectomy or bypass to isolate and exclude the source of emboli.

If severe tissue loss and gangrene are present, amputation is often necessary to prevent further complications. Healing of the surgical wound in these limb salvage cases is particularly likely in patients who have undergone treatment of the underlying disease. Following surgical treatment, medical treatment with anticoagulation and anti-platelets is continued throughout the patient's lifetime.

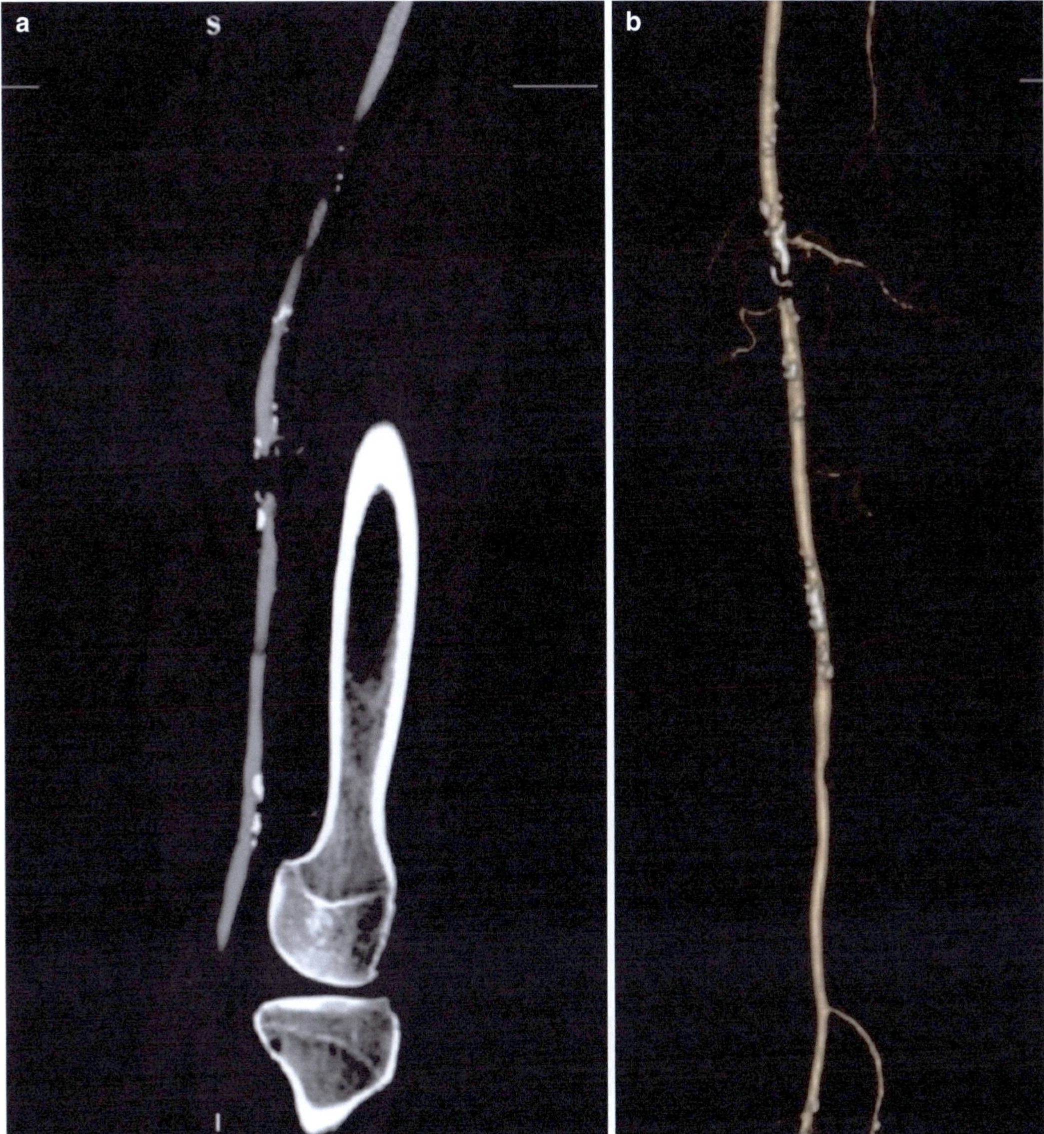

Fig. 6.68 (a) Coronal reformatted images from a computed tomography angiogram (CTA) and (b) 3-dimensional (3D) reconstruction of the same segment demonstrating a focal occlusion of the distal superficial femoral artery, in a patient presenting with blue toe syndrome. Case courtesy by Dr. Alok Bhatt and Dr. Gregg Khodorov

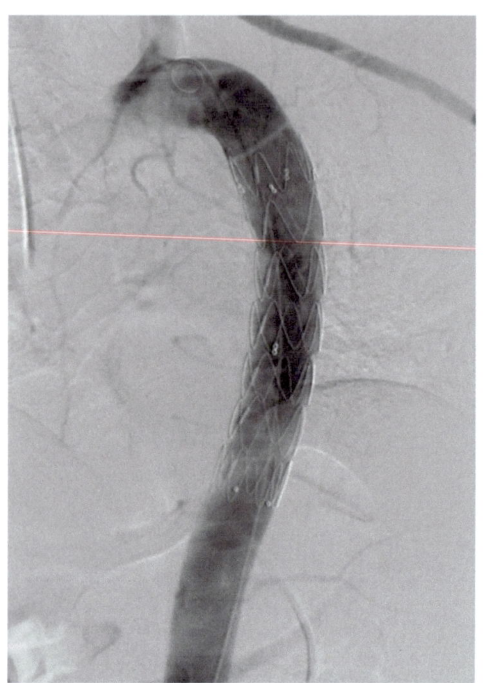

Fig. 6.69 Thoracic aortic endograft placement for treatment of an irregular aortic plaque resulting in peripheral embolization

6.14 Drug-Eluting Technology

Aishwarya Raja and Eric Secemsky

6.14.1 Paclitaxel: Where Are We Now?

6.14.1.1 Introduction to Paclitaxel

Endovascular therapy utilizing traditional uncoated percutaneous transluminal angioplasty (PTA) and bare metal stents (BMS) has been shown to have a restenosis rate as high as 40–60% by 1 year [182]. Inspired by the success of drug-coated devices in percutaneous coronary intervention, researchers have used paclitaxel, a highly lipophilic compound with rapid uptake into tissues and long-term anti-proliferative effects on vascular smooth muscle cells and fibroblasts, to coat peripheral balloons and stents and halt the restenotic process [183].

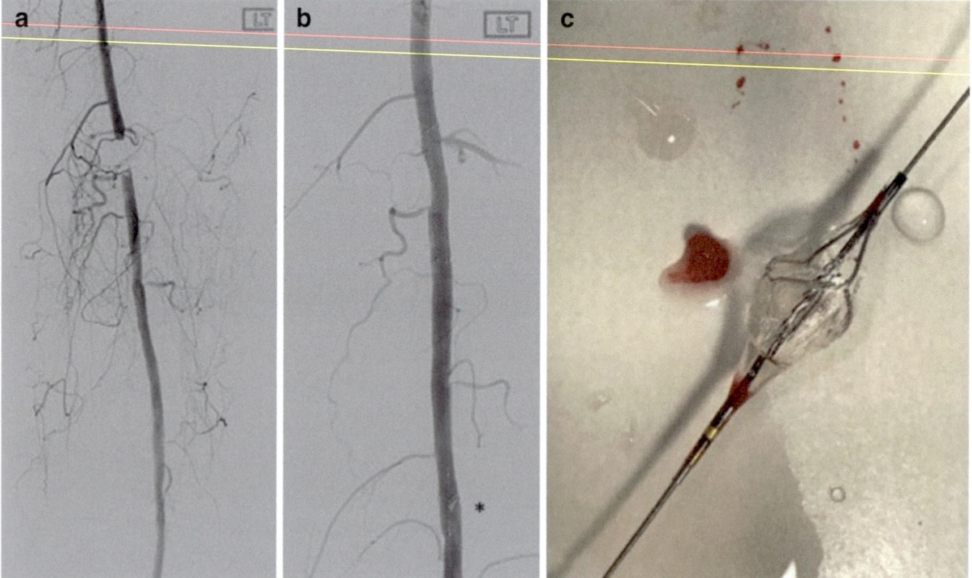

Fig. 6.70 (**a**) Preintervention angiogram of a focal occlusion in a patient with ipsilateral blue toe syndrome (CTA shown in Fig. 6.4); (**b**) endovascular recanalization of the occlusion with angioplasty followed by bare metal stent placement, utilizing a distal embolization protection device (EPD,*) during treatment; (**c**) physical examination of the EPD demonstrates a tiny embolus which is an example of the friability of the offending lesions seen this syndrome. Case courtesy of Dr. Alok Bhatt and Dr. Gregg Khodorov

- The characteristics of paclitaxel make it particularly suitable for use in femoropopliteal artery disease, which is characterized by aggressive atherosclerosis and calcification over a long arterial segment.
- Paclitaxel-coated devices (PCDs) have since emerged as the standard therapy in endovascular revascularization.
- Their use as the definitive treatment of femoropopliteal disease is supported by SCAI consensus guidelines for device selection and the ACC/AHA/SCAI/SIR/SVM Appropriate Use Criteria for Peripheral Artery Intervention [184, 185].

6.14.1.2 Overview of Paclitaxel-Coated Balloons

A scaffold-free approach utilizing balloon angioplasty is often the preferred treatment for the treatment of femoropopliteal artery disease. This is primarily due to the anatomy of this arterial segment, which is uniquely subject to various mechanical stresses, including flexion–extension and torsion. As a result, permanent stents are more prone to in-stent restenosis, displacement, and fracture. Paclitaxel-coated balloons (PCBs) provide the added advantage over other devices of allowing for rapid paclitaxel delivery and arterial wall absorption during a single application, with long-lasting effect on restenosis without necessitating the placement of a scaffold [183, 186].

- The FDA has approved four paclitaxel-coated balloons for femoropopliteal artery disease: the IN.PACT Admiral DCB, the LUTONIX DCB, the Ranger DCB, and the Stellarex DCB. The benefits of PCBs over traditional PTA have been shown in multiple randomized controlled trials (RCTs).
- Tepe *et al.* were the first to compare a PCB to uncoated PTA in a multicenter trial consisting of 48 patients with superficial femoral and popliteal artery disease. The investigators found significant reductions in late lumen loss (0.4 ± 1.2 mm vs 1.7 ± 1.8 mm, $p < 0.001$) and target lesion revascularization (TLR) (4% vs 29%, $P < 0.001$) at 6 months, with findings persisting at 24 months [187].

- Rosenfield *et al.* subsequently compared the Lutonix PCB and non-drug-coated PTA in a larger sample of patients with femoropopliteal artery disease (476 patients at 54 sites) and demonstrated increased primary patency at 12 months (9). Similar findings have been reported in other RCTs with endpoints of 6–24 months [188–190].
- RCTs with longer follow-up periods of 5 years include the THUNDER trial and the IN.PACT SFA trial, in which Schneider et al. found that PCBs had a higher rate of freedom from TLR (Kaplan–Meier estimate of 74.5% vs 65.3%, log-rank $P = 0.02$) among 331 patients with symptomatic femoropopliteal artery lesions [191, 192].

It is important to note that all these initial RCTs primarily compared PCBs to PTA in less complicated lesions (i.e., those less than 10 cm in length with low rates of chronic total occlusions and in-stent restenosis). Since approval, both post-hoc prospective and retrospective analyses have also demonstrated the superiority of PCBs over PTA for more complicated lesions, as well as for patients at higher restenotic risk, including those with advanced PAD (Rutherford 4 and greater) and ages over 75 [193–195]. Overall, the existing evidence supports the benefits of PCBs compared to PTA for patients with femoropopliteal artery lesions over a period of 5 years.

6.14.1.3 Overview of Paclitaxel-Coated Stents

Although balloon angioplasty is often preferred when treating femoropopliteal artery disease, stenting may be selected in certain situations, including for higher complexity lesions, longer lesion lengths, or in the presence of flow-limiting dissections. The FDA has approved two paclitaxel-eluting stents (PESs) for femoropopliteal artery disease: the Zilver PTX and the Eluvia stent. These stents differ in their coating, with the Eluvia stent containing a polymer coating that delivers paclitaxel over a longer period of time, whereas the Zilver PTX stent lacks a polymer. Several RCTs have compared PES with PTA and BMS.

- In a prospective, multicenter RCT, Dake *et al.* randomized 474 patients to PES or PTA; patients who experienced initial PTA failure were subsequently randomized to PES or BMS. The investigators found that initial PES use was associated with higher event-free survival (86.6% vs 77.9%, $P = 0.02$) and patency rates (74.8% vs 26.5%, $P < 0.01$) compared to PTA at 2 years [196].

- In the secondary randomization group, PES was found to have a higher patency rate (83.4% vs 64.1%, $P < 0.01$) compared to BMS. These findings persisted at 5 years.

- In the Imperial trial, a RCT directly comparing Zilver PTX with Eluvia, researchers found the Eluvia PES to be non-inferior to Zilver PTX, although primary patency rates were significantly higher in the Eluvia group [197].

- Additional studies have studied the efficacy of using PES in more complex lesions. In a retrospective analysis of 900 patients with and without patent runoff vessels, Cipollari *et al.* found the rates of freedom from TLR and primary patency to be similar between groups [198]. Another retrospective study of 228 patients with lesions greater than 10 cm in length found that the patency and TLR rates were comparable between PES and PCB at 12 months [199].

- Finally, Bausbeck *et al.* randomly assigned 150 patients with lesions of different lengths and complexity (average lesion length 15 cm, more than half chronic total occlusions) to primary PES or PCB plus bailout stenting over a follow-up time of 36 months [200]. They found comparable effectiveness and safety between these devices at 12 months, with a nonsignificant trend favoring PES at 36 months.

6.14.1.4 Safety of Paclitaxel-Coated Devices

Despite their significant growth and demonstrated superiority in large-scale studies, the long-term safety of these devices eventually came under question. In December 2018, Katsanos et al. published a meta-analysis of randomized clinical trials comparing PCD and non-PCD (PTA/BMS) cohorts and reported a 68% increased risk of mortality at 24 months and a 93% increased risk of mortality at 4–5 years for patients treated with PCDs [201]. They also showed a positive association between the dose of paclitaxel and absolute mortality risk. The publication of this meta-analysis created major ripples in the vascular community. Although PCDs were allowed to remain on the market, the Food and Drug Administration (FDA) issued warnings about the possibility of increased mortality associated with PCDs and recommended their use be restricted to high-risk patients.

- Two major clinical trials (SWEDEPAD 1,2 and BASIL-3) were subsequently halted.

- The FDA convened a large panel to review the available evidence surrounding PCDs. Katsanos *et al.*'s meta-analysis drew criticism for its methodological flaws and biases. This included a significant amount of missing data after endpoints were reached in each RCT, the inclusion of heterogeneous populations with differing baseline characteristics in the pooled RCTs, the lack of an established mechanism for paclitaxel-related mortality, and the variable methods used for paclitaxel coating among devices included in the dose–response analysis.

6.14.1.5 Paclitaxel Dosing and Potential Mechanisms of Harm

At higher concentrations (average doses of 230–300 mg with a single treatment, total doses up to 1200 mg with multiple treatments), paclitaxel has been well-established as a chemotherapeutic drug [202]. It works by interfering with the dynamic reorganization of microtubules and inhibition of cell division. Lower concentrations of paclitaxel (average treatment doses ranging from 1 mg to 20 mg depending on the size of the lesion, number of lesions, and technology utilized) prevent restenosis by inhibiting the secretion of extracellular matrix and migration of smooth muscle cells and fibroblasts [166, 175].

- An important advantage of paclitaxel is that even with short exposure times, it has lasting inhibitory effects on the vasculature. In cell culture and animal models, paclitaxel exposure for 3 min inhibited cell proliferation up to 12 days, with lasting effects up to 60 days [203, 204].
- Additionally, paclitaxel is highly lipophilic and rapidly absorbed into surrounding tissues, concentrating particularly in the arterial intima.
- An important study found that paclitaxel was not detected in the plasma by 24 h after exposure to PCBs [205]. By comparison, chemotherapeutic concentrations of systemic paclitaxel remained in the plasma much longer (half-life of 21 ± 14 h) [206]. Side effects of chemotherapeutic doses of paclitaxel include neutropenia, sensory neuropathy, myalgias, myelotoxicity, cardiovascular effects, alopecia, and nausea.
- The SNAPIST I trial examined systemic nanoparticle paclitaxel administration following deployment of a BMS at doses of 10, 30, 70, and 100 mg/m [207]. Systemic side effects were only reported at the 70 mg/m^2 dose, which is higher than those delivered with FDA-approved PCDs.
- Another postulated mechanism for paclitaxel-related harm is the promotion of microenvironments for tumor growth [175]. However, when analyzing available individual-level data from RCTs, malignancies have not been shown to be a significant cause of mortality among patients receiving PCDs.
- Finally, expanding upon Katsanos *et al.*'s analysis, Schneider *et al.* published a recent study of 1980 patients from 4 prospective studies of PCB stratified into terciles by paclitaxel doses received [175].
  - They found no significant difference in all-cause mortality across terciles over the 5-year period. Additional analyses examining the association between total paclitaxel dose delivered and risk of mortality dispelled any relationship [208].

6.14.1.6   Analyses Published After the Katsanos et al. Meta-Analysis

Since Katsanos et al. published their meta-analysis in 2018, multiple studies have been conducted analyzing clinical outcomes associated with PCD use.

- Schneider *et al.* were the first to perform a survival analysis that showed no significant difference in mortality between patients receiving different doses of paclitaxel from the IN. PACT study program [175].
- Another study that pooled 4 RCTs found no differences in all-cause mortality between patients who received PCBs versus PTA at 24 months (7.9% vs 5.5%, $P = 0.317$) [209]. Multiple device-based analyses have also been performed.
- The LEVANT 2 RCT examining patients treated with the LUTONIX PCB versus PTA reported no difference in mortality at 5 years (14.3% vs 10.6%, $P = 0.198$) [170].
- Similarly, pooled data from the ILLUMENATE RCTs demonstrated no difference in all-cause mortality between 2351 patients treated with PCB versus PTA (9.3% vs 9.9%, $P = 0.93$) [173].
- The Zilver PTX trials, as well as the RANGER SFA trial, also reported similar findings when comparing PES with PTA/BMS and PCB with PTA, respectively [210].
- To further corroborate these findings, Secemsky et al. published two retrospective analyses using Medicare data.
- In the first analysis of 16,560 patients receiving PCDs versus PTA/BMS, they found a reduced all-cause mortality associated with PCDs through 600 days (32.5% vs 34.3%, $P = 0.007$) [211]. In a second analysis comparing PES with BMS among 51,456 patients, they similarly found no difference in mortality through ~4 years (51.7% vs 50.1%, log-rank P-value = 0.16) [212].

Given the growing evidence that PCDs were not associated with greater harm, the FDA convened a panel in June 2019 [213]. The FDA also conducted an internal analysis, which again replicated Katsanos *et al.*'s late mortality signal. However, they were unable to elaborate on the mechanism for paclitaxel-related harm, establish a dose-dependent relationship between paclitaxel and mortality, or confirm that any primary deaths were related to PCD use.

- At this FDA meeting, expanded observational data from over 150,000 patients were also presented by Dr. Secemsky, which demonstrated no evidence of harm associated with PCDs over ~4 years. Additional analyses presented at this meeting originated from the Optum claims database of more than 20,000 patients over 763 days, as well as the Vascular Quality Initiative Peripheral Vascular Intervention Registry of more than 8000 patients over a median of 12.4 months; these studies also showed no association between PCDs and mortality.
- Thus, the FDA panel concluded that although PCDs were associated with a signal of late harm, the mechanism or cause of mortality still remained unclear.

Since this time, several additional prospective and retrospective studies have been published, again all failing to demonstrate long-term harm associated with PTX devices.

- The SWEDEPAD study, a multicenter RCT that randomized 2289 patients to treatment with PCDs or non-coated devices, did not find a difference in mortality between groups during 1 to 4 years of follow-up [214]. This finding persisted even after stratification by intermittent claudication and critical limb-threatening ischemia.
- The VOYAGER PAD sub-analysis of over 4000 patients who underwent EVT found no association between PCDs with mortality or major adverse limb events but did show a reduction in index limb revascularization [215].
- Dihn *et al.* expanded upon the initial Katsanos *et al.* meta-analysis using additional trials and

updated duration of follow-up among those previously included. Among 34 RCTs, they found no evidence of increased risk of all-cause mortality in patients treated with PCDs during 60 months of follow-up [216].

- Finally, in the first analysis of the SAFE-PAD study examining 168,553 Medicare fee-for-service beneficiaries who underwent femoro-popliteal artery revascularization from 2015 through 2018, PCDs were found to be non-inferior for mortality compared to uncoated devices up to 5 years [217].

Figure 6.71 summarizes this updated data, as well as additional studies published since the beginning of the paclitaxel controversy. On the left of the panel, the initial pivotal studies where the harm signal had been detected are shown. Note the attenuating harm signal with inclusion of patients who had been initially missing from follow-up. On the right are both prospective and retrospective studies, none of which have reproduced the harm signal.

6.14.1.7 Conclusions

PCDs offer many key advantages over non-coated devices, including reduced rates of restenosis and clinically driven TLR. However, after a 2018 meta-analysis demonstrated a late mortality signal, there has concerned about the safety of these devices among the vascular community. While it is reassuring that the harm signal has not been replicated in both prospective and retrospective studies, restrictions on PCD use remain in place by the FDA. With new data in hand and the usage of these devices again rising, it is time to reconsider the regulatory action against these devices.

6.14.2 Unmet Needs: Future of Limus-Based Therapy

6.14.2.1 Introduction to Limus-Based Therapy

Paclitaxel-coated devices are widely considered the standard restenotic agent in endovascular therapy (EVT) for peripheral arterial disease

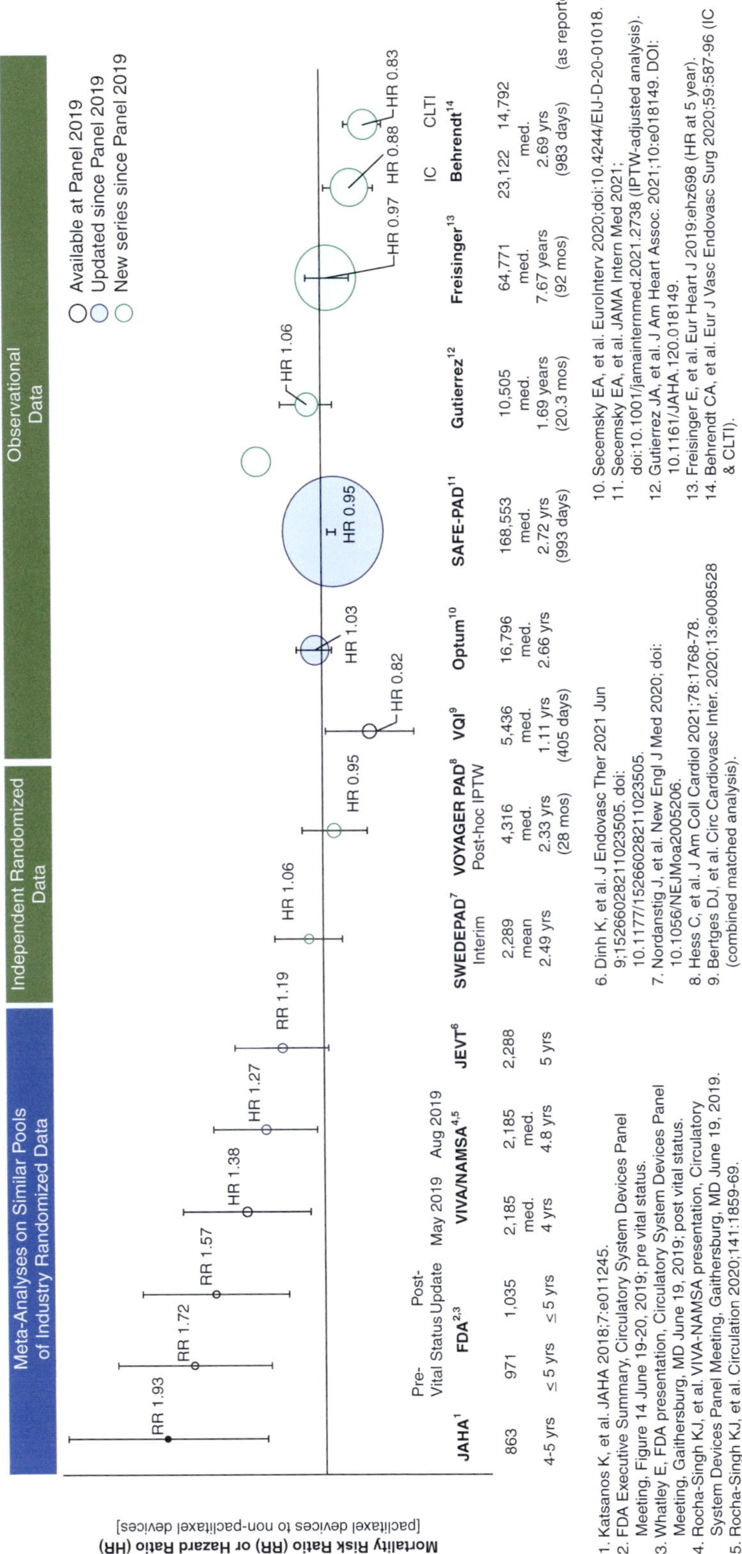

Fig. 6.71 Summary of updated data since publication of Katsanos et al.'s meta-analysis where the initial harm signal has not been reproduced

(PAD). However, against the backdrop of potential harm associated with PCDs, alternative antiproliferative agents are now being explored. Limus-based agents have emerged as a viable option based on their inherent properties and demonstrated efficacy in coronary intervention. This chapter will review the current landscape of limus-based therapies, as well as future directions for these emerging peripheral devices.

6.14.2.2 Differences between Paclitaxel and Limus-Based Compounds

There are significant differences between paclitaxel and limus-based compounds that impact their utilization in peripheral devices.

- First, comparing their mechanism of action, paclitaxel is cytotoxic and works by irreversibly binding to microtubules [218]. This leads to persistent effects on vascular cells, as well as higher potential for toxicity to non-target tissues.
- By comparison, limus-based agents are cytostatic, reversibly binding to the FK506-binding protein and forming a complex with the mammalian target of rapamycin, which results in blocking cell cycle progression [218]. This property ensures that therapeutic tissue levels are maintained over time. Additionally, limus agents have been shown to have a greater effect on preventing restenosis and inflammation, including preventing neutrophilic leukocyte activation and transmigration [219].
- Limus compounds have a wider therapeutic range compared with paclitaxel-coated balloons also making it a desirable agent for endovascular devices [220, 221].
- The primary drawbacks of utilizing limus agents include their relative hydrophilicity, which makes their absorption into tissue and elution from devices more difficult compared to paclitaxel [218]. Limus agents are also less stable and more likely to undergo biologic degradation, thus requiring the drug to be protected following release. These differences are summarized in Table 6.5.

Table 6.5 Differences between paclitaxel and limus-based restenotic agents

Characteristic	Paclitaxel	Limus
Mechanism of action	Cytotoxic	Cytostatic
Margin of safety	Lower	Higher
Tissue absorption and elution	Easier (more lipophilic)	More difficult (more hydrophilic)
Biologic degradation	Lower	Higher
Effect on preventing restenosis	Moderate	Optimal
Therapeutic range	Narrower	Broader

6.14.2.3 Limus-Based Therapy for Coronary Revascularization

Limus-based therapies have become the agent of choice for coronary stents, replacing initial paclitaxel-based stents. The RAVEL trial is one among many RCTs that found superior outcomes associated with limus-based stents, including decreased neointimal proliferation, restenosis, stent thrombosis, and major cardiac events, when compared to BMS use in native coronary arteries [222].

6.14.2.4 Prior Unsuccessful Attempts at Applying Limus-Based Therapy in the Peripheral Endovascular Intervention

Despite the success of limus-based therapies in coronary vessels, applications in the superficial femoral artery have been largely unsuccessful.

- The STRIDES trial, a prospective, non-randomized, multicenter study, evaluated the use of a Dynalink everolimus-eluting stent in 104 patients with symptomatic PAD [223, 224]. Although demonstrating a low restenosis rate of 6% at 6 months, the rate rose to 32% at 12 months, which was much greater than comparator drug-coated devices. Thus, this device was not marketed for use in the United States.
- The SIROCCO randomized controlled trial (RCT) compared a sirolimus-eluting stent with its respective bare metal stent (BMS) counterpart and reported similar findings [224]. After achieving improved patency with

the sirolimus stent at 6 months, the follow-up SIROCCO II trial reported no significant difference in outcomes between groups at 18 months [225, 226].

- Given these disappointing findings, both devices were subsequently abandoned. It is postulated that these differences may be in part due to the inherent differences between the coronary and peripheral vasculatures.
- The femoropopliteal segment faces greater plaque burden and complex mechanical forces across a longer, more elastic, and larger-caliber surface [227]. The time course of femoropopliteal restenosis is also more delayed than its coronary counterpart. Thus, the pharmacokinetics and pharmacodynamics of drug delivery must be adapted accordingly.

6.14.2.5 Optimizing the Formulation and Pharmacokinetics of Limus-Based Therapy

To overcome the challenges discussed above and to achieve therapeutic concentrations of limus-based compounds in the peripheral vascular wall, research has focused on modifying the mode of drug delivery and/or the drug itself. Recent innovation has centered on utilizing nanoparticles to encapsulate sirolimus to improve delivery to target tissues.

- The SELUTION SLR drug delivery system (MedAlliance) is a sirolimus-based drug-coated balloon coupled with four excipients, one of which is a biodegradable polymer that admixes with sirolimus to form nanoparticles that degrade in a regulated fashion [229]. Preclinical models have confirmed the presence of therapeutic levels of sirolimus after SLR application for more than 60 days. Human trials have since applied this technology in both femoropopliteal and tibial artery lesions.
- The SELUTION SFA Study was the first in-human trial to evaluate outcomes of this drug delivery system. They enrolled 50 patients with symptomatic de novo or restenotic superficial femoral artery lesions (Rutherford classes 2–3) across 4 German centers between 2016 and 2017. At 6 months, the mean angiographic late lumen loss was 0.29 ± 0.84 mm ($P < 0.001$) with the sirolimus-based system, a significant reduction from the objective performance goal of 1.04 mm for percutaneous transluminal angioplasty. They also reported significant clinical improvements in Rutherford classification, ankle-brachial index, and walking impairment at 6 months, which were further improved at 12 months and maintained at 24 months. These promising results have paved the way for an investigational device exemption RCT in the United States in the coming years.

- The MagicTouch sirolimus-coated balloon system (Concept Medical) is another nanoparticle-based therapy that received the European CE Mark approval for use in the coronary and peripheral vasculatures [230]. It has been studied in limited registries and small RCTs outside of the United States for applications such as coronary in-stent restenosis, arteriovenous fistula, and peripheral *de novo* disease [231–233].
- Due to demonstrated biological efficacy in these early studies, large-scale RCTs in Europe (SIRONA), Asia (FUTURE SFA/BTK), and the United States are forthcoming [234, 235].

In addition to drug-coated balloons, there has been a reinvestment in developing limus-based peripheral stents for femoropopliteal and tibial artery intervention [236]. For instance, the NiTiDES stent system (Alvimedica) is a device containing sirolimus formulated with an amphiphilic carrier, which is released through an abluminal reservoir technology from a BMS.

- In the first-in-human ILLUMINA trial, this device was associated with a primary patency rate of 83.4% and clinically driven target lesion revascularization rate of 6.9% at 2 years. Functional and clinical benefits were also sustained, including 82.1% of patients being classified as Rutherford category 0 or 1 by the end of the follow-up period [237].

- These results at 2 years are competitive with currently available paclitaxel-based peripheral stents.
- With regards to below-the-knee treatment, several companies are studying limus-coated scaffolds. For example, Abbott Vascular is examining the Espirit everolimus-eluting bioresorbable scaffold for patients with infrapopliteal disease and critical limb ischemia in the LIFE-BTK RCT (NCT04227899).

6.14.2.6 Conclusions

As EVT continues to dominate the peripheral space, the ubiquitous problem of achieving safe, targeted, sustained drug delivery will remain at the forefront. Future research must focus on identifying therapeutics to prevent restenosis, minimize target vessel revascularization, and accelerate the resolution of inflammation and vascular healing. Against the backdrop of concern over paclitaxel-related mortality, limus-based therapies have emerged as a potential agent that can be used to help address many of these unmet needs.

6.15 Popliteal Artery Aneurysm

Pauline Berens and Venita Chandra

6.15.1 Background

Popliteal artery aneurysms (PAAs), while rare, are the most common type of peripheral arterial aneurysm. They are most frequently of atherosclerotic origin, seen in men aged 60 or older with traditional atherosclerotic risk factors, and are associated with concomitant aortic aneurysms (38%) and contralateral PAAs (48%) [238, 239].

Symptoms
- Asymptomatic pulsating mass.
- Pain/pressure behind knee.
- Limb swelling.
- Deep venous thrombosis (DVT).
- Footdrop (from peroneal nerve compression).

- Acute or chronic limb ischemia (can be symptomatic or subclinical).
  - Up to 69% of patients present with only 0–1 patent below-knee vessels [239].

6.15.2 Identification of PAA and Indications for Surgery

- Duplex ultrasound and ankle-brachial indices (ABIs) are excellent initial diagnostic tools.
- Cross-sectional imaging with CTA/MRA or arteriogram needed for operative planning (Fig. 6.72).
- Surgical approach is very dependent on clinical evaluation, in particular the presence or absence of runoff vessels (Fig. 6.73).
- According to the recent clinical practice guidelines from the Society for Vascular Surgery (SVS), asymptomatic PAAs ≥20 mm in diameter should be repaired, with a caveat that repair can be deferred in patients with higher clinical risk until ≥30 mm in diameter, and all symptomatic PAAs should be considered for repair [240].

6.15.3 Treatment

There are three approaches to repair of PAAs: open medial, open posterior, and endovascular (Fig. 6.74). Historically, open surgical repair has been considered the gold standard treatment for PAAs.

- The medial approach involves above- and below-knee exposure, interval ligation of the aneurysm at either end and creation of a bypass around the aneurysmal segment using graft attached with end-to-side anastomoses.
- The posterior approach involves placement of the patient in the prone position and a lazy S incision followed by resection of the aneurysmal artery and reconstruction with an interposition graft using end-to-end anastomoses.
- In either approach, a single piece of vein is preferentially used for graft material, though

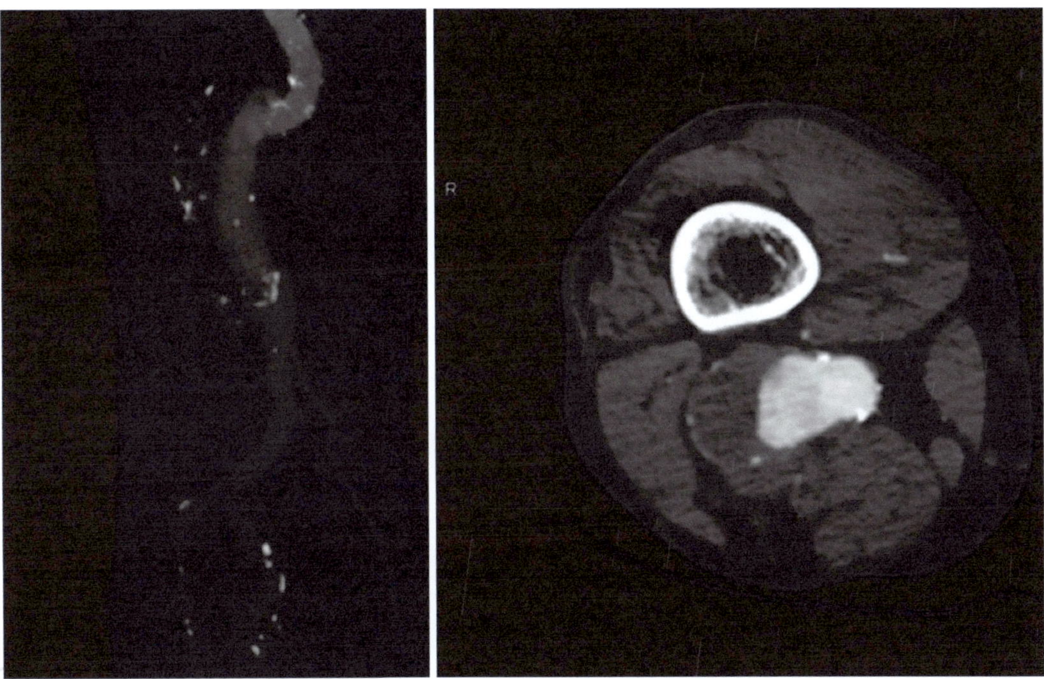

Fig. 6.72 CTA of popliteal aneurysm demonstrating important anatomical features including length, tortuosity and presence of thrombus

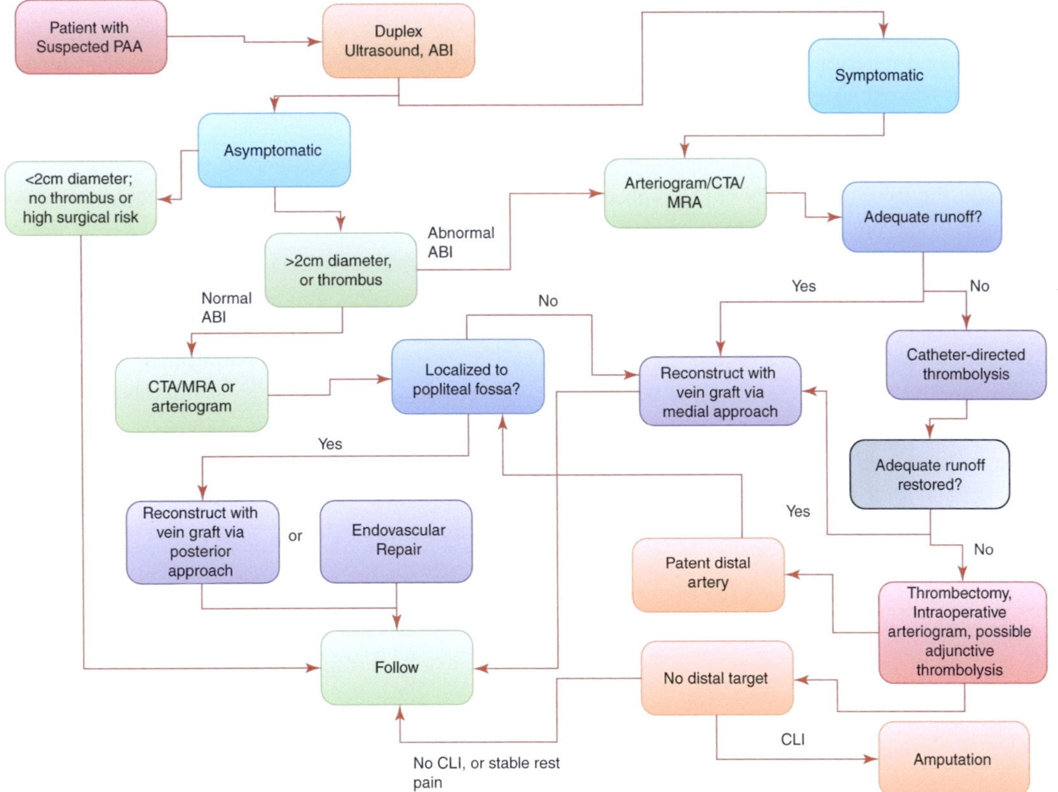

Fig. 6.73 Popliteal Artery Aneurysm Management Algorithm

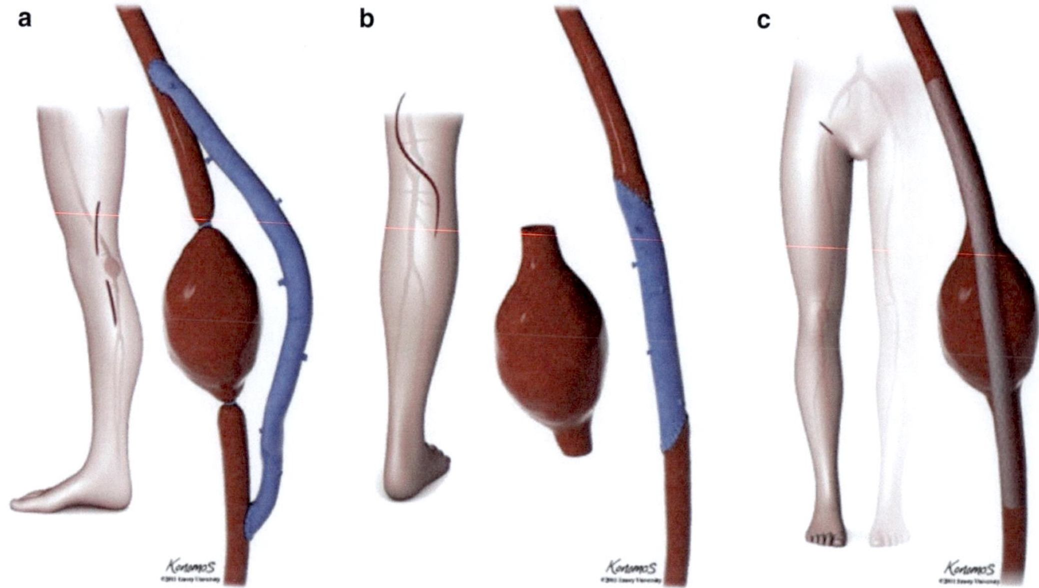

Fig. 6.74 Popliteal aneurysm repairs (**a**) medial approach, (**b**) posterior approach, (**c**) endovascular approach

prosthetic can also be used if adequate vein is not available.

A 2016 meta-analysis found the posterior approach had superior long-term primary patency and aneurysm exclusion, as well as lower rates of limb loss and reoperation. There was no significant difference in long-term secondary patency between the two approaches [241]. The authors speculate that poorer outcomes of the medial approach are in part due to side branches which are not ligated and continue to feed the aneurysm sac, risking further expansion and compression. While these results suggest superiority of a posterior approach when performing open PAA repair, they are based upon seven studies which were retrospective and observational.

Practically, the surgical approach must be tailored based on the patient's unique anatomy.

- For patients with aneurysms extending beyond the popliteal fossa, the medial approach is preferable as it provides more access to the artery.
- For patients who are having compressive symptoms, a posterior approach with complete aneurysm resection is preferable so that the compression may be relieved.

Since 1994, endovascular popliteal aneurysm repair (EPAR) is also a viable method of repairing PAAs.

- EPAR involves covering the aneurysmal section of the artery with a self-expanding covered stent graft.
- Proximal and distal landing zones of 1.5–2 mm are necessary, and adjunctive embolization of aneurysm sac branch vessels is sometimes required to minimize type II endoleak.
- Focal aneurysms are most suitable for EPAR.
- The caliber of the landing zones should be 10–20% smaller than the diameter of the stent graft and free of excessive calcification, thrombus, tortuosity, or angulation.

6.15.4 Surgery Versus Stenting

Several retrospective studies have attempted to compare outcomes of open versus endovascular PAA repair. Only one small prospective RCT

Table 6.6 Results of recent meta-analyses comparing open vs endovascular PAA repair. Equivalent means that there was no statistically significant difference in outcomes of open versus endovascular PAA repair

Recent meta-analyses	Primary patency at one year	Secondary patency at one year	Primary patency at three years	Secondary patency at three years
Leake et al. (2017)	Open > endo	Equivalent	Open > endo	Equivalent
Beuschel et al. (2022)	Open > endo	Equivalent	Equivalent	Not examined

completed in 2003, which included 15 endovascular and 15 open repairs, has directly compared these methods [242]. As such, it must be noted that current recommendations are based on this limited data. Results of two recent meta-analyses comparing outcomes of open versus endovascular approaches are summarized below (Table 6.6) [243, 244].

6.15.4.1 Current SVS Clinical Practical Guidelines

- Recommend open PAA repair for patients with a life expectancy ≥5 years and adequate greater saphenous vein (GSV).
- For patients with diminished life expectancy, recommend considering endovascular repair.
- For patients with inadequate single-segment GSV undergoing open repair, recommend using expanded polytetrafluoroethylene (ePTFE) graft [240].

6.15.4.2 Conclusion

As for most vascular surgical procedures, the decision of open versus endovascular popliteal artery aneurysm repair is a complex one that is dependent on many patient-specific factors. The current evidence directly comparing these methods is limited but favors open repair. For patients who are younger, of lower surgical risk, and have adequate GSV, open repair is the favored method. A posterior approach is preferable when anatomically appropriate, particularly in patients suffering from compressive symptoms. For older patients with significant comorbidities, who do not have compressive symptoms and have adequate landing zones, an endovascular approach is more appropriate. For patients with acute limb ischemia due to thrombosis of a PAA, thrombolysis can be used as an adjunct to open or endovascular repair.

6.16 Common Femoral Artery

6.16.1 Endovascular Versus Surgical

Ankit Mehta and Srini Tummala

6.16.1.1 Introduction

Endovascular therapies have increased over the past decade and many vascular specialists have moved to an endovascular-first strategy when dealing with superficial femoral, popliteal, and tibial artery disease. A notable exception has been common femoral artery (CFA) disease since surgical endarterectomy is the gold standard due to its relative ease and durability. However, many CTLI patients cannot undergo surgery or bypass given comorbidities, lack of suitable vein, and anatomic factors. Although several studies evaluating over 300 common femoral artery endarterectomy (CFE) patients have shown excellent primary patency (PP) rates at 5-, 10-, and 15-years follow-up, there remains a reported complication rate ranging from 6.6%–17.1% with a 3.4% 30-day mortality and a 15% combined mortality and complication rate [245–248]. As a result, less invasive endovascular options have been on the rise for treating CFA disease.

The most common endovascular intervention for CFA disease has always included plain old balloon angioplasty (POBA), but results have not been optimal [249]. More recently, advances in atherectomy, drug-coated balloons (DCBs), and drug-eluting stents (DESs) have shown improved results [250–254].

- For example, the TECCO trial which is the largest randomized controlled trial (RCT) to date, showed that stenting of CFA disease had similar outcomes at two years to that of CFE with decreased periprocedural complications and mortality [255, 256].

Despite these early successful endovascular treatment results, CFA disease is complex and difficult to treat with endovascular strategies due to several factors. These include atherosclerotic plaque that often extends from the CFA into the deep femoral artery (DFA) and proximal superficial femoral artery (SFA), heavy calcification, and biomechanical forces that occur during leg movement including axial compression, twisting, bending, and changes in length [257]. These challenges along with its location on the femoral head at a high flexion zone increase the chance for stent fracture [257].

Newer stents such as the Abbott Supera stent (Fig. 6.75), which have a high crush resistance, have shown promise in the CFA as highlighted by the ongoing prospective VMI-CFA study conducted by Deloose and his colleagues [258]. Other studies are also showing the efficacy of endovascular treatment without stents by employing atherectomy followed by DCB [251]. As a result of newer data and the rise of endovascular CFA interventions throughout the world, an understanding of the current data for endovascular and surgical treatment of the CFA is essential for vascular specialists.

6.16.1.2 CFA: Endarterectomy Data

Common femoral artery endarterectomy (CFE) is currently the gold standard for CFA atheroscle-

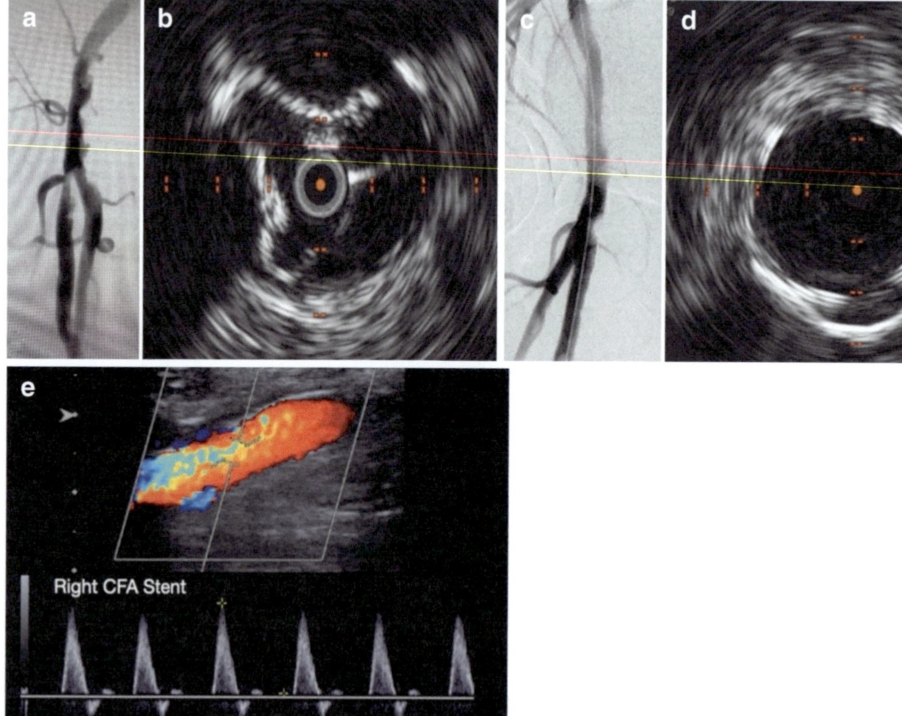

Fig. 6.75 80-yo man presents with lifestyle-limiting claudication and severe CFA disease (**a**). No improvement despite medical management and supervised exercise program. Deemed nonsurgical candidate by multidisciplinary vascular team. CFA was treated with POBA/DCB with significant recoil as seen on IVUS (**b**). After Abbott Supera stent placement, there was an excellent angiographic (**c**) and IVUS (**d**) result with resolution of the patient's symptoms. Follow-up duplex arterial ultrasound at 6 months (**e**) shows patent stent without significant ISR

rotic disease. Endarterectomy is considered to be a technically straightforward and low-risk surgery. In addition, favorable patency and long-term outcomes out to 15 years have been reported.

In 2008, Kechagias and his colleagues conducted a retrospective study involving 111 isolated endarterectomies. They reported favorable patency rates at long-term follow-up with 10- and 15-year primary patency rates of 94% and 85%, respectively. However, the study showed a high complication rate with a 9% hematoma rate, a 17.1% wound infection rate, and a 2% mortality rate [248].

A few years later, Ballotta and his colleagues reported a prospective study on CFE for isolated occlusive atherosclerotic disease in 117 patients [246]. Patients with claudication, rest pain, non-healing ulcer(s)/minor tissue loss and with imaging confirming CFA disease were enrolled. Patients with major tissue loss were excluded.

- They reported primary patency rates of 100%, 99%, 96%, and 96% at 1 year, 3 years, 5 years, and 7 years, respectively.
- Freedom from target lesion revascularization (TLR) and limb salvage (LS) at seven years was 79% and 100%, respectively, with a lower complication rate of 6.6% (mainly lymphatic leaks). No deaths were reported in this study [246].

In 2015, Dufranc and his colleagues conducted a prospective study with 121 patients using the eversion technique during CFE, differing from the studies above which used venous or prosthetic patch closure during CFE [259]. In their study of 121 patients treated with CFE, primary patency was 93% and limb salvage rate was 96% at two-year follow-up.

- They reported an overall complication rate of 8.2% and a 0% mortality rate, suggesting that the eversion technique avoided prosthetic patch complication risks such as pseudoaneurysms and anastomotic rupture [259].

In the same year, Nguyen and his colleagues conducted a retrospective study that reviewed 1843 CFEs between 2005 and 2010 using data from the National Surgical Quality Improvement Program database [260]. Their study focused on postoperative mortality and morbidity occurring before and after hospital discharge.

- They reported a 30-day mortality rate of 3.4% and a combined major complication rate and mortality rate of 15%.
- The study also highlighted an 8.4% wound complication rate with 10% of patients returning to the operating room within 30 days secondary to postoperative bleeding, thrombosis, and infected pseudoaneurysms.
- They concluded that CFE is not a "benign" procedure and careful patient selection is needed prior to CFE [260].

In 2016, Wieker et al. published their data investigating the long-term outcome of CFE in patients with PAD [261]. They retrospectively reviewed 713 vessels in 655 patients who underwent CFE in 2 high-volume centers. 221 patients had CLTI and 434 had intermittent claudication. Below-the-knee runoffs demonstrated 3 patent tibial arteries in 33% of the cohort, 2 patent in 28.3%, 1 patent in 23.4%, and 15.2% had no significant runoff. Hybrid procedures were used to treat 255 limbs (35.8%). The primary end point was PP. Secondary end points were secondary patency (SP), limb salvage, and survival. PP rates were 97%, 90%, and 79% at 6 months, 3 years, and 7 years, respectively. SP rates were 98%, 98%, and 89% at 6 months, 3 years, and 7 years, respectively. Survival rates were 93.9%, 83.0%, 74.1%, and 60.1% at 1, 3, 5, and 7 years, respectively. When PP rates were stratified for non-hybrid (78%) versus hybrid procedures (78%) and CLTI (76%) versus intermittent claudication (79%), there was no significant difference at 7-year ($P = 0.22$ and $P = 0.20$, respectively). A total of 20 major amputations were performed, achieving a limb salvage rate of 92.6%. Procedure-related complications occurred in 11.5% during 7 years of follow-up [261].

6.16.1.3 CFA: Endovascular Treatment Data

Recently endovascular treatment of CFA disease has gained popularity in the vascular community. This is in part due to the endovascular-first approach of many vascular specialists, the reported complication rate of CFE, and the need for an endovascular approach to treat patients with CFA disease who are non-operative candidates.

In 2011, Bonvini and his colleagues evaluated 360 patients with CFA atherosclerotic obstructions and reported their midterm outcomes after endovascular treatment [262]. Of these patients, only 97 patients (26.9%) had isolated CFA disease. Treatment of the CFA and DFA was performed on 93 patients (25.8%) with 60 patients (16.7%) undergoing CFA chronic total occlusions recanalization.

- Patients were treated primarily with POBA, with 36.9% of patients receiving a stent as a bailout per the operator's discretion.
- The one-year PP and TLR rates were 74% and 15.9%, respectively. Patients who received provisional stenting had an increased one-year PP rate and decreased TLR rate without an increased incidence of stent fracture assessed by ultrasound at one-year follow-up.
- Approximately 8.3% of patients had directional atherectomy which showed a trend for lower TLR, but this did not show a statistically significant benefit in terms of one-year PP rate.
- Overall technical success was 92.8% with a major and minor complication rate of 1.4% and 5.0%, respectively [262].

In the same year, Azema and his colleagues published data regarding 36 patients treated with stenting of the CFA for claudication (70%) and CLTI (30%) with mean follow-up of 22 months [263]. CFA lesions were classified into four types:

- Type I lesions involved the external iliac artery (EIA) and extended into the CFA.
- Type II lesions were limited to the CFA.

- Type III lesions involved the CFA and its bifurcation.
- Type IV represented restenosis of a bypass anastomosis.

All lesions were stented with either self-expanding stents (88.3%) or balloon-expandable stents (11.7%). Self-expanding stents included the last generation EverFlex, EV3, Paris; E. Luminexx and FlexStar, Bard, Voisins le Bretonneux. Balloon-expandable stents included Amiia, Cordis, and Issy Les Moulineaux and were used only to treat type III lesions. Primary and secondary patency with sustained clinical improvement at 1 year was 80% and 90%, respectively; TLR cumulative survival was 85% with an in-stent restenosis (ISR) rate of 20%. Only one stent fracture was noted during follow-up [263].

In 2014, Linni et al. reported their results from their RCT comparing endovascular CFA treatment with a bio-absorbable stent (BASI group) versus CFE [264]. The stent used for the study was a balloon-expandable PLLA stent (Remedy; Kyoto Medical Planning Co, Kyoto, Japan). 80 patients were included in the trial. Primary endpoint was surgical site infection, and secondary outcome measures were technical success, hemodynamic improvement, clinical improvement, patency, limb salvage, and survival. Both groups were similar in terms of demographic data, cardiovascular risk factors, and CFA occlusions.

- The BASI group had zero infections vs 7 surgical site infections in the CFE group ($P = 0.002$) and shorter hospital stay at 2 days versus 7 days for the CFE group ($P = 0.001$).
- Technical success rate was 97.5% and 100% for the BASI and CFE groups, respectively. The 30-day PP rate was 92.5% and 100% for the BASI and CFE groups, respectively ($P = 0.038$).
- At 1 year, the PP rate was 80% vs 100% (p = 0.007) and the SP rate was 84% vs. 100% ($P = 0.01$) for BASI and CFE patients, respectively.
- 1-year limb salvage was equivalent and survival rates were 88% and 90% for BASI vs. CFE patients ($P = 0.51$).

Based on these data, the authors concluded that balloon-expandable bioabsorbable stent placement is not an optimal option for CFA occlusion and is a limited option in the setting CFA stenosis. Although clinical and hemodynamic results were comparable between the endovascular and surgical groups, there was an increased rate of redo procedures in the endovascular group which outweighed the lower surgical site infection rates compared to CFE. In addition, short-term patency rates were significantly worse in patients undergoing endovascular treatment with balloon-expandable bioabsorbable stent placement.

In 2016, Nasr and his team further analyzed the Azema data at the same institution [265]. Patients were followed for 5 years in a prospectively maintained database with mean follow-up of 64 months. At 3 and 5 years, PP patency was 77% and 73%, respectively. Freedom from TLR was 79% and the ISR rate was 28% with significant predictors of ISR including DFA stenting ($P = 0.0007$) and type III lesions ($P = 0.014$). Only one stent fracture was reported in the first year of follow-up without clinical consequence.

- Based on their results Nasr and his team concluded that endovascular repair of the CFA and its bifurcation seemed to provide sustained clinical and morphological long-term results and that fear of stent fracture and local complications due to hip mobility were no longer relevant [265].

In the same year, Mehta has his colleagues published their results from a prospectively maintained multicenter database analyzing outcomes in 167 patients who underwent endovascular CFA interventions for Rutherford class 3 to class 6 disease [253]. Treatment included primary POBA, atherectomy + POBA, and stent placement only if needed. Patients were followed out to 7 years. Outcomes included technical failure rate, recurrence, complications, and major or minor amputation rates. Procedure-related complications included one pseudoaneurysm, one thrombosis, one distal embolization, and one death. CFA restenosis occurred in 34 (20%) patients who then underwent additional endovascular (18 patients) or surgical (17 patients) revascularization. Eight patients underwent major and minor amputations.

- The POBA group had a significantly lower patency rate compared to the atherectomy plus POBA group. In addition, patients who underwent provisional stenting had a 100% PP which was significantly better than the PP of the non-stented group which had a combined patency of 77% ($P = 0.0424$) [253].

In 2017, Cioppa and his colleagues prospectively evaluated 30 patients with severely calcified CFA disease [254]. They evaluated the safety, feasibility, and one-year efficacy of endovascular treatment of CFA disease using directional atherectomy (DA) and DCB with provisional stenting for suboptimal results. Procedural success was 100% with provisional stenting in 3 cases (10%). At one year, restenosis and TLR were 6.6% and 3.3%, respectively. The secondary patency rate was 96.7% [254].

Later that year, Siracuse et al. published their retrospective review of 1014 endovascular interventions of the CFA with or without DFA intervention [250]. Data from 2010–2015 were obtained from the Vascular Quality Initiative Registry. Approximately 77% of patients underwent POBA as the primary treatment, 25% of patients had stents placed, and 19.4% of patients had atherectomy. Periprocedural complications were access site hematoma (5.2%), arterial dissection (2.9%), distal embolization (0.7%), access site stenosis/occlusion (0.5%), and arterial perforation (0.6%). Survival was 92.9% at 1 year and 87.2% at 3 years. Amputation-free survival, freedom from loss of patency or death, and reintervention-free survival were 93.5%, 83%, and 87.5% at 1 year, respectively. Thirty-day mortality was 1.6%.

- Based on their analysis, the authors concluded that CFA/DFA interventions are safe with a low complication rate, but that patency was inferior to CFE. Limitations of the study were the lack of DCBs and DESs and the low rate of stenting in most cases [250].

In 2017, the TECCO trial results were published [255]. This RCT was conducted by Goueffic and his colleagues and is *the largest RCT to date comparing stenting of the CFA to CFE with or without patch*. A total of 117 patients at 17 centers with CFA atherosclerotic stenosis were randomized to stenting with the latest generation of self-expanding stents (56 patients) versus surgery (61 patients) and followed for 24 months. The majority of lesions were classified as Azema type 3.

- The primary outcome of the study, which was defined as the perioperative morbidity and mortality rate, was 12.5% (7 of 56 patients) in the stenting group and 26% (16 of 61 patients) in the surgical group ($P = 0.05$).
- There was a significant decrease in the length of hospitalization in the stenting group with an average of 3.2 days versus an average of 6.3 days in the surgical group. This difference was primarily due to paresthesias and delayed wound healing in the surgery group.
- At 24 months, the sustained clinical improvement, PP, and the TLR rates were not significantly different between the two groups. The Rutherford category and the ABI were both significantly improved at 2 years in both groups without a significant difference. There was one stent fracture without restenosis and without the need for reintervention [255].

In 2019, Deloose and his colleagues published the VMI-CFA trial results [258]. This multicenter, prospective study evaluated 100 Rutherford class 2–4 patients with symptomatic CFA disease treated with the Abbott Supera stent. All patients had de novo lesions with greater than 50% stenosis. The majority of the CFA lesions treated were Azema type 2. At 12 months, PP was 95.2% and freedom from TLR was 97.8%. At 24 months, PP was 92.8% and freedom from TLR was 97.8. There was a shift of Rutherford class 3–4 patients toward Rutherford class 0–1

sustained out to 2 years with a survival rate of 85.5%. There were no procedure or device-related adverse events.

- The authors concluded that endovascular treatment of CFA disease with the Abbott Supera stent had good outcomes and safety profile with efficacy that was comparable or higher than CFE [258]. The results of the VMI-CFA trial helped to launch the ongoing SUPERSURG RCT which will include 286 patients comparing treatment of CFA disease with the Abbott Supera stent versus CFE.

In 2020, Shammas and his colleagues published the results from their retrospective study of 89 patients (116 limbs) with CFA disease treated using endovascular techniques [256]. De novo disease was present in 70% of patients. Atherectomy (directional, orbital, rotational, and laser) was used in 104/116 limbs (89.7%), DCB in 15.5%, and stenting in 22.4% of the patients. Embolic protection devices were used in 37.9% of the limbs (Nav-6 by Abbott, 35.3%, Wirion by CSI 1.7%, SpiderFx by Medtronic 0.9%). Using Kaplan–Meier analysis, overall freedom from TLR at 2 years was 72% (50% for POBA, 0% for orbital atherectomy, 29.2% for Jetstream, 36.4% for laser, and 23.1% for SilverHawk/TurboHawk) ($P = 0.0476$). Complications included major bleeding 2.6%, distal embolization 1.7%, dissections 1.7%, and mortality 9% (none related to the procedure) with no unplanned major or minor amputations.

- The authors concluded that atherectomy was safe and successful at treating bulky, calcified, and severe atherosclerotic CFA disease [256].

Currently, the Percutaneous Intervention versus Surgery in the Treatment of Common Femoral Artery Lesions (PESTO-AFC) trial is an ongoing RCT which will enroll 306 patients and compare directional atherectomy plus DCB (stenting only if needed) with CFE with 2 -year follow-up [251].

6.16.1.4 Meta-Analysis Data (Endovascular CFA Treatment Versus CFE)

In 2020, Shammas and his colleagues conducted a meta-analysis evaluating endarterectomy and endovascular treatment for CFA disease [251]. Their meta-analysis focused on prospective studies from the past 10 years. There were 3 studies with 893 patients included for CFE and 8 studies (including the TECCO trial) with 1604 patients included for endovascular treatment of CFA disease [258]. The majority of patients in this review had Azema type II or Azema type III lesions.

CFE data analysis showed a high success rate of 93–100%, sustained PP of 93–96%, and low TLR of 9–18.3% with long-term follow-up. There was a low complication rate, although traditionally CFE is associated with wound infections, hematomas, or seromas affecting >15% of patients [246, 251].

- Analysis of the endovascular data also showed that POBA was not a favorable strategy when compared to CFE [249, 251].
- PP and TLR rates were improved with stenting in the short term (1–2 years); however, restenosis, stent fracture, and TLR favored CFE in the long term. In addition, future percutaneous access of the CFA, covering of the DFA origin, and being able to use the CFA as a future bypass target were all issues after stent placement [251].
- On the other hand, directional atherectomy followed by DCB had a favorable 1-year PP (88–90%) and TLR (6.7–11%) [251, 254].
- Overall, Shammas et al. concluded that the approach to CFA treatment (endovascular treatment vs CFE) is not straightforward and should be a shared decision between the physician and their patient. While endovascular treatment and CFE were comparable in PP and TLR in the short term, CFE was favored over endovascular treatment in the long term. Limitations of the meta-analysis included single-center CFE studies and possible selection bias since all operations were performed by experienced surgeons [251].

In 2021, Bouffi et al. conducted a meta-analysis of endovascular treatment versus open repair for CFA disease [266]. They identified all studies from 2000 to 2018 which reported endovascular treatment (ET), CFE, and comparisons of both techniques. Outcomes measured were 30-day mortality, morbidity, reintervention rates, midterm patency, late reintervention, and restenosis rates. 28 studies were included: 12 ET (1900 patients), 14 CFE (1920 patients), and 2 comparative RCTs (197 patients).

- In the non-comparative studies, the ET cohort had an overall PP of 81.9%, 77.8%, and 75.1% at 1, 2, and 3 years, respectively.
- In the CFE cohort, the overall PP was 93.4%, 91.4%, and 90.5% at 1, 2, and 3 years, respectively. At mean follow-up of 24 months for the ET group and 66 months for the CFE group, the restenosis rate was 14.4% and 4.7%, respectively, with a stent fracture rate of 3.6% [266].
- In the comparative studies, there was no significant difference in 30-day mortality or reintervention rates, but there was decreased 30-day morbidity after ET. At 1 year, the PP and late reintervention rates did not differ between ET and CFE [266].
- Based on these data, the authors concluded that although the PP rate between ET and CFE was comparable in the first year, the long-term PP rate of CFE was much greater. Therefore, ET of CFA disease still required further definition [266]. Limitations of the meta-analysis included a non-consistent methodology of patency in both groups, the fact that newer endovascular treatments were not used in many of the studies, only 2 of the studies were prospective, and 9 of the 14 studies failed to report restenosis or reintervention rates [266].

Of note, there has been growing usage of Lithotripsy in calcified CFA disease which may offset some of the concerns of significant dissections and need for scaffolds, as when utilized appropriately, the increased vessel compliance and subsequent low-pressure PTA may allow use of drug-coated balloons in this critical region. This will require further proper evaluation.

6.16.1.5　Conclusion

While there are favorable limited short-term data regarding endovascular treatment options of CFA disease, long-term outcome data are lacking. Ongoing RCTs including SUPERSURG and PESTO-AFC will add to the growing body of evidence, but given long-term data showing favorable PP, TLR, and efficacy beyond a decade, CFE is still the gold standard for treating CFA disease.

6.16.2　When I Prefer Surgery

Ahmed Kayssi

You are assessing an elderly patient with left leg rest pain and a non-healing forefoot wound. The patient is frail but high-functioning and has a history of end-stage renal disease, diabetes, and hypertension. A Doppler ultrasound study demonstrates a high-grade stenotic lesion in the distal left common femoral artery (CFA), but no other hemodynamically significant arterial lesions in the left lower extremity. A CT angiogram demonstrates the left CFA lesion shown in Fig. 6.76.

There are no other relevant findings on CT. What are your options for managing this patient? If you intervene on the CFA lesion, would you attempt an endovascular approach or arrange for open operative repair?

6.16.2.1　Why Is the Treatment of the CFA Controversial?

The management of CFA disease is a topic that continues to animate vascular specialists and generate much excitement and debate [267–270]. While a more in-depth exploration of this topic will be detailed in the following chapter, it may be useful to go over some of the unique features of the CFA that often make vascular surgeons favor surgical rather than endovascular treatment:

1. The groin is a dynamic area with significant potential for crushing an implanted stent. Flexion and extension of the hip place significant forces on the distal external iliac artery and increase the risk of stent fracture and crushing.
   - (a) Recent studies have shown that the CFA is not mobile and as such may not be subject to as many forces as previously thought [271, 272].
   - (b) However, stents in the CFA will often also include the distal external iliac artery,

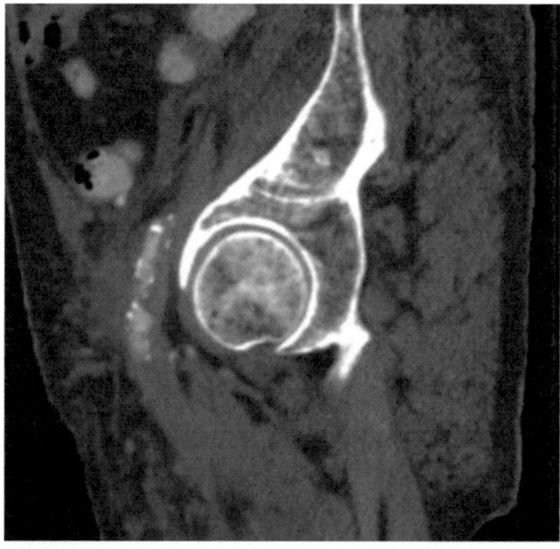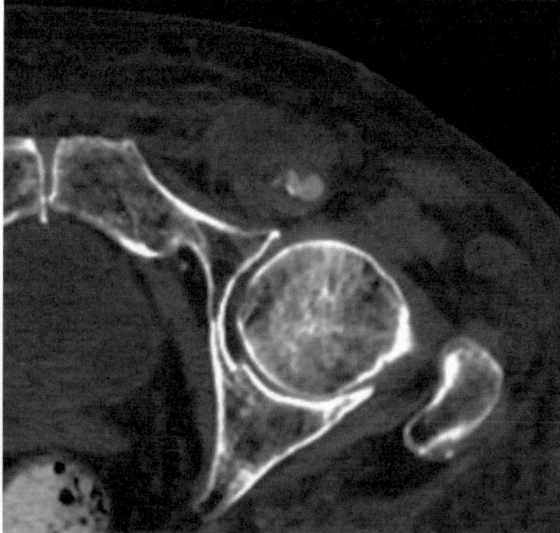

Fig. 6.76 Sagittal and axial plane CT angiogram images of the left common femoral artery demonstrating significant arterial stenosis in a patient with left leg rest pain and a non-healing left forefoot wound

placing them at increased risk of fracture or thrombosis.

2. Surgical repair of any blood vessel requires proximal and distal control. The proximal control of the CFA can be challenging, especially when the distal external iliac artery needs to be clamped because of an occluded stent in the CFA. External iliac artery exposure often requires division of the inguinal ligament and significant retraction that places the patient at an increased risk of complications such as bleeding, vessel re-occlusion, and femoral hernia formation.

3. Acute occlusion of both the superficial femoral and profunda femoris arteries due to CFA dissection post-angioplasty, or a thrombosed CFA stent, significantly increases the risk of catastrophic and irreversible limb ischemia that may lead to limb loss if not treated promptly.

4. The CFA is the most common inflow origin for lower extremity bypass procedures. A stent in the CFA will make it more challenging to use artery for future bypass procedures.

6.16.2.2 When Do I Operate on CFA Disease?

Most commonly, a CFA arterioplasty or patch angioplasty is performed in the following cases:

1. CFA bleeding, pseudoaneurysm, or occlusion as a complication of endovascular therapy or aortoiliac dissection that extends into the CFA.

2. Lower extremity rest pain, night pain, or tissue loss/ulceration with significant ipsilateral CFA disease.

3. In conjunction with other inflow or outflow surgery such as aortic or iliac bypass or popliteal or tibial bypass.

4. Blunt or penetrating trauma to the CFA.

6.16.2.3 What Is My Approach to Surgery on the CFA?

With the exception of hemodynamically unstable patients with severe and life-threatening active medical issues, the majority of patients should be able to tolerate a groin cutdown and CFA repair. In select patients, it can even be performed under local anesthetic with conscious sedation.

The most challenging aspect of CFA surgery is exposure of the proximal CFA and distal external iliac artery due to the reasons previously mentioned. Sometimes, the inguinal ligament needs to be divided and the distal external iliac artery is challenging to clamp due to significant atherosclerotic plaque burden.

Once the proximal CFA or distal external iliac artery is clamped, the distal CFA or the proximal superficial femoral and profunda femoris arteries are then clamped for distal control. An arterioplasty is then performed with prolene sutures if the CFA is bleeding from a small arteriotomy site, or an endarterectomy and patch angioplasty are performed if there is significant plaque burden or the defect in the artery is large. The types of patches available include autologous superficial or deep vein, synthetic (e.g., Polytetrafluoroethylene or Dacron), bovine pericardium, and biologic extracellular matrix. Some vascular surgeons prefer the eversion endarterectomy technique that does not require patch placement [273].

In some cases, such as when it is not possible to remove an occluded or crushed stent, the CFA needs to be bypassed with a graft that connects the distal external iliac artery to the superficial femoral and profunda femoris arteries.

6.16.2.4 What Is the Postoperative Patient Management After CFA Repair?

Depending on patient factors such as body habitus, redo surgery status, and comorbidities such as malnutrition or diabetes, an incisional negative pressure therapy system can be placed on the groin to prevent wound complications [274]. Patients are encouraged to ambulate early and are often discharged home the following day if there are no other active medical or surgical reasons to keep them admitted to hospital. Complications after CFA repair include bleeding, infection, wound dehiscence, and CFA restenosis [275–277].

A typical surveillance protocol after femoral endarterectomy includes a Doppler ultrasound study at 2–4 weeks with the first postoperative clinic visit and then surveillance every 6–12 months with Doppler ultrasound studies.

6.17 The Solo Profunda

Mohamed Nagi, Alison Maringo, and Michele Richard

The profunda femoris artery plays a crucial role in maintaining the viability of the lower extremity. Profunda circulation is frequently spared, even in the setting of severe obliterative disease of both the aortoiliac and femoropopliteal arterial segments. It can serve as an outflow target for suprainguinal bypass and an inflow source for infrainguinal bypass. This chapter will go over indications, techniques, and outcomes of open surgical revascularization of the profunda femoris artery.

6.17.1 Anatomy

The profunda femoris artery (PFA) originates approximately 2 to 5 cm distal to the inguinal ligament as one of two major terminal branches of the common femoral artery (CFA). It arises lateral or posterolateral from the CFA and courses posterolateral and inferior to the sartorius muscle [278].

The PFA has three main branches: medial circumflex femoral artery, lateral circumflex femoral artery, and first through fourth perforating arteries. The PFA terminates in the lower third of the thigh in its fourth perforating branch. Based on its main branches, the PFA can be divided into three anatomical zones (Fig. 6.77):

1. The proximal zone extends from the origin of the PFA to the origin of the lateral circumflex femoral artery.
2. The middle zone extends from the lateral circumflex femoral artery to the second perforating branch lying within the distal femoral triangle.
3. The distal zone extends beyond the second perforating branch, lying distal to the apex of the femoral triangle [278].

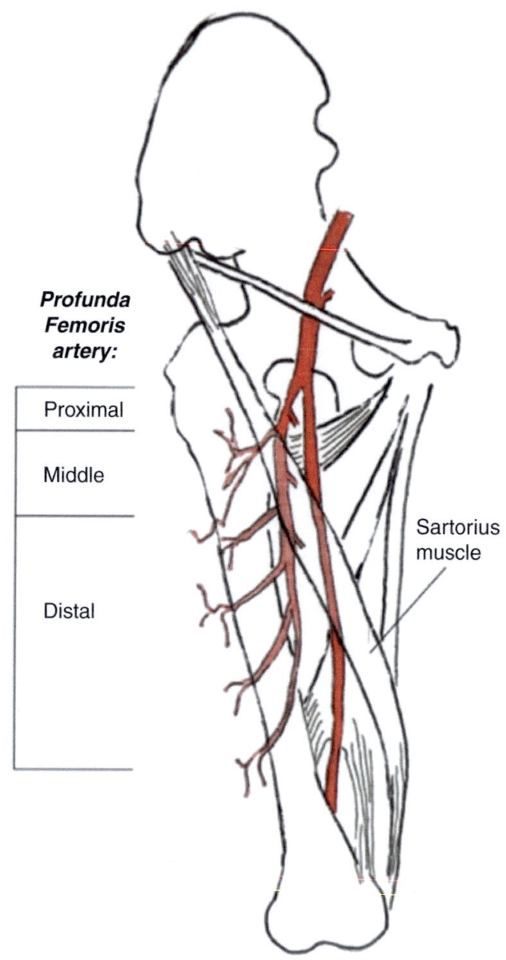

Fig. 6.77 Anatomical division of the profunda femoris artery based on its main perforating branches

6.17.1.1 Surgical Exposure

Conventional Approach
The conventional approach is used to expose the proximal part of PFA. This exposure is useful for common groin procedures, such as femoral endarterectomy and bypass inflow/outflow anastomoses.

The CFA is exposed distal to the inguinal ligament, and dissection is continued to the femoral bifurcation, where the PFA is identified on the lateral or posterior-lateral side of the CFA. The surgeon needs to identify the lateral femoral circumflex vein that crosses the anterior surface of PFA; this vein should be suture-ligated and divided for more distal PFA exposure. Further visualization of the PFA may require division of other crossing veins and lateral retraction of the sartorius muscle [278].

Lateral Approach

The lateral exposure technique allows exposure of the middle and distal zones of PFA. It is helpful when dealing with a redo groin with extensive scar tissue or the presence of infection at the proximal femoral level. It can also be used when a more distal inflow site is necessary to accommodate limited length of venous conduit.

The incision is made parallel to the sartorius muscle, on either the medial or lateral side of the sartorius, depending on the exposure needed based on vessel patency and/or conduit choice. The sartorius muscle is retracted, exposing the dense connective tissue membrane extending from the adductor longus to the vastus medialis. This membrane is longitudinally incised to expose the middle zone PFA. If more distal PFA exposure is required, the adductor longus muscle is divided [278].

Posterior Approach

This approach exposes the middle and distal zones of the PFA.

This unusual and rare exposure is needed when the standard anterior approach is high risk, as in cases of extensive scarring, multiple redo surgeries, infection, or other anatomical/surgical contraindications.

The posterior approach to the PFA is performed with the patient in the prone position. A longitudinal incision is made lateral to the hamstring muscle group, and the muscles are retracted medially in the plane between the biceps femoris and vastus lateralis. The adductor magnus is incised longitudinally, and the adductor brevis is also divided, exposing the PFA. Especially in cases of infection, the adductor longus and its fascial plane should be preserved and not divided, as this isolates the current surgical field from contamination within the subsartorial canal [279].

6.17.2 Profundoplasty

6.17.2.1 Indications

The PFA provides the primary blood supply to the tissues of the thigh and distal leg via genicular collaterals and thus is the most critical collateral vessel in the setting of superficial femoral artery (SFA) occlusion. Atherosclerosis of the PFA is usually focal, involving the origin and the very proximal portion of the artery and sparing the rest of the vessel. This focal atherosclerotic disease can be removed and treated with profundoplasty. An isolated profundaplasty can improve inflow to the lower leg in patients with claudication or rest pain [280]. Adequate profunda perfusion is essential in healing major amputations, specifically below-knee amputations. Thus, by preserving the knee joint, profundoplasty can also result in a high degree of functional rehabilitation for these patients [281].

- However, isolated profundoplasty is not the ultimate revascularization in all vascular patients.

- In patients with critical limb ischemia and significant tissue loss, profundaplasty alone without a concomitant distal bypass is insufficient to provide adequate pulsatile inline flow to the foot.
- Therefore, in certain vascular patients, additional revascularization procedures should be performed on a case-by-case basis [280].

The likelihood of success after profunda intervention can be indirectly measured using the profunda popliteal collateral index (PPCI).

The PPCI indirectly assesses the amount of collateral flow between the profunda and popliteal arteries. With a robust collateral network, improving the profunda perfusion can improve the perfusion to the popliteal artery and more distal vessels, whereas in patients with poorly developed collaterals, increasing the perfusion via the profunda will not significantly impact popliteal/tibial perfusion.

The PPCI is calculated using segmental pressures above and below the knee:

$$PPCI = (AKSP - BKSP) / BKSP$$

where AKSP is above-knee segment pressure, and BKSP is below-knee segment pressure.

A PPCI greater than 0.5 indicates poor collateral development and likely failure of a stand-alone profundaplasty. A PPCI less than 0.2 shows significant collateral formation and likely a good response to stand-alone profundaplasty [282].

6.17.2.2 Technique

Profundaplasty is typically performed in conjunction with femoral endarterectomy. The various techniques will be discussed briefly.

The femoral vessels are exposed (see previous sections), and the SFA, PFA, and CFA vessels are clamped after systemic anticoagulation. A longitudinal arteriotomy is initiated in the mid-CFA and extended proximally toward the external iliac artery (until a soft patent vessel is encountered). The minutia of femoral endarterectomy will not be discussed here. The distal endpoint of the arteriotomy can be extended onto either the SFA or PFA. The PFA should be selected in cases where the SFA is chronically occluded, and PPCI suggests improved distal perfusion with profunda intervention. The arteriotomy onto the PFA should continue until a healthy/patent vessel is identified.

Endarterectomy is then performed, and the plaque is removed from the CFA. The PFA plaque is addressed carefully, where the plaque terminates in a thin, feathered endpoint. Any loose flap is trimmed sharply and/or tacked down with 7–0 Prolene sutures.

The method of arteriotomy closure has many variations. The selection of closure method is influenced by the occlusive pathology, indications for revascularization, and surgeon experi-ence. If a patch closure method is chosen, the patch can be made of Bovine pericardium, Dacron, autogenous vein, or a piece of endarterectomized occluded SFA segment. The latter two are the preferred patch materials in the setting of an infected field. The most common closure methods are summarized below. The ultimate decision in selecting the patch method comes down to surgeon preference and intraoperative findings.

1. *Standard Patch*:

    The patch is cut to length and completed with either one or two running Prolene sutures. The patch extends onto either the PFA or SFA.

    If the patch terminates on the PFA, the SFA can sometimes be transected and ligated, and the remaining posterior wall of the femoral vessel is incorporated into the patch anastomosis, or if the SFA is patent, it can be transected and reattached to the femoral vessel/patch in an end-to-side anastomosis. If the SFA is selected for the distal endpoint of the patch angioplasty, the PFA disease can be addressed in a modified eversion technique.

2. *Bifurcated Patch*:

    Arteriotomy can extend onto both SFA and PFA, and each vessel endpoint is individually endarterectomized. The patch is fashioned with a bifurcated distal endpoint in a "snake tongue" configuration. A wider patch is typically used in this scenario. The anastomosis can be completed using separate running sutures for each patch corner [283].

3. *No Patch, Eversion*:

    The eversion endarterectomy technique commonly described for the carotid artery can also be applied to the femoral vessels. The CFA is transected approximately 1 cm proximal to the femoral bifurcation. The proximal CFA is endarterectomized by the standard eversion technique. The PFA and SFA are addressed with a modified eversion technique. Once the endarterectomy is completed, the CFA is reconnected with an end-to-end anastomosis, using two Prolene sutures, starting first with the back wall [284].

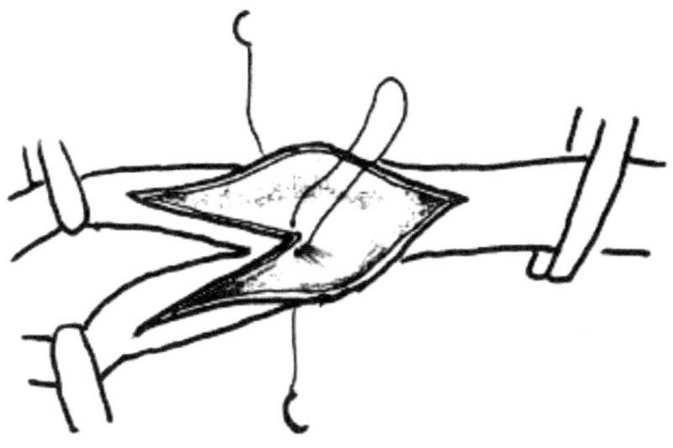

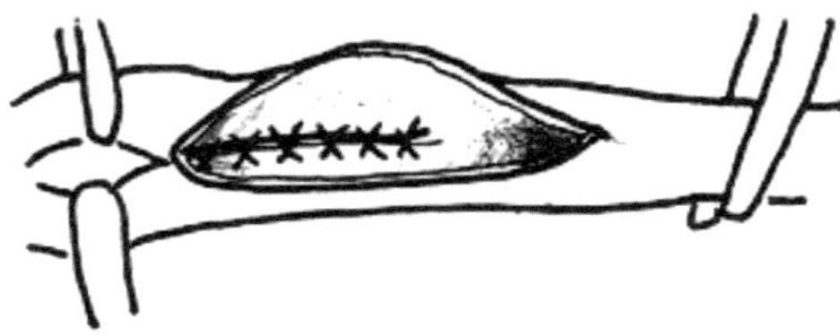

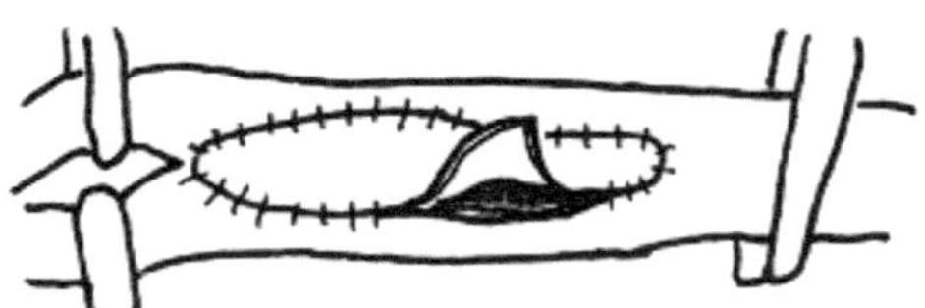

Fig. 6.78 Depiction of "dropped bifurcation" technique for patch angioplasty

4. *Dropped Bifurcation Technique*:

This technique extends onto both PFA and SFA, similar to the bifurcated patch; however, it differs in the suturing technique and only utilizes a simple patch while also elongating the CFA (Fig. 6.78). The arteriotomy extends onto the PFA and SFA, and endarterectomy is performed. The suture begins at the apical junction of the origins of the SFA and PFA with the knot on the outer posterior vessel surface. One arm of this suture is then run distally to unite the posterior edges of these arteries to the distal end of the arteriotomies. This creates a common vessel (extended CFA) that enables the simple placement of a single patch, similar to the standard patch technique [285].

5. *Interposition Graft*:

Rarely femoral interposition grafting may be performed instead of patch angioplasty when arterial wall integrity appears compromised following endarterectomy; PTFE, Dacron, or vein can be used as a conduit. This can be configured in any number of ways:
   (a) Distal anastomosis to syndactylized SFA and PFA.
   (b) Distal anastomosis to the SFA with reimplantation of the deep femoral artery.
   (c) Distal anastomosis to the PFA with reimplantation of SFA.
   (d) Distal anastomosis to the PFA only when the SFA is already occluded.

6.17.3 Profunda Bypass

6.17.3.1 Considerations

In the setting of bypass, the PFA can be used as an inflow or outflow source, depending on the clinical scenario.

1. *Inflow Source*:

The PFA is a particularly useful inflow source for distal bypass if there is inadequate vein length or if exposure to the CFA is challenging (i.e., scar tissue, infection, or prior irradiation). Darling et al. reviewed 2829 infrainguinal reconstructions; 563 (20%) procedures had been performed with the PFA used as the inflow source. The 1- and 5-year secondary patency rates for all bypasses with the PFA were 90.4% and 76.9%, respectively, compared with 88% and 73.3% for CFA-based bypasses [286].

2. *Outflow Source*:

The PFA can be used as outflow for aorto-femoral, axillofemoral, or femoro-femoral bypasses and should be considered in the setting of challenging CFA anatomy or occlusion. The CFA and PFA often require an endarterectomy, and the bypass hood is sewn to both the CFA and the proximal PFA. PFA can be used alone as an outflow source if CFA exposure is problematic or occluded [287, 288]. Both proximal and distal PFA provide a durable outflow source. PFA bypass has results comparable to CFA. Standard aortobifemoral bypass to either CFA or PFA provides cumulative patency and limb salvage exceeding 90% at five years [289].

6.17.3.2 Outcomes of Profunda Revascularization

Bypass

Axillofemoral bypass remains the standard revascularization procedure for aortoiliac occlusive disease in patients who are unsuitable candidates for inline revascularization with aortoiliac or aortofemoral bypass. The reported patency of axillofemoral bypass remains >70% at 5 years [110]. Axillofemoral bypass provides a favorable revascularization option in patients who have significant surgical risk. There are no reported studies comparing patency and outcomes of axillo-PFA bypass compared to CFA.

Profundoplasty

Profundoplasty is a durable, safe, and effective procedure in patients with SFA occlusion and/or CFA stenosis extending to the PFA ostium. For patients with Rutherford category 5 and 6 ischemia, the profundoplasty alone is not considered adequate, and concomitant distal bypass should be planned to improve limb salvage rate. Five-year patency of profundoplasty is excellent and quoted to be >90% [110].

Open Vs. Endovascular

Endovascular treatment of PFA is less durable than profundoplasty but may be an acceptable alternative in selected patients who are at high-risk for surgery or as a secondary intervention to maintain the assisted patency of a bypass graft when the PFA was used either as a bypass outflow target or as an inflow source.

Endovascular intervention access can be approached from a contralateral common femoral access in an "up-and-over" the aortic bifurcation fashion or an ipsilateral radial or brachial access. There is a risk of embolization or occlusion of the patent SFA from the balloon angio-

plasty; placing a "buddy wire" into the SFA should be considered to maintain access to the SFA for rescue interventions if any of these events occur.

Qato et al. reviewed 105,568 lower extremity endovascular interventions. Of those procedures, 361 (0.3%) were performed for isolated PFA occlusive disease. The most common treatment modality was plain balloon angioplasty (58.5%), angioplasty followed by stent (18.6%), drug-coated balloon angioplasty (10.0%), atherectomy (9.4%), and stent graft (3.6%). Overall primary patency at 13 months was 92.9% [290]. Currently, there are no reported data that directly compare endovascular vs open treatment of PFA disease. Endarterectomy remains the standard of care and has consistently demonstrated durable results.

6.18 Don't Mess with the Profunda... Unless

Neal Khurana and Chad Laurich

The profunda femoris artery (PFA), also known as the deep femoral artery, arises posterolaterally from the distal common femoral artery (CFA). Its main branches are the medial and lateral circumflex femoral arteries and three perforating muscular branches. Around the hip, the circumflex branches of the PFA anastomose with branches of the internal and external iliac arteries.

The PFA's primary function is to perfuse the thigh. In the setting of critical limb ischemia (CLI), the PFA becomes more critical as it provides collaterals to the popliteal and infragenicular arteries.

Preservation of the PFA in CLI management is crucial. Profundaplasty during CFA endarterectomy is common. The PFA can also serve as an inflow source for bypass. The PFA can also serve as an inflow source for bypass [291]. The PFA is not commonly treated with endovascular techniques as risk of dissection or occlusion can result in poor clinical outcomes that are complex to manage, as flow to distal PFA

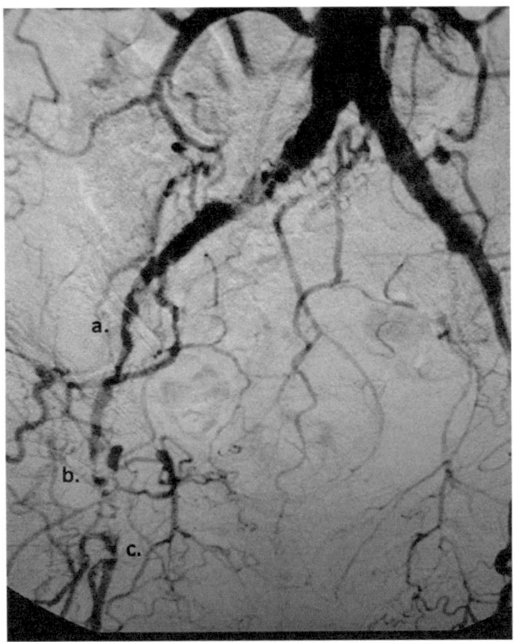

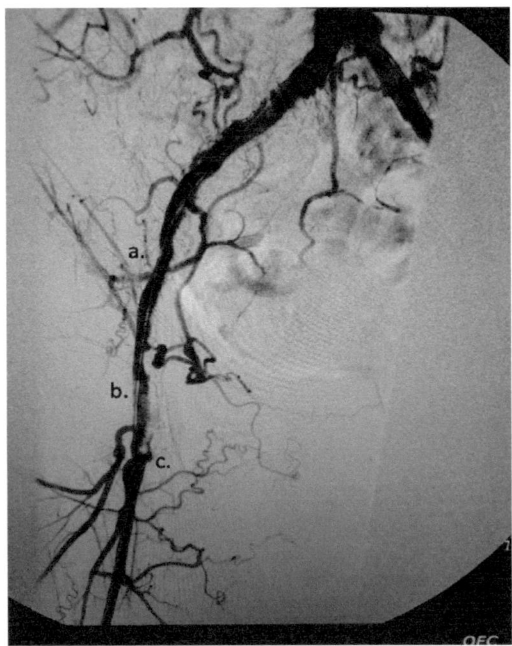

Fig. 6.79 Nonsurgical patient with critical limb ischemia. Pelvic angiogram demonstrates severe stenosis of the *right external iliac artery* (**a**) and chronic occlusions of the *right CFA* (**b**) *and right PFA* (**c**)

Fig. 6.80 Post-treatment angiogram of the *right external iliac artery* (**a**), *right CFA* (**b**), *and origin of the right PFA* (**c**) demonstrates significant luminal gain throughout and inline flow into the right PFA

branches is necessary for stump healing after amputation. However, PFA endovascular intervention can be performed in highly selected cases including patients who have high surgical risk, short life expectancy, or wound-healing considerations.

Endovascular optimization of PFA flow may be the only "bailout" option for limb salvage (Figs. 6.79 and 6.80). Angioplasty alone has shown good long-term patency and limb salvage rates [292]. Drug-coated balloon angioplasty, stenting, and atherectomy of the PFA have all been reported without significant patency rate differences among modalities with 92% patency at 13 months and up to 73% at 24 months [293, 294]. However, reintervention is more likely in patients treated just with plain balloon angioplasty [293]. In regard to stenting, there is significantly higher mean primary patency at 12 months for routine stenting compared to a selective stenting strategy (91.4% versus 75%; $p < 0.05$) [294].

In conclusion, the PFA is an important factor in managing CLI and endovascular treatment is safe and effective in select patients, namely high surgical risk.

6.19   Pedal Surgical Bypass

Samuel Jessula, Claudia Cote, and Anahita Dua

6.19.1 Introduction

The goal of a surgical bypass for treatment of CLTI is to restore pulsatile inline flow to the affected area, typically the foot [295]. Therefore, the distal anastomotic site should be the most proximal outflow target vessel that has at least one continuous runoff artery to the tissue bed in need of revascularization. In patients with occluded tibial vessels and CTLI, hemodynamically significant lesions distal to the popliteal artery and femoral-popliteal bypass would provide insufficient. In such patients, a pedal bypass may provide the optimal perfusion with durable results.

6.19.2 Patient Selection

Indications for pedal bypass include tissue loss or rest pain with or without concomitant infection in the absence of a more proximal outflow target. Patients with diabetes typically present with tibioperoneal occlusions and preserved aortoiliac and femoropopliteal vasculature and thus present ideal candidates for pedal bypass [296].

- Up to 60% of patients with diabetes will heal ulcers after revascularization [297].
- Pedal bypasses are contraindicated in the context of active infection at the site of planned incisions such as ascending foot infections and are very rarely performed for patient with claudication alone without rest pain or tissue loss.

6.19.3 Inflow Selection

Patients with preserved femoral–popliteal flow are candidates for "short bypasses" with inflow targets such as superficial femoral artery or popliteal artery his provides the advantage of avoiding a groin dissection and its associated morbidity, decreasing the length of the surgical incisions, shortening operating time and requiring less length for the conduit, thus increasing the probability of using autologous vein [298]. These advantages provide satisfactory long-term patency, even in the context of worsening superficial femoral disease and may be combined with less invasive procedures to ensure adequate inflow [299–301].

- Prior tibial endovascular interventions should not preclude individuals from being candidates for pedal bypass. Uhl et al. demonstrated that, compared to no prior intervention, previous endovascular intervention was associated with non-statistically significant increased primary patency at 1 year (67 vs 48%) and had no effect on graft occlusions within 1 month or limb salvage within 1 year in patients undergoing pedal bypass [302].

6.19.4 Outflow Selection

Outflow targets are selected based on the distribution of atherosclerosis in the lower extremity vasculature.

- Ideally, a patent continuity of the plantar and pedal arch would be present, thus providing flow to the entire foot; however, this is not mandatory [303].
- In the context of both a patent dorsalis pedis and perimalleolar posterior tibial artery, the dorsalis pedis can be favored as it is an easier anastomosis on the dorsum of the foot.
- In the context of an incomplete plantar arch, if a wound is present on the plantar surface of the foot, the posterior tibial artery may be selected in keeping with the concept of the angiosome, as this vessel will provide direct inline flow to the ischemic area [304].

Of note, angiography alone may underestimate the flow in a pedal vessel and the presence of a Doppler signal should prompt operative exploration (so-called blind exploration) for potential pedal target. Pomposelli et al. performed 6 successful pedal bypasses out of 12 candidates with no angiographic evidence of flow but with a present Doppler signal on physical exam [305]. Similarly, Eiberg et al. completed 5 bypasses on arteriographically occult distal artery targets with only 2 graft occlusions within 1 year, of which one patient remained asymptomatic [306].

6.19.5 Conduit Selection

Similar to femoropopliteal bypasses, the success of pedal bypasses greatly relies on the quality of the conduit [307].

- Autologous vein continues to be the favored conduit for any bypass, and this remains true in the setting of pedal bypass and all efforts should be made to avoid synthetic grafts. Pomposellli et al. described their vast experience with pedal bypasses and techniques to minimize the use of synthetic grafts [308]. Their group prioritized saphenous vein over any conduit, followed by upper extremity vein, and then lesser saphenous vein.
- If the limitation is inadequate length of venous conduit, composite vein can be used or a more distal inflow target, such as superficial femoral or popliteal artery may be selected, even in the context of a diseased artery as long as the lesion is not considered flow limiting.
- Finally, in the absence of any other conduit or bypass configurations, synthetic graft material may be employed although is strongly discouraged [308]. Saphenous vein is associated with improved patency compared to other conduits (other vein and synthetic) (68% vs 46% at 5 years) [309]. As such, the importance of meticulous preoperative vein mapping cannot be understated [310, 311].

When using saphenous vein, it can be employed in the in situ configuration, reversed or non-reversed. In situ has the disadvantage of requiring use of the segment of vein immediately adjacent to the lesion being bypassed, thus limiting which segment of vein can be used. Therefore, transposed saphenous vein is generally preferred. Pomposelli et al. found no statistically significant difference with the use of reversed vs non-reversed saphenous vein [309]. On meta-analysis, the reversed configuration displayed slightly higher primary patency (83% vs 78% at 1 year and 66% vs 59% at 5 years) and secondary patency (88% vs 84% at 1 year and 73% vs 67% at 5 years); however, this was not statistically significant [307].

6.19.6 Operative Technique

The patient is placed supine on the operating room table and general or regional anesthesia is induced. Inflow exposure is performed in routine fashion. Briefly, the common femoral artery is approached through a vertical incision under the inguinal ligament in the groin. The superficial femoral artery can be identified as the continuation of the femoral artery and the same incision can be lengthened as needed. The supra and infragenicular popliteal artery can be exposed through medial incisions above or below the knee, respectively.

Outflow exposure remains quite simple, emphasizing the elegance of a pedal bypass. As the dorsalis pedis is very superficial, the dissection is relatively easy compared to other vascular beds. The dorsalis pedis artery is the continuation of the anterior tibial artery and lies medial to the extensor hallucis longus tendon down to the proximal space between the first and second metatarsals on the dorsum of the foot [312]. Doppler identification is important prior to incising as significant variability exists in how lateral the dorsalis pedis artery lies [313, 314]. A longitudinal incision is performed slightly lateral to the Doppler signal of the artery on the dorsum of the foot, between the first and second metatarsal, allowing for a small skin flap [305]. The dorsal branch of the superficial peroneal nerve is identified and retracted laterally, underneath which the deep fascia is incised to expose the neurovascular bundle. The extensor hallucis longus and brevis are separated and the dorsalis pedis is identified lateral to the deep peroneal nerve [312]. Care is taken to preserve the medial and lateral tarsal branches of the dorsalis pedis [313, 314].

The distal posterior tibial artery lies posterior to the medial malleolus, between the flexor digitorum longus tendon and the flexor hallucis longus muscle before passing under the flexor retinaculum to enter the foot [312]. To expose it, the patient's leg is externally rotated and flexed 60° at the knee. A vertical incision is performed 1 cm posterior to the distal tibia and curved around the medial malleolus. The flexor retinaculum is then divided exposing the neurovascular bundle in a groove formed by the tendons of the flexor digitorum longus and the flexor hallucis longus. The posterior tibial artery is found anterior to the tibial nerve [312].

Once the inflow and outflow arteries are exposed, the graft is tunneled as needed and the patient receives systemic heparin. The anastomoses are performed in a standard fashion with continuous permanent monofilament suture. Completion angiography or angioscopy can be performed selectively at case completion to confirm adequacy of bypass [303, 315]. All incisions are closed primarily.

- Postoperatively, patients are administered 81 mg of aspirin daily for life and prophylactic heparin while in hospital.
- Postoperative foot edema is common, and best treated with leg elevation and elastic wrapping [309].
- Patients are instructed to avoid weight bearing on the operative foot for 2–7 days.

6.19.7 Outcomes

In the largest series of pedal bypasses, operative mortality was <1% with a 4.2% 30-day graft failure rate, of which one third were successfully revised [309]. Primary patency was 57% and 38%, while secondary patency was 63% and 41% at 5 and 10 years, respectively.

- Limb salvage was 78% at 5 years and 58% at 10 years. On multivariable analysis, increased length of stay (OR 0.95, 95% CI 0.93 to 0.98) and graft occlusion as indication (OR 0.38, 95% CI 0.17 to 0.89) were significantly predictive of graft failure at 1 year, while use of the saphenous vein as conduit was protective (OR 1.82, 95% CI 1.25–2.65) [309].
- On meta-analysis of over 2320 pedal bypasses, 30-day mortality had a weighted average 2.6%, and 1-year mortality was 13%. 1-month outcomes demonstrated primary patency of 93%, secondary patency of 95%, and foot preservation rate of 95%.
- 5-year outcomes demonstrated primary patency of 63%, secondary patency 71%, and limb preservation of 78% [307].

On meta-analysis, compared to dorsalis pedis bypass, tibial bypass was favored for primary patency (86% vs 77% at 1 year, 69% vs 57% at 5 years), secondary patency (90% vs 81% at 1 year, 76% vs 65% at 5 years), and foot preservation at 5 years (80% vs 76%) [307]. However, the meta-analysis did not comment on whether the tibial artery target was proximal or distal, thus rendering a true comparison between distal/perimalleolar tibial artery vs dorsalis pedis artery difficult.

6.19.8 Alternatives to Pedal Bypass

Tibial angioplasty would provide an alternative to short pedal bypass for lesions isolated to the tibial vessels. Ferraresi et al. reported the largest series of 107 isolated tibial angioplasties with a procedural success rate of 94%, a restenosis rate of 42%, and a limb salvage rate of 93% at a median follow-up of 1.4 years [316].

- In the event of an occluded dorsalis pedis and paramalleolar posterior tibial artery, revascularization to a more distal target, such as to a plantar or tarsal vessel, is feasible.
- Hughes et al. report successful bypass of 77 plantar and 21 tarsal arteries in patients of which 18 had previous revascularization including 5 previous dorsalis pedis bypasses [317].

  - 30-day mortality was 1% and 30-day graft occlusion occurred in 11%.
  - Primary, secondary patency, and limb salvage rates were 67%, 70%, and 75% in 1 year and 41%, 50% and 69% in 5 years, respectively [317].

Although not technically considered a pedal vessel, the peroneal artery can be an alternative outflow target if patent on preoperative imaging. Darling et al. reported a series of 159 patients with bypasses to the distal peroneal artery, demonstrating a primary patency of 86% at 30 days, 82% at

1 year, and 69% at 5 years [318]. The secondary patency was 86% at 1 year and 75% at 5 years, with a limb salvage rate of 87% at 5 years [318].

- When compared to tibial and pedal bypass, peroneal bypass has increased secondary patency (55% vs 67%) but decreased limb salvage (33% vs 46%) at 2 years [319].

6.19.9 Target Limitations

Pedal bypasses cannot be performed if there is active infection over the intended incision for the distal anastomosis and thus cannot be performed in the context of an active, ascending infection of the foot. Furthermore, the poor outcomes of synthetic grafts in pedal bypasses limit the applicability of the procedure in patients with absent vein conduit. If a pedal bypass fails, a redo pedal bypass may be considered; however, it requires the availability of another vein conduit and patency is poor, especially if failure was within 30 days [320]. Finally, although pedal bypass has demonstrated robust durability, endovascular technologies are rapidly progressing and may at some point outperform bypasses. To date, no trials comparing the two techniques have been published.

6.19.10 Conclusion

Pedal bypass is a straightforward, reliable technique for revascularization of CTLI with acceptable long-term patency and limb salvage rates. It should be considered in patients with ischemia and a distal pedal Doppler signal or angiographic flow.

Pearls:
- Ensure adequate preoperative vein mapping and prioritize saphenous vein conduits when feasible.
- Consider exploration of any artery with a Doppler signal on physical exam, even in the absence of angiographic evidence of flow.

Pitfalls:
- Avoid prosthetic conduits at all costs.

6.20 Intravascular Ultrasound-Based Femoropopliteal Atherectomy Selection

Bryan Fischer

The popliteal segment represents one of the most difficult vascular beds to treat for multiple reasons, the most striking being the stress placed on the vessel during knee extension and flexion. This has been illustrated by the historical failure of traditional scaffolding secondary to fracture and further supported by a relative paucity of devices that are considered on label for this segment. As with the SFA, popliteal occlusive disease is often treated with vessel preparation followed by definitive therapy (DCB/scaffold). Modification and/or plaque debulking with atherectomy is often part of the toolbox aimed at reducing the disease burden before moving on to the next step.

A wide variety of atherectomy devices are approved in the USA, and this number continues to grow despite a relative paucity of high-quality data to support its use [321, 322]. However, in the real-world setting, interventionalists across each of the vascular interventional specialties have found atherectomy to be a helpful tool in their toolbox. The decision of which device to use lies with the interventionalists comfort level/expertise and the ability to apply the appropriate treatment to address a particular disease morphology based on intraprocedural findings. This is the most important component of a successful treatment algorithm and reiterates the need to have a selective and personalized approach to each individual patient.

Identifying the type of lesion is a key to choosing the appropriate atherectomy device in the popliteal space. Luminal size and landing zone planning are also key to procedural success. For this reason, advanced intraprocedural imaging is paramount to achieving the desired end result for treating symptomatic occlusive disease in the popliteal artery. Angiography, while widely accepted as a reliable reference of vessel characteristics, has been shown to be inadequate [323].

The use of either EVUS/IVUS has proven to be reliable in such cases. Once IVUS-based assessment of the underlying lesion morphology, intervention can be planned [323].

Rather than discussing a given morphology type and the resulting choice of atherectomy device, it may be more helpful to know where devices have known limitations. Few scenarios dwarf the morbidity of complications that ensue when a device is chosen for the wrong disease morphology. For instance, some devices are almost certain to cause distal embolization in very soft plaque or luminal thrombus. Each has its strengths and weaknesses that will be addressed.

6.20.1 Calcified Plaque

Calcified disease is the disease morphology for which most atherectomy devices perform poorly with regard to luminal gain or plaque modification. The appearance of calcium is obvious with IVUS interrogation and can often be appreciated in less detail with fluoroscopy [323].

- Traditionally, orbital atherectomy has done well by sanding the lesion in a controlled fashion. While some routinely use distal protection, deliberate escalation of rotation speeds and advancing in a slow but steady fashion is effective at mitigating embolization risk. Laser is not traditionally thought of as first-line treatment for bulky calcified disease; however, several operators have demonstrated an ability to successfully cross calcium-rich lesions and modify less dense calcified dis-

ease. Again, a slow and deliberate approach is necessary and achieved by allowing the device to vaporize plaque with steady forward pressure. Though it takes several passes with escalating energy, many operators are surprised by the luminal gain achieved that can be seen clearly with intravascular ultrasound.

- Other atherectomy devices like phoenix and directional atherectomy are capable of achieving luminal gain by plaque removal but have been known to require a higher skillset for successful operation. Knowing the device and being facile with its use is key [324, 325].

6.20.2 Fibrous Plaque

Fibrous disease morphology represents an altogether different type of challenge with regard to atherectomy effectiveness.

- While orbital atherectomy does well with calcified disease, other devices tend to perform better here [326].
- Directional atherectomy has tremendous upside with the ability to debulk lesions in a deliberate fashion. The resultant luminal gain combined with the appropriate definitive therapy can lead to a good result and the return of pulsatile inflow to the tibial vessels.
- Most use distal protection in the event of distal embolization, a known but accepted risk given the upside of successful debulking [327].
- Laser also performs well here, and luminal gain is readily apparent with IVUS. Dissections are often seen with laser, the extent of which can vary based on energy delivery and number of passes [328].
- Luminal gain is less efficient than directional atherectomy but can still be achieved.
- Hybrid devices like phoenix are also effective here when operators can effectively apply device deflection with an enlarging radius.

- Finally, rotational atherectomy is often successful in this space as well.

6.20.3 Soft Plaque

Soft plaque and intraluminal thrombus represent a unique challenge for even the most skilled operator. Distal embolization is a constant intraprocedural risk that only increases with passage of each wire or device. Atherectomy in this scenario can potentially increase this risk when the wrong device is chosen.

- Devices that actively aspirate in addition to plaque modification perform well in this space.
- Rotarex combines an aggressive rotational mechanism combined with the ability to draw debris and soft plaque thrombus into an attached receptacle. The benefits increase when the 8-Fr device is used, though its application is limited by vessel diameter [329].

- Jetstream works well here as well, but often necessitates the use of distal embolic protection.
- Laser may occasionally be applied here, especially if there is soft thrombus.
- Orbital atherectomy is often avoided here due to the relative high risk of embolic complications.

The decision to utilize any atherectomy device in the popliteal artery should be made with careful consideration. Kinetic forces make this vascular bed challenging even for the most experienced proceduralist. The choice of atherectomy device is important to allow for efficient vessel preparation which in turn lays the foundation for a durable result. Many tools exist that can assess disease morphology, but real-time ultrasound interrogation can provide valuable detailed information and help guide device selection. Based on findings from EVUS/IVUS, the skilled technician is better equipped to tackle a wide variety of disease morphologies while limiting the risk of complications like vessel occlusion or distal embolization.

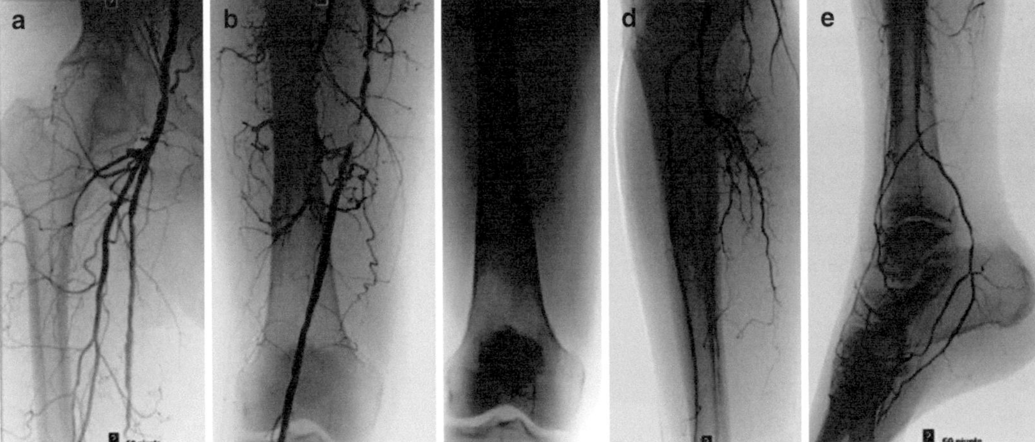

Fig. 6.81 Diagnostic angiogram of the RLE showing ISR/occlusion of the stent (**a–c**). There was primary anterior tibial artery runoff (**d**) with a reconstituted peroneal artery at the level of the ankle which continues to the foot as a hypertrophied posterior tibial artery and plantar circulation

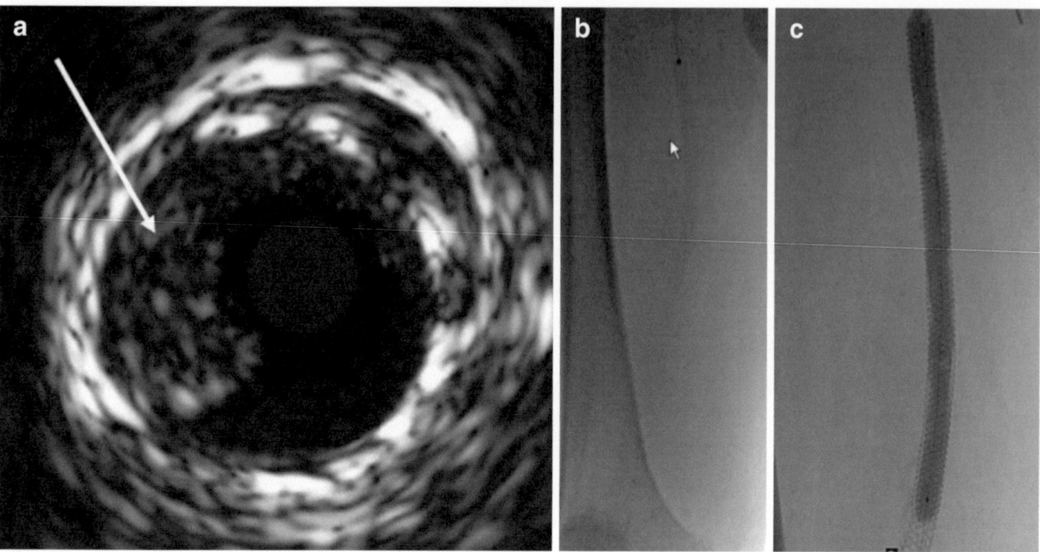

Fig. 6.82 IVUS catheter was used to delineate the ISR contents which appears to be nonthrombotic (white arrow) and more consistent with hyperplasia/soft plaque (**a**). Laser atherectomy was performed after placement of EPD filter to catch potential debris (**b**). Scoring balloon angioplasty was then performed (**c**)

6.20.4 Case Example

6.20.4.1 Courtesy of Sreekumar Madassery, MD

75-year-old patient with history of prior RLE bare metal stenting for progressive claudication 18 months prior. Patient presented with 3–4 weeks of worsening symptoms and subsequently developed rest pain. Diagnostic angiogram was done showing ISR/occlusion of the stent (Fig. 6.81a–c). There was primary anterior tibial artery runoff to the ankle with reconstituted peroneal artery that continued to the foot as a hypertrophied posterior tibial artery and plantar circulation (Fig. 6.81d, e). IVUS catheter was used to delineate the in-stent restenosis which appeared to be nonthrombotic and more consistent with hyperplasia/soft plaque (Fig. 6.82a). Laser atherectomy was performed in the area and scoring balloon angioplasty was then done (Fig. 6.82b, c). Drug-coated balloon angioplasty was then done of the area. Percutaneous old balloon angioplasty was done of the anterior tibial artery and peroneal artery, with completion angiogram demonstrating two-vessel runoff to the ankle with improved perfusion to the forefoot (Fig. 6.83).

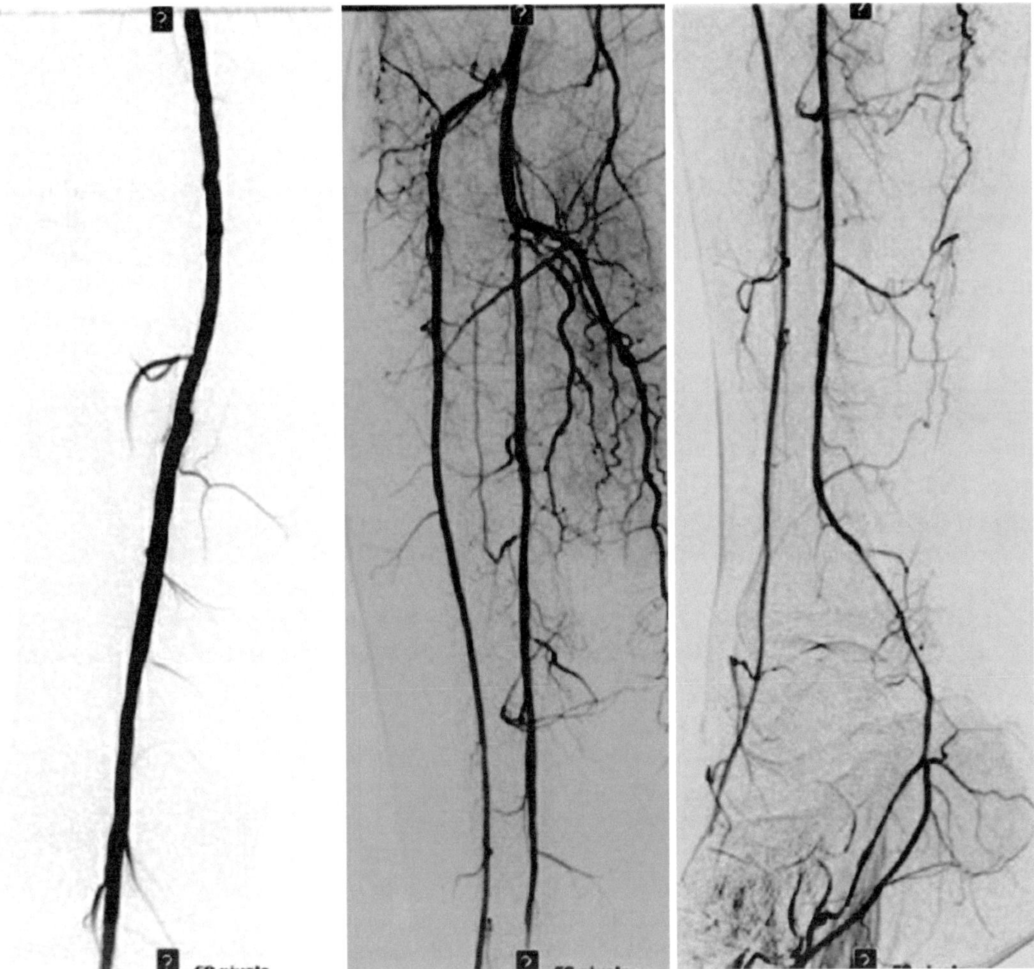

Fig. 6.83 Completion angiogram after scoring balloon angioplasty and drug-coated balloon angioplasty of the ISR and POBA of the peroneal and anterior tibial arteries demonstrated two-vessel runoff and adequate perfusion to the forefoot

6.21 Below-the-Ankle Atherectomy

Bret Wiechmann

The "last frontier" of endovascular intervention in critical limb ischemia (CLI) involves the pedal arch and plantar vessels. Maintenance of outflow through the lateral plantar, medial plantar, and metatarsal branches may have significant impact on endovascular intervention in the tibial vessels in this challenging patient group. Patients with small artery disease (SAD) may indeed have poor outcomes due to this lack of outflow [330]. The inherently small diameter of the pedal vessels in general combined with the presence of extensive calcification (particularly within the media and common in patients with diabetes and chronic kidney disease) makes establishing outflow through the plantar vessels and/or establishing a patent pedal arch critical in many CLI patients.

Percutaneous transluminal angioplasty (PTA) is certainly the mainstay of endovascular therapy. While adjunctive therapy such as atherectomy and stenting in the femoropopliteal segment has been frequently studied and in general is a widely adopted practice among vascular interventional-ists, the atherectomy and stenting options below the knee are limited and the evidence base to support its routine use is even more limited. While there are large data sets supporting atherectomy in the tibial vessels, including a recently published study of over 36,000 patients showing excellent limb salvage rate and lower 4-year mortality with use of atherectomy in conjunction with angioplasty, other studies have not produced the same conclusion [331].

- The published data on use of atherectomy as adjunctive therapy in the below ankle levels are even more sparse.
- A PubMed search of "below-the-ankle atherectomy" yields only one single-center, retrospective study. In this study by Palena, 317 patients with diabetes and CLI underwent orbital atherectomy plus drug-coated balloon angioplasty. Patients were followed at 30 days and 6 months. The limb salvage rate was 100% at 6 months with an amputation-free survival (AFS) of 50% at 6 months. No major amputations and six minor amputations were noted at 6 months. Freedom from clinically driven target lesion revascularization (fCDTLR) was 100% at 30 days and 91.7% at six months. There were no major adverse cardiovascular or limb events (MACE/MALE) and no evidence of perforation, dissection, or embolization [332].

Considerations regarding use of atherectomy in the below-the-ankle vessels revolve around deliverability and safety. The profile of certain FDA-approved atherectomy devices likely preclude their delivery into these vessels that are typically less than 3 mm. The lowest profile atherectomy devices are the Nexcimer Laser System (Philips, Amsterdam, Netherlands), the Auryon Laser System (AngioDynamics, Latham, NY), the Rotablator (Boston Scientific, Maple Grove, MN), and the Stealth 360 orbital atherectomy system (Cardiovascular Systems Inc., St. Paul, MN). Beyond and perhaps more important than deliverability, however, is the safety of these devices in this arterial segment; to date, peer-reviewed publications have not established their safety other than the one small study noted above. It is worth noting that these data were produced at a center that is well known for its technical expertise and outstanding clinical outcomes. The applicability of this approach on a broader scale and the reproducibility of its clinical efficacy remain uncertain.

Consideration of adjunctive atherectomy in the below ankle/pedal vessels, as in the Palena study, is typically performed in those patients in whom crossing of a standard balloon catheter is not successful. The inability to cross with a low-profile balloon suggests that the atherosclerotic burden, particularly calcification, is extensive which is known to be associated with poor angioplasty results due to recoil and dissection. Since stenting through this area is neither recommended nor proven, and with no approved scaffolds/stents for this segment, optimal angioplasty is desired and debulking these lesions may indeed make intuitive sense.

When performing atherectomy in these vessels, methodical attention to detail is paramount. Complications in this area can be devastating and potentially limb-threatening.

- The idea of using one of these devices just because it *can be* delivered to the target vessel does not mean that it *should be* done.
- A slow cadence is used with laser systems.
- With orbital/rotational systems, low speed is used. Without a definable endpoint, knowing when to stop is critical.
- Negotiating these devices through the pedal arch has resulted in well-known cases of getting them stuck and requiring surgical removal.
- Remembering that below-the-ankle atherectomy is *adjunctive* therapy in order to optimize angioplasty is the key to safety.

Much of endovascular treatment in the lower extremity for peripheral arterial disease is proven therapy and has repeatable, reproducible outcomes. The complexity of CLI patients with multiple comorbidities and a high short-term mortality rate makes this a very challenging population to treat in general. Enrolling patients in CLI trials has proven to be difficult, and therefore, obtaining definitive treatment strategies and algorithms has been elusive. As a result, tremendous treatment variation exists, which further confounds the ability to develop consensus. This is perhaps no more apparent than in the infrapopliteal vessels including the pedal/plantar vessels.

- There is extensive data to support the use of PTA in the pedal/below ankle vessels due to improved wound outcomes in those with a patent pedal arch, but clear, definitive data regarding the use of BTA atherectomy are yet to be produced [333–335].

- Therefore, while it may be intuitive, conventional wisdom suggests it should only be performed in unique situations with caution.

6.21.1 Case Courtesy of Sreekumar Madassery, MD

68-yo patient with ESRD, DM, CAD, and non-healing wounds of the right second and third digits with noninvasive imaging consistent with popliteal and infrapopliteal significant stenotic disease. ABI on the RLE was 0.6, TBI of 0.3. Procedural images as below (Figs. 6.84, 6.85, 6.86, and 6.87). Successful antegrade crossing of calcified distal anterior tibial artery and dorsalis

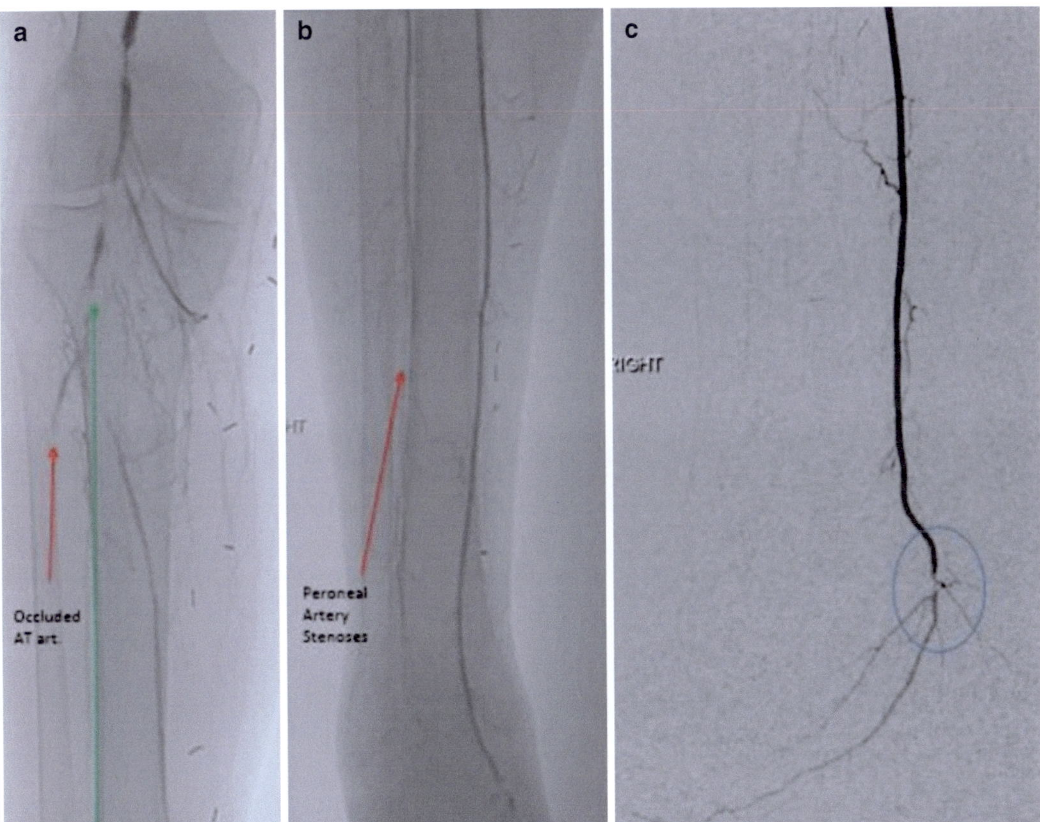

Fig. 6.84 (**a**) Diagnostic angiogram demonstrated multifocal stenosis in the previously stented popliteal artery (green arrow) and chronically occluded anterior tibial artery (red arrow), with additional TP trunk disease. (**b**) Additionally, there is peroneal artery stenosis at the level of mid-calf (red arrow). (**c**) There is primarily posterior tibial artery inflow with an area of focal stenosis at the bifurcation into plantar arteries (blue circle)

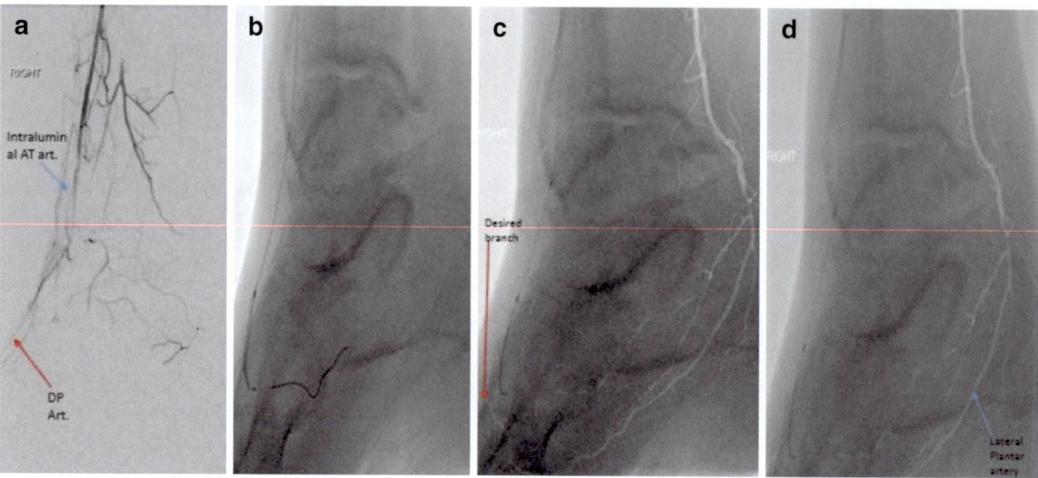

Fig. 6.85 (**a**) After recanalization of the anterior tibial artery, intraluminal injection demonstrated a small whisp of a dorsalis pedis artery (red arrow). (**b**) There was initial difficulty traversing the pedal loop into the lateral plantar artery. (**c**) DSA roadmap was done with groin sheath injection which demonstrates the wire in lateral tarsal branch (red arrow). (**d**) Wire was subsequently advanced into the desired branch to traverse the lateral plantar artery (blue arrow)

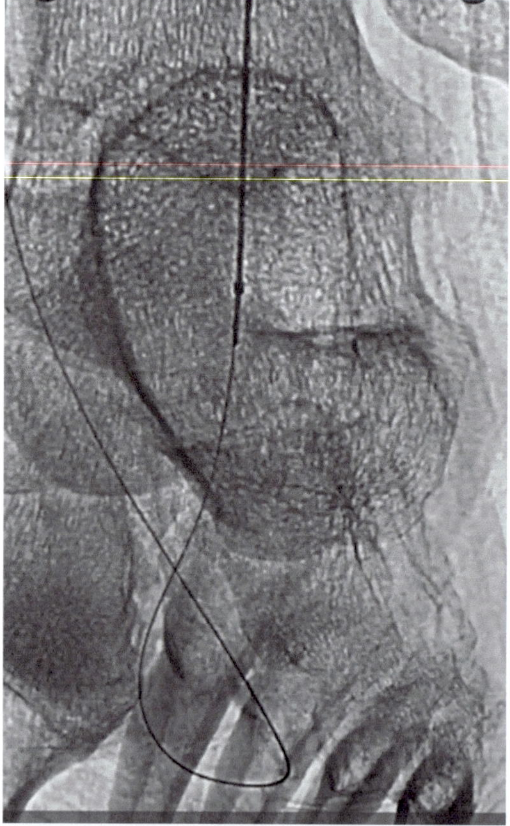

Fig. 6.86 Decision was made to perform orbital atherectomy of the DP into the pedal loop to increase compliance

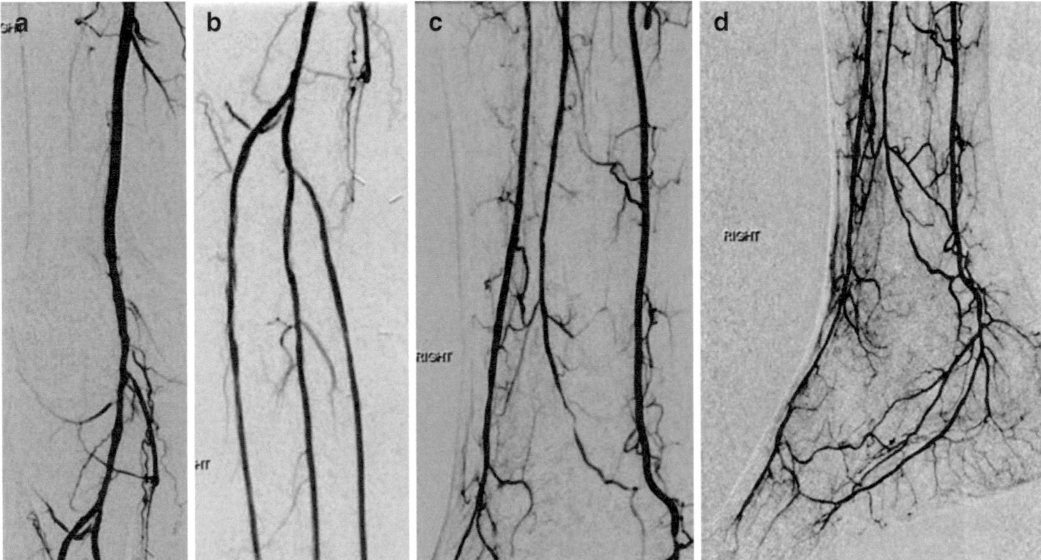

Fig. 6.87 Completion angiogram after plain and drug-coated balloon angioplasty of popliteal artery stenosis shows three-vessel runoff both proximally (**a**, **b**) and distally (**c**). Completion angiogram of the foot shows three-vessel runoff at the ankle with now an intact pedal loop (**d**)

pedis artery, through the Pedal loop and retrograde into the distal posterior tibial artery, thus completing the loop. The loop was ideal to increase perfusion after intervention to the watershed areas of the digits and also to be able to treat the focal distal posterior tibial artery stenosis (as below) with the same access. Post-procedure, after several weeks of continued wound care, the digits were able to be healed with debridement, and without amputation.

6.22 What Is My Endpoint on Angiogram?

Abhishek Kumar

An estimated 150,000 amputations occur due to critical limb ischemia (CLI) in the United States each year, with a large number of primary amputations being performed without diagnostic angiograms and attempts at revascularization [336]. In 2016, the American Heart Association/American College of Cardiology released a Class I recommendation stating that an evaluation for revascularization options should be considered with imaging or an angiogram prior to amputation [337]. More recently, the CLI global society published an expert recommendation statement recommending use of digital subtraction angiography (DSA) for evaluation of revascularization in patients with CLI prior to amputation [338]. The primary goal of revascularization is to improve wound perfusion to allow healing. Equally important is tissue perfusion when an amputation is performed. While considerable debate still exists on angiographic endpoints for endovascular therapy, an understanding of angiographic patterns needed for successful healing of amputation levels is necessary for the endovascular specialist.

1. Toe Amputation Versus Trans-Metatarsal Amputation (TMA):

    A wound blush (WB) on angiogram after revascularization has been associated with high rates of wound healing [339]. For healing of toe or partial ray amputations, it is usually necessary to have a patent pedal arch and sufficient angiographic perfusion to the wound. Figure 6.88 illustrates a poorly healing partial ray amputation that healed after successful tibial revascularization.

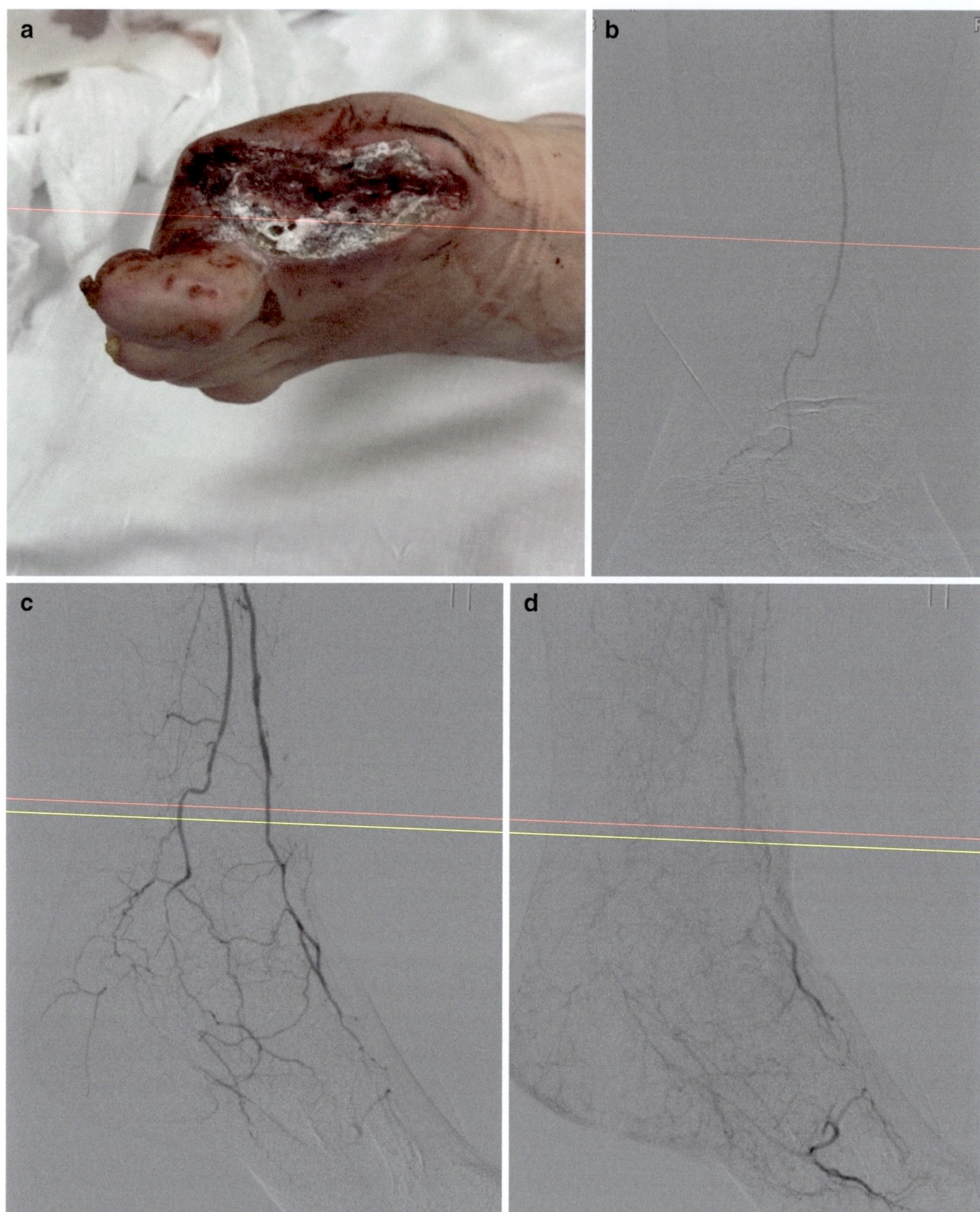

Fig. 6.88 (**a**) Status post-first ray amputation with poor wound healing, (**b**) digital subtraction angiography of the below-knee vessels shows occlusion of anterior tibial and posterior tibial arteries with single-vessel runoff to the ankle, and (**c**) DSA at the level of the lower leg after endovascular revascularization of the anterior tibial artery and peroneal arteries shows improved supply to the foot. (**d**) Delayed image from a foot angiogram after revascularization demonstrates a "wound blush" leading to adequate wound healing

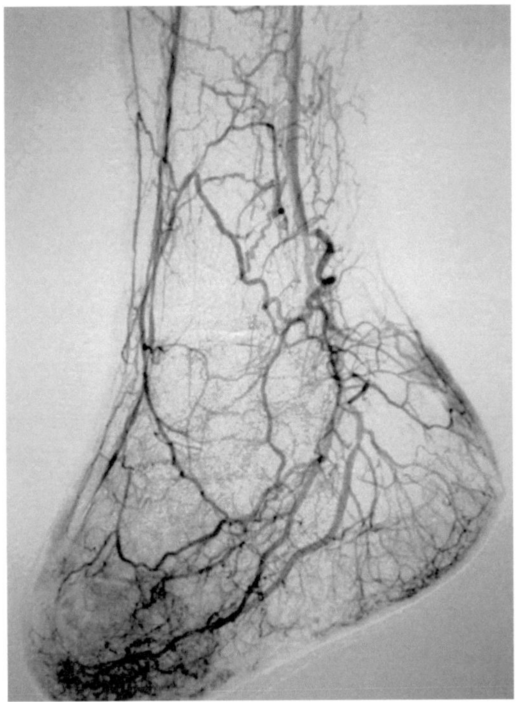

Fig. 6.89 Digital subtraction angiogram showing wound blush and adequate supply to a TMA

Healing at a TMA requires patency of one or more infrapopliteal vessels with inline flow to the foot. A patent pedal arch has been associated with higher rates of healing after TMAs. When possible, a patent pedal arch is desirable. Figure 6.89 illustrates an angiogram with ample supply to heal a TMA.

2. Symes:

A symes amputation or an ankle disarticulation is an alternative to below-knee amputation. Advantages include a more comfortable stump and a more functional gait. Studies have shown that compared to BKA or AKA, the symes amputation results in decreased morbidity, early weight bearing without the need for gait training, and a better gait pattern.

A patent posterior tibial artery is necessary for healing of a symes amputation.

3. Above-knee vs below-knee amputation (AKA vs BKA).

A BKA is a transtibial amputation that involves removing the foot, ankle joint, and distal tibia and fibula with related soft tissue structures. It is preferred over an AKA because it has better functional and long-term outcomes. A popliteal artery pressure of 50 mmhg is considered adequate for healing a BKA [340].

On angiography, occlusion of the distal superficial femoral and popliteal artery is usually an indication that a BKA would be difficult to heal.

6.23 Orphan Heel

Farnaz Dadrass and Sreekumar Madassery

6.23.1 Introduction

Heel ulcers are commonly seen in PAD patients with diabetes. These are frequently the result of trauma from constant pressure in the setting of ischemia and/or neuropathy. Heel ischemia results from disease of the posterior tibial and peroneal arteries, with a subset of these patients being diagnosed with orphan heel syndrome. Orphan heel syndrome (OHS) is defined as an ischemic heel ulcer seen with a compilation of three disease processes that result in a characteristic pathological triad of:

1. Poorly controlled diabetes mellitus.
2. Chronic kidney disease/renal failure.
3. Occlusive PAD of the peroneal artery and posterior tibial artery.

These ulcers are notoriously difficult to treat, likely due to arterial insufficiency, neuropathy, high levels of inflammation, decreased expression of various growth factors and increased apoptosis [341]. This compartmentalization of the blood flow to the heel becomes compromised, resulting in ischemia. Orphan heel syndrome is also difficult to diagnose as conventional measures can be misleading. The angiosome-based model of revascularization is often used to target the ischemic areas and has been shown to be effective [342–344]. The calcaneal branch of the

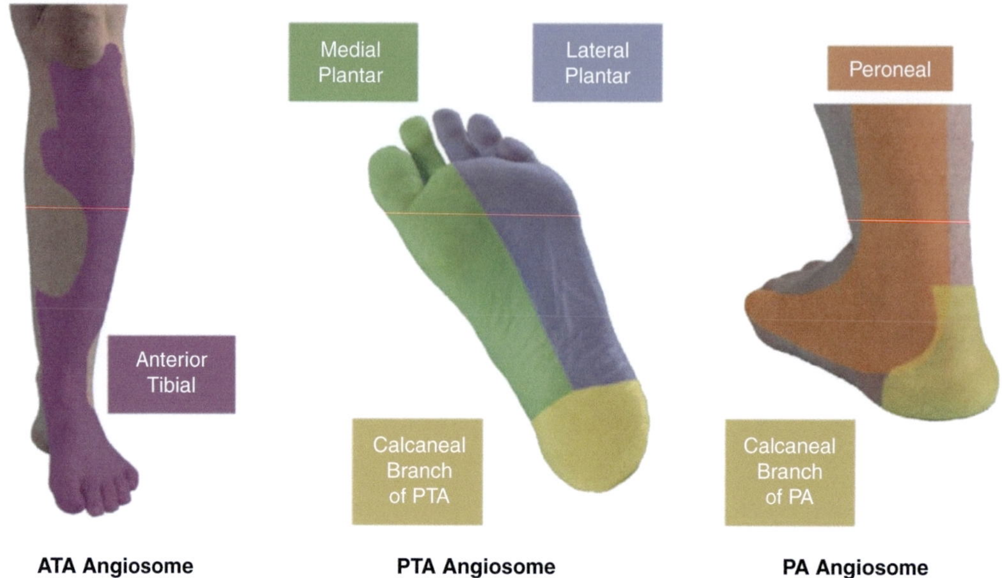

Fig. 6.90 This figure is a representation of the angiosome concept. Reproduced from Iida et al. [343]. There are six angiosomes total in the foot, broken down into different coloring per angiosome. The three source arteries that feed the six angiosomes include the anterior tibial artery (ATA), posterior tibial artery (PTA), and peroneal artery (PA). The ATA supplies the dorsalis pedis artery (DPA), which supplies the dorsum of the foot. The PTA has three branches: the medial plantar artery to the medial sole of the foot, the lateral plantar artery to the lateral midfoot, and the forefoot calcaneal branch to the heel. The PA branches off into the anterior perforating branch of the PA, which supplies the lateral border of the ankle and the calcaneal branch which supplies the outside of the heel

posterior tibial artery (PTA) supplies the heel. The calcaneal branch of the peroneal artery (PA) also supplies the heel (Fig. 6.90).

Multiple collaterals exist between the tibial arteries and their branches to supply all six angiosomes, as a protective measure should one of the arteries become compromised. These arterial–arterial connections are referred to as "choke vessels." Occlusion of a main source artery frequently changes angiosome locations for patients with PAD [345]. Compensation with collateral vessels allow for this process to take place in chronic ischemic patients rather than acute limb patients as "choke vessels" require four to ten days to become patent after an ischemic event [345]. This results in the branches of main source arteries getting their supply from proximal arteries, rather than the main source arteries themselves. The reliance on collateral circulation over time ultimately causes a mismatch between arterial occlusion with wound angiosome location.

Ischemic ulceration of the heel can be understood in terms of the angiosome concept. As a source vessel is compromised from calcification secondary to atherosclerosis, the corresponding skin at that angiosome can become ischemic and necrotic. The compensatory mechanisms of pedal choke vessels may be severely compromised by atherosclerosis secondary to both DM and ESRD, predisposing patients to the ischemic heel ulceration seen in the triad of OHS [345, 346].

6.23.2 Diagnosis

Orphan heel syndrome stems from occlusive peripheral arterial disease of the PTA and PA, both of which have branching calcaneal arteries supplying blood to the heel. Once the compartmentalized flow to the heel becomes compromised, the heel can become ulcerated and necrotic. The compensatory choke vessels are

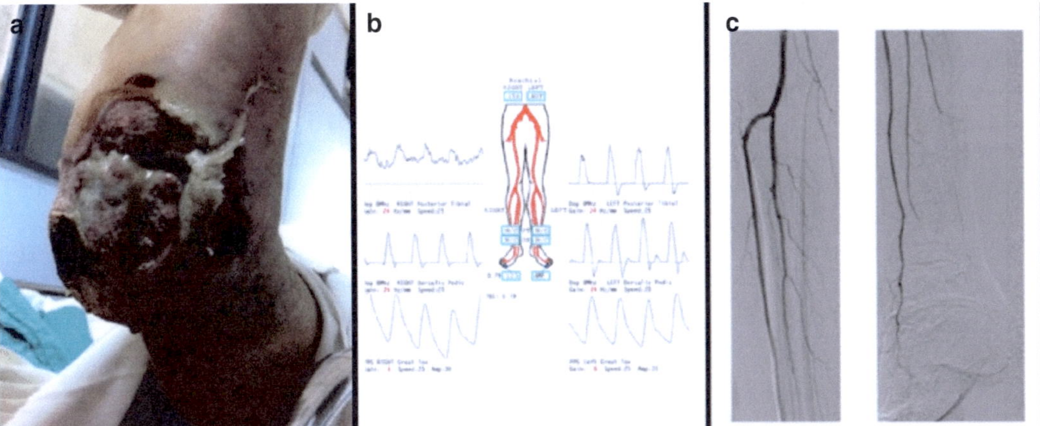

Fig. 6.91 (**a**) Gross image of ischemic ulcer as seen in orphan heel syndrome (OHS); (**b**) noninvasive Doppler with waveforms and pressures. Characteristic blunted PTA waveforms with normal DP waveforms as the ATA is not characteristically involved; (**c**) angiography demonstrating patent ATA with occlusive disease of both the PTA and posterior perforating branch of the PA prior to intervention. Images courtesy of Miguel-Montero Baker MD

also often compromised due to pedal atherosclerosis from DM and ESRD [345].

The heel ischemia seen in OHS is characteristically difficult to diagnose as the vascular compromise is frequently underestimated. This is thought to be due to a typically well-perfused forefoot. Noninvasive imaging with arterial Doppler provides ankle–brachial pressure indices (ABI) and toe-brachial pressure indices (TBI) that do not accurately represent the extent of heel ischemia, overvaluing the healing potential of the wound [345, 346]. Because these values use the best ankle pressure reading, which in these patients comes from the ATA, ABI and TBI can artificially imply normal or acceptable perfusion to the foot (Fig. 6.91).

Alternative noninvasive testing like transcutaneous oxygen tension (tcPO2) and skin perfusion pressure (SPP) can more accurately assess vascular perfusion to the heel. Monitoring the dissemination of IV indocyanine green (ICG) injection into the tissues under florescent angiography, a slightly more invasive modality to evaluate ischemia in these patients, is also shown to be effective. Another method for assessment is through bio-compatible implantable luminescent oxygen microsensors, which serve to evaluate foot vessels for the purposes of revascularization planning.

6.23.3 Treatment

Treatment for OHS is similar to treating other ulcers in that it is usually multi-faceted and includes a combination of debridement, offloading pressure, infection control, local wound care, and either surgical or endovascular revascularization [342]. Angiography is an important diagnostic and therapeutic tool that provides detailed evaluation of the foot circulation and in turn allows for direct revascularization of the targeted vessels supplying the ischemic angiosome [344–347].

Revascularization for critical limb ischemia can be either direct or indirect.

- Direct revascularization (DR) is when the target artery is a source for the affected angiosome.
- Indirect revascularization (IR) is when intervention is on the arteries in the surrounding angiosome.

While IR can be effective when there are strong collaterals supporting the area, DR with angiosome-based infrapopliteal angioplasty has been associated with better wound healing and higher rates of limb salvage in diabetic foot ischemia [348]. There remains some controversy regarding which method of revascularization is most effective when there are strong collaterals, with a few studies showing IR and DR to be equivocal [342, 345]. An advantage of endovascular repair, when compared to surgical intervention with bypass grafting, is the ability to treat more than one vessel (combined revascularization).

The development of OHS usually indicates poor prognosis in terms of their PAD, despite multi-specialty treatment plans and successful revascularization [342]. ESRD on dialysis has already been described as a high-risk factor for limb amputation, with the outcomes of OHS shown to be more severe [342, 345]. The collaterals between the perfused forefoot angiosome to the ischemic heel are usually compromised for this patient population. A theory for this is the strong prevalence of microvascular disease negatively affecting luminal caliber and/or physiological flow, hindering choke vessels, and in turn collateral flow from neighboring angiosomes [344, 345]. This is what "orphans" heel with occlusive disease of the peroneal artery and posterior tibial artery. This process occurs regardless of DPA pulse with an intact ATA, rendering DR more successful than IR in these patients [344, 345].

OHS patients are frequently poor surgical candidates as they have high-risk comorbid conditions, inadequate target artery, or vein conduit. This makes an endovascular approach the preferred therapy. After revascularization is completed, it is critical to reassess perfusion to the foot as adequate reperfusion is not guaranteed. A wound blush from contrast opacification of the vessels around the wound on angiography has been associated with higher rates of limb salvage in patients with critical limb ischemia [349].

6.24 Deep Vein Arterialization

6.24.1 When to Consider DVA?

Fakhir Elmasri, August Ysa,
and Sreekumar Madassery

In patients with CLTI, we are often faced with challenging cases of distal tibial arterial occlusions. We try repetitively to recanalize the occluded distal tibial arteries and, on many occasions, still have no success. The reason for this failure is usually the lack of reconstituted tibial and pedal arteries. The reconstituted tibial arteries, dorsalis pedis, or plantar arteries act as a target point for antegrade recanalization or serve as a direct access for retrograde recanalization. This condition, when the tibial arteries are occluded and there is no reconstitution of any named distal arteries in the foot (i.e. only collaterals), is referred to as a "Desert foot." These patients are also not candidates for surgical bypass, since there is no target vessel for distal anastomosis. Before DVA, these patients were considered as "no option."

Percutaneous deep venous arterialization (p-DVA) emerged several years ago as a viable option for patients with "desert foot," who have previously had no other option. Over the last few years, the terms for venous arterialization include DVA, p-DVA, dDVA, TADV, and simply "venous arterialization."

- All of these refer to the same end goal, with the only caveat being that dDVA is a "distal" DVA creation, which is described below.

There have also been several different technical approaches in DVA creation, mainly with varying equipment, approach, stent types, valve lysis, etc., which makes it impossible to completely cover all the methods. However, the examples and descriptions in this book should provide a relatively comprehensive guide.

- It should be noted that the concept of using the disease-free venous bed as an alternative conduit for perfusion of the peripheral tissues with arterial blood flow is not new.
- This was first described in surgical literature and published by Halstead and Vaughan in 1912 [350].
- That was followed by multiple iterations of surgically created deep venous arterialization.
- Some of these surgical approaches were plagued by valves, which are a hindrance to blood flow and would need to be made incompetent. In addition, numerous draining venous

collaterals would "steal back" the blood flow from the ischemic foot.

- A fully percutaneous approach, p-DVA, simplified the procedure, making it less morbid and less invasive. Mastering this procedure is critical for any interventionalist treating CLTI patients.

6.24.2   Advent of Percutaneous DVA

The first description of a totally percutaneous venous arterialization (p-DVA) was reported in 2015 by S. Kum et al. in Singapore [350]. The authors designed a dedicated device (LimFlow) based on an ultrasound-guided puncture to establish the arteriovenous (AV) communication (AVF). A tapered crossover-covered stent is thereafter deployed between the artery and the vein to redirect flow distally. This stent is extended with multiple self-expanding covered stents to the ankle level, to serve as a conduit, hence focalizing flow toward the foot and avoiding bleeding off from venous collaterals. Finally, an ancillary antegrade valvulotomy is performed to render the valves in the foot veins incompetent in order to increase forefoot perfusion.

6.24.2.1   Patient Selection/Evaluation

Subjectively, the patient should have an ejection fraction (EF) of at least 20% or above. This is important for two reasons.

- First, DVA may increase the hyperdynamic circulation, which might put some stress on the heart and push patients with weak hearts into heart failure. Beware of patients already on hemodialysis.
- Second, a poor ejection fraction with slow blood flow will not be able to maintain the patency through the long synthetic stents in the distal leg.
- Clearly, the patient should still have a viable leg to be a candidate. In a patient with Rutherford 5/6, the necrosis has to be in the toes or forefoot, with a healthy hindfoot/midfoot to sustain toes or midfoot amputation (TMA). A patient with ischemia or necrosis of

the stump of a midfoot amputation undergoing debridement is still a candidate.

- Nevertheless, if the amputation is recent, the swelling following the DVA might require decompression surgery.
- CLTI patients with rest pain can benefit greatly from this procedure. Some of these patients are in so much pain that they get addicted to painkillers.

Inflow to the TPT and PT has to be open. If the inflow arteries are occluded, they have to be recanalized prior to creating the DVA. Ultrasound of the venous system of the lower leg and foot with a tourniquet in place to evaluate the veins is often performed prior to the procedure. The good news is that the veins are usually paired, so one can pick the larger one of the medial or lateral PTV. Patency and size of the common plantar vein and medial and lateral plantar veins are critical to the success of the procedure.

6.24.2.2   Two Types of DVA

Proximal DVA: This is by far the most common approach, and most people refer to it as just DVA. After the creation of the arteriovenous Fistula (AVF), covered stent grafts are used to stent from the proximal tibial artery through the tibial vein, all the way to the ankle, in order to prevent blood flow going into the multiple draining veins.

- The most common and preferable location for creating the DVA fistula is between the proximal to mid-posterior tibial artery (PTA) and the posterior tibial vein (PTV).
- It can also be created from the tibioperoneal trunk (TPT) if the PTA is occluded. Although creating the fistula between the proximal anterior tibial artery and the anterior tibial vein is technically possible, it is not preferred, since the stents must be extended to the ankle and tends to have higher occlusion rates, as it cannot be extended into the dorsalis pedis artery due to the angulation.

Proximal DVA fistula creation is performed using re-entry devices, to connect the proximal

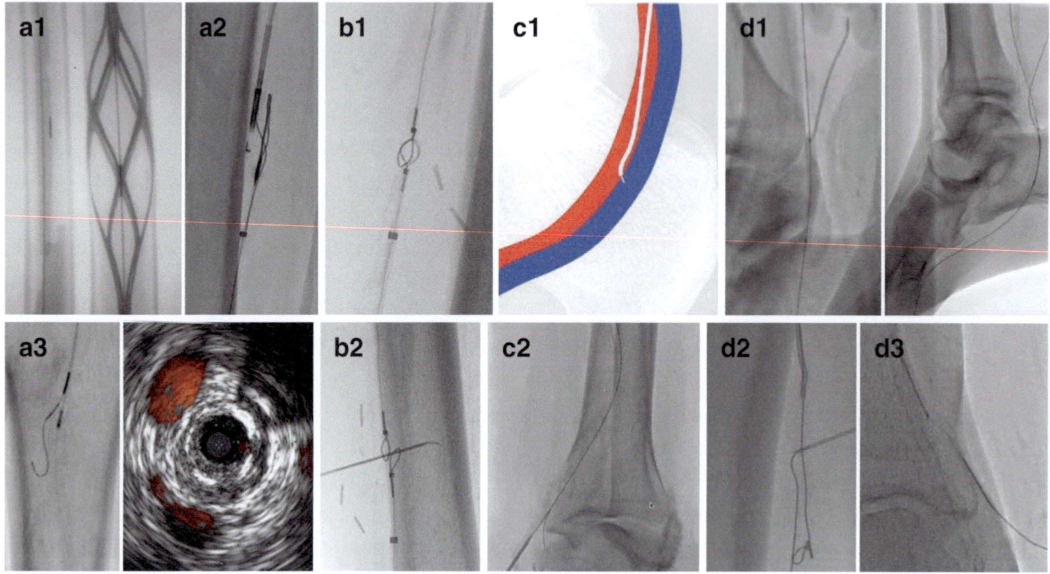

Fig. 6.92 Various DVA techniques including the use of (**a**) re-entry devices, (**b**) gun-sight technique, (**c**) Gandini's use of tibial vessel anatomy, and (**d**) the Spear technique

Fig. 6.93 Diagram of different types of percutaneous DVA

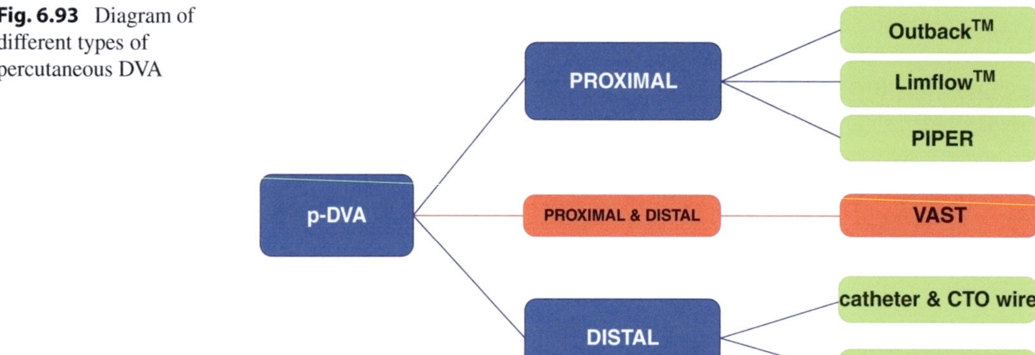

PTA to one of the two proximal PTVs. LimFlow (LimFlow, Santa Clara, CA) is the only FDA-approved device system for this procedure currently and in trials only, although others are in the works.

- Re-entry devices such as Outback Elite (Cordis, Santa Clara, CA) (Fig. 6.92A1–2) and Pioneer Plus (Philips Volcano) (Fig. 6.92A3) are being used to create the AVF, which are not FDA approved for this purpose [351, 352].
  - They are used mainly because the LimFlow device has a high cost and is not readily available at the time of this publication. This restriction resulted in various physicians globally developing different techniques, using "off-the-shelf" devices to create their own DVAs (Fig. 6.93).
- The targeting methods for AVF creation with re-entry devices vary, with some using an inflated balloon or a snare as a landmark in the vein, and to facilitate the capture of the deployed wire from the arterial side into the vein. In fact, this strategy has also recently been adopted by the LimFlow system.
- The gun-sight technique another approach, which is placing two snares, one in the PTA

placed through the antegrade common femoral artery (CFA) sheath, and the second snare placed in one of the PTVs, through retrograde access in the ankle, and subsequently advancing a needle percutaneously through both snares with a single guidewire (Fig. 6.92B1–2).

- The PIPER technique described by B. Migliara allows one to clearly visualize, which is the best venous target, and avoids the necessity of creating a distal venous access [352]. The increased profile and stiffness of the catheters used, and the difficulty to perforate the arterial wall by the embedded hollow crossing needle of the devices must be considered when dealing with small diameter, tortuous, or heavily calcified arteries.

- **Distal DVA:** This technique is in its infancy, and there are spurs of cases and data to support it currently. The fistula is created distally, at or just above the ankle, between the distal PTA and the PTV. As the AV connection is created distally, with less flow, this has been reported to have less swelling of the foot, and less burden on the heart, which are both advantageous.

  - One additional value of distal DVA approach is that, even if the mid- to distal aspect of planned inflow tibial artery is occluded, as long as a subintimal tract can be created down to the level of desired distal AV connection site, the DVA can still be performed.

  - Also, since the DVA is at the ankle, it is claimed that it has better perfusion of the foot, expediting healing to 2–4 weeks compared to 6–8 weeks for a proximal DVA, anecdotally.

- A distal DVA technique utilized by some operators is to perform the double gun-sight approach with two snares located just above the ankle, while a percutaneous needle is advanced through both snares, followed by a single wire that gets externalized. This is followed by angioplasty and ideally, no stent placement.

  - Some interventionalists place short coronary stents at the distal DVA to prevent the fistula from collapsing and closing. This

procedure can only be achieved by using the gun-sight technique.

- R. Gandini based on the anatomical disposition of the tibial vessels around the ankle (double veins with the arteries lying in between) uses the arterial calcification as a landmark to steer a curved catheter toward its wall and thereafter breaks into the vein with a CTO wire (Fig. 6.92C1) [353].

  - This is an inexpensive technique since all the required material is usually already on the table in any standard below-the-knee revascularization procedure.

  - The main downside of this relatively "blind maneuver" is the related 22% failure rate due to the inability to cross heavily calcified arteries or precisely locate the vein, although the latter could be overcome using a wire in the vein as a landmark as reported by M. Palena (Fig. 6.92C2).

- For improved venous access, there is an alternative approach which is preferred, with access into the lateral plantar vein, in the lateral aspect of the sole of the foot, at the level of the fourth metatarsal head.

  - Lateral plantar vein access can help track along the plantar and tibial vein valves with ease, which is sometimes difficult in the other direction.

  - This may have benefits to avoid stent graft infection.

- The so-called "Spear Techniques" was simultaneously described by M Montero-Baker, M. Manzi, and S. Ichihashi [354].

  - The authors perform an ultrasound-guided percutaneous puncture of either the vein or the artery. Once the first vessel is pierced, the needle is steered toward the second one and placed within it. A wire is progressed and thereafter externalized using a snare, a balloon, or a needle itself. A support catheter is generally used to reverse the tip of the withdrawn wire, and finally, both the catheter and the wire are simultaneously retrieved until the latter reaches the target vessel lumen. Once the wire is clearly within it, the access is secured by simple balloon dilation (Fig. 6.92D1–3).

- The "Spear Techniques" are also quite inexpensive and permit a distal location of the DVA.
- They have a substantial increased needle penetration power when dealing with calcified vessels.
- The US-guided access significantly decreases the radiation exposure.
- The technical demand of the Spear procedure is somewhat increased, which could sometimes limit its reproducibility.

- Based on the "gun-sight" approach, the author's group has described the venous arterialization simplified technique (VAST) [355, 356].

  - The AV connection is made by aligning two snares (one in each vessel) that are percutaneously pierced by a 21G needle.
  - The VAST technique is no longer a blind maneuver compared to Gandini's curved catheter and CTO wire approach.
  - Although this is not a codified technique, its technical difficulty is fairly low since the utilization of snares streamlines the overall procedure and the needle penetration power is also clearly increased.
  - Due to its universal availability and low cost, the main advantage of this technique is that it permits either a proximal LimFlow like p-DVA or a distal p-DVA using common "off-the-shelf" devices.

So far, there are no studies to validate these anecdotal claims and small patient samples; thus far, more studies are needed.

There is still an ongoing unsolved controversy whether it is better to perform a proximal or distal DVA since distal AVF usually generate lower flows than the proximal ones. The significance of this finding is however unclear as the limb salvage and wound-healing rates are equivalent for both proximal and distal p-DVA [357–359]. On the other hand, due to its location and enlarged flow rates there seems to be a general agreement that proximal DVAs are more prone to develop an increased systemic effect, of the so-called "storm after DVA" where one can see heart overload, swelling, cyanosis, pain secondary to arterial steal syndrome, etc.

6.24.2.3 Detailed Technique Description

Anesthesia: General anesthesia (GA) is preferred, but a significant number of patients do not get cleared for GA, so be prepared to do it under conscious sedation. In the first couple of cases, GA is recommended due to the learning curve. Patients with inability to remain still can be detrimental to this procedure.

Prep: Scrub the entire leg from the groin to the toes. Cover the toes with a sterile cover. Place a sterile tourniquet under the calf ready to be tied later on for tibial vein access.

Access: Gain antegrade access of the ipsilateral CFA and perform a runoff documenting patent inflow arteries to the proximal PTA (most patients already have prior angiograms). Place a 6F sheath, 45 cm in length with the tip in the popliteal artery, and select the PTA. Then, access the PTV at the ankle in a retrograde fashion. If the veins are small, use the tourniquet and pick the lager vein of the two PTVs. Place a 4F slender or regular sheath.

- Several operators prefer accessing the lateral plantar vein under the midfoot and using a tapered small caliber sheath, which can be beneficial to make navigating venous valves easier and safer.

Creation: Create the AVF between the proximal PTA and the bigger PTV using the LimFlow device if it is available to you, otherwise you can use the re-entry device, or gun-sight approach.

- Inflating a balloon in the PTV will facilitate the entry into the vein by creating a body to the vein, and a sturdy visible target to puncture using the re-entry devices. The wire can be pushed into the punctured and collapsed balloon and used to externalize the wire out of the venous access site.
- Another option is to place a snare in the PTV as a fluoroscopic target for the re-entry device.
- The author of this section has used all of these methods but now uses the gun-sight technique exclusively, because it is cheap and very effective. As described earlier, place the two snares in the PTA and PTV. Gain access percutane-

ously through both snares aided by two orthogonal views.

- After confirming that the micropuncture needle went through both snares, place a microwire (e.g., V18 wire, 300 cm in length) and remove the needle. Most of the time, the wire goes first through the arterial snare and the tip is at the venous snare.
- If this is the case, there are many techniques to be used here, but the simplest one is to externalize the tip through the 4F venous sheath by snaring the tip and pulling the wire while someone is feeding it from the calf to reduce the tension and friction until there is an equal length out of the calf and out of the venous sheath.
- Now pull the arterial snare and you will start pulling a loop through the 6F arterial sheath, while your assistant should be feeding the two ends of the wire, the one percutaneously through the calf, and the one through the PTV sheath to reduce friction. Have a clamp at the distal tip of the wire out of the PTV sheath.
- Once you externalize the loop from the 6F arterial sheath pull on each limb of the loop to determine which one is entering the calf percutaneously, and that is the one you need to pull out and externalize through the 6F arterial sheath.
- At this point, the back of the wire is out of the CFA arterial sheath and the tip is exiting the venous sheath in the ankle.
- Advance a catheter over the V18 from the 6F arterial sheath all the way through the 4F sheath in the PTV.
- A 5F catheter will not come out through the 4F sheath, which is fine. Take out the old wire, and it is probably beaten badly by now. Place a new V18 wire, then pull back the catheter intravascularly, and place the 4F slender back over the new V18.
- Pull the V18 back out of the 4F sheath into the PTV and then advance it around the sheath into the foot veins.
- In a minority of cases the reverse happens, and the wire goes through the venous snare first and the tip is at the arterial snare. In this case, snare out the tip through the 6F

arterial sheath. Do not loop it into the venous sheath because it is small and will not come out through it. Instead, advance a 4F or 5F catheter to the snare on the venous side. Then, advance a second V18 wire through the 4F sheath keeping the calf wire as a buddy wire. The new V18 wire will pass into the PTV and then advance to the foot beside the 4F sheath into the distal PTV.

In both scenarios, you will end up with a microwire through the 6F CFA sheath, through the AVF PTA/PTV, and with the floppy tip in the distal PTV or preferably plantar veins.

From this point, the procedure is the same regardless of what device or technique you use.

Dilate the AVF using a 4 mm balloon to facilitate the passage of the 5x25 mm Gore Viabahn stent (or similar graft outside of USA). Most patients will need to extend stent graft to the ankle level, based on location of valves. The author of this chapter used to previously place a Viabahn stent just distal to the AVF and a coronary stent into the PTA. Currently, the author just extends the Viabahn stent to the proximal PTA.

- This is unless the PT is occluded and the TPT was used instead, and then, the Viabahn is placed just distal to the AVF, and a coronary stent is placed into the TPT to keep the peroneal artery patent.

A long 5 mm balloon can be used throughout the PTV to prep the vein prior to stenting and to destroy the valves. Alternatively, initially the PTV can be stented, followed by high-pressure balloon venoplasty to fully open the two coaxial stents to the level of the ankle. An angiogram is then performed to demonstrate the patent AVF and stented PTV filling the arterialized venous bed of the foot.

- There is an invariable valve at the mid-calcaneus level, which needs to be destroyed, often performed with a 4- or 5-mm balloon.
- Next, try to pass a V18 (or similar) wire carefully through the pedal venous arch and balloon

any narrowing using a 3 mm balloon. It is recommended to not be aggressive in this step, so as not to cause a venous perforation.

6.24.2.4 Dealing with Stubborn Valves

One of the most cumbersome aspects once your wire has reached the calcaneal segment, while performing a p-DVA, is to cross and destroy the remaining valves of the foot. To overcome this issue, it is essential to be familiar with the venous foot anatomy so that one can locate the pathway to the plantar venous arch. A curved catheter and a 0.035 glide wire can be used to cross the valves (by looping the tip of the wire and gently pocking into them).

- Alternatively, R. Ferraresi described his "dancing wire" maneuver, where the catheter is constantly rotated to change the direction of the wire until the wire crossed the valve tips, and the catheter was then further advanced [360].
- On the other hand, many interventionalists usually prefer to gain direct distal venous access of the venous plantar arch as this bidirectional approach streamlines the overall crossing maneuver.
- Similarly, both the GSV and the LSV can be used as alternative retrograde routes to facilitate the passage of the wire (Fig. 6.94a–c).

There are several ways to render the remaining venous valves of the foot incompetent either using a dedicated antegrade valvulotome (LimFlow system) or "off-the-shelf" devices (Fig. 6.95).

- The most common maneuver is still using plain old balloon angioplasty (POBA) (Fig. 6.94d) to destroy the valves.
- In case of stubborn residual valve stenosis, ancillary techniques can be used such as ultra-non-compliant balloon angioplasty, cutting/scoring balloons (Fig. 6.94e), double wire maneuvers, or excimer laser, or even the "Pierce" technique by S. Ichihashi [361] (Fig. 6.94f).

Following the "escape from the fortress" concept reported by R. Ferraresi, once in the venous plantar arch, it is highly advisable to gain access and destroy the remaining valves into the first metatarsal vein (main drainage source to the forefoot) in order to avoid a roundabout effect of the flow through the venous plantar arch (Fig. 6.94g–i) [360].

6.24.2.5 How Low Can I Stent?

In the PROMISE and ALPS trials, the stents were generally extended to above the upper border of the calcaneus following the recommendations of S. Kum (developer of the LimFlow concept) [362, 363]. Oppositely, B. Migliara recommends overpassing the retinaculum ligament to avoid vein compression at that spot (Fig. 6.94j) [352]. Moreover, within the ALPS trial, "beyond the graft" distal extensions (Supera stents or DES) were sometimes used to overcome stent graft occlusions/restenosis on the venous side of the DVA during the follow-up.

6.24.3 Post-DVA Considerations

Reuben PerezAhmad Omar Hallak, and Zola N'Dandu

6.24.3.1 Antiplatelet and Anticoagulation Medications

There is no consensus on the optimal postprocedural antiplatelet and anticoagulation regimen. Most published deep venous arterialization (DVA) cases used a single antiplatelet agent indefinitely with full dose anticoagulation for 3–6 months, with some operators opting for dual antiplatelets for at least 3 months [364–371]. The decision on anticoagulation regimen should be tailored to individual patient comorbidities and risks for bleeding and thrombosis.

6.24.3.2 Restenosis and Reintervention

In a study that prescribed dual antiplatelets for at least 3 months, a reintervention rate of 14% at 6 months was reported compared to the other

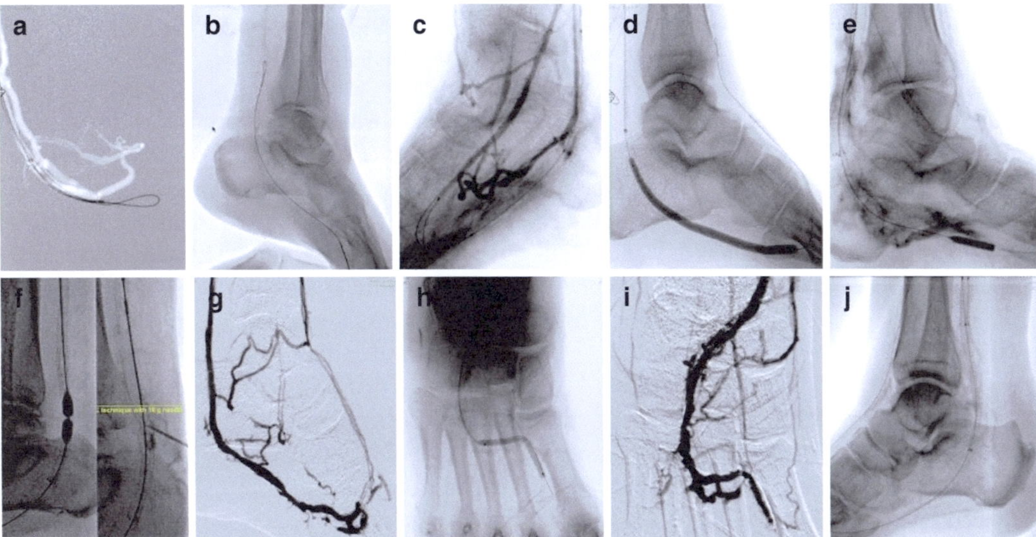

Fig. 6.94 Examples of dealing with stubborn venous valves during a DVA including (**a–c**) retrograde routes such as the saphenous veins, (**d**) POBA, or (**e**) cutting/scoring balloons to destroy the valves, or the (**f**) PIERCE technique. Once in the venous plantar arch, it is advised to (**g–i**) destroy the remainder of the valves. (**j**) It is recommended to stent passed the retinaculum ligament to avoid vein compression at that spot

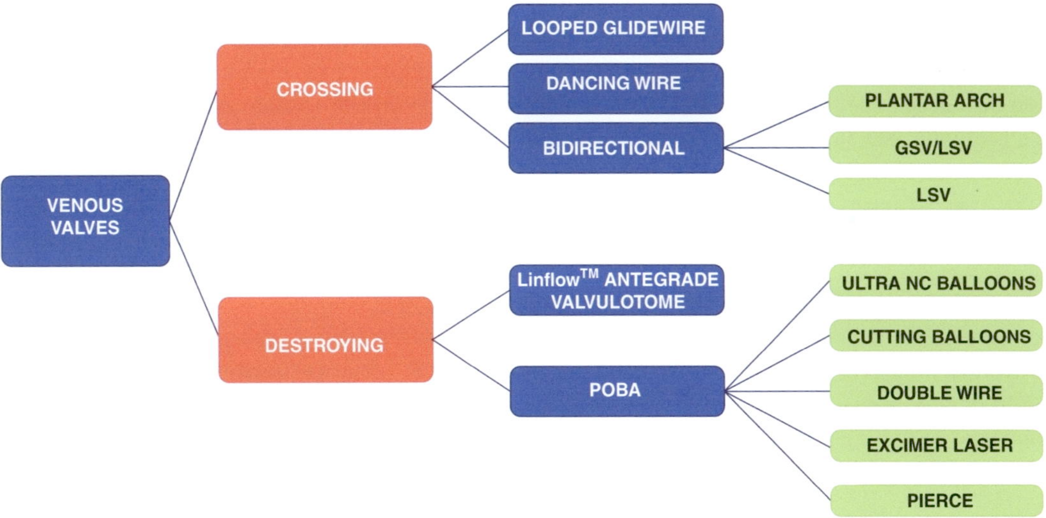

Fig. 6.95 Various methods to deal with stubborn valves during a DVA

studies with single antiplatelet agent with or without anticoagulation, which ranged between 25 and 86%. Interestingly, in AV fistula studies for vascular access in dialysis patients, the use of antiplatelets or anticoagulation has not been shown to reduce thrombosis rates or improve maturation [372]. Restenosis has been reported to be approximately 65% at six months, and the rate of reintervention history has been reported up to 15% at six months. Reintervention of inflow lesions, circuit, and outflow lesions have been reported.

6.24.3.3 Pharmacological Viewpoint

Arterial thrombosis is known to consist of clotted thrombocytes due to activation of the clotting cascade from damaged endothelium. This necessitates the use of antiplatelet therapy to prevent this cascade. Venous thrombosis typically involves fibrin, which can be inhibited by anticoagulation. Occlusions in DVA patients may be attributed to arterial thrombosis, venous thrombosis, or a combination of both. As mentioned previously, however, antiplatelets and anticoagulants have not been shown to reduce thrombosis or improve maturation in patients with AV fistulas for dialysis.

6.24.3.4 Covered Stents

Currently available self-expanding covered stents are Viabahn (Gore), Covera (BD, Fluency (BD), and dedicated LimFlow (LimFlow) covered stents (not commercially available). Some operators use balloon-expandable covered stents across the fistula for their radial strength and then overlap with self-expanding stents to the foot.

6.24.3.5 Skin Changes: Edema, Cyanosis, and Necrosis

Edema is very common after percutaneous or surgical deep venous arterialization. It is usually self-limiting and improves after 1 to 2 weeks. Some experts have used gentle diuresis and leg elevation. Cyanosis or deep purple discoloration has been reported due to venous hypertension. It usually resolves within a week but requires close monitoring as it could also be a sign of occlusion or excessive arterial steal from the fistula. Necrosis may initially get worse post-procedurally because of the initial arterial steal and reperfusion injury. It improves as the demarcation of the distal forefoot occurs.

6.24.3.6 Pain Management

Pain management is critical after DVA. Warn the patient about the throbbing pain and consider utilization of narcotics in addition to non-narcotic pain relievers such as tramadol, Neurontin, Lyrica, Cymbalta, and Elavil. NSAIDs are discouraged due to high risk of bleeding in the setting of dual antiplatelet therapy and/or anticoagulation. Pain improves as the circuit matures and delivers more oxygenated blood to the tissue indicative of an above healing thresh-

old TcPO2 of at least 40 mm Hg. Pain resolution can vary from 1 to 6 weeks.

6.24.3.7 Patency Assessment/Duplex Ultrasound

Close follow-up ultrasound surveillance is important to evaluate for early thrombosis, which can be re-vascularized with TPA and mechanical thrombectomy. If the thrombus is older than 6 to 8 weeks, it usually cannot be thrombectomized or lysed; however, the patient may have developed collaterals and still have better perfusion than prior to DVA creation in some patients where the DVA shutdown the wounds are already healed and then you have to evaluate the benefit/risk ration for reintervention. Also, some operators wait 4–6 weeks after creation to consider collateral embolization or other adjunctive techniques to assist wound healing.

Elevation in peak systolic velocity greater than 500 cm/s or doubling between two consecutive segments is concerning for high-grade stenosis. It is best obtained in the arterial inflow or proximal part of the circuit. Flow volume of less than 200 cc/min is also concerning for stenotic disease. Baseline duplex ultrasound can be obtained 48 to 72 h after the index procedure and then monthly thereafter until the wound is healed. A low threshold for angiography and intervention should be part of the strategy to maintain the patency of the circuit.

6.24.3.8 Reinterventions and Techniques

Interventions include angioplasty of outflow and inflow lesions, thrombectomy of the graft in case of thrombosis, and stenting to reline the graft or treat inflow or outflow lesions.

6.24.3.9 Amputation Strategies

It takes nearly 6 to 8 weeks to reach a healing threshold according to the ALPS registry. Delaying any major surgeries to allow for maturation of the circuit and remodeling of the vascular distribution is crucial for limb salvage. A guillotine amputation in cases to drain severe infection has been suggested with the definitive treatment six to eight weeks later. Preference is for open TMA amputation if it is being considered in the early weeks after DVA creation.

6.24.3.10 Wound Care

Wound care for DVA patients requires a dedicated team that ideally includes an angiologist, cardiologist, radiologist, vascular interventionalist, plastic surgeon, endocrinologist, podiatrist, social worker, a home health team, a nurse navigator, infectious disease expert, nephrologist, primary care physician, and family support for successful outcomes. The team should be able to provide *tension-free debridement* and *amputation without using tourniquets* to prevent occlusion of the circuit and the arterialized veins. Utilization of dermal substitutes, split thick skin grafts, allografts, vacuum-assisted therapy, and rotational skin flaps can improve and accelerate wound healing after revascularization.

6.24.4 When to Never Perform Deep Venous Arterialization

Reuben Perez McCon, RT Ahmad Omar Hallak, MDZola N'Dandu, MD

6.24.4.1 Patient Selection Process

DVA should be considered for no-option CLTI patients who have had multiple failed interventions whether surgical or endovascular without an available standard revascularization option to perfuse a desert foot. The *foot should not be severely infected to salvage a functional limb.*

Appropriate patient selection is critical for the successful outcome of DVA. Not every critical limb ischemia patient is a candidate for DVA.

- DVA should not be performed on a patient with extensive infection where the foot cannot be salvaged or whenever a patient cannot tolerate antiplatelet therapy or anticoagulation, which is required for the patency of the conduit.
- Additionally, it should not be performed on a patient with less than one-year life expec-

tancy. DVA should not be offered to patients who continue to smoke.

- Lastly it cannot be performed on a patient with thrombosed pedal veins.

6.24.4.2 Clinical Experience and Expert Opinion

The goal of DVA is limb salvage to improve both longevity and quality of life as compared to patients who would otherwise undergo amputation. While this procedure has the potential to save limbs, it is not without significant sacrifice including healthcare cost and resource utilization and prolonged radiation exposure to the vascular specialist and support staff. Since many factors contribute to positive outcomes following deep venous arterialization, a comprehensive evaluation of all determinants of health should be utilized to enhance patient selection and overall success.

6.24.5 What I Wish I Knew About DVA

Reuben Perez McConRT, Ahmad Omar Hallak and Zola N'Dandu

6.24.5.1 New Information/Lack of Information

Although currently dual integrated therapy or oral anticoagulation is used, there is no consensus thus far on the ideal or proven post-procedure regimen. With the worldwide interest in providing advanced treatment options for end-stage critical limb ischemia and more clinical trials, hopefully there will be more evidence-based information needed to perform these procedures with successful outcomes.

6.24.5.2 Clinical Experience and Expert Opinion

Not everyone involved in post-patient care will know the dos and don'ts of postoperative DVA care. Education on the concepts of DVA is important to both the patient/family and the entire team of providers caring for no-option CLTI patients.

6.24.6 What to Tell the Patient, Family Member, and/or Referring Provider

Sreekumar Madassery

Percutaneous deep vein arterialization (p-DVA, DVA, TADV) is still in its infancy, and clear understanding of long-term effects, outcomes, and how to optimize it are still yet to be clarified. However, as a growing body of evidence that it provides yet another limb preservation option, many operators have adopted this procedure. With that, it is important to have a frank and honest discussion with the patient, family, and other providers based on the short-term understandings noted thus far.

When discussing the potential for DVA option, it is important to bring the topic early in the discussions with any CLI/CLTI patient and family, so that they have heard the term in their journey of limb preservation. They should be told that if it is found that there is microvascular disease pattern on angiogram in the foot, also referred to as SAD (small arterial disease), DVA may be the only option for them if revascularization is needed. The following should also be considered:

- It must be stated that the long-term outcomes, the sequelae of true cardiac impact, venous complications, and other matters are not well understood. It is known that small subset of patients may develop high-output cardiac failure, which is a reason why DVA should not offered to patients with severe heart failure, or potentially the DVA may need to be embolized/ligated.
- Patients with significant preexisting venous insufficiency and edema may have negative impact from the venous hypertension that develops with DVA, which is why some operators try to perform distal DVA(dDVA) in these patients or avoid the procedure.
- All involved must be told that creation of DVA could hasten the time to major amputation, which may be due to increased venous hypertension causing blistering wounds and pro-

gression of infection, or with the process turning stable gangrene into wet gangrene.

- If there is an underlying infection, there is concern with infecting the implanted stent grafts that are used in DVA procedures, so this must be discussed as well.
- It is important to clearly inform that from what is known thus far, the true benefits of the arterialization may take 6–8 weeks to be realized. Therefore, everyone involved must be aware that pain relicf and wound healing will not be immediate, and the wound needs to be stable and continually monitored during this time. It has been noted that some wounds may appear worsened (especially with a recent TMA), before it starts improving.
  - However, it is not uncommon for some wound healing to be seen in the early weeks post-DVA, with granulation seen during wound care, and with pain improvement.
- Once the DVA is created, it is possible that repeat interventions may be needed, to treat stenoses, thrombosis, collateral vein embolization, etc., until maturation is achieved. Therefore, giving patients this warning is prudent to prevent any surprises.
- Patients and teams should understand that if the DVA occludes after the initial few months, the operator may choose to leave it alone, as the arterialization should have already commenced and shown its benefit. It could be futile to perform an exhaustive attempt to revascularize the DVA.

  - This does not hold true for the first two months, where it seems beneficial to address any issues noted on noninvasive imaging, physical examination, or direct angiogram.

Additional concerns to keep in mind are that minor amputation, particularly TMAs, should be delayed, if possible, until the DVA has had time to mature. The best estimates are between 4 and 8 weeks and based on thorough evaluation by the operator in follow-up. If the amputation is necessary in the interim, recommend tension-free amputation to allow the tissue to progressively heal.

In the end, as long as an upfront and honest conversation is had between the operator and the patient and family, with clear setting of expectations and unknowns, this procedure can be very successful technique to save limbs. Giving constant updates to the other providers only helps to improve outcomes, as the operator will be made aware of any important changes that happen, so timely intervention can be performed.

6.25 Hybrid Deep Vein Arterialization

Jill SommersetJorge Miranda, and Miguel Montero Baker

6.25.1 Definition of No Option

In the treatment of CLTI, the therapeutic goal is restoration of blood flow and perfusion; however, there is a segment of the CLTI population where standard surgical and endovascular revascularization attempts do not suffice, leaving no option for further treatment. The term "no-option CLTI" is an evolving concept that lacks a standardized definition by scientific consensus. Broadly speaking, no-option CLTI represents patients, which have no viable options for arterio-arterial reconstructions. Objective definitions and classification have been proposed in the past and include patients with extensive tissue loss, "desert foot" pedal anatomy, and the inability to revascularize the limb, but there is not yet broad adoption of any one definition by the medical community [373, 374].

6.25.2 MAC Classification

The main histopathological driver of no-option CLTI is severe below-the-ankle calcium burden. This burden can be graded via medial artery calcification (MAC) scoring. Ferraresi et al. proposed a risk classification of MAC, which divides patients into three groups based on distribution of MAC as evaluated by plain radiographic study of the foot [375]. The higher the MAC score, the worse the clinical results, including vascular and podiatric unplanned reinterventions and major adverse limb events.

6.25.3 Venous Arterialization

Though conventional revascularization approaches have been unsuccessful in no-option CLTI, the concept of venous arterialization as a solution has been hypothesized and attempted in various iterations for the last century. As previously discussed, arterialization of the veins retroperfuses the capillary bed in the ischemic foot by diverting oxygenated blood flow from diseased artery into non-diseased vein. The results have been heterogeneous and difficult to compare owing to the drastic differences in technical approaches and advances in technology. The absence of consistency has led to limited reported cohorts and poor adoption of the procedure.

Miranda et al. have shown clinical success with two main techniques: Transcatheter deep venous arterialization (TADV, aka deep vein arterialization/DVA) and hybrid superficial venous arterialization (HYSA) [376].

6.25.3.1 Selecting TADV vs HYSA

- TADV/DVA is a purely endovascular procedure that involves placing PTFE-covered stents across an anastomosis from the posterior tibial artery (ideally) to the posterior tibial vein and lining the PTV to divert arterial flow into the lateral plantar vein, where the venous valves have been lysed.
- Hybrid endovascular and surgical approach to this procedure is also performed. The HYSA procedure involves making an in situ open surgical anastomosis from the *greater saphenous vein to the popliteal artery* followed by valve lysis and distal endovascular focalization of flow.

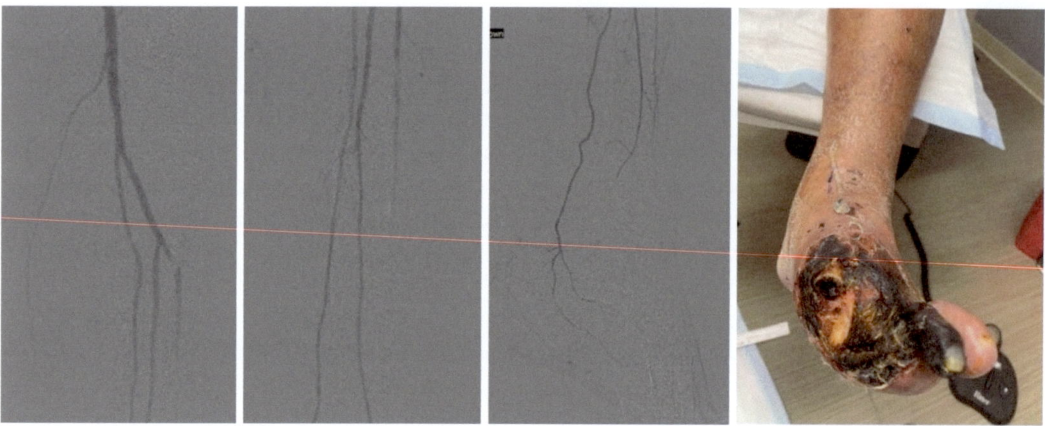

Fig. 6.96 Occlusive pattern of the forefoot. This pattern is best suited to perform a HSYA. During a HYSA procedure, there is no disruption of the PTA inflow as the anastomosis is done end-to-side

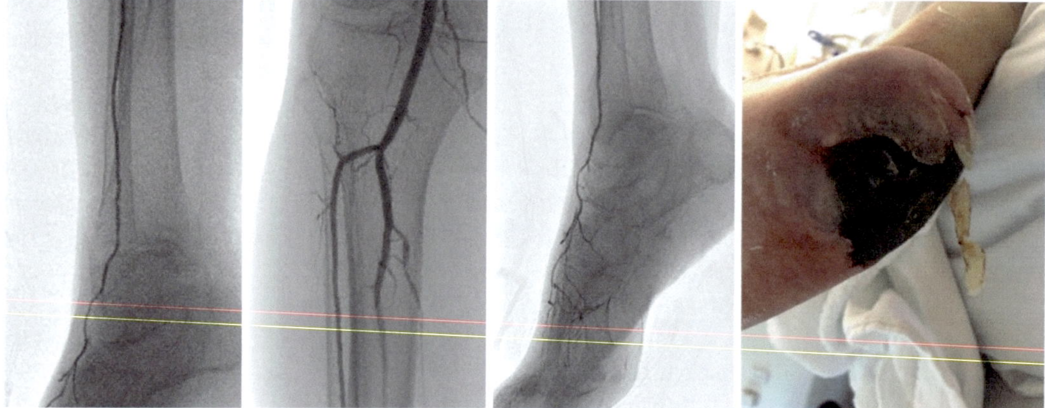

Fig. 6.97 Occlusive pattern of the hindfoot, also called orphan heel. This pattern is best suited to perform a TADV. Using the PTA as inflow would not alter baseline hemodynamics

- The decision to perform either primarily depends on the anatomical distribution of disease: In patients with an occluded anterior tibial artery and suitable GSV (>3.0 mm), HYSA is preferred. On the contrary, patients with an (Fig. 6.96) occluded posterior tibial artery regardless of GSV status, TADV/DVA is more suitable (Fig. 6.97).

6.25.3.2 Data

There is a growing body of evidence for both approaches, as technical advances allow for increased availability of appropriate devices for performing the procedures and as the procedure continues to be standardized.

- Early prospective studies of HYSA have shown very promising results, with Ferraresi et al. reporting limb salvage of 69% and wound healing in 44% of limbs at a mean follow-up of 10.8 months in a 35-patient cohort of no-option CLTI patients [377].
- TADV/DVA results in no-option CLTI patients have been reported in several patient cohorts including the experience of Kum et al., Del Giudice et al., Clair et al., and Schmidt et al., all of which reported consistent amputation-free survival rates at 12 months of 57–74% [370, 378–380].
- In addition to fully percutaneous TADV/DVA, Miranda et al. reported 81% limb salvage in a

cohort of 41 patients who underwent HYSA or TADV/DVA [376].

6.25.4 LimFlow System for Venous Arterialization

Sreekumar Madassery

LimFlow (LimFlow Inc.) system for deep vein arterilization(DVA) is a proprietary system used currently only in trials globally. The system has the necessary main components for DVA creation including ultrasound-based arterial and venous catheters to create the AV fistula, tapered covered stent graft, and an over-the-wire valvulotome.

LimFlow has thus far underdone two trials:

- PROMISE I, which had 32 patients followed for 1 year, reported in 2020, with 70% amputation-free survival (AFS) and 75% wounds healed/healing at 12 months.
- PROMISE II, which followed 105 patients, and the 6-month follow-up results were released on October 2022 at VIVA conference.
- The recent results were very promising, with 66% AFS (compared to 54% in the general population performance goal in these patients), and 76% limb salvage rate with >75% of wounds healed/healing at 6 months [381].

The results of these trials are incredibly promising, as these are the most complex and limb-threatening cohorts in the PAD population. While the proprietary system in under trials and awaiting commercial use, many operators globally have been performing DVA off the shelf for several years. The data for this are very difficult to generalize as there is no standardization of the techniques, and only retrospective reviews are currently reported. Recently, there was a retrospective review of 42 patient non-LimFlow DVA review, with 33 successful arterializations, and overall AFS at 6 months was ~61% for 25 patients, and 16 patients with minor amputations [382]. There will be far more retrospective studies reported in the coming years and hopefully more prospective and randomized studies so that a better understanding can be attained in this complex patient population. In the meantime, for patients truly with no options, and ambulatory status, venous arterialization may be the only option that still exists and still better than major amputation if avoidable.

6.26 No-Option Aortoiliac Patients Still Have Options

Murat Osman and Bulent Arslan

Historically, aortoiliac occlusive disease has been primarily managed with an open surgical approach. However, over the past several decades advents in interventional techniques and tools have allowed for hybrid and completely interventional/endovascular options to become possible. Open repair of aortoiliac disease is associated with higher operative mortality/morbidity, net cost, and longer length of stay when compared to hybrid and/or completely interventional repair [383, 384]. Hybrid and percutaneous approaches are especially better suited for patients who are deemed high risk for open surgery. Ultimately, appropriate selection of management should be based on center experience with open and endovascular procedures and patient factors such as age, comorbidities, and vascular anatomy.

We present a 77-year-old man with severe lifestyle-limiting claudication (> 50 feet) involving bilateral thighs and calves for approximately 15 years. He has a complex medical history including 40+ pack year smoking history, systolic heart failure s/p CABG in 1999 with two occluded coronary bypass grafts (LIMA to LAD patent), and previously placed bilateral external iliac artery (EIA) and renal artery stents. The patient was offered open only surgical revascularization at several major academic institutions, with a high mortality/morbidity risk due to his comorbidities. He declined those options and presented to our institution for a "fifth" opinion. Pertinent physical examination findings include non-palpable femoral, popliteal, dorsalis pedis (DP), and posterior tibial (PT) pulses bilaterally.

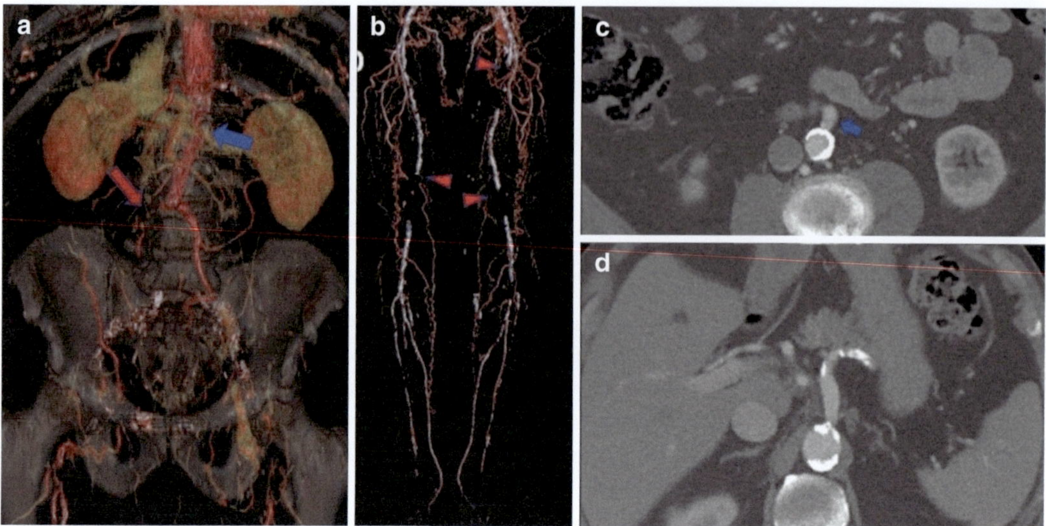

Fig. 6.98 Preprocedure coronal CTA 3D rendering (**a, b**) and axial planes (**a, b**) of the abdomen and pelvis demonstrate multilevel atherosclerotic disease and multilevel aortoiliac occlusions. (**a**) Note critical stenosis of the infrarenal aorta (blue arrow) and occlusion of the bilateral CIA stents and occluded EIA (red arrow). (**b**) Coronal 3D runoff demonstrates dominant high-grade atherosclerotic stenosis in the bilateral common and superficial femoral arteries (arrowheads), with one vessel runoff to the R foot via a reconstituted PT and L foot via reconstituted AT and PT arteries. (**c**) There is post-stenotic dilation of the IMA (blue arrow) and occlusive stenosis of the celiac origin (**d**), with complete occlusion of the SMA (not shown)

Initial ABI study was notable for ABI/TBI of 0.26/0.21 on the right and 0.29/0.12 on the left with biphasic PT/DP bilaterally. CTA of the abdomen/pelvis with runoffs demonstrated occlusion of the distal aorta below the IMA, bilateral common iliac (CIA), external iliac (EIA), common (CFA), and superficial femoral arteries (SFA) (Fig. 6.98a). Only the bilateral deep femoral branches and tibial arteries were patent, which were primarily fed by collaterals (Fig. 6.98b). The SMA and celiac artery were occlusive and were reconstituted through IMA collaterals (Fig. 6.98c, d). The bilateral renal artery stents were patent. Preprocedural aortography from a left brachial artery approach confirmed these findings (Fig. 6.99).

After considering patient's preference on forgoing any open abdominal surgery, a hybrid approach was planned, which aimed at recanalizing the distal aorta, L CIA/EIA arteries into the occlusive L CFA. This would be followed by immediate surgical repair of the bilateral CFAs and placement of a femoral–femoral bypass graft in one procedural setting.

Case Technical Description:

- First, left groin dissection with exposure of the left CFA was performed and access was obtained directly into the occlusive L CFA with a micropuncture system. Then, a 5 Fr pinnacle sheath was advanced with its tip into the occlusive EIA.
  - Through this sheath, an 0.035″ GLIDEWIRE and a Berenstein catheter were used to cross the occlusive segments to access the patent segment of the distal aorta.
- Then, the GLIDEWIRE was exchanged with an Amplatz wire, and over the wire, a 12 Fr introducer sheath was placed. Initial aortogram was performed (Fig. 6.100a) and angioplasty of the L CIA and EIA was performed (Fig. 6.100b).
- A 10 mm x15cm Viabahn stent was advanced and placed from the mid-portion of the L CIA extending into the proximal CFA segment (Fig. 6.100c).

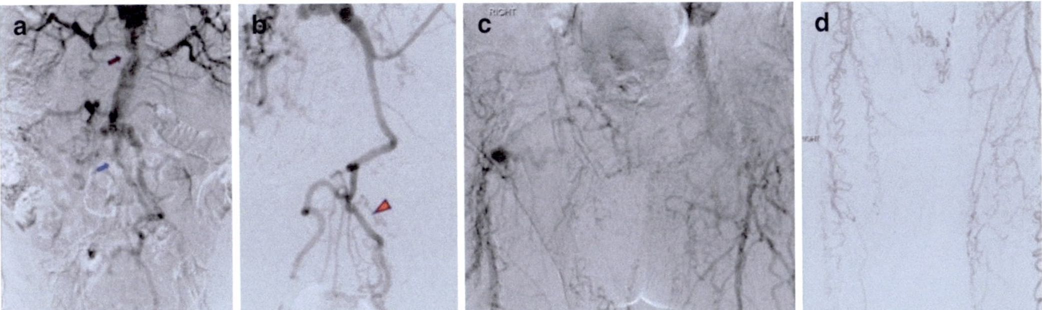

Fig. 6.99 Preprocedure aortogram (**a**) performed via L brachial access confirms findings of preprocedure CTA, with multilevel stenosis of the aorta just below the level of the renal arteries (red arrow) and occlusion of the aorta below the IMA (blue arrow). The bilateral renal artery stents are patent; however, no significant filling of the proximal celiac artery was visualized. Selective angiography (**b**) demonstrates hypertrophic IMA with large rectal artery collaterals (arrowhead). Pelvic and lower extremity angiography (**c**, **d**) demonstrates occlusions of the bilateral CIA, EIA, and CFA, and SFAs with prominent collaterals

- – This would allow the surgeon to access the distal stent and suture it into the surgically created femoral patch (i.e., conduit).
- At the proximal end of the stent construct, a Viabahn VBX balloon-expandable stent was placed to bridge the self-expanding Viabahn stents and the patent aorta (Fig. 6.100d). During placement of the VBX balloon-expendable stent, attention was paid not to push the plaque to the origin of the IMA.
  - – The restricted space in the distal aorta at the origin of the IMA was also a reason to recanalize only the left iliac system instead of both right and left.
- Post-deployment angiography demonstrated re-established arterial inflow to the L CFA; however, the IMA was no longer visualized (Fig. 6.100e). This was due to displacement of atherosclerotic plaque near the IMA ostium by the VBX stent graft.
- Subsequently, the VBX stent was pulled down a few millimeters by inflating a balloon inside it and applying a downward force (images not available). Repeat angiogram demonstrated improved flow to the IMA but persistent, suboptimal flow (Fig. 6.100f).
- Steps were then taken to ensure optimal flow to the IMA. A steerable sheath was advanced and positioned near the origin of the IMA (Fig. 6.101a). Using a Berenstein catheter with a 0.018 wire was advanced, and the IMA was successfully catheterized. Over the 0.018 wire, angioplasty of the IMA was performed, which resulted in rupture of the balloon (Fig. 6.101b, c).
  - – A snare was advanced over the existing system to retrieve the ruptured balloon fragment (Fig. 6.102a). After this, it was recognized that the balloon separated into two pieces.
- Although the proximal fragment was successfully removed, the distal fragment migrated into the distal IMA, adjacent to the arc of Riolan (Fig. 6.102b). To retrieve the distal fragment and optimize the IMA flow, first a 5 mm × 2.2 cm drug-eluting stent was deployed into the origin of the IMA (Fig. 6.102c). Through the stent, a snare was advanced, and the distal balloon was retrieved (Fig. 6.102d).
  - – After retrieval, residual spasm was noted secondary to instrumentation, which slowly resolved (Fig. 6.102e).
- Subsequently, a 10 mm × 4 cm balloon was inflated left within the stented L EIA to temporarily obstruct flow and allow for repair of bilateral CFA and placement of a fem-fem bypass graft (Fig. 6.102f), which was successfully completed.

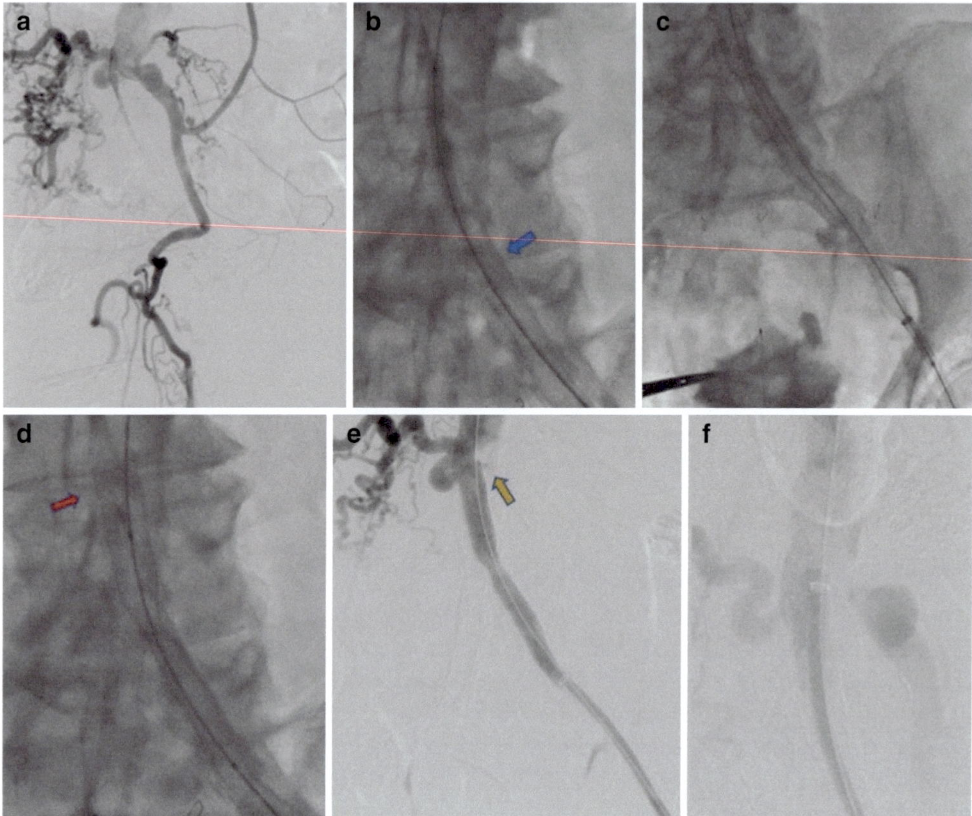

Fig. 6.100 Sequential fluoroscopic images demonstrating recanalization of the occluded left CIA. After obtaining initial aortogram (**a**), fluoroscopic image demonstrates serial dilation of the previous chronically occluded L EIA stent (arrow) and occlusive segments (**b**) prior to placement of Viabahn stent grafts extending to the proximal L CFA (**c**). Deployment of the proximal VBX stent graft (**d**) with post-dilation of the stent construct. Following deployment of the VBX stent, repeat angiogram (**e**) demonstrates diminished flow to the IMA (arrow). Following attempts to mechanically pull down the VBX stent with a balloon (**f**) and flow through the IMA improved however suboptimal flow persisted

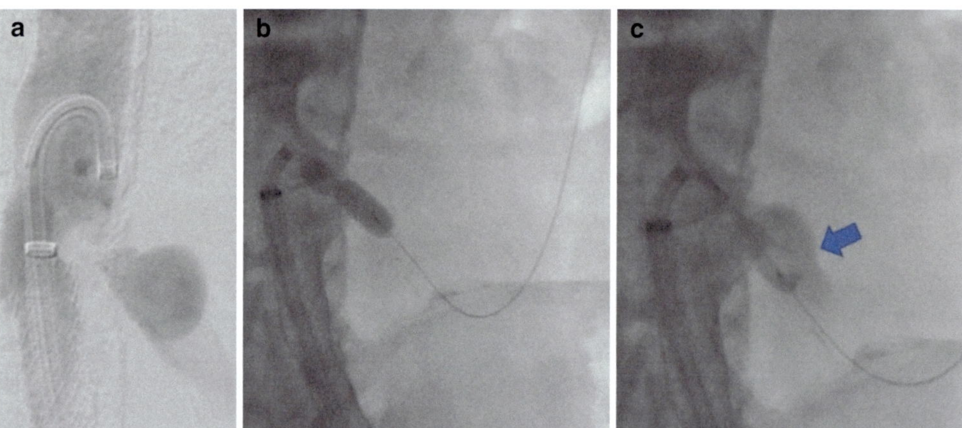

Fig. 6.101 Sequential fluoroscopic images demonstrating angioplasty of stenotic IMA origin and balloon rupture. Angiogram (**a**) demonstrating advancement of a steerable sheath with redemonstrated diminished flow. Sequential fluoroscopic images (**b** and **c**) demonstrate rupture of the balloon during inflation, as demonstrated by presence of contrast leaking outside the contours of the balloon (blue arrow)

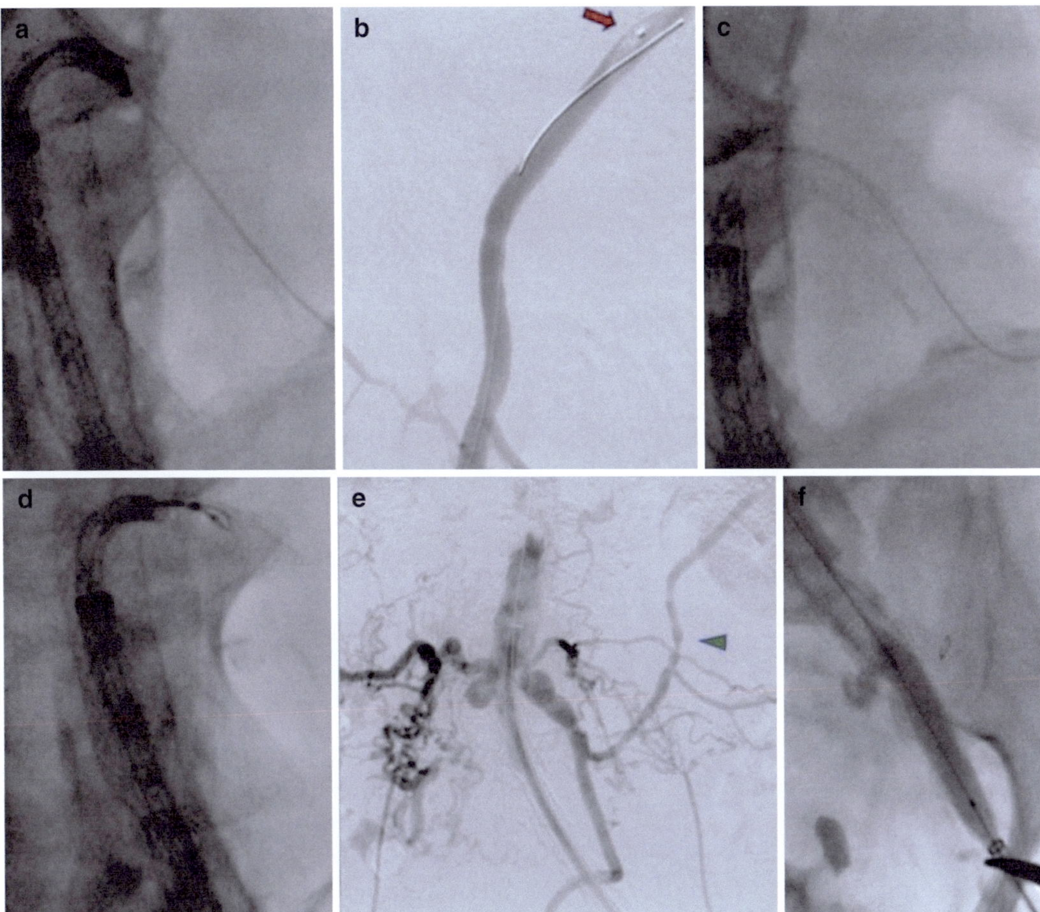

Fig. 6.102 Sequential fluoroscopic images demonstrating retrieval of the ruptured balloon. A snare was advanced through the existing system, and the retained balloon was successfully retrieved (**a**). Following snare retrieval, repeat angiography of the IMA demonstrates a radio-opaque density and surrounding filling defect in the distal IMA (**b**), representing an embolized fragment of the balloon. A drug-eluting stent was first deployed at the IMA origin (**c**) followed by retrieval of the distal balloon fragment with a snare (**d**). Subsequent aortography demonstrates improved and patent flow through the proximal and distal IMA (**e**). Note residual spasms of the mid-distal IMA (green arrow). At the end of the case, a balloon was left inflated within the stented L EIA to aid in the placement of a surgical bifemoral bypass (**f**)

The patient was ultimately discharged on POD #7. The patient's claudication symptoms resolved on one-month follow-up, with follow-up ABI demonstrating improved ABI/TBI bilaterally 0.60/0.43 on the right and 0.59/0.43 on the left with improved biphasic DP/PT waveform and palpable bilateral common femoral arteries. Several follow-up CTA studies at two months through 4 years demonstrate continued patency of the IMA, stent graft construct, and bifemoral bypass with no recurrence of claudication symptoms (Fig. 6.103).

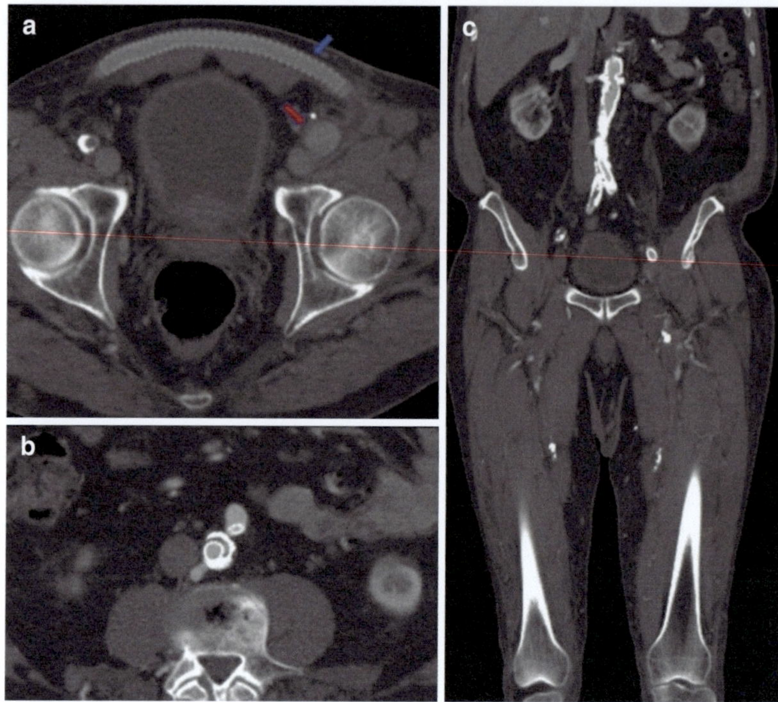

Fig. 6.103 Four-year follow-up CTA of the abdomen/pelvis with runoff in the axial plane (**a**, **b**) and 3D volume rendering (**c**) demonstrate patent bifemoral bypass graft (blue arrow) and surgical changes related to endarterectomy and patch angioplasty of the L EIA to the CFA bifurcation (red arrow). The stented IMA is patent (**b**)

6.27 Inequalities in Limb Preservation

Jordan Taylor, Nicole Keefe, Gloria Salazar and Maureen Kohi

6.27.1 Introduction

Peripheral artery disease affects an extensive and diverse patient population both domestically and abroad in the global health setting. There is strong evidence that supports major gaps in equality regarding the affected population and the involved diagnosis, treatment, and management. These gaps result in racial and gender disparities that increase the disease burden, severity at initial presentation, and ultimately result in a greater number of lower extremity amputations. This section will address racial, gender, and geographic disparities. The majority of the literature available focuses on Black Americans and non-Hispanic Whites. The current studies evaluating gender disparities focus on white females with a limited amount of data involving black females.

There is a paucity of data available on Hispanic Americans, Native Americans, Asian Americans, and other races within the USA. Lastly, this section will explore the differences in disease burden and demographics in the global health setting, understanding that each country and geographical landscape provide vastly different epidemiological data and management is usually limited by the infrastructure available to these countries.

The authors of this chapter recognize that race and ethnicity are a social construct without a biological basis with somewhat arbitrary official definitions, which continue to change over time. With that understanding, the authors have based conclusions using racial guidelines defined by the US Census Bureau, the US Office of Management and Budget, and the World Health Organization Racial and Ethnic Categories.

6.27.2 Racial Disparities in PAD

The overall prevalence of peripheral artery disease (PAD) among individuals over age 40 in the

United States is between 3 and 4% with the lowest rate among Asian Americans [385].

- There is an approximately 50% greater likelihood of PAD among Black Americans; this is likely underrepresented as 40% of patients present with severe disease, disproportionally affecting Black Americans [386].

While race is often reported as an independent risk factor for PAD[3], evaluation of the management and treatment of the cardiovascular risk factors such as hypertension, diabetes, metabolic disease, and chronic kidney disease reveal disparities that can, in part, account for these differences [387–389].

- Hypertension results in a greater than twofold increase in stroke and five times increase in end-stage renal disease in both Black men and women [390].
- Overall, the increased prevalence of tobacco use, diabetes, hypertension, and hyperlipidemia in Black Americans leads to a population-wide increased 30-year mortality [391–393]. While concerted efforts are made to reduce these risk factors in the overall population, Black Americans are less likely to receive adequate treatment and management.

Tobacco use is the most important risk factor associated with PAD; there is a direct dose–response relationship between smoking and atherosclerotic disease burden [394]. Smoking contributes to the pathophysiology of PAD by inducing endothelial cell dysfunction, remodeling of smooth muscle, and macrophage phenotype transformation leading to inflammation and atherosclerosis of vessel walls [395]. Estimates place the prevalence of smoking among patients with PAD at approximately 80% [396]. It is well established that the PAD progression can be slowed or even halted with smoking cessation [397].

- Unfortunately, Black Americans have lower rates of smoking cessation [398, 399]. Varying explanations are offered for this phenomenon and mainly pertain to increased socioeconomic pressures, lower rates of health insurance, which limit pharmacological aids, higher rates of traumatic experiences, especially in the urban setting, increased number of macro and microaggressions, and living in physically and socially impoverished areas [399, 400].
- Lastly, Black Americans are more likely to smoke mentholated cigarettes over non-Hispanic Whites (NHW); use of mentholated cigarettes is associated with decreased smoking cessation when compared to non-mentholated cigarettes among Black Americans [401, 402]. Special attention should be provided in the clinical setting to make construed efforts toward Black American patients who have experienced difficulty with smoking cessation; to gain a holistic understanding of the individual and create a clear roadmap for success in order to eliminate the most highly impactful modifiable risk factor.

Other modifiable risk factors that disproportionately affect Black Americans include pharmacological management of hyperlipidemia and hypertension. It has been well established that statin therapy not only reduces the rate of cardiovascular and cerebrovascular disease, but also leads to a reduction in limb amputations in patients with PAD [403].

- There exists an underutilization of guideline-appropriate statin therapy among the Black American community when compared to NHWs [404].

Blood pressure management faces a similar challenge: Undermedication and poor control are most prevalent among Black Americans [405]. These combined risk factors lead to an overall increase in PAD and critical limb ischemia. The underlying factors involved in this discrepancy are complex. Proposed ideas involve socioeconomic, belief-related, and clinician differences, all of which are a part of the larger more complex story of structural racism that afflicts these American communities.

Lastly, diabetes is a major risk factor in the development of PAD.

- Black Americans are more likely to have type 2 diabetes, have less awareness of the disease, and ultimately have poorer glycemic control [406]. While there has been no direct link between the mainstays of treatment such as sodium–glucose co-transporter 2 (SGLT2) and glucagon-like peptide 1 agonists (GLP1) agents and decreasing rates of PAD, their effect on decreasing cardiovascular risk is enough to include them in treatment plans [407].

When medical management fails to limit the progression of PAD, revascularization via endovascular or operative treatment serves as limb salvage therapy before amputation. There are robust disparities between NHWs, Black Americans, and Hispanics.

- Black Americans in particular are less commonly offered limb revascularization and four times more likely to undergo amputation, while Hispanic Americans have a 50% increased risk, when compared to NHWs [408–411]. This extends to additional treatment modalities as well including inpatient medical management and wound debridement [409].
- Additionally, Black Americans who are offered limb salvage have worse outcomes including a higher 30-day mortality rate, lower successful limb salvage rates, and higher hospital costs [412–414]. Overall, these trends lead to worse outcomes for Black and Hispanic Americans even when controlled for severity of presentation, rates of diabetes, and level of comorbidity.

Racial disparities in the management and outcomes of critical limb ischemia are widely accepted to disproportionally affect Black and Hispanic Americans when compared to NWHs.

- Black Americans in particular have a higher prevalence and severity of presentation of PAD. Black Americans have a higher prevalence of risk factors for PAD such as tobacco use, diabetes, and hypertension, which are often not well controlled.
- Lastly, Black and Hispanic Americans have a higher risk of undergoing amputation versus revascularization.

Addressing these racial disparities is essential to addressing the growing PAD population, especially as endovascular treatment improves in efficacy and availability.

6.27.3 Gender Disparities in PAD

The US population gender-related differences in critical limb ischemia are growing as a crucial area of concern.

- While the incidence of PAD in men and women is the same, women outlive men and prevalence is higher in the aging female population [415].
- In addition, there is a growing rate of women initially presenting with critical limb ischemia, the most advanced presentation of PAD [416].
- Lastly, there is an overall lack of awareness of PAD in women and underrepresentation in clinical trials [417, 418].
- Diagnosis of PAD in women tends to occur at a later age and with more advanced disease [419]. Proposed explanations for this difference include differences in risk factors and higher asymptomatic disease presentations [420].
- It is postulated that estrogen may serve as a protective barrier to the development of PAD, which may explain why women present at a later age. The traditional risk factors for developing PAD such as smoking, hypertension, dyslipidemia, and diabetes are typically higher among men [421].
- There are also women-specific comorbidities such as hypothyroidism, arthritis, osteoporosis, and inflammation that occur more often in women with PAD [422]. Lack of knowledge of these comorbidities may contribute to lower

identification of early PAD. Women also tend to present more often with asymptomatic disease [422, 423].

- Prior evidence has demonstrated that less than half of women with an ABI less than 0.91 will present with typical PAD symptoms and instead present with atypical symptoms such as slower walking velocity, poorer standing balance, slower time to arise, and fewer steps per week [424, 425].

Dissemination of this knowledge is critical to the identification of early PAD, especially in the primary care setting where prevalence is high [426]. Furthermore, early intervention can lead to decreased rates of critical limb ischemia (CLI) as evidence has not shown differences in treatment outcomes between sexes [427, 428].

- The available data suggest women tend to undergo revascularization more often than amputation [429].
- Of those who undergo intervention, women tend to undergo endovascular over open surgical revascularization [430].
- Women also tend to have a higher technical success rate and higher patency rate following endovascular treatment [431].
- However, there is a limited yet growing body of evidence to suggest that women experience higher complication rates, treatment failure, and eventual limb loss [431–434].

Overall, there remains a paucity of data on the sex differences between males and females with PAD.

- Women tend to present with advanced disease, with asymptomatic and atypical presentations.
- There is a preference for endovascular treatment with higher technical success rates and patency rate. This is despite a growing body of evidence that women experience higher complications and treatment failure rates, with the underlying reasons not yet well understood.
- Finally, women are underrepresented in PAD clinical trials, which limit evidence-based outcomes that can further inform clinicians on the best treatment modalities to address these sex-based differences.

6.27.4 Regional and Global Inequalities of PAD

Inequalities in peripheral arterial disease differ geographically both domestically and globally. In the United States, there is regional variation in patient factors that lead to the development of PAD. These include the prevalence of diabetes, cardiovascular disease, and tobacco use; these risk factors tend to be more prevalent in the Southeastern United States [435]. Furthermore, there are significant disparities between the treatments of critical limb ischemia.

- There is strong evidence that rural populations have higher amputation rates than their urban counterparts [436, 437].
- In addition, Black Americans within the Southeastern United States, especially those with diabetes, are at increased risk of amputation over endovascular revascularization, underscoring the importance in providing equitable care to this very high-risk population [438–440].

There is limited research on the global health burden of PAD. It is understood that global prevalence of PAD continues to rise and affects approximately 236 million people worldwide [441]. Risk factors such as age, smoking, hypertension, and diabetes are associated with an increased prevalence of PAD and vary throughout the world, particularly affecting low-to-middle-income countries [441].

- A total of 15 countries account for two-thirds of the global PAD burden; China had the highest level of PAD in low-to-middle-income countries [441].
- The lowest rates of PAD were in Africa though there is debate as to if there is actually a high prevalence of PAD in sub-Saharan Africa [442].

- In lower-income countries, PAD was noted to affect younger patients, as compared to older men and women in high-income countries [443]. Possible explanations for this discordant disease development include a younger generation, which has grown up in a less health-promoting environment with increased exposure to cardiovascular disease risk factors, and smoking in particular is of upmost concern.
- Younger patients are also more likely to be asymptomatic, a point at which disease modification and treatment will have the largest impact.
- Furthermore, in more affluent countries, disease presentation may occur at an older age due to better control of modifiable risk factors.
- Future global health efforts should focus on low-to-middle-income countries to identify and treat PAD before there is an inevitable increase in CLI within these countries.

Conclusion: Inequalities in PAD must be addressed via outreach, treatment, and research. PAD and CLI disproportionally affect Black and Hispanic Americans leading to ultimately higher rates of amputation. Women face substantial inequalities via atypical and asymptomatic presentations, lack of awareness, and higher complication/treatment failure rates. Lastly, the global burden of PAD is expected to increase in young patients of low- and middle-income countries; identifying these patients and then instituting public health risk modifications strategies can lead to a decrease burden of CLI.

6.28 BEST-CLI Trial: in Limb Preservation

Sreekumar MadasseryBrian Schiro, and Carlos Bechara

As readers have hopefully understood from the expansive material covered in the arterial chapter of this book, the growth of endovascular and surgical approaches in limb preservation has been immense. One of the difficulties often encountered is to know whether a surgical, endovascular, or hybrid approach is best suited for these patients, and to muddy the waters even more, who is best suited to treat these patients. While the latter cannot be answered since operator experience and technical success, practice environments, patient populations, and other variables will never be standardized, there are efforts to explore if certain approaches have better outcomes than others. While it is difficult to standardize patients into a truly randomized controlled study, a very recent study (BEST-CLI), had just completed and results published/presented at the time of this book completion, so we felt it would be amiss if its findings and operator perspectives were not included in this book. Additionally, and perhaps more importantly, a brief understanding of how this study has impacted varying physician practice patterns. Since its first presentation at the end of 2022 at the AHA annual meeting, as well as more and more readers dissect through this valiant effort of a study, many varying interpretations, questions, and disagreements have ensued. This must be expected with such a big undertaking of a study, for which all involved should be commended for completing, and many more questions and thoughts will come in the future.

We felt that it would only do proper justice to at least have the thoughts and opinions from the perspective of a highly experienced vascular surgeon, as well as nonsurgical limb preservation endovascular specialist.

6.28.1 An Endovascular Specialist's Thoughts

The long-awaited results from the BEST-CLI trial were published with modest fanfare in the New England Journal of Medicine in December 2022 [444]. Although this was a large, international trial, it fell short of the target enrollment of 2100 patients (enrolling 1830) due to reported "difficulties with enrollment." Nonetheless, it was a prospective, randomized, open-label, multicenter, superiority trial in patients with

Rutherford 4 or greater critical limb-threating ischemia. Patients were randomized to undergo open surgery versus endovascular therapy and were assigned to two surgical cohorts: Cohort 1 (1434 patients) had a single segment of great saphenous vein as a bypass conduit, while cohort 2 (396 patients) required an alternative conduit for bypass. Interestingly, 19% of the surgical patients were found to have a single segment of great saphenous vein as a bypass conduit at the time of surgery.

Endovascular interventions were performed by a heterogeneous group of operators, including vascular surgeons (73%), cardiologists (15%), and interventional radiologists (13%) with no specific requirement for validation of skillset or experience. While this is not unique to other trials of surgical and endovascular therapy, it is important to consider the potential for bias toward the surgical groups without knowing the operators' endovascular skill sets. Moreover, early technical failure rates were high in the endovascular group (15% and 19.4% in Cohorts 1 and 2, respectively) as were major reinterventions (23.5%). This compares with little to no technical failures in the surgical groups (2% and 0% in Cohorts 1 and 2, respectively) and low major reinterventions (9.2%). One could deduce, from these dichotomous outcomes, suboptimal endovascular skills and excellent surgical skills in the collective group of operators. Furthermore, it is interesting that patients initially without a suitable great saphenous vein were found to have a single-segment, adequate vein in 19%, yet no difference in outcome was found in the open versus endovascular cases in Cohort 2. Could this have instigated a bias toward more dedication to the endovascular procedure, knowing there were limited bailout surgical options? Lastly, it is also worthwhile to consider the rapid evolution of tools and techniques in the endovascular realm, which may also outpace the relevance of procedures performed in the early years of this study. While drug-coated and drug-eluting devices were used, these devices were placed on hold in the latter years of the study due to concerns for an increased mortality signal, thus limiting state-of-the-art devices even during the study period.

The primary outcome of major adverse limb events or death occurred in 42.6% and 42.8% of the surgical groups and 57.4% and 47.7% of the endovascular groups in Cohort 1 (hazard ratio, 0.68; 95% confidence interval [CI], 0.59 to 0.79; $P < 0.001$) and Cohort 2 (hazard ratio, 0.79; 95% CI, 0.58 to 1.06; $P = 0.12$), respectively. From these data, the following conclusions were drawn: In patients with a good-quality great saphenous vein, surgery-first strategy is associated with a 32% lower risk of major adverse limb events or death over endovascular therapy; those without a suitable single-segment great saphenous vein have similar efficacy and safety between surgical and endovascular treatments. It is important to consider what patients were enrolled in this trial. During the follow-up period, only 40.3% of patients had a major adverse cardiovascular event. This is historically low in patients with CLTI, which may suggest a healthier patient population [445].

Most patients with CLTI have extensive comorbidities that often preclude them from undergoing general anesthesia or open surgery. The true number of patients not enrolled due to lack of surgical candidacy is not known but likely speaks to the slow recruitment for the trial (note that most sites enrolled less than 10 patients). Perhaps it would have been interesting to compare these patients' endovascular outcomes with those of the trial patients. Irrespective, endovascular treatments should not be withheld from this patient population in concordance with discussions on this trial. As expected, serious adverse events, perioperative death, and length of stay favored the endovascular group; this is particularly important in the sicker patient populations. Also, the reported higher quality-of-life responses favored endovascular repair in Cohort 1 despite inferior outcomes.

While the BEST-CLI trial has brought to light several important points on treatment of patients with CLTI, the unusually healthy patient population, unknown skillset of operators, and rapidly evolving endovascular techniques bring into question the applicability of the data to everyday patients. As of now, we do not know anatomical patterns or complexity of vascular disease, predictors of technical failure, full effect on quality of life, cost analysis, or role of patient preference, and subgroup analyses are underway to determine, which may impact treatment strategies. Until then, we will continue to offer endovascular first as the primary treatment strategy in the majority of CLTI patients.

## 6.28.2	A Vascular Surgeon's Thoughts

This is a great randomized study published in the prestigious New England Journal of Medicine, but in my humble opinion did not answer, nor will it change my practice as an academic vascular surgeon. Here is why: We already know that nothing is better than a bypass using a single-segment greater saphenous vein. Now, for patients who do not have a single-segment greater saphenous vein, both surgery and endovascular therapy were similar in overall efficacy and safety. In my mind, a prosthetic bypass with a Linton patch is second best for CLI patients, but I will focus on the endovascular group. Before I do that, bypass surgery is tedious, but the principle is easy, do the bypass from a healthy inflow vessel to a healthy target vessel. However, endovascular therapy is not that simple or easy, despite following the same principle going from healthy to healthy. When faced with a long-segment occlusion, finding and using the right endovascular tools is heterogeneous and dependent on both operator preference and the patient's anatomy (i.e., length of occlusion, calcifications, and tortuosity). This probably explains why the BEST-CLI study had a technical failure rate for endovascular therapy of 15.3% [444].

Another heterogeneous practice exclusive to endovascular therapy and not open surgical bypass is the type of intervention, which could lead to suboptimal or less durable results. Tools like using re-entry devices, crossing devices, atherectomy, different balloon angioplasties, lithotripsy, and stenting are very operator-dependent, even within the same institution. Even when we successfully cross a lesion, the therapy is variable too. When I perform balloon angioplasty, I use

2- to 3-min inflation and usually with 2.5–3.5 mm diameter balloons to treat tibial lesions, whereas sometimes I see operators using <2 mm balloon with only a few seconds of inflation time. In my opinion, that is not durable.

Hence, this heterogeneous practice in endovascular therapy for limb salvage led to 42.5% reintervention rate within 30 days in the endovascular group [444]. At the end of the day, our patients with tissue loss will only benefit from a multidisciplinary discussion among surgeons, interventionalists, podiatric surgeons, infectious disease, and other specialties involved in limb preservation.

References

1. Sincos IR, da Silva ES, Ragazzo L, Belczak S, Nascimento LD, Puech-Leão P. Chronic thrombosed abdominal aortic aneurysms: a report on three consecutive cases and literature review. Clinics (Sao Paulo). 2009;64(12):1227–30.
2. Lotto CE, Sharma G, Walsh JP, Shah SK, Nguyen LL, Ozaki CK, Menard MT, Belkin M. The impact of combined iliac occlusive disease and aortic aneurysm on open surgical repair. J Vasc Surg. 2020;71(6):2021–2028.e1.
3. Wolf YG, Otis SM, Schwend RB, Bernstein EF. Screening for abdominal aortic aneurysms during lower extremity arterial evaluation in the vascular laboratory. J Vasc Surg. 1995;22(4):417–21. discussion 421-3
4. Tuna Katırcıbaşı M, Güneş H, Çağrı Aykan A, Aksu E, Özgül S. Comparison of ultrasound guidance and conventional method for common femoral artery cannulation: a prospective study of 939 patients. Acta Cardiol Sin. 2018;34(5):394–8.
5. Arko F, McCollough R, Manning L, Buckley C. Use of intravascular ultrasound in the endovascular management of atherosclerotic aortoiliac occlusive disease. Am J Surg. 1996;172(5):546–9. discussion 549-50
6. Pescatori LC, Tacher V, Kobeiter H. The use of re-entry devices in aortoiliac occlusive disease. Front Cardiovasc Med. 2020;7:144.
7. Price LZ, Safir SR, Faries PL, McKinsey JF, Tang GHL, Tadros RO. Shockwave lithotripsy facilitates large-bore vascular access through calcified arteries. J Vasc Surg Cases Innov Tech. 2020;7(1):164–70.
8. Bosch JL, Hunink MG. Meta-analysis of the results of percutaneous transluminal angioplasty and stent placement for aortoiliac occlusive disease. Radiology. 1997;204(1):87–96.
9. Mwipatayi BP, Thomas S, Wong J, Temple SE, Vijayan V, Jackson M. Burrows SA; Covered

Versus Balloon Expandable Stent Trial (COBEST) Co-investigators. A comparison of covered vs bare expandable stents for the treatment of aortoiliac occlusive disease. J Vasc Surg. 2011;54(6):1561–70.

10. Mwipatayi BP, Sharma S, Daneshmand A, Thomas SD, Vijayan V, Altaf N, Garbowski M, Jackson M, COBEST co-investigators. Durability of the balloon-expandable covered versus bare-metal stents in the Covered versus Balloon Expandable Stent Trial (COBEST) for the treatment of aortoiliac occlusive disease. J Vasc Surg. 2016;64(1):83–94.e1.

11. Mwipatayi BP, Ouriel K, Anwari T, Wong J, Ducasse E, Panneton JM, de Vries JPM, Dave R. A systematic review of covered balloon-expandable stents for treating aortoiliac occlusive disease. J Vasc Surg. 2020;72(4):1473–1486.e2.

12. Van Haren RM, Goldstein LJ, Velazquez OC, Karmacharya J, Bornak A. Endovascular treatment of TransAtlantic Inter-Society Consensus D aortoiliac occlusive disease using unibody bifurcated endografts. J Vasc Surg. 2017;65(2):398–405.

13. Jean-Baptiste E, Brizzi S, Bartoli MA, Sadaghianloo N, Baqué J, Magnan PE, Hassen-Khodja R. Pelvic ischemia and quality of life scores after interventional occlusion of the hypogastric artery in patients undergoing endovascular aortic aneurysm repair. J Vasc Surg. 2014;60(1):40–9. 49.e1

14. Kalteis M, Gangl O, Huber F, Adelsgruber P, Kastner M, Lugmayr H. Clinical impact of hypogastric artery occlusion in endovascular aneurysm repair. Vascular. 2015;23(6):575–9. https://doi.org/10.1177/1708538114560462. Epub 2014 Nov 20

15. Smith AH, Dash S, Driscoll EC, Kirksey L, Rowse J, Hardy D, Lyden SP, Caputo FJ, Smolock CJ. Outcomes of hypogastric coverage and occlusion during endovascular treatment of aortoiliac occlusive disease. Ann Vasc Surg. 2021;77:116–26.

16. Goverde PC, Grimme FA, Verbruggen PJ, Reijnen MM. Covered endovascular reconstruction of aortic bifurcation (CERAB) technique: a new approach in treating extensive aortoiliac occlusive disease. J Cardiovasc Surg. 2013;54(3):383–7.

17. Taeymans K, Goverde P, Lauwers K, Verbruggen P. The CERAB technique: tips, tricks and results. J Cardiovasc Surg. 2016;57(3):343–9. Epub 2016 Mar 24

18. Kruszyna, Lukasz & Staniśić, Michał-Goran & Dzieciuchowicz, Lukasz & Krasiński, Zbigniew. (2019). Results of the Covered Endovascular Repair of the Aortic Bifurcation (CERAB) Technique With BeGraft Balloon Expandable Covered Stent for Endovascular Treatment of Complex Aortoiliac Lesions. Eur J Vasc Endovasc Surg. 58:e813–e814.

19. Taeymans K, Groot Jebbink E, Holewijn S, Martens JM, Versluis M, Goverde PCJM, Reijnen MMPJ. Three-year outcome of the covered endovascular reconstruction of the aortic bifurcation technique for aortoiliac occlusive disease. J Vasc Surg. 2018;67(5):1438–47.

20. Antonello M, Squizzato F, Piazza M. The Viabahn balloon expandable stent for endovascular reconstruction of the infrarenal aorta and its bifurcation in cases of severe obstructive disease. Vascular. 2021;29(1):40–4.

21. Dijkstra ML, Goverde PC, Holden A, Zeebregts CJ, Reijnen MM. Initial experience with covered endovascular reconstruction of the aortic bifurcation in conjunction with chimney grafts. J Endovasc Ther. 2017;24(1):19–24.

22. Shiloh AL, et al. Ultrasound-guided catheterization of the radial artery: a systematic review and meta-analysis of randomized controlled trials. Chest. 2011;139(3):524–9.

23. Seto AH, et al. Real-time ultrasound guidance facilitates femoral arterial access and reduces vascular complications: FAUST (Femoral Arterial Access With Ultrasound Trial). JACC Cardiovasc Interv. 2010;3(7):751–8.

24. Randolph AG, et al. Ultrasound guidance for placement of central venous catheters: a meta-analysis of the literature. Crit Care Med. 1996;24(12):2053–8.

25. Hind D, et al. Ultrasonic locating devices for central venous cannulation: meta-analysis. BMJ. 2003;327(7411):361.

26. Abu-Fadel MS, et al. Fluoroscopy vs. traditional guided femoral arterial access and the use of closure devices: a randomized controlled trial. Catheter Cardiovasc Interv. 2009;74(4):533–9.

27. Adam DJ, et al. Bypass versus angioplasty in severe ischaemia of the leg (BASIL): multicentre, randomised controlled trial. Lancet. 2005;366(9501):1925–34.

28. Edelman SK, editor. Understanding ultrasound physics : fundamentals and exam review. 2nd ed. Houston, TX: ESP; 1994. p. 391.

29. Saab F, et al. Chronic total occlusion crossing approach based on plaque cap morphology: the CTOP classification. J Endovasc Ther. 2018;25(3):284–91.

30. Mustapha JA, et al. Comparison between angiographic and arterial duplex ultrasound assessment of tibial arteries in patients with peripheral arterial disease: on behalf of the Joint Endovascular and Non-Invasive Assessment of LImb Perfusion (JENALI) Group. J Invasive Cardiol. 2013;25(11):606–11.

31. Hua WR, Yi MQ, Min TL, Feng SN, Xuan LZ, Xing J. Popliteal versus tibial retrograde access for subintimal arterial flossing with antegrade-retrograde intervention (SAFARI) technique. Eur J Vasc Endovasc Surg. 2013;46(2):249–54.

32. Ye M, Zhang H, Huang X, Shi Y, Yao Q, Zhang L, Zhang J. Retrograde popliteal approach for challenging occlusions of the femoral-popliteal arteries. J Vasc Surg. 2013;58(1):84–9.

33. Fanelli F, Lucatelli P, Allegritti M, Corona M, Rossi P, Passariello R. Retrograde popliteal access in the supine patient for recanalization of the superficial femoral artery: initial results. J Endovasc Ther. 2011;18(4):503–9.

34. Sheth RA, Ganguli S. Closure of alternative vascular sites, including axillary, brachial, popliteal, and surgical grafts. Tech Vasc Interv Radiol. 2015;18(2):113–21.

35. Ballı Ö, Çakır V, Coşkun M, Pekçevik R, Gür S. Implementation of the EXOSEAL vascular closure device in the transpopliteal arterial approach. J Vasc Interv Radiol. 2018;29(8):1180–6.

36. Noory E, Rastan A, Sixt S, Schwarzwälder U, Leppännen O, Schwarz T, Bürgelin K, Hauk M, Branzan D, Hauswald K, Beschorner U, Nazary T, Brantner R, Neumann FJ, Zeller T. Arterial puncture closure using a clip device after transpopliteal retrograde approach for recanalization of the superficial femoral artery. J Endovasc Ther. 2008;15(3):310–4.

37. Barbetta I, van den Berg JC. Access and hemostasis: femoral and popliteal approaches and closure devices-why, what, when, and how? Semin Intervent Radiol. 2014;31(4):353–60.

38. Pezold M, Blumberg S, Sadek M, Maldonado T, Cayne N, Jacobowitz G, James H, Berland T. Antegrade superficial femoral artery access for lower extremity arterial disease is safe and effective in the outpatient setting. Ann Vasc Surg. 2021;72:175–81.

39. Kweon M, Bhamidipaty V, Holden A, Hill AA. Antegrade superficial femoral artery versus common femoral artery punctures for infrainguinal occlusive disease. J Vasc Interv Radiol. 2012;23(9):1160–4.

40. Zenunaj G, Traina L, Acciarri P, Mucignat M, Scian S, Alesiani F, Serra R, Gasbarro V. Superficial femoral artery access for infrainguinal antegrade endovascular interventions in the hostile groin: a prospective randomized study. Ann Vasc Surg. 2022:S0890-5096(22)00200-X.

41. Gutzeit A, Schoch E, Sautter T, Jenelten R, Graf N, Binkert CA. Antegrade access to the superficial femoral artery with ultrasound guidance: feasibility and safety. J Vasc Interv Radiol. 2010;21(10):1495–500.

42. Avraham E, Natour M, Obaid W, Karmeli R. Superficial femoral artery access for endovascular aortic repair. J Vasc Surg. 2020;71(5):1538–45.

43. Schmidt A, Bausback Y, Piorkowski M, Werner M, Bräunlich S, Ulrich M, Varcoe R, Friedenberger J, Schuster J, Botsios S, Scheinert D. Retrograde recanalization technique for use after failed antegrade angioplasty in chronic femoral artery occlusions. J Endovasc Ther. 2012;19(1):23–9.

44. Palena LM, Manzi M. Direct stent puncture technique for intraluminal stent recanalization in the superficial femoral and popliteal arteries in-stent occlusion: outcomes from a prospective clinical analysis of diabetics with critical limb ischemia. Cardiovasc Revasc Med. 2013;14(4):203–6.

45. Aprigliano G, Giupponi L, Palloshi A, Glavina F, Morici N. Sheathless use of Supera stent minimizes access complications in antegrade femoral puncture: technical note with case series. J Vasc Access. 2021;16:11297298211050480.

46. Titano JJ, Biederman DM, Zech J, Korff R, Ranade M, Patel R, et al. Safety and outcomes of transradial access in patients with international normalized ratio 1.5 or above. J Vasc Interv Radiol. 2018;29(3):383–8.

47. Posham R, Young LB, Lookstein RA, Pena C, Patel RS, Fischman AM. Radial access for lower extremity peripheral arterial interventions: do we have the tools? Semin Interv Radiol. 2018;35(5):427–34.

48. Sher A, Posham R, Vouyouka A, Patel R, Lookstein R, Faries PL, et al. Safety and feasibility of transradial infrainguinal peripheral arterial disease interventions. J Vasc Surg. 2020;72(4):1237–46.e1.

49. Uhlemann M, Möbius-Winkler S, Mende M, Eitel I, Fuernau G, Sandri M, et al. The Leipzig prospective vascular ultrasound registry in radial artery catheterization: impact of sheath size on vascular complications. JACC Cardiovasc Interv. 2012;5(1):36–43.

50. van Leeuwen MAH, Hollander MR, van der Heijden DJ, van de Ven PM, Opmeer KHM, Taverne Y, et al. The ACRA Anatomy Study (Assessment of Disability After Coronary Procedures Using Radial Access): a comprehensive anatomic and functional assessment of the vasculature of the hand and relation to outcome after transradial catheterization. Circ Cardiovasc Interv. 2017;10(11):e005753.

51. Shoji S, Kohsaka S, Kumamaru H, Sawano M, Shiraishi Y, Ueda I, et al. Stroke after percutaneous coronary intervention in the era of transradial intervention. Circ Cardiovasc Interv. 2018;11(12):e006761.

52. Patel VG, Brayton KM, Kumbhani DJ, Banerjee S, Brilakis ES. Meta-analysis of stroke after transradial versus transfemoral artery catheterization. Int J Cardiol. 2013;168(6):5234–8.

53. Pancholy SB, Karuparthi PR, Gulati R. A novel nonpharmacologic technique to remove entrapped radial sheath. Catheter Cardiovasc Interv. 2015;85(1):E35–8.

54. Ying L, Xu K, Gong X, Liu X, Fan Y, Zhao H, et al. Flow-mediated dilatation to relieve puncture-induced radial artery spasm: a pilot study. Cardiol J. 2018;25(1):1–6.

55. Satti SR, Sivapatham T, Eden T. Radial artery neuro guide catheter entrapment during mechanical thrombectomy for acute ischemic stroke: Rescue brachial plexus block. Interv Neuroradiol. 2020;26(5):681–5.

56. Repanas T, Christopoulos G, Brilakis ES. Administration of ViperSlide™ for treating severe radial artery spasm: case report and systematic review of the literature. Cardiovasc Revasc Med. 2015;16(4):243–5.

57. Fidone E, Price J, Gupta R. Use of ViperSlide lubricant to extract entrapped sheath after severe radial artery spasm during coronary angiography. Tex Heart Inst J. 2018;45(3):186–7.

58. Raje V, Christopher S, Hopkinson DA, Kania DA, Jovin IS. Administration of Rotaglide™ solution for treating refractory severe radial artery spasm: a case report. Cardiovasc Revasc Med. 2018;19(8s):56–7.

59. Sciahbasi A, Cuono A, Marrangoni A, Rigattieri S. Papaverine use for radial artery sheath entrapment. Anatol J Cardiol. 2019;22(1):44–5.

60. Nazir S, Nesheiwat Z, Syed MA, Gupta R. Severe radial artery spasm causing entrapment of the Terumo radial to peripheral destination slender sheath: a case report. Eur Heart J Case Rep. 2020;4(2):1–4.

61. Dawson K, Jones TL, Kearney KE, McCabe JM. Emerging role of large-bore percutaneous axillary vascular access: a step-by-step guide. Interv Cardiol. 2020;15:e07.

62. Yufa A, Mikael A, Gautier G, Yoo J, Vo TD, Tayyarah M, et al. Percutaneous axillary artery access for peripheral and complex endovascular interventions: clinical outcomes and cost benefits. Ann Vasc Surg. 2022;83:176–83.

63. Harris E, Warner CJ, Hnath JC, Sternbach Y, Darling RC 3rd. Percutaneous axillary artery access for endovascular interventions. J Vasc Surg. 2018;68(2):555–9.

64. Rudnick MR, Leonberg-Yoo AK, Litt HI, Cohen RM, Hilton S, Reese PP. The controversy of contrast-induced nephropathy with intravenous contrast: what is the risk? Am J Kidney Dis. 2020;75(1):105–13. https://doi.org/10.1053/j.ajkd.2019.05.022.

65. Rundback JH, Nahl D, Yoo V. Contrast-induced nephropathy. J Vasc Surg. 2011;54:575–9.

66. Gupta RK, Bang TJ. Prevention of contrast-induced nephropathy (CIN) in interventional radiology practice. Semin Interv Radiol. 2010;27(4):348–59. https://doi.org/10.1055/s-0030-1267860.

67. Davenport MS, Cohan RH, Caoili EM, Ellis JH. Repeat contrast medium reactions in premedicated patients: frequency and severity. Radiology. 2009;253(2):372–9.

68. Sharafuddin MJ, Marjan AE. Current status of carbon dioxide angiography. J Vasc Surg. 2017;66(2):618–37.

69. Cho KJ. Carbon dioxide angiography: scientific principles and practice. Vasc Specialist Int. 2015;31(3):67–80. https://doi.org/10.5758/vsi.2015.31.3.67.

70. Caridi JG, Cho KJ, Fairia C, Eghbalieh N. Carbon dioxide digital subtraction angiography (CO_2 DSA): a comprehensive user guide for all operators. Vasc Dis Manag. 2014;11:E221–56.

71. Kozlov DB, Lang EV, Barnhart W, Gossler A, De Girolami U. Adverse cerebrovascular effects of intraarterial CO_2 injections: development of an in vitro/in vivo model for assessment of gas-based toxicity. J Vasc Interv Radiol. 2005;16:713–26.

72. Thomas RP, Viniol S, König AM, Portig I, Swaid Z, Mahnken AH. Feasibility and safety of automated CO_2 angiography in peripheral arterial interventions. Medicine. 2021;100(2):e24254. https://doi.org/10.1097/MD.0000000000024254.

73. Palena LM, Diaz-Sandoval LJ, Candeo A, Brigato C, Sultato E, Manzi M. Automated carbon dioxide angiography for the evaluation and endovascular treatment of diabetic patients with critical limb ischemia. J Endovasc Ther. 2016;23:40–8.

74. Kawarada O, Sakamoto S, Harada K, Ishihara M, Yasuda S, Ogawa H. Contemporary crossing techniques for infrapopliteal chronic total occlusions. J Endovasc Ther. 2014;21(2):266–80.

75. DeMartini TJ. Retrograde dissection reentry for coronary chronic total occlusions. Interv Cardiol Clin. 2012;1(3):339–44.

76. Joyal D, Thompson CA, Grantham JA, Buller CE, Rinfret S. The retrograde technique for recanalization of chronic total occlusions: a step-by-step approach. JACC Cardiovasc Interv. 2012;5(1):1–11.

77. Tepe G, Beschorner U, Ruether C, et al. Drug-eluting balloon therapy for femoropopliteal occlusive disease: predictors of outcome with a special emphasis on calcium. J Endovasc Ther. 2015;22(5):727–33.

78. Fanelli F, Cannavale A, Gazzetti M, et al. Calcium burden assessment and impact on drug-eluting balloons in peripheral arterial disease. Cardiovasc Intervent Radiol. 2014;37(4):898–907.

79. Zeller T, Langhoff R, Rocha-Singh KJ, et al. Directional atherectomy followed by a paclitaxel-coated balloon to inhibit restenosis and maintain vessel patency: twelve-month results of the DEFINITIVE AR study. Circ Cardiovasc Interv. 2017;10(9):e004848.

80. Kokkinidis DG, Jawaid O, Cantu D, et al. Two-year outcomes of orbital atherectomy combined with drug-coated balloon angioplasty for treatment of heavily calcified femoropopliteal lesions. J Endovasc Ther. 2020;27(3):492–501.

81. Foley TR, Cotter RP, Kokkinidis DG, Nguyen DD, Waldo SW, Armstrong EJ. Mid-term outcomes of orbital atherectomy combined with drug-coated balloon angioplasty for treatment of femoropopliteal disease. Catheter Cardiovasc Interv. 2017;89(6):1078–85.

82. Tepe G, Brodmann M, Werner M, et al. Intravascular lithotripsy for peripheral artery calcification: 30-day outcomes from the randomized disrupt PAD III trial. JACC Cardiovasc Interv. 2021;14(12):1352–61.

83. Brodmann M, Werner M, Holden A, et al. Primary outcomes and mechanism of action of intravascular lithotripsy in calcified, femoropopliteal lesions: Results of Disrupt PAD II. Catheter Cardiovasc Interv. 2019;93(2):335–42.

84. Ichihashi S, Shibata T, Fujimura N, Nagatomi S, Yamamoto H, Kyuragi R, Adachi A, Iwakoshi S, Bolstad F, Saeki K, Obayashi K, Kichikawa K. Vessel calcification as a risk factor for in-stent restenosis in complex femoropopliteal lesions after Zilver PTX paclitaxel-coated stent placement. J Endovasc Ther. 2019;26(5):613–20.

85. Tepe G, Brodmann M, Bachinsky W, Holden A, Zeller T, Mangalmurti S, Nolte-Ernsting C, Virmani R, Parikh S, Gray W, For the Dirupt PAD III Investigators. Intravascular lithotripsy for peripheral artery calcification: mid-term outcomes from the

randomized disrupt PAD III trial. JSCAI. Original Research. 2022;1(4):100341.

86. Disrupt BTK II. CTG Labs - NCBI https://beta.clinicaltrials.gov/study/NCT05007925

87. Schillinger M, Minar E. Percutaneous treatment of peripheral artery disease: novel techniques. Circulation. 2012;126(20):2433–40. https://doi.org/10.1161/CIRCULATIONAHA.111.036574.

88. Neville RF, Sidawy AN. Myointimal hyperplasia: basic science and clinical considerations. Semin Vasc Surg. 1998;11(3):142–8.

89. Dias-Neto M, Matschuck M, Bausback Y, Banning-Eichenseher U, Steiner S, Branzan D, Staab H, Varcoe RL, Scheinert D, Schmidt A. Endovascular treatment of severely calcified femoropopliteal lesions using the "Pave-and-Crack" technique: technical description and 12-month results. J Endovasc Ther. 2018;25(3):334–42. https://doi.org/10.1177/1526602818763352. Epub 2018 Mar 20

90. Stanek F. Laser angioplasty of peripheral arteries: basic principles, current clinical studies, and future directions. Diagn Interv Radiol. 2019;25(5):392–7. https://doi.org/10.5152/dir.2019.18515.

91. Dippel EJ, Makam P, Kovach R, George JC, Patlola R, Metzger DC, Mena-Hurtado C, Beasley R, Soukas P, Colon-Hernandez PJ, Stark MA, Walker C, EXCITE ISR Investigators. Randomized controlled study of excimer laser atherectomy for treatment of femoropopliteal in-stent restenosis: initial results from the EXCITE ISR trial (EXCImer Laser Randomized Controlled Study for Treatment of FemoropopliTEal In-Stent Restenosis). JACC Cardiovasc Interv. 2015;8(1 Pt A):92–101. https://doi.org/10.1016/j.jcin.2014.09.009. Epub 2014 Dec 10

92. Herzog A, Bogdan S, Glikson M, Ishaaya AA, Love C. Selective tissue ablation using laser radiation at 355 nm in lead extraction by a hybrid catheter; a preliminary report. Lasers Surg Med. 2016;48(3):281–7. https://doi.org/10.1002/lsm.22451. Epub 2015 Dec 22

93. Stavroulakis K, Argyriou A, Watts M, Varghese JJ, Estes BA, Torsello G, Bisdas T, Huasen B. How to deal with calcium in the superficial femoral artery. J Cardiovasc Surg (Torino). 2019;60(5):572–81. https://doi.org/10.23736/S0021-9509.19.11038-5. Epub 2019 Jun 21

94. Adams G, Subramanian V. Optimizing laser atherectomy for different lesion morphologies. J Crit Limb Ischem. 2021;1(1):E27–33.

95. Mustapha JA, Diaz-Sandoval LJ, Saab F. Tibioperoneal CTOs in patients with critical limb ischemia. Endovasc Today May 2014.

96. Banerjee S, Shishehbor MH, Mustapha JA, Armstrong EJ, Ansari M, Rundback JH, Fisher B, Peña CS, Brilakis ES, Lee AC, Parikh S. A Percutaneous crossing algorithm for femoropopliteal and tibial artery chronic total occlusions (PCTO Algorithm). J Invasive Cardiol. 2019;31:111–9.

97. Thomas R, Sarode K, Mohammad A, Sethi S, Baig MS, Gigliotti OS, Ali MI, Klein A, Abu-Fadel MS, Shammas NW, Prasad A, Brilakis ES. Crossing of infrainguinal peripheral arterial chronic total occlusion with a blunt microdissection catheter. J Invasive Cardiol. 2014;26:363–9.

98. Bosiers M, Diaz-Cartelle J, Scheinert D, Peeters P, Dawkins KD. Revascularization of lower extremity chronic total occlusions with a novel intraluminal recanalization device: results of the ReOpen study. J Endovasc Ther. 2014;21:61–70.

99. Laird JR, Mathews SJ, Brodmann M, Soukas PA, Schmidt A, Wing-It Trial Investigators. Performance of the Wingman catheter in peripheral artery chronic total occlusions: short-term results from the international Wing-It trial. Catheter Cardiovasc Interv. 2021;97:310–6.

100. Laird J, Joye J, Sachdev N, Huang P, Caputo R, Mohiuddin I, Runyon J, Das T. Recanalization of infrainguinal chronic total occlusions with the crosser system: results of the PATRIOT trial. J Invasive Cardiol. 2014;26:497–504.

101. Gur I, Lee W, Akopian G, Rowe VL, Weaver FA, Katz SG. Clinical outcomes and implications of failed infrainguinal endovascular stents. J Vasc Surg. 2011;53:658–66. discussion 667

102. Dippel E, Makam P, Kovach R, et al. Randomized control study of Excimer Laser atherectomy for treatment of femoropopliteal In-Stent restenosis. J Am C CardiolInt. 2015;8:92–101.

103. Ho K, Owens C. Diagnosis, classification and treatment of femoropopliteal artery in-stent restenosis. J Vasc Surg. 2017;65:545–54.

104. Tosaka A, et al. Classification and clinical impact of restenosis after femoropopliteal stenting. J Am Coll Cardiol. 2012;59:16–23.

105. Sabeti D, Mlekusch S, et al. Conventional balloon angioplasty versus peripheral cutting balloon angioplasty for treatment of femoropopliteal artery in-stent restenosis: initial experience. Radiology. 2008;248:297–302.

106. Krakenberg H, Tubler T, et al. Drug Coated balloon versus standard balloon for superficial femoral artery in-stent restenosis. The randomized Femoral Artery In-Stent restenosis (FAIR) trial. Circulation. 2015;132:2230–6.

107. Virga V, Stabile E, et al. Drug-Eluting balloons for treatment the superficial femoral artery In-stent restenosis. J Am Coll Cardiol. 2014;7:411–5.

108. Boisers M, Deloose K, et al. Superiority of stent-grafts for in-stent restenosis in the superficial femoral artery: twelve month results from a multicenter randomized trial. J Endovasc Ther. 2015;22(1):1–10.

109. Zeller T, Dake M, et al. Treatment of femoropopliteal in-stent restenosis with paclitaxel-eluting stents. J Am Coll Cardiol Int. 2013;6:274–81.

110. Blaisdell FW. Development of femoro-femoral and axillo-femoral bypass procedures. J Vasc Surg. 2011;53(2):540–4.

111. Mishall PL, Matakas JD, English K, Allyn K, Algava D, Howe RA, Downie SA. Axillobifemoral bypass: a brief surgical and historical review. Einstein J Biol Med. 2016;31(1–2):6–10.
112. Samson RH, Showalter DP, Lepore MR Jr, Nair DG, Dorsay DA, Morales RE. Improved patency after axillofemoral bypass for aortoiliac occlusive disease. J Vasc Surg. 2018;68(5):1430–7.
113. Tadros RO, Vouyouka AG, Ting W, et al. A review of superficial femoral artery angioplasty and stenting. J Vasc Med Surg. 2015;3:183.
114. Goodney PP, Beck AW, Nagle J, et al. National trends in lower extremity bypass surgery, endovascular interventions, and major amputations. J Vasc Surg. 2009;50(1):54–60.
115. van de Weijer MA, Kruse RR, Schamp K, et al. Morbidity of femoropopliteal bypass surgery. Semin Vasc Surg. 2015;28(2):112–21.
116. Krievins DK, Halena G, Scheinert D, Savlovskis J, Szopiński P, Krämer A, Ouriel K, Nair K, Holden A, Schmidt A. One-year results from the DETOUR I trial of the PQ Bypass DETOUR System for percutaneous femoropopliteal bypass. J Vasc Surg. 2020;72(5):1648–1658.e2.
117. Halena G, Krievins DK, Scheinert D, Savlovskis J, Szopiński P, Krämer A, Ouriel K, Schmidt A, Zdunek M, Lyden SP. Percutaneous femoropopliteal bypass: 2-year results of the DETOUR system. J Endovasc Ther. 2022;29(1):84–95.
118. Usman HU, Varghese V, Janzer S, George JC. Histopathologic characterization of chronic total occlusions by directional atherectomy: the HIPACT study. J Invasive Cardiol. 2021;33(6):E443–50.
119. Zhang F, Zhang H, Luo X, Liang G, Feng Y, Zhang WW. Catheter-directed thrombolysis-assisted angioplasty for chronic lower limb ischemia. Ann Vasc Surg. 2014;28(3):590–5.
120. Scheer F, Lüdtke CW, Kamusella P, Wiggermann P, Vieweg H, Schlöricke E, Lichtenberg M, Andresen R, Wissgott C. Combination of rotational atherothrombectomy and Paclitaxel-coated angioplasty for femoropopliteal occlusion. Clin Med Insights Cardiol. 2015;8(Suppl 2):43–8.
121. Shammas NW. JETSTREAM atherectomy: a review of technique, tips, and tricks in treating the femoropopliteal lesions. Int J Angiol. 2015;24(2):81–6.
122. Teymen B, Aktürk S. Chronic femoropopliteal occlusions: comparison of drug-eluting balloon angioplasty with or without prior rotational thrombectomy. Acta Cardiol Sin. 2020;36(2):118–24.
123. Shammas NW, Weissman NJ, Coiner D, Shammas GA, Dippel E, Jerin M. Treatment of subacute and chronic thrombotic occlusions of lower extremity peripheral arteries with the excimer laser: a feasibility study. Cardiovasc Revasc Med. 2012;13(4):211–4.
124. Warkentin TE. Heparin-induced thrombocytopenia: a ten-year retrospective. Annu Rev Med. 1999;50(1):129–47.
125. Smythe MA, Koerber JM, Mattson JC. The incidence of recognized heparin-induced thrombocytopenia in a large, tertiary care teaching hospital. Chest [Internet]. 2007;131(6):1644–9. https://doi.org/10.1378/chest.06-2109.
126. Nand S, Wong W, Yuen B, Yetter A, Schmulbach E, Fisher SG. Heparin-induced thrombocytopenia with thrombosis: Incidence, analysis of risk factors, and clinical outcomes in 108 consecutive patients treated at a single institution. Am J Hematol. 1997;56(1):12–6.
127. Cuker A, Arepally GM, Chong BH, Cines DB, Greinacher A, Gruel Y, et al. American Society of Hematology 2018 guidelines for management of venous thromboembolism: heparin-induced thrombocytopenia. Blood Adv. 2018;2(22):3360–92.
128. Ouriel K. A history of thrombolytic therapy. J Endovasc Ther. 2004;11(SUPPL. 2):128–33.
129. Morrison HL. Catheter-directed thrombolysis for acute limb ischemia. Semin Interv Radiol. 2006;23(3):258–69.
130. Ouriel K, Veith FJ, Sasahara AA, Whittemore AD, Roon AJ, Braithwaite BD, et al. Thrombolysis or peripheral arterial surgery: Phase I results. J Vasc Surg. 1996;23(1):64–75.
131. Ouriel K, Shortell CK, DeWeese JA, Green RM, Francis CW, Azodo MVU, et al. A comparison of thrombolytic therapy with operative revascularization in the initial treatment of acute peripheral arterial ischemia. J Vasc Surg. 1994;19(6):1021–30.
132. Kaufman C, Kinney T, Quencer K. Practice trends of fibrinogen monitoring in thrombolysis. J Clin Med. 2018;7(5):111.
133. Shammas NW, Torey JT, Shammas WJ, Jones-Miller S, Shammas GA. Intravascular ultrasound assessment and correlation with angiographic findings demonstrating femoropopliteal arterial dissections post atherectomy: results from the idissection study. J Invasive Cardiol. 2018;30(7):240–4.
134. Spiliopoulos S, Karamitros A, Reppas L, Brountzos E. Novel balloon technologies to minimize dissection of peripheral angioplasty. Expert Rev Med Devices. 2019;16(7):581–8.
135. Poncyljusz W, Falkowski A, Safranow K, Rać M, Zawierucha D. Cutting-balloon angioplasty versus balloon angioplasty as treatment for short atherosclerotic lesions in the superficial femoral artery: randomized controlled trial. Cardiovasc Intervent Radiol. 2013;36(6):1500–7. https://doi.org/10.1007/s00270-013-0603-5. Epub 2013 Apr 11
136. AngioSculpt Test Plan ST-1197 (2008), on file at AngioScore, Inc.
137. Scheinert D, Peeters P, Bosiers M, O'Sullivan G, Sultan S, Gershony G. Results of the multicenter first-in-man study of a novel scoring balloon catheter for the treatment of infra-popliteal peripheral arterial disease. Catheter Cardiovasc Interv. 2007;70(7):1034–9.

138. Bosiers M, Deloose K, Cagiannos C, Verbist J, Peeters P. Use of the AngioSculpt scoring balloon for infrapopliteal lesions in patients with critical limb ischemia: 1-year outcome. Vascular. 2009;17(1):29–35.

139. Sirignano P, Mansour W, d'Adamo A, Cuozzo S, Capoccia L, Speziale F. Early experience with a new concept of angioplasty nitinol-constrained balloon catheter (Chocolate®) in severely claudicant patients. Cardiovasc Intervent Radiol. 2018;41(3):377–84.

140. Bouras G, Lansky A, McClure J, et al. TCT-778 outcomes from the chocolate BAR: a large, multicenter, prospective, post-market study on use of the chocolate percutaneous transluminal angioplasty (PTA) balloon. J Am Coll Cardiol. 2016;68(18_Supplement):B314. https://doi.org/10.1016/j.jacc.2016.09.809.

141. Holden A. The use of intravascular lithotripsy for the treatment of severely calcified lower limb arterial CTOs. J Cardiovasc Surg. 2019;60(1):3–7.

142. Holden A, Hill A, Walker A, Buckley B, Merrilees S, Nowakowski P, Krzanowski M, Brodmann M. PRELUDE prospective study of the serranator device in the treatment of atherosclerotic lesions in the superficial femoral and popliteal arteries. J Endovasc Ther. 2019;26(1):18–25.

143. Holden A, Lichtenberg M, Nowakowski P, Wissgott C, Hertting K, Brodmann M. Prospective study of serration angioplasty in the infrapopliteal arteries using the serranator device: PRELUDE BTK study. J Endovasc Ther. 2021;20:15266028211059917.

144. Rocha-Singh KJ, Jaff M, Joye J, et al. Major adverse limb events and wound healing following infrapopliteal artery stent implantation in patients with critical limb ischemia: the XCELL trial. Catheter Cardiovasc Interv. 2012;80(6):1042–51.

145. Scheinert D, Katsanos K, Zeller T, et al. A prospective randomized multicenter comparison of balloon angioplasty and infrapopliteal stenting with the sirolimus-eluting stent in patients with ischemic peripheral arterial disease: 1-year results from the ACHILLES trial. J Am Coll Cardiol. 2012;60(22):2290–5.

146. Rastan A, Brechtel K, Krankenberg H, et al. Sirolimus-eluting stents for treatment of infrapopliteal arteries reduce clinical event rate compared to bare-metal stents: long-term results from a randomized trial. J Am Coll Cardiol. 2012;60:587–91.

147. Kok HK, Prabhudesai SG, Ahmed I, Karunanithy N, Abisi S, Katsanos K, Diamantopoulos A. Techniques for infrapopliteal arterial bifurcation stenting. Ann Vasc Surg. 2018;50:288–96.

148. Bosiers M, Scheinert D, Peeters P, et al. Randomized comparison of everolimus-eluting versus bare-metal stents in patients with critical limb ischemia and infrapopliteal arterial occlusive disease. J Vasc Surg. 2012;55:390–8.

149. Siablis D, Kitrou PM, Spiliopoulos S, et al. Paclitaxel-coated balloon angioplasty versus drug-eluting stenting for the treatment of infrapopliteal long-segment arterial occlusive disease: the IDEAS randomized controlled trial. JACC Cardiovasc Interv. 2014;7:1048–56.

150. Sawaya FJ, Lefèvre T, Chevalier B, Garot P, Hovasse T, Morice M-C, Rab T, Louvard Y. Contemporary approach to coronary bifurcation lesion treatment. J Am Coll Cardiol Intv. 2016;9(18):1861–78. https://doi.org/10.1016/j.jcin.2016.06.056.

151. Biondi-Zoccai GG, Sangiorgi G, Lotrionte M, et al. Infragenicular stent implantation for below-the-knee atherosclerotic disease: clinical evidence from an international collaborative meta-analysis on 640 patients. J Endovasc Ther. 2009;16:251–60.

152. Huizing E, Kum S, Ipema J, et al. Mid-term outcomes of an everolimus-eluting bioresorbable vascular scaffold in patients with below-the-knee arterial disease: a pooled analysis of individual patient data. Vasc Med. 2021;26:195–9.

153. Ochoa Chaar CI, Shebl F, Sumpio B, Dardik A, Indes J, Sarac T. Distal embolization during lower extremity endovascular interventions. J Vasc Surg. 2017;66(1):143–50.

154. Shammas NW, Shammas GA, Dippel EJ, Jerin M, Shammas WJ. Predictors of distal embolization in peripheral percutaneous interventions: a report from a large peripheral vascular registry. J Invasive Cardiol. 2009;21(12):628–31.

155. Shrikhande GV, Khan SZ, Hussain HG, Dayal R, McKinsey JF, Morrissey N. Lesion types and device characteristics that predict distal embolization during percutaneous lower extremity interventions. J Vasc Surg. 2011;53(2):347–52.

156. Fukagawa T, Hirano K, Mori S, Yamawaki M, Kobayashi N, Tsutsumi M, Honda Y, Makino K, Ito Y. Efficacy of the novel technique HIRANODOME in preventing distal embolization during endovascular treatment of femoropopliteal lesions. Catheter Cardiovasc Interv. 2021;97(5):E697–703.

157. Jalal S, Mustapha JA, Rosman HS, Mehta RH, Davis TP. Distal cuff occlusion: a novel, simple approach for distal embolic protection in peripheral vascular intervention. J Invasive Cardiol. 2017;29(9):297–300.

158. Krishnan P, Tarricone A, Purushothaman KR, Purushothaman M, Vasquez M, Kovacic J, Baber U, Kapur V, Gujja K, Kini A, Sharma S. An algorithm for the use of embolic protection during atherectomy for femoral popliteal lesions. JACC Cardiovasc Interv. 2017;10(4):403–10.

159. Czihal M, Findik Z, Bernau C, Seidensticker M, Ricke J, Hoffmann U, Treitl M, Treitl KM. Embolic protection in complex femoropopliteal interventions: safety, efficacy and predictors of filter macroembolization. Cardiovasc Intervent Radiol. 2021;44(5):700–8.

160. Boc A, Blinc A, Boc V. Distal embolization during percutaneous revascularization of the lower extremity arteries. Vasa. 2020;49(5):389–94.

161. Cannavale A, Santoni M, Gazzetti M, Catalano C, Fanelli F. Current status of distal embolization in femoropopliteal endovascular interventions. Vasc Endovasc Surg. 2018;52:440–7.
162. Farhat-Sabet AA, Tolaymat B, Voit A, Drucker CB, Santini-Dominguez R, Ucuzian AA, Toursavadkohi SA, Nagarsheth KH. Successful treatment of acute limb ischemia secondary to iatrogenic distal embolization using catheter directed aspiration thrombectomy. Front Surg. 2020;7:22.
163. Applebaum RM, Kronzon I. Evaluation and management of cholesterol embolization and the blue toe syndrome. Curr Opin Cardiol. 1996;11(5):533–42.
164. O'Keeffe ST, Woods BO, Breslin DJ, Tsapatsaris NP. Blue toe syndrome. Causes and management. Arch Intern Med. 1992;152(11):2197–202.
165. Karmody AM, Powers SR, Monaco VJ, Leather RP. "Blue toe" syndrome. An indication for limb salvage surgery. Arch Surg. 1976;111(11):1263–8.
166. Flory CM. Arterial occlusions produced by emboli from eroded aortic atheromatous plaques. Am J Pathol. 1945;21(3):549–65.
167. Hoye SJ, Teitelbaum S, Gore I, Warren R. Atheromatous embolization; a factor in peripheral gangrene. N Engl J Med. 1959;261(3):128–31.
168. Matchett WJ, McFarland DR, Eidt JF, Moursi MM. Blue toe syndrome: treatment with intra-arterial stents and review of therapies. J Vasc Interv Radiol. 2000;11(5):585–92.
169. Khafif RA, DeLima C, Silverberg A, Frankel R. Calciphylaxis and systemic calcinosis. Collective review. Arch Intern Med. 1990;150(5):956–9.
170. Ridker PM, Michel T. Streptokinase therapy and cholesterol embolization. Am J Med. 1989;87(3):357–8.
171. Feder W, Auerbach R. "Purple toes": an uncommon sequela of oral coumarin drug therapy. Ann Intern Med. 1961;55:911–7.
172. Conn DL, Tompkins RB, Nichols WL. Glucocorticoids in the management of vasculitis--a double edged sword? J Rheumatol. 1988;15(8):1181–3.
173. Al Aboud A, Abrams M, Mancini AJ. Blue toes after stimulant therapy for pediatric attention deficit hyperactivity disorder. J Am Acad Dermatol. 2011;64(6):1218–9.
174. Borovoy M, Beresh AS. Transient vasospasm. The blue toe. J Am Podiatr Med Assoc. 1985;75(12):656–7.
175. Foley WD, Stonely T. CT angiography of the lower extremities. Radiol Clin N Am. 2010;48(2):367–96. ix
176. Ma T, Zhou B, Hsiai TK, Shung KK. A review of intravascular ultrasound-based multimodal intravascular imaging: the synergistic approach to characterizing vulnerable plaques. Ultrason Imaging. 2016;38(5):314–31.
177. Brewer ML, Kinnison ML, Perler BA, White RI Jr. Blue toe syndrome: treatment with anticoagulants and delayed percutaneous transluminal angioplasty. Radiology. 1988;166(1 Pt 1):31–6.
178. Renshaw A, McCowen T, Waltke EA, Wattenhofer SP, Tahara RW, Baxter BT. Angioplasty with stenting is effective in treating blue toe syndrome. Vasc Endovasc Surg. 2002;36(2):155–9.
179. Dolmatch BL, Rholl KS, Moskowitz LB, Dake MD, van Breda A, Kaplan JO, et al. Blue toe syndrome: treatment with percutaneous atherectomy. Radiology. 1989;173(3):799–804.
180. Clugston RA, Eisenhauer AC, Matthews RV. Atherectomy of the distal aorta using a "kissing-balloon" technique for the treatment of blue toe syndrome. AJR Am J Roentgenol. 1992;159(1):125–7.
181. Kumpe DA, Zwerdlinger S, Griffin DJ. Blue digit syndrome: treatment with percutaneous transluminal angioplasty. Radiology. 1988;166(1 Pt 1):37–44.
182. Johnston KW. Femoral and popliteal arteries: reanalysis of results of balloon angioplasty. Radiology. 1992;183(3):767–71.
183. Ng VG, Mena C, Pietras C, Lansky AJ. Local delivery of paclitaxel in the treatment of peripheral arterial disease. Eur J Clin Investig. 2015;45(3):333–45.
184. Feldman DN, Armstrong EJ, Aronow HD, Gigliotti OS, Jaff MR, Klein AJ, et al. SCAI consensus guidelines for device selection in femoral-popliteal arterial interventions. Catheter Cardiovasc Interv. 2018;92(1):124–40.
185. Bailey SR, Beckman JA, Dao TD, Misra S, Sobieszczyk PS, White CJ, et al. ACC/AHA/SCAI/SIR/SVM 2018 Appropriate Use Criteria for Peripheral Artery Intervention: A Report of the American College of Cardiology Appropriate Use Criteria Task Force, American Heart Association, Society for Cardiovascular Angiography and Interventions, Society of Interventional Radiology, and Society for Vascular Medicine. J Am Coll Cardiol. 2019;73(2):214–37.
186. Gray WA, Granada JF. Drug-coated balloons for the prevention of vascular restenosis. Circulation. 2010;121(24):2672–80.
187. Tepe G, Zeller T, Albrecht T, Heller S, Schwarzwalder U, Beregi JP, et al. Local delivery of paclitaxel to inhibit restenosis during angioplasty of the leg. N Engl J Med. 2008;358(7):689–99.
188. Rosenfield K, Jaff MR, White CJ, Rocha-Singh K, Mena-Hurtado C, Metzger DC, et al. Trial of a paclitaxel-coated balloon for femoropopliteal artery disease. N Engl J Med. 2015;373(2):145–53.
189. Werk M, Albrecht T, Meyer DR, Ahmed MN, Behne A, Dietz U, et al. Paclitaxel-coated balloons reduce restenosis after femoro-popliteal angioplasty: evidence from the randomized PACIFIER trial. Circ Cardiovasc Interv. 2012;5(6):831–40.
190. Fanelli F, Cannavale A, Boatta E, Corona M, Lucatelli P, Wlderk A, et al. Lower limb multilevel treatment with drug-eluting balloons: 6-month results from the DEBELLUM randomized trial. J Endovasc Ther. 2012;19(5):571–80.
191. Brodmann M, Werner M, Meyer DR, Reimer P, Kruger K, Granada JF, et al. Sustainable antirestenosis effect with a low-dose drug-coated balloon:

the ILLUMENATE European randomized clinical trial 2-year results. JACC Cardiovasc Interv. 2018;11(23):2357–64.

192. Tepe G, Schnorr B, Albrecht T, Brechtel K, Claussen CD, Scheller B, et al. Angioplasty of femoropopliteal arteries with drug-coated balloons: 5-year follow-up of the THUNDER trial. JACC Cardiovasc Interv. 2015;8(1 Pt A):102–8.

193. Schneider PA, Laird JR, Doros G, Gao Q, Ansel G, Brodmann M, et al. Mortality not correlated with paclitaxel exposure: an independent patient-level meta-analysis of a drug-coated balloon. J Am Coll Cardiol. 2019;73(20):2550–63.

194. Schmidt A, Piorkowski M, Gorner H, Steiner S, Bausback Y, Scheinert S, et al. Drug-coated balloons for complex femoropopliteal lesions: 2-year results of a real-world registry. JACC Cardiovasc Interv. 2016;9(7):715–24.

195. Ott I, Cassese S, Groha P, Steppich B, Voll F, Hadamitzky M, et al. ISAR-PEBIS (paclitaxel-eluting balloon versus conventional balloon angioplasty for in-stent restenosis of superficial femoral artery): a randomized trial. J Am Heart Assoc. 2017;6(7):e006321.

196. Dake MD, Ansel GM, Jaff MR, Ohki T, Saxon RR, Smouse HB, et al. Sustained safety and effectiveness of paclitaxel-eluting stents for femoropopliteal lesions: 2-year follow-up from the Zilver PTX randomized and single-arm clinical studies. J Am Coll Cardiol. 2013;61(24):2417–27.

197. Gray WA, Keirse K, Soga Y, Benko A, Babaev A, Yokoi Y, et al. A polymer-coated, paclitaxel-eluting stent (Eluvia) versus a polymer-free, paclitaxel-coated stent (Zilver PTX) for endovascular femoropopliteal intervention (IMPERIAL): a randomised, non-inferiority trial. Lancet. 2018;392(10157):1541–51.

198. Cipollari S, Yokoi H, Ohki T, Kichikawa K, Nakamura M, Komori K, et al. Long-term effectiveness of the zilver PTX drug-eluting stent for femoropopliteal peripheral artery disease in patients with no patent tibial runoff vessels-results from the Zilver PTX Japan post-market surveillance study. J Vasc Interv Radiol. 2018;29(1):9–17. e1

199. Zeller T, Rastan A, Macharzina R, Tepe G, Kaspar M, Chavarria J, et al. Drug-coated balloons vs. drug-eluting stents for treatment of long femoropopliteal lesions. J Endovasc Ther. 2014;21(3):359–68.

200. Bausback Y, Wittig T, Schmidt A, Zeller T, Bosiers M, Peeters P, et al. Drug-eluting stent versus drug-coated balloon revascularization in patients with femoropopliteal arterial disease. J Am Coll Cardiol. 2019;73(6):667–79.

201. Katsanos K, Spiliopoulos S, Kitrou P, Krokidis M, Paraskevopoulos I, Karnabatidis D. Risk of death and amputation with use of paclitaxel-coated balloons in the infrapopliteal arteries for treatment of critical limb ischemia: a systematic review and meta-analysis of randomized controlled trials. J Vasc Interv Radiol. 2020;31(2):202–12.

202. Horwitz SB. Mechanism of action of taxol. Trends Pharmacol Sci. 1992;13(4):134–6.

203. Gongora CA, Shibuya M, Wessler JD, McGregor J, Tellez A, Cheng Y, et al. Impact of paclitaxel dose on tissue pharmacokinetics and vascular healing: a comparative drug-coated balloon study in the familial hypercholesterolemic swine model of superficial femoral in-stent restenosis. JACC Cardiovasc Interv. 2015;8(8):1115–23.

204. Axel DI, Kunert W, Goggelmann C, Oberhoff M, Herdeg C, Kuttner A, et al. Paclitaxel inhibits arterial smooth muscle cell proliferation and migration in vitro and in vivo using local drug delivery. Circulation. 1997;96(2):636–45.

205. Freyhardt P, Zeller T, Kroncke TJ, Schwarzwaelder U, Schreiter NF, Stiepani H, et al. Plasma levels following application of paclitaxel-coated balloon catheters in patients with stenotic or occluded femoropopliteal arteries. Rofo. 2011;183(5):448–55.

206. Rowinsky EK, Donehower RC. Paclitaxel (taxol). N Engl J Med. 1995;332(15):1004–14.

207. Margolis J, McDonald J, Heuser R, Klinke P, Waksman R, Virmani R, et al. Systemic nanoparticle paclitaxel (nab-paclitaxel) for in-stent restenosis I (SNAPIST-I): a first-in-human safety and dose-finding study. Clin Cardiol. 2007;30(4):165–70.

208. Rocha-Singh KJ, Duval S, Jaff MR, Schneider PA, Ansel GM, Lyden SP, et al. Mortality and paclitaxel-coated devices: an individual patient data meta-analysis. Circulation. 2020;141(23):1859–69.

209. Albrecht T, Ukrow A, Werk M, Tepe G, Zeller T, Meyer DR, et al. Impact of patient and lesion characteristics on drug-coated balloon angioplasty in the femoropopliteal artery: a pooled analysis of four randomized controlled multicenter trials. Cardiovasc Intervent Radiol. 2019;42(4):495–504.

210. Sachar R, Soga Y, Ansari MM, Kozuki A, Lopez L, Brodmann M, et al. 1-year results from the RANGER II SFA randomized trial of the ranger drug-coated balloon. JACC Cardiovasc Interv. 2021;14(10):1123–33.

211. Secemsky EA, Kundi H, Weinberg I, Jaff MR, Krawisz A, Parikh SA, et al. Association of survival with femoropopliteal artery revascularization with drug-coated devices. JAMA Cardiol. 2019;4(4):332–40.

212. Secemsky EA, Kundi H, Weinberg I, Schermerhorn M, Beckman JA, Parikh SA, et al. Drug-eluting stent implantation and long-term survival following peripheral artery revascularization. J Am Coll Cardiol. 2019;73(20):2636–8.

213. FDA Executive Summary. https://www.fda.gov/media/127698/download. Accessed April 24, 2022.

214. Nordanstig J, James S, Andersson M, Andersson M, Danielsson P, Gillgren P, et al. Mortality with paclitaxel-coated devices in peripheral artery disease. N Engl J Med. 2020;383(26):2538–46.

215. Hess CN, Patel MR, Bauersachs RM, Anand SS, Debus ES, Nehler MR, et al. Safety and effectiveness of paclitaxel drug-coated devices in peripheral

artery revascularization: insights From VOYAGER PAD. J Am Coll Cardiol. 2021;78(18):1768–78.

216. Dinh K, Limmer AM, Chen AZL, Thomas SD, Holden A, Schneider PA, et al. Mortality rates after paclitaxel-coated device use in patients with occlusive femoropopliteal disease: an updated systematic review and meta-analysis of randomized controlled trials. J Endovasc Ther. 2021;28(5):755–77.

217. Secemsky EA, Shen C, Schermerhorn M, Yeh RW. Longitudinal assessment of safety of femoropopliteal endovascular treatment with paclitaxel-coated devices among medicare beneficiaries: the SAFE-PAD study. JAMA Intern Med. 2021;181(8):1071–80.

218. di Palma G, Sanchez-Jimenez EF, Lazar L, Cortese B. Should paclitaxel be considered an old generation DCB? The limus era. Rev Cardiovasc Med. 2021;22(4):1323–30.

219. Blaich R, Rupprecht W. Comparative chromatographic studies on arthropod cocoons. Naturwissenschaften. 1968;55(6):300–1.

220. Ferreira LT, Figueiredo AC, Orr B, Lopes D, Maiato H. Dissecting the role of the tubulin code in mitosis. Methods Cell Biol. 2018;144:33–74.

221. Herdeg C, Oberhoff M, Baumbach A, Blattner A, Axel DI, Schroder S, et al. Local paclitaxel delivery for the prevention of restenosis: biological effects and efficacy in vivo. J Am Coll Cardiol. 2000;35(7):1969–76.

222. Regar E, Serruys PW, Bode C, Holubarsch C, Guermonprez JL, Wijns W, et al. Angiographic findings of the multicenter Randomized Study With the Sirolimus-Eluting Bx Velocity Balloon-Expandable Stent (RAVEL): sirolimus-eluting stents inhibit restenosis irrespective of the vessel size. Circulation. 2002;106(15):1949–56.

223. Lammer J, Bosiers M, Zeller T, Schillinger M, Boone E, Zaugg MJ, et al. First clinical trial of nitinol self-expanding everolimus-eluting stent implantation for peripheral arterial occlusive disease. J Vasc Surg. 2011;54(2):394–401.

224. Lammer J, Scheinert D, Vermassen F, Koppensteiner R, Hausegger KA, Schroe H, et al. Pharmacokinetic analysis after implantation of everolimus-eluting self-expanding stents in the peripheral vasculature. J Vasc Surg. 2012;55(2):400–5.

225. Duda SH, Pusich B, Richter G, Landwehr P, Oliva VL, Tielbeek A, et al. Sirolimus-eluting stents for the treatment of obstructive superficial femoral artery disease: six-month results. Circulation. 2002;106(12):1505–9.

226. Duda SH, Bosiers M, Lammer J, Scheinert D, Zeller T, Tielbeek A, et al. Sirolimus-eluting versus bare nitinol stent for obstructive superficial femoral artery disease: the SIROCCO II trial. J Vasc Interv Radiol. 2005;16(3):331–8.

227. Duda SH, Bosiers M, Lammer J, Scheinert D, Zeller T, Oliva V, et al. Drug-eluting and bare nitinol stents for the treatment of atherosclerotic lesions in the superficial femoral artery: long-term results from the SIROCCO trial. J Endovasc Ther. 2006;13(6):701–10.

228. Li J, Tzafriri R, Patel SM, Parikh SA. Mechanisms underlying drug delivery to peripheral arteries. Interv Cardiol Clin. 2017;6(2):197–216.

229. Zeller T, Brechtel K, Meyer DR, Noory E, Beschorner U, Albrecht T. Six-month outcomes from the first-in-human, single-arm SELUTION sustained-limus-release drug-eluting balloon trial in femoropopliteal lesions. J Endovasc Ther. 2020;27(5):683–90.

230. Lemos PA, Farooq V, Takimura CK, Gutierrez PS, Virmani R, Kolodgie F, et al. Emerging technologies: polymer-free phospholipid encapsulated sirolimus nanocarriers for the controlled release of drug from a stent-plus-balloon or a stand-alone balloon catheter. EuroIntervention. 2013;9(1):148–56.

231. El-Mokdad R, di Palma G, Cortese B. Long-term follow-up after sirolimus-coated balloon use for coronary artery disease. Final results of the Nanolute study. Catheter Cardiovasc Interv. 2020;96(5):E496–500.

232. Tang TY, Soon SXY, Yap CJQ, Chan SL, Tan RY, Pang SC, et al. Early (6 months) results of a pilot prospective study to investigate the efficacy and safety of sirolimus coated balloon angioplasty for dysfunctional arterio-venous fistulas: MAgicTouch Intervention Leap for Dialysis Access (MATILDA) Trial. PLoS One. 2020;15(10):e0241321.

233. BLearning Peripheral. LINC 2020: XTOSI study interim findings suggest "highly promising" safety and efficacy of sirolimus DCB. https://blearning.net/sirolimus-dcb-safety. Accessed 31 August 2020.

234. Sirolimus- vs. Paclitaxel-Drug Coated Balloons in Patients With Peripheral Artery Disease (SIRONA). NCT04475783. Clinicaltrials.gov website. https://clinicaltrials.gov/ct2/show/NCT04475783. Accessed 31 August 2021.

235. Sirolimus Coated Balloon Versus Standard Balloon for SFA and Popliteal Artery Disease (FUTURE-SFA). Clinicaltrials.gov website. Accessed 31 August 2021.

236. Secemsky EA, Kochar A. Illuminating the path for novel peripheral drug-eluting stents. JACC Cardiovasc Interv. 2022;15(6):627–9.

237. Steiner S, Honton B, Langhoff R, Chiesa R, Kahlberg A, Thieme M, et al. 2-year results with a sirolimus-eluting self-expanding stent for femoropopliteal lesions: the first-in-human ILLUMINA study. JACC Cardiovasc Interv. 2022;15(6):618–26.

238. Dawson I, Sie RB, van Bockel JH. Atherosclerotic popliteal aneurysm. BJS Br J Surg. 1997;84:293–9.

239. Tsilimparis N, Dayama A, Ricotta JJ. Open and endovascular repair of popliteal artery aneurysms: tabular review of the literature. Ann Vasc Surg. 2013;27:259–65.

240. Farber A, Angle N, Avgerinos E, et al. The Society for Vascular Surgery clinical practice guidelines on popliteal artery aneurysms. J Vasc Surg. 2022;75:109S–20S.

241. Phair A, Hajibandeh S, Hajibandeh S, Kelleher D, Ibrahim R, Antoniou GA. Meta-analysis of posterior versus medial approach for popliteal artery aneurysm repair. J Vasc Surg. 2016;64:1141–1150.e1.

242. Antonello M, Frigatti P, Battocchio P, Lepidi S, Cognolato D, Dall'Antonia A, Stramanà R, Deriu GP, Grego F. Open repair versus endovascular treatment for asymptomatic popliteal artery aneurysm: results of a prospective randomized study. J Vasc Surg. 2005;42:185–93.

243. Leake AE, Segal MA, Chaer RA, Eslami MH, Al-Khoury G, Makaroun MS, Avgerinos ED. Meta-analysis of open and endovascular repair of poplitcal artery aneurysms. J Vasc Surg. 2017;65:246–256.e2.

244. Beuschel B, Nayfeh T, Kunbaz A, Haddad A, Alzuabi M, Vindhyal S, Farber A, Murad MH. A systematic review and meta-analysis of treatment and natural history of popliteal artery aneurysms. J Vasc Surg. 2022;75:121S–125S.e14.

245. Nguyen BN, Amdur RL, Abugideiri M, et al. Postoperative complications after common femoral endarterectomy. J Vasc Surg. 2015;61:1489–94.

246. Ballotta E, Gruppo M, Mazzalai F, Da Giau G. Common femoral artery endarterectomy for occlusive disease: an 8-year single-center prospective study. Surgery. 2010;147:268–74.

247. Kang JL, Patel VI, Conrad MF, Lamuraglia GM, Chung TK, Cambria RP. Common femoral artery occlusive disease: contemporary results following surgical endarterectomy. J Vasc Surg. 2008;48:872–7.

248. Kechagias A, Ylonen K, Biancari F. Long-term outcome after isolated endarterectomy of the femoral bifurcation. World J Surg. 2008;32:51–4.

249. Bonvini RF, Rastan A, Sixt S, et al. Endovascular treatment of common femoral artery disease: medium-term outcomes of 360 consecutive procedures. J Am Coll Cardiol. 2011;58:792–8.

250. Siracuse JJ, Van Orden K, Kalish JA, et al. Vascular Quality Initiative. Endovascular treatment of the common femoral artery in the Vascular Quality Initiative. J Vasc Surg. 2017;65:1039–46.

251. Shammas N, Doumet AA, Karia R, Khalafallah R. An overview of the treatment of symptomatic common femoral artery lesions with a focus on endovascular therapy. Vasc Health Risk Manag. 2020;16:67–73.

252. Deloose, Koen Full Cohort 24-Month Safety and Efficacy Results of the VMI-CFA Trial. VIVA: 2019.

253. Mehta M, Zhou Y, Paty PS, Teymouri M, Jafree K, Bakhtawar H, Hnath J, Feustel P. Percutaneous common femoral artery interventions using angioplasty, atherectomy, and stenting. J Vasc Surg. 2016;64(2):369–79.

254. Cioppa A, Stabile E, Salemme L, Popusoi G, Pucciarelli A, et al. Combined use of directional atherectomy and drug-coated balloon for the endovascular treatment of common femoral artery disease: immediate and one-year outcomes. EuroIntervention. 2017;12:1789–94.

255. Gouëffic Y, Schiava ND, Thaveau F, Rosset E, Favre J-P, et al. Stenting or surgery for de novo common femoral artery stenosis (TECCO Trial). J Am Coll Cardiol Intv. 2017;10(13):1344–54.

256. Shammas N, Shammas GA, Karia R, Khalafallah R, Jones-Miller S, et al. Two-year outcomes of endovascular interventions of the common femoral artery: a retrospective analysis from two medical centers. Cardiovasc Revasc Med. 2021;24:72–6.

257. Klein AJ, James Chen S, Messenger JC, Hansgen AR, Plomondon ME, et al. Quantitative assessment of the conformational change in the femoropopliteal artery with leg movement. Catheter Cardiovasc Interv. 2009;74(5):787–98.

258. Deloose K. Full Cohort 24-month safety and efficacy results of the VMI-CFA Trial. VIVA: 2019.

259. Dufranc J, Palcau L, Heyndrickx M, Gouicem D, Coffin O, Felisaz A, et al. Technique and results of femoral bifurcation endarterectomy by eversion. J Vasc Surg. 2015;61(3):728–33.

260. Nguyen B-N, Amdur RL, Abugideiri M, Rahbar R, Neville RF, et al. Postoperative complications after common femoral endarterectomy. J Vasc Surg. 2015;61:1489–94.

261. Carola Marie Wieker MD, Eva Schönefeld MD, Nani Osada DRM, Christina Lührs MD, Roland Beneking MD, et al. Results of common femoral artery thromboendarterectomy evaluation of a traditional surgical management in the endovascular era. J Vasc Surg. 2016;64:995–1001.

262. Bonvini RF, Rastan A, Sixt S, Noory E, Schwarz T, et al. Endovascular treatment of common femoral artery disease: medium-term outcomes of 360 consecutive procedures. J Am Coll Cardiol. 2011;58:792–8.

263. Azéma L, Davaine JM, Guyomarch B, Chaillou P, Costargent A, et al. Endovascular repair of common femoral artery and concomitant arterial lesions. Eur Soc Vasc Surg. 2011;41:1078–5884.

264. Linni K, Ugurluoglu A, Hitzl W, Aspalter M, ThomasHo l. Bioabsorbable stent implantation vs common femoral artery endarterectomy: early results of a randomized trial. J Endovasc Ther. 2014;21:493–502.

265. Nasr B, Kaladji A, Vent P-A, Chaillou P, Costargent A, et al. Long-term outcomes of common femoral artery stenting. Ann Vasc Surg. 2017;40:10–8.

266. Boufi M, Ejargue M, Gaye M, Boyer L, Alimi Y, et al. Systematic review and meta-analysis of endovascular versus open repair for common femoral artery atherosclerosis treatment. J Vasc Surg. 2021;73:1445–55.

267. Siracuse JJ, Van Orden K, Kalish JA, Eslami MH, Schermerhorn ML, Patel VI, et al. Endovascular treatment of the common femoral artery in the Vascular Quality Initiative. J Vasc Surg. 2017;65(4):1039–46.

268. Halpin D, Erben Y, Jayasuriya S, Cua B, Jhamnani S, Mena-Hurtado C. Management of isolated atherosclerotic stenosis of the common femoral artery:

a review of the literature. Vasc Endovasc Surg. 2017;51(4):220–7.

269. Dattilo PB, Tsai TT, Kevin Rogers R, Casserly IP. Acute and medium-term outcomes of endovascular therapy of obstructive disease of diverse etiology of the common femoral artery. Catheter Cardiovasc Interv. 2013;81(6):1013–22.

270. Drachman DE, Armstrong EJ. Stenting the common femoral artery: crossing the rubicon of endovascular treatment? JACC Cardiovasc Interv. 2017;10(13):1355–6.

271. Tijani Y, Burgaud M, Hamel A, Raux M, Nasr B, Goueffic Y. The common femoral artery is a fixed arterial segment. Ann Vasc Surg. 2021;73:51–4.

272. Ni Ghriallais R, Heraty K, Smouse B, Burke M, Gilson P, Bruzzi M. Deformation of the femoropopliteal segment: effect of stent length, location, flexibility, and curvature. J Endovasc Ther. 2016;23(6):907–18.

273. Esposito A, Menna D, Baiano A, Benedetto P, Di Leo F, Cappiello AP. Eversion endarterectomy of the femoral bifurcation: technique, results and potential advantages. Ann Vasc Surg. 2020;66:580–5.

274. Kwon J, Staley C, McCullough M, Goss S, Arosemena M, Abai B, et al. A randomized clinical trial evaluating negative pressure therapy to decrease vascular groin incision complications. J Vasc Surg. 2018;68(6):1744–52.

275. Sapienza P, Napoli F, Tartaglia E, Venturini L, Sterpetti AV, Brachini G, et al. Infection of prosthetic patches after femoral endarterectomy: an unreported complication. Ann Vasc Surg. 2019;56:11–6.

276. Uhl C, Gotzke H, Woronowicz S, Betz T, Topel I, Steinbauer M. Treatment of lymphatic complications after common femoral artery endarterectomy. Ann Vasc Surg. 2020;62:382–6.

277. Nguyen BN, Amdur RL, Abugideiri M, Rahbar R, Neville RF, Sidawy AN. Postoperative complications after common femoral endarterectomy. J Vasc Surg. 2015;61(6):1489–94. e1

278. Nunez AA, Veith FJ, Collier P, Ascer E, Flores SW, Gupta SK. Direct approaches to the distal portions of the deep femoral artery for limb salvage bypasses. J Vasc Surg. 1988;8(5):576–81. https://doi.org/10.1067/mva.1988.avs0080576.

279. Bertucci WR, Marin ML, Veith FJ, Ohki T. Posterior approach to the deep femoral artery. J Vasc Surg. 1999;29(4):741–4.

280. Taurino M, Persiani F, Ficarelli R, Filippi F, Dito R, Rizzo L. The role of the profundoplasty in the modern management of patient with peripheral vascular disease. Ann Vasc Surg. 2017;45:16–21. https://doi.org/10.1016/j.avsg.2017.05.018. Epub 2017 May 24

281. Rollins DL, Towne JB, Bernhard VM, Baum PL. Isolated profundaplasty for limb salvage. J Vasc Surg. 1985;2(4):585–90.

282. Boren CH, Towne JB, Bernhard VM, Salles-Cunha S. Profundapopliteal collateral index. A guide to successful profundaplasty. Arch Surg. 1980;115(11):1366–72.

283. Khwaja HA, Omotoso PO. Bifurcated Dacron patch for simultaneous superficial femoroplasty and profundoplasty: a case report. J Med Case Rep. 2009;3:9294. https://doi.org/10.1186/1752-1947-3-9294.

284. Dufranc J, Palcau L, Heyndrickx M, Gouicem D, Coffin O, Felisaz A, Berger L. Technique and results of femoral bifurcation endarterectomy by eversion. J Vasc Surg. 2015 Mar;61(3):728–33.

285. Bernik T, Montoya M, Ibrahim I, Dardik H. Dropped bifurcation technique for femoral endarterectomy. Ann Vasc Surg. 2019;54:316–7.

286. Darling RC 3rd, Shah DM, Change BB, Lloyd WE, Leather RP. Can the deep femoral artery be used reliably as an inflow source for infrainguinal reconstruction? Long-term results in 563 procedures. J Vasc Surg. 1994;20(6):889–94. discussion 894-5

287. Kontopodis N, Lioudaki S, Chronis C, Kalogerakos P, Lazopoulos G, Papaioannou A, Ioannou CV. The use of the profunda femoral artery as the sole target vessel to bypass aortoiliac disease in patients with critical limb ischemia and concomitant unreconstructable infrainguinal disease. Ann Vasc Surg. 2018;48:45–52.

288. Balasundaram N, Whitrock JN, Braet DJ, Vogel TR, Bath JM. Importance of the profunda femoris upon patency following aortoiliac procedures. J Vasc Surg. 2022;S0741-5214(22)00410-4. https://doi.org/10.1016/j.jvs.2022.02.043. Epub ahead of print.

289. Prendiville EJ, Burke PE, Colgan MP, Wee BL, Moore DJ, Gregor Shanik D. The profunda femoris: a durable outflow vessel in aortofemoral surgery. J Vascu Surg. 1992;16(1):23–9.

290. Qato K, Nguyen N, Bouris V, Conway A, Ehidom C, Leung T, Giangola G, Carroccio A. Outcomes of endovascular management of isolated profunda femoris artery occlusive disease. Ann Vasc Surg. 2021;72:244–52.

291. Darling RC 3rd, Shah DM, Change BB, Lloyd WE, Leather RP. Can the deep femoral artery be used reliably as an inflow source for infrainguinal reconstruction? Long-term results in 563 procedures. J Vasc Surg [Internet]. 1994;20(6):889–94. discussion 894-5.

292. Donas KP, Pitoulias GA, Schwindt A, Schulte S, Camci M, Schlabach R, et al. Endovascular treatment of profunda femoris artery obstructive disease: nonsense or useful tool in selected cases? Eur J Vasc Endovasc Surg [Internet]. 2010;39(3):308–13.

293. Qato K, Nguyen N, Bouris V, Conway A, Ehidom C, Leung T, et al. Outcomes of endovascular management of isolated profunda femoris artery occlusive disease. Ann Vasc Surg [Internet]. 2021;72:244–52.

294. Bath J, Avgerinos E. A pooled analysis of common femoral and profunda femoris endovascular interventions. Vascular [Internet]. 2016;24(4):404–13.

295. Conte MS, Bradbury AW, Kolh P, White JV, Dick F, Fitridge R, et al. Global vascular guidelines on the management of chronic limb-threatening ischemia. J Vasc Surg. 2019;69(6):3S–125S.e40.

296. Lowry D, Saeed M, Narendran P, Tiwari A. A review of distribution of atherosclerosis in the lower limb arteries of patients with diabetes mellitus and peripheral vascular disease. Vasc Endovasc Surg. 2018;52(7):535–42.

297. Woelfie KD, Lange G, Mayer H, Bruijnen H, Loeprecht H. Distal vein graft reconstruction for isolated tibioperoneal vessel occlusive disease in diabetics with critical foot ischaemia-does it work? Eur J Vasc Surg. 1993;7(4):409–13.

298. Veith FJ, Gupta SK, Samson RH, Flores SW, Janko G, Scher LA. Superficial femoral and popliteal arteries as inflow sites for distal bypasses. Surgery. 1981;90(6):980–90.

299. Rosenbloom MS, Walsh JJ, Schuler JJ, Meyer JP, Schwarcz TH, Eldrup-Jorgensen J, et al. Long-term results of infragenicular bypasses with autogenous vein originating from the distal superficial femoral and popliteal arteries. J Vasc Surg. 1988;7(5):691–6.

300. Ascer E, Veith FJ, Gupta SK, White SA, Bakal CW, Wengerter K, et al. Short vein grafts: a superior option for arterial reconstructions to poor or compromised outflow tracts? J Vasc Surg. 1988;7(2):370–8.

301. Schneider PA, Caps MT, Ogawa DY, Hayman ES. Intraoperative superficial femoral artery balloon angioplasty and popliteal to distal bypass graft: an option for combined open and endovascular treatment of diabetic gangrene. J Vasc Surg. 2001;33(5):955–62.

302. Uhl C, Hock C, Betz T, Töpel I, Steinbauer M. Pedal bypass surgery after crural endovascular intervention. J Vasc Surg. 2014;59(6):1583–7.

303. Davidson JT, Callis JT. Arterial reconstruction of vessels in the foot and ankle. Ann Surg. 1993;217(6):699–710.

304. Hendawy K, Fatah MA, Ismail OAO, Ismail O, Essawy MG, Kader MA. Revascularization of a specific angiosome for limb salvage: does the target artery matter? Egypt J Radiol Nucl Med. 2019;50(1):84.

305. Pomposelli FB, Jepsen SJ, Gibbons GW, Campbell DR, Freeman DV, Miller A, et al. Efficacy of the dorsal pedal bypass for limb salvage in diabetic patients: Short-term observations. J Vasc Surg. 1990;11(6):745–52.

306. Eiberg JP, Hansen MA, Jørgensen LG, Rasmussen JBG, Jensen F, Schroeder TV. In-situ bypass surgery on arteriographically invisible vessels detected by Doppler-ultrasound for limb salvage. J Cardiovasc Surg. 2004;45(4):375–9.

307. Pereira CE, Albers M, Romiti M, Brochado-Neto FC, Pereira CAB. Meta-analysis of femoropopliteal bypass grafts for lower extremity arterial insufficiency. J Vasc Surg. 2006;44(3):510–517.e3.

308. Pomposelli FB, Jepsen SJ, Gibbons GW, Campbell DR, Freeman DV, Gaughan BM, et al. A flexible approach to infrapopliteal vein grafts in patients with diabetes mellitus. Arch Surg-chicago. 1991;126(6):724–9.

309. Pomposelli FB, Kansal N, Hamdan AD, Belfield A, Sheahan M, Campbell DR, et al. A decade of experience with dorsalis pedis artery bypass: analysis of outcome in more than 1000 cases. J Vasc Surg. 2003;37(2):307–15.

310. Seeger JM, Schmidt JH, Flynn TC. Preoperative saphenous and cephalic vein mapping as an adjunct to reconstructive arterial surgery. Ann Surg. 1987;205(6):733–9.

311. Wengerter KR, Veith FJ, Gupta SK, Ascer E, Rivers SP. Influence of vein size (diameter) on infrapopliteal reversed vein graft patency. J Vasc Surg. 1990;11(4):525–31.

312. Valentine J, Wind GG. Anatomic exposures in vascular surgery. 4th ed. Alphen aan den Rijn: Wolters Kluwer; 2021.

313. Chepte AP, Ambiye MV. Study of branching pattern of dorsalis pedis artery and its clinical significance. Anat Physiol Curr Res. 2018;8(3):1–5.

314. Yamada T, Gloviczki P, Bower TC, Naessens JM, Carmichael SW. Variations of the arterial anatomy of the foot. Am J Surg. 1993;166(2):130–5.

315. Miller A, Marcaccio EJ, Tannenbaum GA, Kwolek CJ, Stonebridge PA, Lavin PT, et al. Comparison of angioscopy and angiography for monitoring infrainguinal bypass vein grafts: results of a prospective randomized trial. J Vasc Surg. 1993;17(2):382–98.

316. Ferraresi R, Centola M, Ferlini M, Ros RD, Caravaggi C, Assaloni R, et al. Long-term outcomes after angioplasty of isolated, below-the-knee arteries in diabetic patients with critical limb ischaemia. J Vasc Surg. 2009;49(3):815.

317. Hughes K, Domenig CM, Hamdan AD, Schermerhorn M, Aulivola B, Blattman S, et al. Bypass to plantar and tarsal arteries: an acceptable approach to limb salvage. J Vasc Surg. 2004;40(6):1149–57.

318. Darling RC, Shah DM, Chang BB, Lloyd WE, Paty PSK, Leather RP. Arterial reconstruction for limb salvage: is the terminal peroneal artery a disadvantaged outflow tract? Surgery. 1995;118(4):763–7.

319. Elliott BM, Robison JG, Brothers TE, Cross MA. Limitations of peroneal artery bypass grafting for limb salvage. J Vasc Surg. 1993;18(5):881–8.

320. Domenig CM, Hamdan AD, Holzenbein TJ, Kansal N, Aulivola B, Skillman JJ, et al. Timing of pedal bypass failure and its impact on the need for amputation. Ann Vasc Surg. 2005;19(1):56–62.

321. Pelka M, Dieter RS. The Jury is still out on atherectomy. Cardiovasc Revasc Med. 2020;21(5):682–3. https://doi.org/10.1016/j.carrev.2020.05.024.

322. Gandini R, Pratesi G, Merolla S, Scaggiante J, Chegai F. A single-center experience with phoenix atherectomy system in patients with moderate to heavily calcified femoropopliteal lesions. Cardiovasc Revasc Med. 2020;21(5):676–81. https://doi.org/10.1016/j.carrev.2019.08.019. Epub 2019 Aug 23

323. Arthurs ZM, Bishop PD, Feiten LE, Eagleton MJ, Clair DG, Kashyap VS. Evaluation of peripheral atherosclerosis: a comparative analysis of angiography and intravascular ultrasound imaging. J Vasc

Surg. 2010;51(4):933–8. https://doi.org/10.1016/j.jvs.2009.11.034. Epub 2010 Jan 15. discussion 939

324. Cioppa A, Stabile E, Popusoi G, Salemme L, Cota L, Pucciarelli A, Ambrosini V, Sorropago G, Tesorio T, Agresta A, Biamino G, Rubino P. Combined treatment of heavy calcified femoro-popliteal lesions using directional atherectomy and a paclitaxel coated balloon: one-year single centre clinical results. Cardiovasc Revasc Med. 2012;13(4):219–23. https://doi.org/10.1016/j.carrev.2012.04.007. Epub 2012 May 25

325. Schwarzwälder U, Zeller T. Debulking procedures: potential device specific indications. Tech Vasc Interv Radiol. 2010;13(1):43–53. https://doi.org/10.1053/j.tvir.2009.10.006.

326. Babaev A, Halista M, Bakirova Z, Avtushka V, Matsumura M, Maehara A. Directional versus orbital atherectomy of femoropopliteal artery lesions: angiographic and intravascular ultrasound outcomes. Catheter Cardiovasc Interv. 2022; https://doi.org/10.1002/ccd.30339.

327. Gupta R, Siada S, Lai S, Al-Musawi M, Malgor EA, Jacobs DL, Malgor RD. Critical appraisal of the contemporary use of atherectomy to treat femoropopliteal atherosclerotic disease. J Vasc Surg. 2022;75(2):697–708.e9. https://doi.org/10.1016/j.jvs.2021.07.106. Epub 2021 Jul 22

328. Shammas NW, Torey JT, Shammas WJ, Jones-Miller S, Shammas GA. Intravascular ultrasound assessment and correlation with angiographic findings of arterial dissections following auryon laser atherectomy and adjunctive balloon angioplasty: results of the idissection auryon laser study. J Endovasc Ther. 2022;29(1):23–31. https://doi.org/10.1177/15266028211028200. Epub 2021 Jun 28

329. Pan T, Tian SY, Liu Z, Zhang T, Li C, Ji DH. Combination of Rotarex®S rotational athero-thrombectomy and drug-coated balloon angioplasty for femoropopliteal total in-stent occlusion. Ann Vasc Surg. 2022;80:213–22. https://doi.org/10.1016/j.avsg.2021.08.058. Epub 2021 Nov 5

330. Ferraresi R, Mauri G, Losurdo F, Troisi N, Brancaccio D, Caravaggi C, et al. BAD trans-mission and SAD distribution: a new scenario for critical limb ischemia. J Cardiovasc Surg. 2018;59(5):655–64.

331. Mustapha JA, Katzen BT, Neville RF, Lookstein RA, Zeller T, Miller LE, et al. Propensity score-adjusted comparison of long-term outcomes among revascularization strategies for critical limb ischemia. Circ Cardiovasc Interv. 2019;12(9):e008097.

332. Palena LM, Saad PF, Piccolo E, et al. Below the ankle orbital atherectomy in chronic limb-threatening ischemia patients as a bailout strategy for limb salvage: Early Clinical Experience, Article in Press, published on line ahead of print. Cardiovasc Revasc Med.

333. Iashimori A, Iida O, Yamauchi Y, Kawasaki D, Nakamura M, Soga Y, et al. Outcomes of one straight-line flow with and without pedal arch in patients with critical limb ischemia. Catheter Cardiovasc Interv. 2016;87(1):129–33.

334. Manzi M, Fusaro M, Ceccacci T, Erente G, Dalla Paola L, Brocco E. Clinical results of below-the knee intervention using pedal-plantar loop technique for the revascularization of foot arteries. J Cardiovasc Surg. 2009;50(3):331–7.

335. Palena LM, Brocco E, Manzi M. The clinical utility of below-the-ankle angioplasty using "transmetatarsal artery access" in complex cases of CLI. Catheter Cardiovasc Interv. 2014;83(1):123–9.

336. Hirsch AT, Duval S. The global pandemic of peripheral artery disease. Lancet. 2013;382(9901):1312–4.

337. Gerhard-Herman MD. 2016 AHA/ACC Guideline on the Management of Patients With Lower Extremity Peripheral Artery Disease: A Report of the American College of Cardiology/American Heart Association Task Force on Clinical Practice Guidelines (vol 135, pg e726, 2017). Circulation. 2017;135(12):E791–E2.

338. Mustapha JA, Saab FA, Martinsen BJ, Pena CS, Zeller T, Driver VR, et al. Digital subtraction angiography prior to an amputation for critical limb ischemia (CLI): an expert recommendation statement from the CLI global society to optimize limb salvage. J Endovasc Ther. 2020;27(4):540–6.

339. Utsunomiya M, Takahara M, Iida O, Yamauchi Y, Kawasaki D, Yokoi Y, et al. Wound blush obtainment is the most important angiographic endpoint for wound healing. JACC Cardiovasc Interv. 2017;10(2):188–94.

340. Kozlow JH, Zwyghuizen AM, Wakefield TW. Chapter 39: Below- and above-the-knee amputation. In: Minter RM, Doherty GM, editors. Current procedures: surgery. New York: The McGraw-Hill Companies; 2010.

341. Park TH, Anand A. Management of diabetic foot: brief synopsis for busy orthopedist. J Clin Orthop Trauma. 2015;6(1):24–9. https://doi.org/10.1016/j.jcot.2014.10.003. Epub 2014 Nov 14

342. Miguel M, Bernadino Castelo Branco R, David GA, Kay RG, John M, Joseph L, Mills S. Diagnosis and endovascular management of segmental heel ischemia. Int. J Clin Cardiol. 2018;5(2) https://doi.org/10.23937/2378-2951/1410117.

343. Iida O, Soga Y, Hirano K, Kawasaki D, Suzuki K, Miyashita Y, Terashi H, Uematsu M. Long-term results of direct and indirect endovascular revascularization based on the angiosome concept in patients with critical limb ischemia presenting with isolated below-the-knee lesions. J Vasc Surg. 2012;55(2):363–370.e5. https://doi.org/10.1016/j.jvs.2011.08.014. Epub 2011 Nov 1

344. Söderström M, Albäck A, Biancari F, Lappalainen K, Lepäntalo M, Venermo M. Angiosome-targeted infrapopliteal endovascular revascularization for treatment of diabetic foot ulcers. J Vasc Surg. 2013;57(2):427–35. https://doi.org/10.1016/j.jvs.2012.07.057. Epub 2012 Dec 7

345. Slawinski C, Kim I, Ahmad N. Orphan heel syndrome: a vascular perspective article points. Diabet Foot J. 2017;20:250–2

346. Dilaver N, Twine CP, Bosanquet DC. Editor's Choice - direct vs. indirect angiosomal revascularisation of infrapopliteal arteries, an updated systematic review and meta-analysis. Eur J Vasc Endovasc Surg. 2018;56(6):834–48. https://doi.org/10.1016/j.ejvs.2018.07.017. Epub 2018 Aug 24

347. Fujii M, Terashi H. Angiosome and tissue healing. Ann Vasc Dis. 2019;12(2):147–50. https://doi.org/10.3400/avd.ra.19-00036.

348. Ji D, Zhang T, Li C, Liu Y, Wang F. Evaluation of angiosome-targeted infrapopliteal endovascular revascularization in critical diabetic limb ischemia. J Interv Med. 2019;1(3):176–81. https://doi.org/10.19779/j.cnki.2096-3602.2018.03.08.

349. Utsunomiya M, Nakamura M, Nakanishi M, Takagi T, Hara H, Onishi K, Yamada T, Sugi K. Impact of wound blush as an angiographic end point of endovascular therapy for patients with critical limb ischemia. J Vasc Surg. 2012;55(1):113–21. https://doi.org/10.1016/j.jvs.2011.08.001. Epub 2011 Sep 22

350. Kum S, Tan YK, Schreve MA, et al. Midterm outcomes from a pilot study of percutaneous deep vein arterialization for the treatment of no-option critical limb ischemia. J Endovasc Ther. 2017;24:619–26.

351. Béland M, Méthot M, Bradette S, et al. Venous arterialization with common endovascular devices. J Vasc Interv Radiol. 2019;30:570–1.

352. Migliara B, Cappellari TF. A novel technique to create an arteriovenous fistula during total percutaneous deep foot venous arterialisation using an IVUS guided catheter. Eur J Vasc Endovasc Surg. 2018;55:735.

353. Gandini R, Merolla S, Scaggiante J, et al. Endovascular distal plantar vein arterialization in dialysis patients with no-option critical limb ischemia and posterior tibial artery occlusion: a technique for limb salvage in a challenging patient subset. J Endovasc Ther. 2018;25:127–32.

354. Ichihashi S, Shimohara Y, Bolstad F, et al. Simplified endovascular deep venous arterialization for non-option CLI patients by percutaneous direct needle puncture of tibial artery and vein under ultrasound guidance (AV Spear Technique). Cardiovasc Intervent Radiol. 2020;43:339–43.

355. Ysa A, Lobato M, Mikelarena E, et al. Homemade device to facilitate percutaneous venous arterialization in patients with no-option critical limb ischemia. J Endovasc Ther. 2019;26:213–8.

356. Ysa A, Lobato M. Reply to "Regarding: Homemade device to facilitate percutaneous venous arterialization in patients with no-option critical limb ischemia". J Endovasc Ther. 2019;26:427–8.

357. Ho VT, Gologorsky R, Kibrik P, Chandra V, Prent A, Lee J, et al. Open, percutaneous, and hybrid deep venous arterialization technique for no-option foot salvage. J Vasc Surg. 2020;71:2152–60.

358. Ysa A, Lobato M. Complete update of the "state of the art" of percutaneous venous arterialization. J Vasc Surg. 2020;71:2185–7.

359. Nakama T, Ichihashi S, Ogata K, Kojima S, Muraishi M, Obunai K, Watanabe H. Twelve-month clinical outcomes of percutaneous deep venous arterialization with alternative techniques and ordinary endovascular therapy devices for patients with chronic limb-threatening ischemia: results of the DEPARTURE Japan study. Cardiovasc Intervent Radiol. 2022; https://doi.org/10.1007/s00270-022-03095-1.

360. Ferraresi R, Casini A, Losurdo F, Caminiti M, Ucci A, Longhi M, et al. Hybrid foot vein arterialization in no-option patients with critical limb ischemia: a preliminary report. J Endovasc Ther. 2019;26(1):7–17.

361. Ichihashi S, Sato T, Iwakoshi S, Itoh H, Kichikawa K. Technique of percutaneous direct needle puncture of calcified plaque in the superficial femoral artery or tibial artery to facilitate balloon catheter passage and balloon dilation of calcified lesions. J Vasc Interv Radiol. 2014;25:784–8.

362. Clair DG, Mustapha JA, Shishehbor MH, Schneider PA, Henao S, Bernardo NN, Deaton DH. PROMISE I: Early feasibility study of the LimFlow System for percutaneous deep vein arterialization in no-option chronic limb-threatening ischemia: 12-month results. J Vasc Surg. 2021;5:1626–35.

363. Schmidt A, Schreve MA, Huizing E, Del Giudice C, Branzan D, Ünlü Ç, et al. Midterm outcomes of percutaneous deep venous arterialization with a dedicated system for patients with no-option chronic limb-threatening ischemia: the ALPS multicenter study. J Endovasc Ther. 2020;27:658–65.

364. Alexandrescu V, Ngongang C, Vincent G, Ledent G, Hubermont G. Deep calf veins arterialization for inferior limb preservation in diabetic patients with extended ischaemic wounds, unfit for direct arterial reconstruction: preliminary results according to an angiosome model of perfusion. Cardiovasc Revasc Med. 2011;12(1):10–9.

365. Ysa A, Lobato M, Mikelarena E, Arruabarrena A, Gómez R, Apodaka A, Metcalfe M, Fonseca JL. Homemade device to facilitate percutaneous venous arterialization in patients with no-option critical limb ischemia. J Endovasc Ther. 2019;26(2):213–8.

366. Gandini R, Merolla S, Scaggiante J, Meloni M, Giurato L, Uccioli L, Konda D. Endovascular distal plantar vein arterialization in dialysis patients with no-option critical limb ischemia and posterior tibial artery occlusion: a technique for limb salvage in a challenging patient subset. J Endovasc Ther. 2018;25(1):127–32.

367. Schmidt A, Schreve MA, Huizing E, Del Giudice C, Branzan D, Ünlü Ç, Varcoe RL, Ferraresi R, Kum S. Midterm outcomes of percutaneous deep venous arterialization with a dedicated system for patients with no-option chronic limb-threatening ischemia: the ALPS multicenter study. J Endovasc Ther. 2020;27(4):658–65.

368. Schreve MA, Huizing E, Kum S, de Vries JPP, de Borst GJ, Ünlü Ç. Volume flow and peak systolic velocity of the arteriovenous circuit in patients after percutaneous deep venous arterialization. Diagnostics. 2020;10(10):760.

369. Cangiano G, Corvino F, Giurazza F, De Feo EM, Fico F, Palumbo V, Amodio F, Silvestre M, Corvino A, Niola R. Percutaneous deep foot vein arterialization IVUS-guided in no-option critical limb ischemia diabetic patients. Vasc Endovasc Surg. 2021;55(1):58–63.

370. Del Giudice C, Van Den Heuvel D, Wille J, Mirault T, Messas E, Ferraresi R, Kum S, Sapoval M. Percutaneous deep venous arterialization for severe critical limb ischemia in patients with no option of revascularization: early experience from two European centers. Cardiovasc Intervent Radiol. 2018;41(10):1474–80.

371. Kum S, Huizing E, Schreve MA, Unlu C, Ferraresi R, Samarakoon LB, van den Heuvel DA. Percutaneous deep venous arterialization in patients with critical limb ischemia. J Cardiovasc Surg. 2018;59(5):665–9.

372. Schmidli J, Widmer MK, Basile C, de Donato G, Gallieni M, Gibbons CP, Haage P, Hamilton G, Hedin U, Kamper L, Lazarides MK, Lindsey B, Mestres G, Pegoraro M, Roy J, Setacci C, Shemesh D, JHM T, van Loon M, Committee EG, Kolh P, de Borst GJ, Chakfe N, Debus S, Hinchliffe R, Kakkos S, Koncar I, Lindholt J, Naylor R, Vega de Ceniga M, Vermassen F, Verzini F, Reviewers EG, Mohaupt M, Ricco JB, Roca-Tey R. Editor's choice–vascular access: 2018 clinical practice guidelines of the European Society for Vascular Surgery (ESVS). Eur J Vasc Endovasc Surg. 2018;55(6):757–818.

373. Sprengers RW, Teraa M, Moll FL, de Wit GA, van der Graaf Y, Verhaar MC, JUVENTAS Study Group; SMART Study Group. Quality of life in patients with no-option critical limb ischemia underlines the need for new effective treatment. J Vasc Surg. 2010;52:843–9.e1.

374. Kim TI, Vartanian SS, Schneider PA. A review and proposed classification system for the no-option patient with chronic limb- threatening ischemia. J Endovasc Ther. 2021;28:183–93.

375. Ferraresi R, Ucci A, Pizzuto A, Losurdo F, Caminiti M, Minnella D, et al. A novel scoring system for small artery disease and medial arterial calcification is strongly associated with major adverse limb events in patients with chronic limb-threatening ischemia. J Endovasc Ther. 2021;28:194–207.

376. Miranda J, Pallister Z, Sharath S, Ferrer L, Chung J, Lepow B, Mills J, Montero-Baker M. Early experience with venous arterialization for limb salvage in no-option patients with chronic limb-threatening ischemia. J Vasc Surg. 2022:1–10.

377. Ferraresi R, Casini A, Losurdo F, Caminiti M, Ucci A, Longhi M, Schreve M, Lichtenberg M, Kum S, Clerici G. Hybrid foot vein arterialization in no-option patients with critical limb ischemia: a preliminary report. J Endovasc Ther. 2019;26(1):7–17.

378. Kum S, Tan YK, Schreve MA, Ferraresi R, Varcoe RL, Schmidt A, Scheinert D, Mustapha JA, Lim DM, Ho D, Tang TY, Alexandrescu VA, Mutirangura P. Midterm outcomes from a pilot study of percutaneous deep vein arterialization for the treatment of no-option critical limb ischemia. J Endovasc Ther. 2017;24(5):619–26.

379. Clair DG, Mustapha JA, Shishehbor MH, Schneider PA, Henao S, Bernardo NN, Deaton DH. PROMISE I early feasibility study of the LimFlow System for percutaneous deep vein arterialization in no-option chronic limb-threatening ischemia 12-month results. J Vasc Surg. 2021 May 18:S0741-5214(21)00737-0.

380. Schmidt A, Schreve MA, Huizing E, Del Giudice C, Branzan D, Ünlü Ç, Varcoe RL, Ferraresi R, Kum S. Midterm outcomes of percutaneous deep venous arterialization with a dedicated system for patients with no-option chronic limb-threatening ischemia: the ALPS multicenter study. J Endovasc Ther. 2020 Aug;27(4):658–65.

381. Second Round of Late-Breaking Clinical Trials Announced at VIVA 2022. https://viva-foundation.org/news-article?id=159162. Nov 2022.

382. Saab F, Mustapha J, Ansari M, Pupp G, Madassery S, N'Dandu Z, Wiechmann B, Bernstein R, Mize A, Pliagas G. Percutaneous deep vein arterialization: treatment of patients with end-stage plantar disease. JSCAI. 2022; https://doi.org/10.1016/j.jscai.2022.100437.

383. Indes JE, Mandawat A, Tuggle CT, Muhs B, Sosa JA. Endovascular procedures for aorto-iliac occlusive disease are associated with superior short-term clinical and economic outcomes compared with open surgery in the inpatient population. J Vasc Surg. 2010;52(5):1173–9. 1179.e1

384. Kashyap VS, Pavkov ML, Bena JF, Sarac TP, O'Hara PJ, Lyden SP, Clair DG. The management of severe aortoiliac occlusive disease: endovascular therapy rivals open reconstruction. J Vasc Surg. 2008;48(6):1451–7. https://doi.org/10.1016/j.jvs.2008.07.004. 1457.e1–3. Epub 2008 Sep 19

385. Shu J, Santulli G. Update on peripheral artery disease: Epidemiology and evidence-based facts. Atherosclerosis. 2018;275:379–81.

386. Hughes K, Seetahal S, Oyetunji T, et al. Racial/ethnic disparities in amputation and revascularization: a nationwide inpatient sample study. Vasc Endovasc Surg. 2014;48(1):34–7.

387. Collins TC, Johnson M, Henderson W, Khuri SF, Daley J. Lower extremity nontraumatic amputation among veterans with peripheral arterial disease: is race an independent factor? Med Care. 2002;40(1 Suppl):I106–16.

388. Carnethon MR, Pu J, Howard G, et al. Cardiovascular health in African Americans: a scientific statement from the American Heart Association. Circulation. 2017;136(21):e393–423.

389. Lackland DT. Racial differences in hypertension: implications for high blood pressure management. Am J Med Sci. 2014;348(2):135–8.

390. Ford ES. Trends in mortality from all causes and cardiovascular disease among hypertensive and non-hypertensive adults in the United States. Circulation. 2011;123(16):1737–44.

391. Lackland DT, Keil JE, Gazes PC, Hames CG, Tyroler HA. Outcomes of black and white hypertensive individuals after 30 years of follow-up. Clin Exp Hypertens N Y N 1993. 1995;17(7):1091–105.

392. Huen KH, Chowdhury R, Shafii SM, et al. Smoking cessation is the least successful outcome of risk factor modification in uninsured patients with symptomatic peripheral arterial disease. Ann Vasc Surg. 2015;29(1):42–9.

393. Mensah GA. Cardiovascular diseases in African Americans: fostering community partnerships to stem the tide. Am J Kidney Dis. 2018;72(5 Suppl 1):S37–42.

394. Willigendael EM, Teijink JAW, Bartelink ML, et al. Influence of smoking on incidence and prevalence of peripheral arterial disease. J Vasc Surg. 2004;40(6):1158–65.

395. Wang W, Zhao T, Geng K, Yuan G, Chen Y, Xu Y. Smoking and the pathophysiology of peripheral artery disease. Front Cardiovasc Med. 2021;8. https://www.frontiersin.org/article/10.3389/fcvm.2021.704106 (Accessed April 9, 2022).

396. Smith GD, Shipley MJ, Rose G. Intermittent claudication, heart disease risk factors, and mortality. The whitehall study. Circulation. 1990;82(6):1925–31.

397. General USPHSO of the S, Health NC for CDP and HP (US) O on S and. The Health Benefits of Smoking Cessation. US Department of Health and Human Services; 2020. https://www.ncbi.nlm.nih.gov/books/NBK555590/. Accessed 9 April 2022.

398. Caraballo RS, Kruger J, Asman K, et al. Relapse among cigarette smokers: the CARDIA longitudinal study – 1985–2011. Addict Behav. 2014;39(1):101–6.

399. Kulak JA, Cornelius ME, Fong GT, Giovino GA. Differences in quit attempts and cigarette smoking abstinence between whites and African Americans in the United States: literature review and results from the international tobacco control US survey. Nicotine Tob Res. 2016;18(Suppl. 1):S79–87.

400. Keith VM, Nguyen AW, Taylor RJ, Mouzon DM, Chatters LM. Microaggressions, discrimination, and phenotype among African Americans: a latent class analysis of the impact of skin tone and BMI. Sociol Inq. 2017;87(2):233–55.

401. Munro HM, Tarone RE, Wang TJ, Blot WJ. Menthol and nonmenthol cigarette smoking: all-cause deaths, cardiovascular disease deaths, and other causes of death among blacks and whites. Circulation. 2016;133(19):1861–6.

402. Delnevo CD, Gundersen DA, Hrywna M, Echeverria SE, Steinberg MB. Smoking-cessation prevalence among U.S. smokers of menthol versus non-menthol cigarettes. Am J Prev Med. 2011;41(4):357–65. https://doi.org/10.1016/j.amepre.2011.06.039.

403. Arya S, Khakharia A, Binney ZO, et al. Association of statin dose with amputation and survival in patients with peripheral artery disease. Circulation. 2018;137(14):1435–46.

404. Nanna MG, Navar AM, Zakroysky P, et al. Association of patient perceptions of cardiovascular risk and beliefs on statin drugs with racial differences in statin use: insights from the patient and provider assessment of lipid management registry. JAMA Cardiol. 2018;3(8):739–48.

405. Fields LE, Burt VL, Cutler JA, Hughes J, Roccella EJ, Sorlie P. The burden of adult hypertension in the United States 1999 to 2000: a rising tide. Hypertens Dallas Tex 1979. 2004;44(4):398–404.

406. Golden SH, Brown A, Cauley JA, et al. Health disparities in endocrine disorders: biological, clinical, and nonclinical factors--an Endocrine Society scientific statement. J Clin Endocrinol Metab. 2012;97(9):E1579–639.

407. Schubert M, Hansen S, Leefmann J, Guan K. Repurposing antidiabetic drugs for cardiovascular disease. Front Physiol. 2020;11:568632.

408. Durazzo TS, Frencher S, Gusberg R. Influence of race on the management of lower extremity ischemia: revascularization vs amputation. JAMA Surg. 2013;148(7):617–23.

409. Holman KH, Henke PK, Dimick JB, Birkmeyer JD. Racial disparities in the use of revascularization before leg amputation in Medicare patients. J Vasc Surg. 2011;54(2):420–6. 426.e1

410. Rizzo JA, Chen J, Laurich C, et al. Racial disparities in PAD-related amputation rates among native americans and non-hispanic whites: an HCUP analysis. J Health Care Poor Underserved. 2018;29(2):782–800.

411. Loja MN, Brunson A, Li CS, et al. Racial disparities in outcomes of endovascular procedures for peripheral arterial disease: an evaluation of California hospitals, 2005–2009. Ann Vasc Surg. 2015;29(5):950–9.

412. Selvarajah S, Black JH, Haider AH, Abularrage CJ. Racial disparity in early graft failure after infrainguinal bypass. J Surg Res. 2014;190(1):335–43.

413. Gandjian M, Sareh S, Premji A, et al. Racial disparities in surgical management and outcomes of acute limb ischemia in the United States. Surg Open Sci. 2021;6:45–50.

414. Nejim B, Beaulieu RJ, Alshaikh H, Hamouda M, Canner J, Malas MB. A unique All-payer rate-setting system controls the cost but not the racial disparity in lower extremity revascularization procedures. Ann Vasc Surg. 2018;52:116–25.

415. Hirsch AT, Allison MA, Gomes AS, et al. A call to action: women and peripheral artery disease: a scientific statement from the American Heart Association. Circulation. 2012;125(11):1449–72.

416. Ortmann J, Nüesch E, Traupe T, Diehm N, Baumgartner I. Gender is an independent risk factor for distribution pattern and lesion morphology in chronic critical limb ischemia. J Vasc Surg. 2012;55(1):98–104.

417. Hirsch AT, Murphy TP, Lovell MB, et al. Gaps in public knowledge of peripheral arterial disease: the first national PAD public awareness survey. Circulation. 2007;116(18):2086–94.

418. Hamburg NM. Clinical outcomes of women with PAD. J Am Coll Cardiol. 2020;75(6):618–9.

419. Vouyouka AG, Egorova NN, Salloum A, et al. Lessons learned from the analysis of gender effect on risk factors and procedural outcomes of lower extremity arterial disease. J Vasc Surg. 2010;52(5):1196–202.

420. Schramm K, Rochon PJ. Gender differences in peripheral vascular disease. Semin Interv Radiol. 2018;35(1):9–16.

421. Grenon SM, Cohen BE, Smolderen K, Vittinghoff E, Whooley MA, Hiramoto J. Peripheral arterial disease, gender, and depression in the Heart and Soul Study. J Vasc Surg. 2014;60(2):396–403.

422. Barochiner J, Aparicio LS, Waisman GD. Challenges associated with peripheral arterial disease in women. Vasc Health Risk Manag. 2014;10:115–28.

423. Hooi JD, Kester AD, Stoffers HE, Overdijk MM, van Ree JW, Knottnerus JA. Incidence of and risk factors for asymptomatic peripheral arterial occlusive disease: a longitudinal study. Am J Epidemiol. 2001;153(7):666–72.

424. McDermott MM, Fried L, Simonsick E, Ling S, Guralnik JM. Asymptomatic peripheral arterial disease is independently associated with impaired lower extremity functioning: the women's health and aging study. Circulation. 2000;101(9):1007–12.

425. McDermott MM, Greenland P, Liu K, et al. Sex differences in peripheral arterial disease: leg symptoms and physical functioning. J Am Geriatr Soc. 2003;51(2):222–8.

426. Hirsch AT, Criqui MH, Treat-Jacobson D, et al. Peripheral arterial disease detection, awareness, and treatment in primary care. JAMA. 2001;286(11):1317–24.

427. Pande RL, Hiatt WR, Zhang P, Hittel N, Creager MA. A pooled analysis of the durability and predictors of treatment response of cilostazol in patients with intermittent claudication. Vasc Med Lond Engl. 2010;15(3):181–8.

428. Lundgren F, Dahllöf AG, Lundholm K, Scherstén T, Volkmann R. Intermittent claudication--surgical reconstruction or physical training? A prospective randomized trial of treatment efficiency. Ann Surg. 1989;209(3):346–55.

429. Egorova N, Vouyouka AG, Quin J, et al. Analysis of gender-related differences in lower extremity peripheral arterial disease. J Vasc Surg. 2010;51(2):372–378.e1.

430. Freisinger E, Malyar NM, Reinecke H, Unrath M. Low rate of revascularization procedures and poor prognosis particularly in male patients with peripheral artery disease – a propensity score matched analysis. Int J Cardiol. 2018;255:188–94.

431. Gallagher KA, Meltzer AJ, Ravin RA, et al. Gender differences in outcomes of endovascular treatment of infrainguinal peripheral artery disease. Vasc Endovasc Surg. 2011;45(8):703–11.

432. Jackson EA, Munir K, Schreiber T, et al. Impact of sex on morbidity and mortality rates after lower extremity interventions for peripheral arterial disease: observations from the Blue Cross Blue Shield of Michigan Cardiovascular Consortium. J Am Coll Cardiol. 2014;63(23):2525–30.

433. Hernández Mateo MM, Martínez López I, Revuelta Suero S, et al. Clinical outcomes after endovascular treatment failure in patients with femoropopliteal occlusive disease. Ann Vasc Surg. 2016;30:299–304.

434. Lee MS, Choi BG, Hollowed J, et al. Assessment of sex differences in 5-year clinical outcomes following endovascular revascularization for peripheral artery disease. Cardiovasc Revasc Med Mol Interv. 2020;21(1):110–5.

435. Margolis DJ, Hoffstad O, Nafash J, et al. Location, location, location: geographic clustering of lower-extremity amputation among medicare beneficiaries with diabetes. Diabetes Care. 2011;34(11):2363–7.

436. Skrepnek GH, Mills JL, Armstrong DG. A diabetic emergency one million feet long: disparities and burdens of illness among diabetic foot ulcer cases within emergency departments in the United States, 2006–2010. PLoS One. 2015;10(8):e0134914.

437. McGinigle KL, Minc SD. Disparities in amputation in patients with peripheral arterial disease. Surgery. 2021;169(6):1290–4.

438. Goodney PP, Travis LL, Nallamothu BK, et al. Variation in the use of lower extremity vascular procedures for critical limb ischemia. Circ Cardiovasc Qual Outcomes. 2012;5(1):94–102.

439. Goodney PP, Holman K, Henke PK, et al. Regional intensity of vascular care and lower extremity amputation rates. J Vasc Surg. 2013;57(6):1471–1480.e3.

440. Soden PA, Zettervall SL, Deery SE, et al. Black patients present with more severe vascular disease and a greater burden of risk factors than white patients at time of major vascular intervention. J Vasc Surg. 2018;67(2):549–556.e3.

441. Song P, Rudan D, Zhu Y, et al. Global, regional, and national prevalence and risk factors for peripheral artery disease in 2015: an updated systematic review and analysis. Lancet Glob Health. 2019;7(8):e1020–30.

442. Johnston LE, Stewart BT, Yangni-Angate H, et al. Peripheral arterial disease in sub-saharan Africa: a review. JAMA Surg. 2016;151(6):564–72.

443. Kengne AP, Echouffo-Tcheugui JB. Differential burden of peripheral artery disease. Lancet Glob Health. 2019;7(8):e980–1.

444. Farber A, Menard MT, Conte MS, Kaufman JA, Powell RJ, Choudhry NK, Hamza TH, Assman SF, Creager MA, Cziraky MJ, Dake MD, for the BEST-CLI Investigators, Jaff MR, et al. Surgery or endovascular therapy for chronic limb-threatening ischemia. N Engl J Med. 2022;387:2305–16.

445. Teraa M, Conte MS, Moll FL, Verhaar MC. Critical limb ischemia: current trends and future directions. J AHA. 2016;5:e002938.

Syed Samaduddin Ahmed, Adam Said,
Osman Ahmed, Patrick Lee, Sreekumar Madassery,
Ron Winokur, Brian P. Holly, Mark Lessne,
Shin Mei Chan, Kush R. Desai, Jordan C. Tasse,
Griffin Mcnamara, Jillian Drogin, and Keith Pereira

7.1 Primary Treatment Strategy in Superficial and Deep Venous Disease

Syed Samaduddin Ahmed, Adam Said,
and Osman Ahmed

The original version of this chapter was revised. The correction to this chapter can be found at https://doi.org/10.1007/978-3-031-36480-8_12

7.1.1 Work-up

Clinical evaluation is the initial step in management of a patient with lower extremity edema. Past medical and family histories are valuable in the assessment of the underlying cause. Non-

S. S. Ahmed
Midwestern University Chicago College of Osteopathic Medicine, Downers Grove, IL, USA

A. Said
University of Illinois at Urbana-Champaign, University of Chicago, Chicago, IL, USA
e-mail: adamys2@illinois.edu

O. Ahmed
Department of Radiology, Section of Interventional Radiology, Chicago, IL, USA

P. Lee · R. Winokur
Department of Radiology, Division of Interventional Radiology, Thomas Jefferson University Hospital, Philadelphia, PA, USA
e-mail: patrick.lee@jefferson.edu;
Ronald.Winokur@jefferson.edu

S. Madassery (✉) · J. C. Tasse
Department of Vascular and Interventional Radiology, Rush University Medical Center, Chicago, IL, USA
e-mail: jordan_c_tasse@rush.edu

B. P. Holly
Department of Radiology and Radiologic Sciences, Division of Vascular and Interventional Radiology, John Hopkins Medical Institute, Baltimore, MD, USA
e-mail: bholly3@jhmi.edu

M. Lessne
Vascular and Interventional Specialists, North Carolina, IL, USA

S. M. Chan
Yale University School of Medicine, New Haven, CT, USA
e-mail: shinmei.chan@yale.edu

K. R. Desai
Northwestern University Feinberg School of Medicine, Chicago, IL, USA
e-mail: kdesai007@northwestern.edu

G. Mcnamara · J. Drogin
Saint Louis University School of Medicine, St. Louis, MO, USA
e-mail: griffin.mcnamara@health.slu.edu;
jillian.drogin@health.slu.edu

K. Pereira
Department of Vascular and Interventional Radiology, Saint Louis University, St. Louis, MO, USA
e-mail: keith.pereria@health.slu.edu

venous causes of edema must also be considered, such as congestive heart failure, or kidney disease.

The first line diagnostic imaging tool used is duplex ultrasound as it is useful in the assessment of venous reflux as well as thrombosis in both superficial and deep venous systems.

- Reflux is defined as reversed flow >0.5 s for superficial veins, and >1.0 s for deep veins [1]. In patients with a concern for more central or compressive etiology of edema, additional imaging may be warranted.
- Contrast-enhanced venous phase CT or MRI can help evaluate for compression of IVC or iliac veins (i.e., May-Thurner syndrome).
- Furthermore, invasive diagnostic tools, such as venography and intravascular ultrasound, can be used to assess deep veins. However, these are typically used only when there is high clinical suspicion for compression and intervention will be performed upon a positive finding.

Multiple classification systems are available to assist with assessment and standardization of venous disease, in order to determine appropriate treatment. The CEAP (Clinical-Etiology-Anatomy-Pathophysiology) classification system includes Clinical severity, Etiology, Anatomical distribution, and Pathophysiological dysfunction (Table 7.1) [1]. It is used to describe patients at a single point in time whereas the Venous Clinical Severity Score (VCSS) can be used to follow patients longitudinally (Table 7.2). VCSS scores

Table 7.1 Clinical classes of CEAP classification

Class	Description
C0	Heavy legs, pain in the legs, pruritus No clinical or palpable signs of venous disease
C1	Telangiectasia or reticular veins
C2	Visible and palpable varicose veins
C3	Venous edema (without trophic changes)
C4	Trophic changes of venous origin (a) Pigmentation or eczema (b) Lipodermatosclerosis or atrophie blanche
C5	Healed ulcer with trophic changes
C6	Venous ulcer

Table 7.2 Venous clinical severity score

Attribute	Absent = 0	Mild = 1	Moderate = 2	Severe = 3
Pain	None	Occasional, not restricting daily activity	Daily, interfering but not preventing daily activity	Daily, limits most daily activity
Varicose veins	None	Few, isolated branch varices or clusters, corona phlebectatica (ankle flare)	Confined to calf or thigh	Includes calf and thigh
Venous edema	None	Limited to foot and ankle	Extends above the ankle but below knee	Extends to knee and above
Skin Pigmentation	None or Focal	Limited to perimalleolar	Diffuse over lower third of calf	Wider distribution above lower third of calf
Inflammation	None	Mild cellulitis, ulcer margin limited to perimalleolar	Diffuse over lower third of calf	Wider distribution above lower third of calf
Induration	None	Limited to perimalleolar	Diffuse over lower third of calf	Wider distribution above lower third of calf
Active Ulcer Number	0	1	2	>3
Active Ulcer Duration	N/A	<3 months	>3 months but <1 year	Not healed for >1 year
Active Ulcer Size	N/A	Diameter <2 cm	Diameter 2–6 cm	Diameter >6 cm
Use of Compression Therapy	0; Not used	1; Intermittent use of stockings	2; Wears stockings most days	3; Full compliance of stockings

Table 7.3 Villalta score for post thrombotic syndrome

Symptoms	None	Mild	Moderate	Severe
Pain	0 points	1 point	2 points	3 points
Cramps	0 points	1 point	2 points	3 points
Heaviness	0 points	1 point	2 points	3 points
Paresthesia	0 points	1 point	2 points	3 points
Pruritus	0 points	1 point	2 points	3 points
Clinical Signs	None	Mild	Moderate	Severe
Pretibial edema	0 points	1 point	2 points	3 points
Skin induration	0 points	1 point	2 points	3 points
Hyperpigmentation	0 points	1 point	2 points	3 points
Redness	0 points	1 point	2 points	3 points
Venous ectasia	0 points	1 point	2 points	3 points
Pain on calf compression	0 points	1 point	2 points	3 points
Venous ulcer	Absent			Present

9 clinical characteristics and is useful in monitoring treatment outcomes. Other classification systems include the Villalta score which is widely used for patients with post-thrombotic syndrome (Table 7.3) and the Venous Segmental Disease Score which grades venous segments based on presence of reflux and/or obstruction and relies exclusively on venous imaging [2].

7.2 Superficial Venous Disease

Patrick Lee, Sreekumar Madassery, and Ron Winokur

7.2.1 Introduction

Chronic venous insufficiency (CVI) describes a spectrum of signs and symptoms that occur secondary to venous hypertension usually due to obstruction, or valvular incompetence, in the deep and/or superficial venous system [3]. Incompetent perforator veins (IPV), communications between the deep and superficial veins, and tributary veins are another potential sources of pathology.

- Most commonly, in the superficial venous system, valvular incompetence at the saphenofemoral (SFJ) or saphenopopliteal junction (SPJ) results in retrograde flow of blood (reflux), from the deep veins into the superficial veins, causing elevated venous pressures.
- Early symptoms of CVI include lower extremity pain ("venous claudication"), achiness, heaviness, and edema with varicose veins and skin changes (hyperpigmentation and lipodermatosclerosis) occurring later [3].

The most advanced and debilitating presentation of CVI are venous leg ulcerations (VLU). The incidence of VLU is estimated at approximately 500,000 annually, with higher estimates up to 1% of the population [3, 4]. Unfortunately, poor healing and recurrent ulceration are common with conservative management. The cost of caring for VLU is estimated at $3 billion in the United States alone, making early treatment critical in improving patient outcomes and limiting costs [3].

- Average healing time of VLU with conservative management is reported at 12 weeks [4].
- However, early endovenous interventions can bring this down to 8 weeks while also prolonging time to recurrence [5].
- An understanding of superficial venous disease is especially important as superficial venous reflux is the etiology of VLU in more than half of limbs. Less commonly, disorders of the deep venous system are contributory in VLU [6].

7.2.1.1 Clinical Evaluation

A thorough history and physical examination are necessary to understand the impact of venous hypertension as an underlying etiology of VLU.

- This can occur independent of, or in addition to, peripheral arterial disease.
- Documentation of location, size, characteristics, and evidence of active ulceration and/or bleeding is important for the initial patient assessment.
- Photographs and measurements of the lower extremities should be stored in the electronic medical record. Wounds can be monitored and evaluated at each dressing change or at each follow-up visit.
- Classically, VLU are shallow with an irregular base with the most characteristic locations occurring at the medial malleolus and along the medial ankle (Fig. 7.1). Bleeding from the wound occurs more commonly with VLU than arterial ulcers [7].

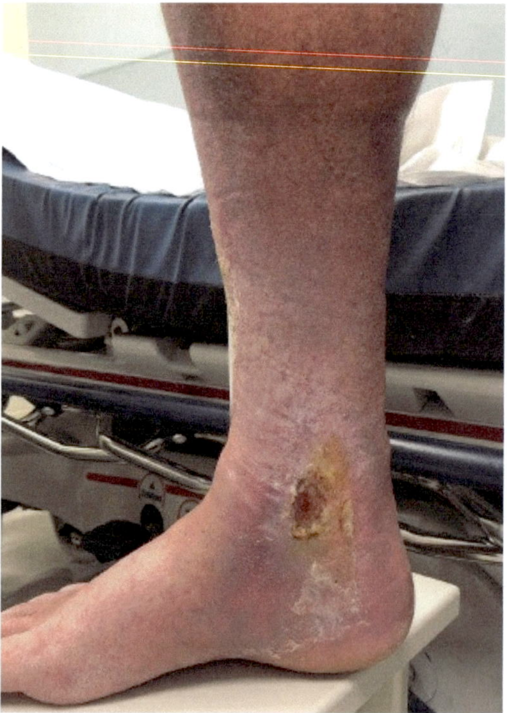

Fig. 7.1 Image demonstrating a typical Venous Leg Ulceration (VLU)

- The aforementioned classification systems exist to standardize clinical evaluations. Using the CEAP classification system, a C6 or C6r describes an active or recurrent VLU.

A thorough ultrasound evaluation of the venous system is important to assess the specific vein(s) underlying the cause of VLU. This should include a complete assessment of the superficial and deep venous anatomy of the lower extremity, which will differentiate superficial venous insufficiency from deep venous obstruction or post-thrombotic change as the underlying etiology of VLU.

- In the case of superficial venous insufficiency, the pathologic veins that are the source of reflux and resultant venous hypertension should be delineated.
- The axial segments of the superficial system such as the great saphenous vein (GSV), anterior accessory great saphenous vein (AA-GSV), and small saphenous vein (SSV) are usually affected.
- IPV or tributary veins adjacent to the VLU should also be noted, as reflux in these veins can contribute to VLU or even be the sole cause [7].

7.2.1.2 Treatment Strategies

Conservative Care.

Conservative management of VLU consists of local wound care and compression therapy. Local wound care was previously discussed. Compression therapy is inexpensive and has been shown to increase healing rates of VLU [8].

- Multicomponent systems with an elastic bandage have favorable results compared to single-component systems [8].
- Two-layer compression bandages can be applied in the office with frequent dressing changes every 7 days or as specified by each brand. However, some authors argue that inelastic bandages are more effective in reducing venous hypertension due to exertion of higher pressures [9].

– For example, the Unna boot (Coban, 3M, St. Paul, MN) is an inelastic low-cost compression system that is proven to increase rates of VLU healing [10].
– Several other multilayer options exist which have variations in compression degree and can be utilized in a step-wise approach based on response and comfort.

- It is important to ensure that patients do not have concomitant PAD with inadequate arterial perfusion through history/exam and non-invasive arterial evaluation (i.e., ensure ABI > 0.5 or ankle pressure 50 mmHg). These patients can have significant complications if aggressive compression therapy is undertaken if PAD is undiagnosed or not addressed first.

Endovascular Intervention

Early endovenous intervention is associated with faster wound healing and prolonged time to recurrent ulceration [5]. The main objective in treating superficial venous insufficiency is causing irreversible occlusion of the incompetent vein. This most commonly involves the axial venous segments, which can be detected in the clinical work-up, using duplex ultrasound as described previously.

- Reflux is assessed in the standing position, following augmentation with greater than 0.5 s of retrograde flow in one of the superficial axial veins being diagnostic.
- Perforator and tributary vein incompetence is also important to assess in VLU patients as localized incompetent perforators may be the source of VLU despite normal axial vein segments.
- Reflux greater than 0.5 s in a tributary or perforator vein is considered significant [11].

Figure 7.2 summarizes a typical approach to treating superficial venous disease with VLU [7]. If there is concurrent obstruction of the deep venous system, this will need to be addressed separately. Patients with a combination of superficial and deep reflux are generally not good candidates for ablation as there is a high recurrence rate of varicose veins, typically due to coexisting conditions and generalized venous hypertension. The priority of treating iliac vein obstruction before or after superficial venous insufficiency has not been clearly delineated, although anecdotally, operators do prefer to address the deep system prior to the superficial system.

Numerous commercially available systems exist to treat pathologic reflux of axial vein segments. Endovenous valvular closure consists of the insertion of a catheter from the most peripheral site of incompetence with advancement to the SFJ or SPJ. Table 7.1 summarizes the major differences among the most used systems. Broadly, these are divided into thermal and non-thermal techniques.

- Ablation works by promoting thrombus formation via endothelial and vein wall damage, leading to the closure of that vein, and thus reducing or eliminating reflux.
- Thermal ablation is the oldest and most frequently used approach including endovenous laser therapy (EVLT) and radiofrequency ablation (RFA). This intervention requires the addition of tumescent anesthetic to prevent heat-related injury to adjacent structures as demonstrated in Fig. 7.3.
- Non-thermal ablation allows for vein closure utilizing cyanoacrylate glue or sclerosant-mediated closure using either Venaseal, Clarivein, or Varithena.

The diameter, depth, tortuosity, length, location, and presence of deep vein communication must always be considered when deciding on which of the above methods is most suitable.

For diseases involving smaller veins, endovenous sclerotherapy may be considered as an alternative to RFA/EVLA. Sclerotherapy is similar to the former treatment modalities, however, uses a chemical sclerosing agent. According to the ACR Appropriateness Criteria, sclerotherapy is primarily used to treat telangiectasias, in addition to small veins [12]. Additionally, ultrasound-guided foam sclerotherapy (UGFS) is a lower-cost alternative for sclerosis of axial venous segments.

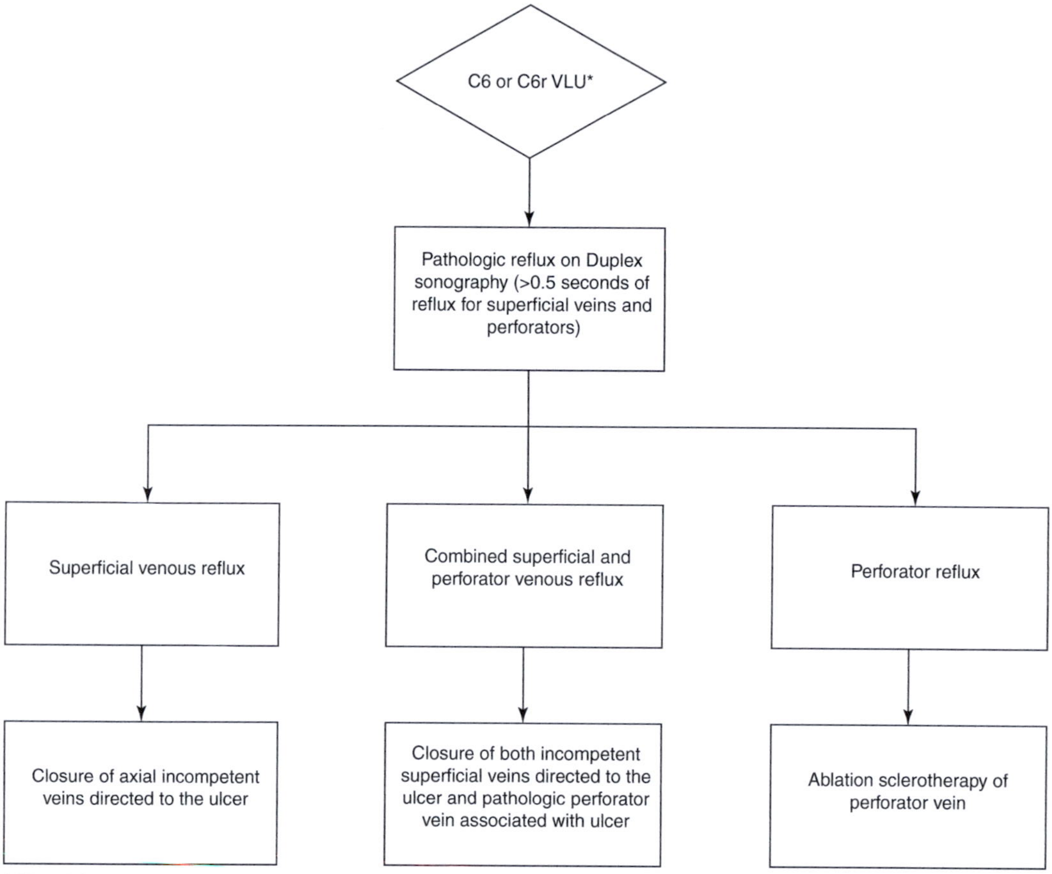

C6 or C6r VLU*

Pathologic reflux on Duplex sonography (>0.5 seconds of reflux for superficial veins and perforators)

Superficial venous reflux

Combined superficial and perforator venous reflux

Perforator reflux

Closure of axial incompetent veins directed to the ulcer

Closure of both incompetent superficial veins directed to the ulcer and pathologic perforator vein associated with ulcer

Ablation sclerotherapy of perforator vein

*C6 and C6r = active and recurrent venous leg ulceration in the CAP classification system respectively

Fig. 7.2 Flowchart summarizing a typical approach in treating superficial venous disease in the setting of VLU

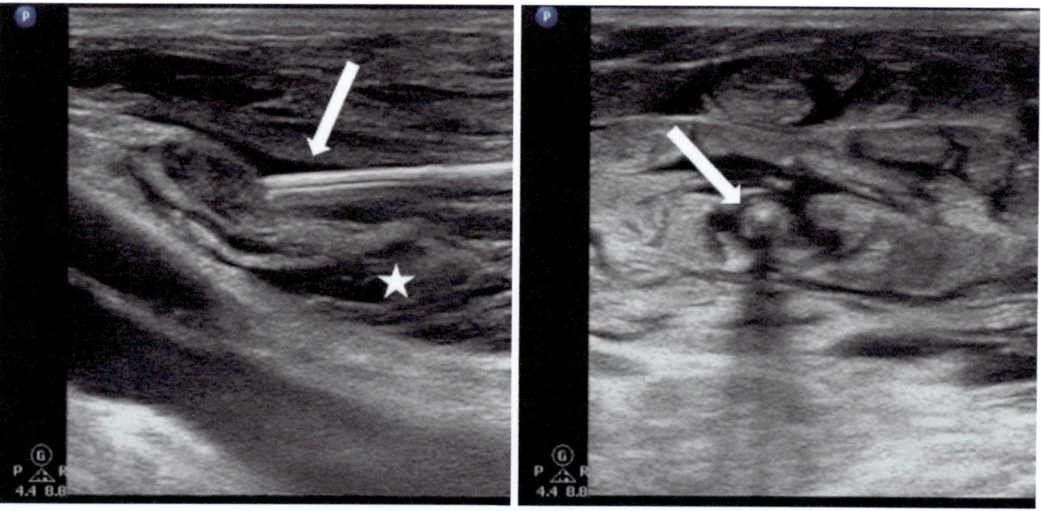

Fig. 7.3 Ultrasound images of the great saphenous vein during endovenous laser therapy show the tip of the device in the central GSV (Arrow) and tumescent anesthetic in the perivascular space (Star)

- UGFS is performed by obtaining access to the target vein with a 21–25 gauge needle. Sclerosant is then injected under ultrasound guidance to ensure sclerosant does not enter the deep system.
- Central compression with the ultrasound probe to prevent reflux into the deep system and dorsiflexion of the foot can occlude the calf perforator veins in some instances.
- Foam is relatively easy to create by mixing sclerosant with room air. Ratios can vary, but the Tessari method using 1:4 liquid to room air via a 3-way stopcock is popular [13]. Currently, the FDA has approved sodium tetradecyl sulfate (STS) and polidocanol (POL) for sclerosis of lower extremity veins. A rule of thumb is that the lowest concentration of sclerosant should be used that will achieve endoluminal fibrosis to minimize potential complications.
- Alternatively, Varithena is a relatively new system that contains a preloaded dose of POL ensuring a consistent delivery (Table 7.4).

Foam sclerotherapy has been shown to be more efficacious than liquid sclerosants in the ablation of lower extremity vein [14].

If IPV or tributary veins are identified in conjunction with reflux in the axial veins, follow-up ablation or sclerosis of these segments can be performed on the same day or in subsequent sessions using the same techniques as previously described. Isolated perforator incompetence can be treated alone if it is underlying the site of VLU or leading to superficial tributaries and the VLU. Figure 7.4 demonstrates ultrasound images of an IPV. The standard treatment for pathologic venous tributaries and perforators is sclerosis, but endovenous ablation has become another option.

- Studies have shown higher rates of perforator closure and ulcer healing with ablation compared to UGFS [11, 15].

Outcomes

The Early Venous Reflux Ablation (EVRA) trial compared early endovenous intervention with deferred intervention as an adjunct to compression therapy for superficial venous reflux in the setting of VLU.

- The trial demonstrated the benefits of intervention with significantly shorter ulcer healing time (median 56 days versus 82 days) and prolonged recurrent ulceration (306 days versus 278 days) for early intervention versus deferred intervention, respectively.
- The authors highlight that an even stronger effect is likely in clinical practice given the strict adherence to compression therapy that is unlikely to be replicated in the real world during the trial [5].

EVRA was the first large randomized-controlled trial to show the benefits of endovenous ablation in VLU healing but did not clarify the optimal treatment method. Interventions were left to the discretion of the treating physician and outcomes were analyzed as a composite. Interventions included UGFS (most common), endovenous laser or radiofrequency ablation, non-thermal (cyanoacrylate glue or mechanochemical ablation), or a combination.

- Notably, on sub-group analysis, EVLT did show healing advantage compared to other modalities, but this was not statistically significant [5]. While prior studies have shown lower occlusion rates using UGFS compared to other ablation methods, it is unclear if this impacts ulcer healing. Future studies investigating the optimal ablative method for treating VLU are warranted.

Complications

Most complications following endovenous interventions are minor, self-limited, and managed conservatively (Table 7.4).

- Thermal injury is specific to thermal ablative methods but occurs in less than 1% of patients [16]. Symptoms include dysesthesias and skin burns.
- Deep vein thrombosis (DVT) has been reported with thermal ablation and Varithena [17]. Skin changes can occur following

Table 7.4 Comparison of thermal axial ablation therapy, non-thermal axial ablation therapy, and ultrasound-guided foam sclerotherapy in treatment of the GSV

Technique	Cost [25, 26]	Mechanism	Technique (for GSV) [27]	Advantages	Complications [20, 22–24]	Occlusion rate at 1-year (or greater)
Thermal						
Laser	$$	Heat transfer	• Position catheter tip 2 cm from the SFJ beyond the superficial epigastric vein • Pull back at a rate for a goal of 80–100 J/cm of energy deposition • Thigh-high compression stockings (30–40 mmHg) are typically used	• Robust long-term data	• Cutaneous (soreness, bruising, tenderness, and induration) • Superficial phlebitis • Thermal: nerve injury and skin burns (rare) • DVT (rare)	93–97% [28, 29]
Radiofrequency (ClosureFAST)	$$	Heat-induced thrombosis	• Position catheter tip 2 cm from the SFJ • Pullback 7 cm for the first cycle • Advance catheter and repeat 7 cm pullback for a "double cycle" • Pullback 6.5 cm/cycle for the remainder of the vein • Thigh-high compression stockings (30–40 mmHg) are typically used	• Robust long-term data	• Cutaneous (soreness, bruising, tenderness, and induration) • Superficial phlebitis • Thermal: nerve injury and skin burns (rare) • DVT (rare)	94% [30]

	Cost	Mechanism	Technique	Advantages	Complications	Occlusion rate
Non-thermal						
Cyanoacrylate glue (VenaSeal)	$$$	Polymerization with blood	• Position catheter tip 5 cm peripheral from the SFJ • Manually compress centrally with US probe • Push trigger for 3 s to deliver first dose • Pull back 1 cm and apply a second dose • Compress treated vein for 3 min after first dose • Subsequently pull back every 3 cm/dose and compress for 30 s	• Post-procedure compression not required • No tumescent anesthesia	• Cutaneous (pain and ecchymosis) • Superficial phlebitis • Allergic reaction	97% [31]
Mechanochemical (ClariVein)	$$$	Mechanical rotating wire and chemical detergent	• Position catheter tip 1 cm peripheral to the SFJ • Activate wire rotation at ~3500 rpm for 2–10 s to induce venospasm • Engage motor trigger while simultaneously injecting sclerosant and pulling back at a rate of 1.5 mm/s every 3 s • Thigh-high compression stockings for 2 weeks	• No tumescent anesthesia • Dual modality	• Cutaneous (induration and ecchymosis) • Superficial phlebitis	94% [32]
Polidocanol (Varithena)	$$$	Detergent	• Attach canisters to generate foam • Detach canisters and attach syringe to transfer unit at the top of the polidocanol canister and waste 3 mL • Elevate leg 45° • Inject in aliquots of 5 mL for maximum of 15 mL • Apply pressure at GSV once microfoam reaches SFJ • Thigh-high compression stockings for 2 weeks	• No tumescent anesthesia • Fixed pre-determined concentration • Fills incompetent perforators	• Pain • Superficial phlebitis • DVT	73% [33]
Ultrasound-guided foam sclerotherapy	$	Detergent	• Mix 1–1.5% STS or 2–3% POL with room air or CO_2 in a preferred ratio dependent on vessel size • Inject in aliquots of 3–5 mL limiting to under 10 mL per session	• No tumescent anesthesia • Inexpensive	• Hyperpigmentation • Ulceration • Matting	72% [34]

Cost: $ = <$500, $$ = 500–1000, $$$ > 1000 in U.S. dollars.

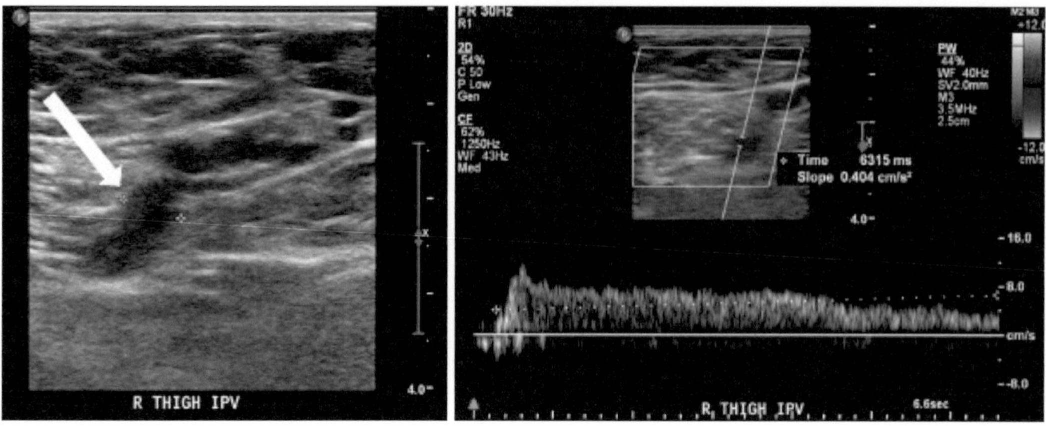

Fig. 7.4 Ultrasound images demonstrate a dilated perforator vein in the thigh (Arrow) and reflux for greater than 0.5 s

UGFS. It is important that patients be aware prior to treatment.

- Extravasation of sclerosant is the most feared complication of UGFS and can result in ulceration secondary to tissue necrosis. Treatment consists of local wound care.

Peri-Ulcer Varices Management

It is not uncommon to find that there are patients with VLU and venous insufficiency by examination, however, noninvasive studies are inconclusive or disgruent. In these patients, it is prudent to perform a more detailed direct ultrasound evaluation of the wound area, which may demonstrate varices around and coursing from the ulcer. In these situations, percutaneous foam sclerotherapy of these varices under ultrasound (can be combined with fluoroscopy to ensure no deep vein reflux) guidance. In doing this, it is possible to accelerate VLU healing.

Case Example

Courtesy of Sreekumar Madassery, MD

A 72-year-old female with long-term wound care management of bilateral painful VLUs, despite compressive therapy, arterial evaluation, wound care including skin substitutes and other conservative approaches. After percutaneous sclerotherapy of peri-ulcer varices, there was rapid VLU healing with eventual wound closure (Fig. 7.5).

Conclusion

A thorough understanding of the pathophysiology of superficial venous disease that results in venous hypertension and VLU is essential. Prompt evaluation, diagnosis, and endovenous intervention can improve the time to ulcer healing and prevent significant morbidity. The optimal treatment should be directed at the intended source of venous hypertension, which can be mixed between superficial venous reflux and deep vein obstruction. While early endovenous intervention is beneficial in shortening healing time, it is important to remember that recurrent ulceration is common and continued follow-up of patients with prior VLU is important.

Finally, it should be noted that superficial venous closure has grown in abundance over the years, often for cosmetic reasons, as well as for symptomatic grounds. This is a vital conduit for other vascular beds in patients such as those with CAD and PAD, thus it should be considered with some caution in all comers. For patients with VLU, many operators will choose to intervene on patients that have significant varicosities in the venous distribution of the wound and those that demonstrate peri-wound varices, as these anecdotally can have a greater healing result, compared to patients with less obvious reflux-related sequelae.

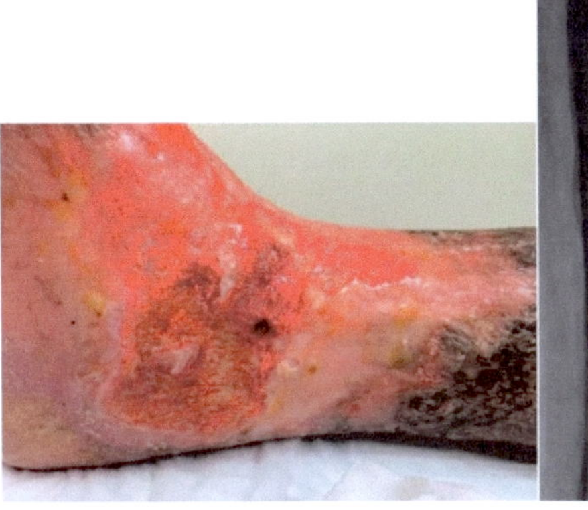
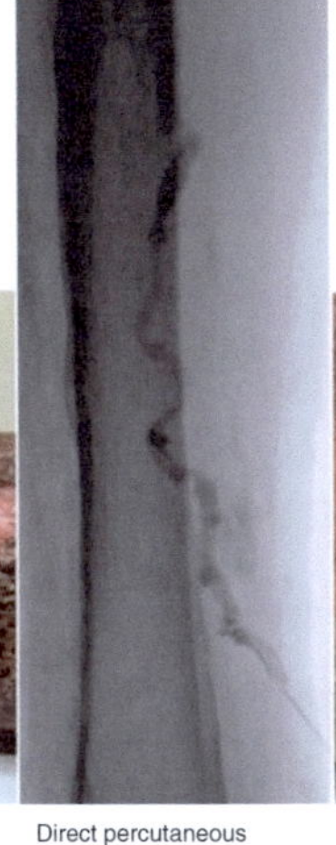
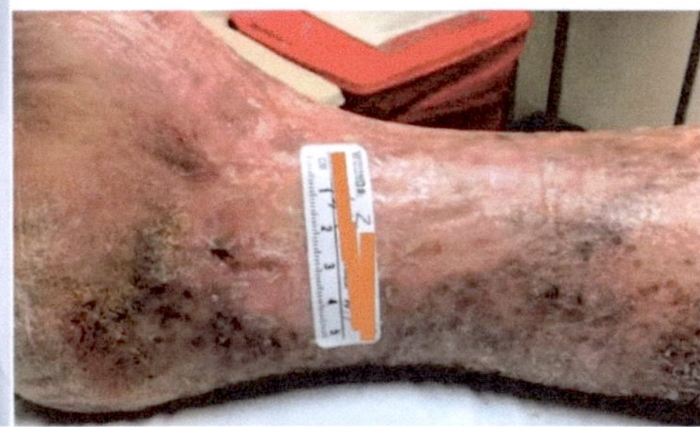

Long standing (>1 year) LLE distal leg and ankle venous non healing ulcers despite wound care, compression therapy, skin substitutes, and attempts at increased ambulation. Noninvasive venous studies showed relatively small caliber and insignificant areas of GSV and SSV reflux.

Direct percutaneous sclerotherapy of abnormal peri-ulcer varices, with tourniquet applied just below the knee.

2 months after embolization and continued wound care, rapid VLU healing was noted, with eventual wound closure as well as pain relief.

Fig. 7.5 Case example of nonhealing VLU that improved after endovenous intervention

7.3 Deep Venous Disease

Brian P. Holly and Mark Lessne

7.3.1 Introduction

Deep venous disease can be categorized as acute, subacute, or chronic with symptoms resulting from deep venous reflux or obstruction. The exact categorization of the chronicity may be difficult, however, many consider >4 weeks into the chronic phase. Acute venous disease rarely leads to limb loss outside of phlegmasia cerulea dolens, which is an extensive, occlusive venous thrombosis leading to venous gangrene in 40–60% of patients [18, 19]. Even chronic deep venous disease resulting from venous stenosis/ occlusion or from compression syndromes rarely results in limb loss. Causes of obstruction or compression may include occlusion from thrombosis, compression from a mass, post-thrombotic syndrome, or non-thrombotic causes. However, venous leg ulcers account for 70% of all chronic leg ulcers and are associated with high recurrence rates. As discussed in previous sections, it is estimated that billions of dollars are spent each year on venous leg ulcers worldwide with direct medical costs per patient averaging over $5000 (USD) per year [20]. Therefore, preventing ulcer formation is the main goal of treatment. This section will review indications for deep venous disease treatment, including stent placement and techniques to maximize patient safety and efficacy.

7.3.1.1 When to Treat Deep Veins

The presence of deep venous disease is not, by itself, an indication for treatment as many patients with deep venous reflux, venous stenosis, or compression may be entirely asymptomatic depending on the anatomic distribution, compensatory collateralization, and patient condition. For example, seemingly significant (>50%) left common iliac vein compression can be found not uncommonly in healthy subjects or those without lower extremity symptoms [21–23]. Therefore, confirmation of clinically significant and correlative signs and symptoms of deep venous disease is mandatory prior to intervention. The previously mentioned classification systems are available to assist with this assessment.

In patients with deep vein obstruction, post-thrombotic syndrome (PTS) develops in 20–50% of patients and presents as lower extremity swelling, abdominal fullness or bloating (in the setting of IVC occlusion), lower extremity heaviness, fatigue, and/or paresthesias.

- Venous stasis changes are also seen including lipodermatosclerosis, skin bronzing, dilated varicose, spider, or reticular veins, and in severe cases, ulcerations [24].

Many signs and symptoms of superficial venous disease may overlap with those of deep venous disease. It is an important principle that when patients' symptoms can be ameliorated by treating the superficial venous reflux alone, this should be pursued first and exclusively.

- Treatment of deep venous disease, almost always requires implantation of a permanent stent in the iliac veins and should be reserved for those patients in whom symptoms are predominately related to deep venous obstruction.
- Additionally, while conservative management is often the first-line therapy for mild venous disease—including weight loss, exercise, lower extremity compression, and leg elevation—for patients with venous ulcers related to deep vein disease, a trial of conservative management is not always required and more aggressive interventional therapies early on may be warranted.
- Early endovenous treatment has been shown beneficial for superficial venous disease and likely holds true for symptomatic deep venous disease in the setting of severe symptoms, as well [5]. Medical management can and should, however, still be offered concurrently with intervention for venous stasis ulcers: aside from wound care and compression, pentoxifylline has been found to be a more effective therapy for venous wounds than compression alone [25].
- Primary patency for iliac vein stenting in non-thrombotic disease is reported to be 90%—100% and 74%–89% in post-thrombotic disease [26].

- Additional indications for recanalization or reconstruction include deep vein occlusion secondary to recurrent DVT, post-thrombotic syndrome, and thrombosis of the IVC, all leading to lifestyle limitations.
- Surgical treatments are rarely utilized and reserved for cases refractory to stenting.

7.3.1.2 Work-Up

A thorough history and physical are essential to the diagnosis, and should evaluate for:

- Signs and Symptoms of venous obstruction.
- Prior vascular interventions (including venous catheterizations as a neonate and child), history of surgery, infections, and/or radiotherapy that may have compromised the deep venous system.
- Personal and family history of VTE and relevant details (anatomic location, recurrence, provoking factors, genetic disorders).

Typically, some imaging is performed for patients with clinical suspicion of deep venous disease.

- Duplex ultrasound to evaluate the superficial and deep venous system is almost always the first imaging test.
- Depending on the patient's body habitus and skill set of the sonographer, ultrasound can be very useful to depict iliac vein compressions and even IVC patency.
  - Even when the pelvic veins cannot be imaged, deep venous reflux or loss of phasicity and augmentation in the common femoral vein may be indirect signs of iliac vein or caval obstruction and may warrant cross-sectional or catheter-based venography and intravascular ultrasound for further evaluation.
- Lab work for systemic causes of lower extremity swelling should also be considered in the appropriate clinical context.
- Etiologies with the suspicion of inferior vena cava or iliac vein involvement are typically diagnosed via CT or MRI.

Iliac Vein Compression

Acute or chronic deep vein thrombosis (DVT) of the inferior vena cava (IVC) and iliac veins, otherwise known as iliocaval thrombosis, can lead to lower extremity edema, pain, and other limb-threatening occlusive symptoms. Iliocaval thrombectomy, recanalization, and/or reconstruction (i.e., angioplasty/stenting) are accepted treatment options in management of this disease.

Non-thrombotic iliac vein lesions (NIVL) may lead to May-Thürner disease commonly caused by an obstructive anatomical variant that can lead to occlusion of the left iliac vein due to compression from the right iliac artery as it crosses over the vein. Some other causes include compression by a pelvic mass (tumor, fibroids, etc.), pregnancy, or retroperitoneal fibrosis. Initial diagnosis requires evaluation for DVT. Once DVT has been ruled out, then further work-up for May-Thurner syndrome (MTS) includes imaging evidence to suggest compression.

Imaging Findings Suggestive of Iliac Vein Compression

- Duplex ultrasound—sluggish venous outflow, venous reflux, poor
- augmentation.
- CT/MR Venography—Generally very sensitive and specific (>95%) for diagnosing iliac vein compression [27].
- Catheter venography—Filling defects, compression was seen in multiple projections, transvenous (hemodynamic) pressure measurements.
- Intravascular Ultrasound (IVUS)—Now considered by many to be the gold standard to diagnose iliac vein compression with improved sensitivity and specificity relative to catheter venography alone [28]. IVUS can accurately measure normal vessel diameter, percent stenosis, identify exact location of stenosis, and aid in planning stent placement.

Treatment (When to Stent)

- Stent placement is an established treatment for symptomatic NIVL with excellent long-term patency. Stent placement should be considered for symptomatic patients with venographic and IVUS findings demonstrating a significant flow-limiting stenosis.
- Thrombolysis can be used if necessary.
- Stent diameter should be sized according to the diameter of the normal vessel adjacent to the stenotic segment. The stent must cover the stenosis entirely.

Figure 7.6 demonstrates left common iliac vein compression by the overlying right common iliac artery, findings are consistent with non-thrombotic MTS. Figure 7.7 demonstrates restored flow of the left common iliac vein via stent placement.

Case courtesy of Osman Ahmed, MD

Iliac Vein Occlusion

Iliac vein occlusion (ILVO) most often is the result of an iliac vein thrombus that failed to adequately recanalize. Patients presenting with ILVO often have similar symptoms to those with iliac vein compression, however, symptoms are often worse. Post-thrombotic syndrome (PTS) in these patients can be severe and debilitating.

Treatment (When to Stent)

- Any patient with an ILVO, in whom the occlusion can be crossed with a wire, will require stent placement.
- Stent should be sized according to the closest segment of patent/healthy vein. The stent must have good venous inflow and extend into an open outflow vein.

Stent Placement Below the Inguinal Ligament

In the case of ILVO, often the diseased segment of vein extends below the inguinal ligament.

- It is mandatory to stent from healthy vein to healthy vein, as this gives the stented portion of the vein the best chance of maintaining long-term patency, by creating good inflow and outflow. This may also require extending the stent below the inguinal ligament into the femoral vein.
    - Stenting below the inguinal ligament has been considered controversial as some

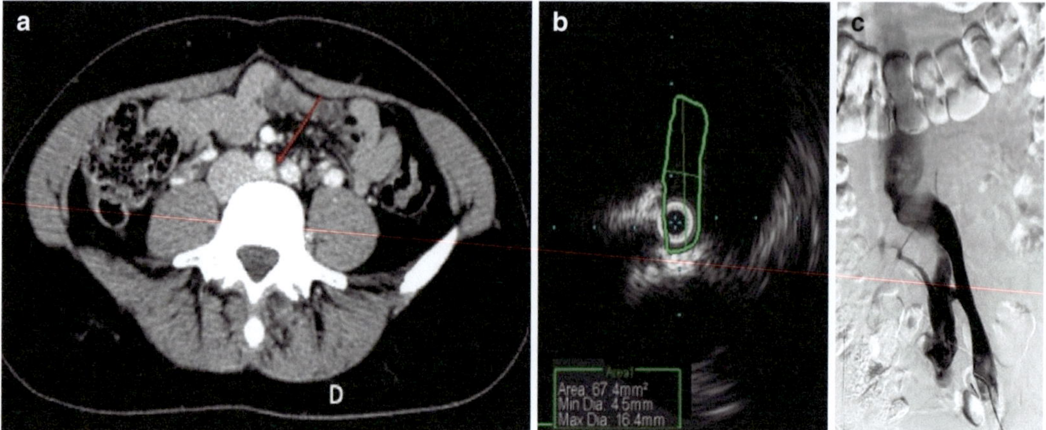

Fig. 7.6 Pre-intervention contrast CT pelvis (**a**), intravascular ultrasound (**b**), and venogram (**c**), all demonstrate compression of the iliac vein by the overlying right common iliac artery. These findings are compatible with non-thrombotic May-Thurner syndrome

Fig. 7.7 Post-stent placement intravascular ultrasound (**a**) and fluoroscopy X-ray (**b**) demonstrate restored flow of the left common iliac vein. Coils can also be noted in Fig. 7.2b as gonadal vein embolization was concurrently for pelvic congestion

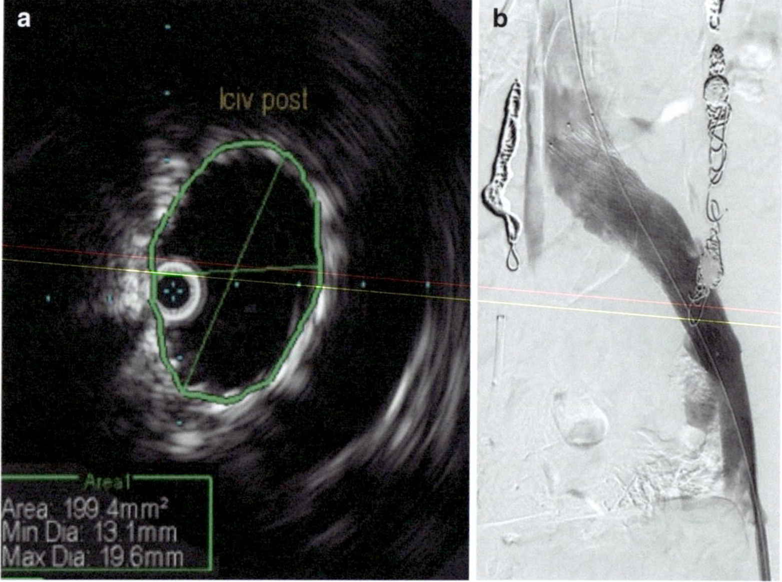

report decreased patency rates when extending the stent below the inguinal ligament. However, more recent reports demonstrate similar patency rates and rates of clinical improvement when extending the stent below the inguinal ligament if required to cover all diseased segments [29].

Tips and Tricks

Note: It is expected that the interventionalist caring for the patient with deep vein disease possesses basic and fundamental skills in endovascular techniques including catheter and wire crossing, stent deployment, radiation safety, as well as mitigation of and therapy for complications. A list of "tips and tricks" cannot replace formal and proper training through an accredited interventional/endovascular program.

IVC and Iliofemoral Occlusions

Since all deep venous disease must start and end with a healthy vessel to establish normal inflow and normal outflow, the segments of diseased veins must be carefully delineated prior to intervention in order to guide appropriate access.

- Avoid accessing a vein that will limit the ability to treat the entire segment of diseased vein. Common femoral vein access may be appropriate for isolated iliac vein or IVC obstruction but may hinder treatment of disease extending to distal external iliac and common femoral vein.
  - In this case, a mid-femoral vein, popliteal vein, or greater saphenous vein access may be preferred.
- As discussed above, it is mandatory for stents to bridge from normal vessel to normal vessel. Iliofemoral stents may be placed down to but ideally never beyond the lesser trochanter.
  - It is critical to maximize inflow into the stent by ensuring adequate flow is present from the deep femoral and/or femoral veins.

Equipment

- Micropuncture or single wall needle for access.
- Guidewires:
  - Crossing Wires: 0.035 and 0.018 stiff hydrophilic wires and weighted wires (30 g tip load).
  - Working wires: Super stiff Amplatz wire.
- Sheath: ≥8 or 9 Fr sheath (to allow for IVUS catheter and venous stents, respectively), 7 Fr MPA guide catheter for extra support; Alternatively, prefabricated support systems such as Triforce (Cook, Bloomington IN).
- Catheters: Angled diagnostic or support catheters.
- Balloons: Noncompliant, high-pressure balloons.

- Stents: Dedicated venous stents; Wallstents or Z-stents (less commonly); covered stents available for bailout in case of complications.
- Intravascular Ultrasound: 0.035 compatible IVUS catheters.
- Niche devices: Trans-septal needle, Chiba needle, RF Power Wire, snares.

Venous Recanalization Procedure Steps

1. Access site selection: Internal/external jugular, brachial/basilic, common femoral, femoral, popliteal, and posterior tibial veins are all viable access options.
2. Robust support, such as triaxial system with sheath, guide catheter, and crossing catheter is mandatory. The system should be placed close to the occlusion ("take the fight to the sight"). Attempt crossing using glidewire and support catheter. Rotate the wire while applying minimal forward pressure in an Archimedes screw type fashion clockwise and then counterclockwise—do not let wire prolapse into a J shape.

   Tip: For chronic total occlusions, keep catheter closely behind tip of wire and cross incrementally, advancing catheter to wire tip, millimeter by millimeter if necessary.
3. Once successfully crossed, repeat venogram to confirm expected, intraluminal position.

   Tip: Can further confirm with lateral view and cone beam CT (ideal), as there can be inadvertent spinal canal crossing if not cautious.
4. Place stiff working wire, such as Amplatz wire.
5. Intravascular ultrasound (IVUS) has been shown to be more sensitive in detecting stenotic lesions compared to venography and is critical to aid with proper vessel sizing, confirmation of stent expansion, and evaluation of residual disease.
   (a) IVUS is used complimentary with venography, which demonstrates hemodynamic obstruction, such as filling of venous collaterals or poor contrast washout.

Tip: With IVUS in a suspected compressive lesion, leave the IVUS catheter at the site over multiple respiratory cycles to confirm the lesion is fixed and not a "pseudo stenosis," that should not be treated (Fig. 7.8). Patient leg positioning can also fix pseudo stenotic lesions.

6. Angioplasty and/or stent according to clinical scenario (see tips above).

Tip: While IVUS and venography are essential tools for optimal stent positioning, bony landmarks can also be used, including the right vertebral pedicle and spinous process for left iliac vein stent placement [30].

Stenting the ILIAC Venous Confluence

There are four main techniques employed when stent reconstruction of the bilateral iliac veins and iliac venous confluence is required (Fig. 7.9):

1. Double barrel: Self-expanding stents are placed extending from the IVC into the iliac veins in parallel fashion.
2. Fenestrated Inverted Y: A single stent is placed extending from the IVC to one of the iliac veins, jailing the contralateral iliac vein. The interstices of that stent are then crossed from the contralateral side and dilated, allowing for placement of another stent through the dilated interstice and into the contralateral iliac vein.
3. T-stent: A single stent is placed extending from the IVC to one of the iliac veins, jailing the contralateral iliac vein. A second stent is placed in the contralateral iliac vein up to and abutting the first stent, but not crossing into it.
4. Coaxial IVC-double barrel: A single, large stent is placed in the IVC, followed by parallel stents placed into the IVC stent and extending into the iliac veins.

In general, fenestrated inverted Y and T-stent techniques are strongly discouraged and there is data to support that these techniques lead to worse patency [31]. The fenestrated inverted Y technique, however, is the only option when presented with a patient who requires iliac vein stent placement on a side jailed by a previously placed iliocaval venous stent (Fig. 7.10).

Complications

1. Failure: The most common "complication" of recanalization procedures is the inability to cross the lesion. If this occurs, consider alternative access, obliquities, techniques, or imaging to delineate the geometry of the

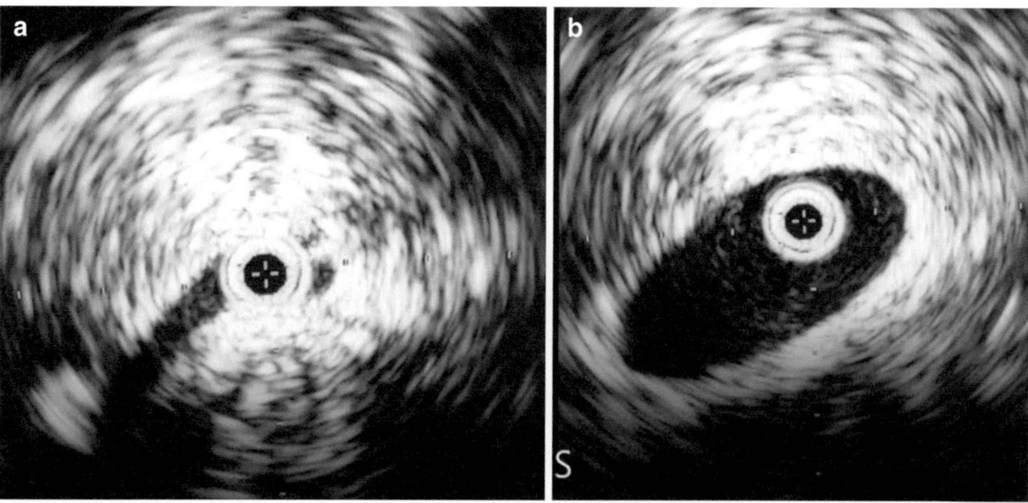

Fig. 7.8 (a) Initial IVUS image demonstrates venous stenosis. (b) Later in the respiratory cycle the stenosis is shown to be a normal, well-expanded vein, not a fixed lesion ("pseudo stenosis")

Fig. 7.9 Techniques of Iliac Confluence Stent Placement: (**a**) Double Barrel—two stents have been placed parallel from the iliac veins to the IVC (**b**) T stent- Right iliac vein stent abuts a left iliocaval venous stent (this is strongly discouraged) (**c**) Coaxial—a large IVC stent is placed, and (**d**) two double barrel stents have been placed coaxial from the iliac veins into the IVC stent

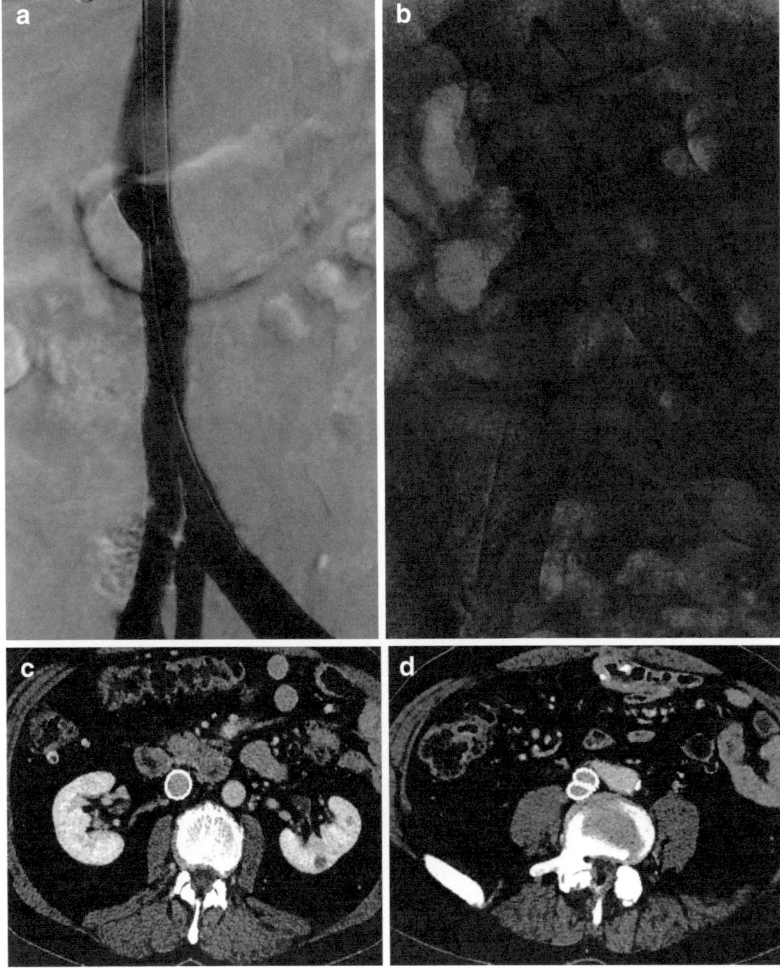

occlusion better. Alternatively, consider referral to a center with more expertise and experience.

2. Vessel perforation: Contrast extravasation outside the vein wall is usually asymptomatic if resulting from a wire perforation. It is the failure to recognize an extraluminal wire and subsequent balloon dilation that can have catastrophic consequences. Always confirm the wire position before proceeding with intervention. If extravasation persists, balloon tamponade, and reversal of anticoagulation usually seal the leak; however, covered stents should be readily available during all vascular procedures.

   Tip: Bleeds from the IVC are usually well-tamponaded in the retroperitoneum. Extra care and caution should be taken in patients who have had prior surgical violation of their retroperitoneum in whom this protective effect may be lost. Likewise, patients with a history of radiation to the abdomen or pelvis may be at higher risk for vessel perforation or rupture.

3. Intraprocedural thrombosis: Adequate inflow and outflow across a vein is essential to maintain patency. Intraprocedural thrombosis may be a result of poor inflow, outflow, or inadequate anticoagulation. This can initially be treated with additional anticoagulation and pharmacomechanical thrombectomy. However, an exhaustive search for the etiology of the thrombosis is warranted with venography and IVUS.

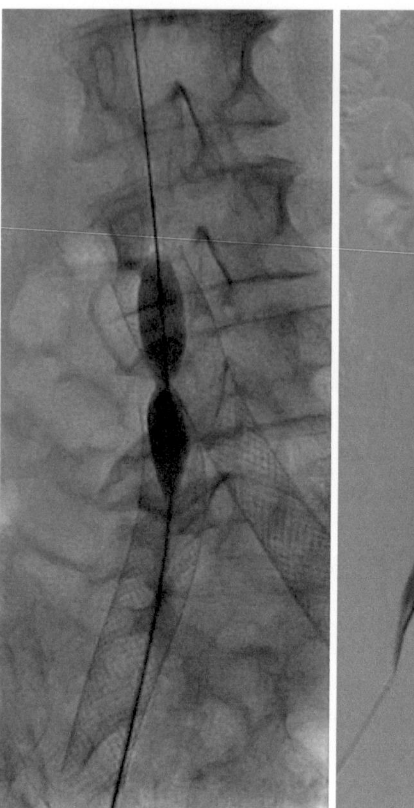
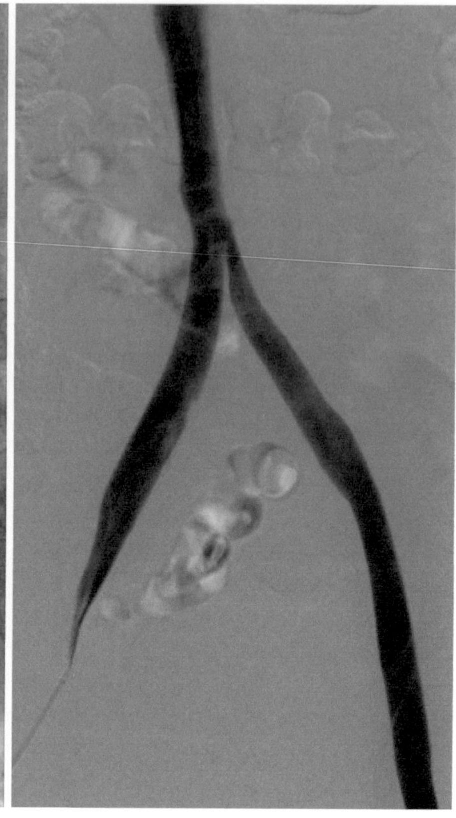

Fig. 7.10 Salvage of a T-stent configuration: The interstices of the previously placed iliocaval stent have been crossed and dilated, allowing for extension of the contralateral stent, forming the fenestrated, inverted Y configuration

4. Access site hematoma: This risk is mitigated with ultrasound-guided access. Consider purse string suture for venous access >16 Fr.

7.4 Reconstruction of Chronic Iliocaval Occlusion

Shin Mei Chan and Kush Desai

7.4.1 Introduction

Deep venous obstruction is split into non-thrombotic, acute thrombotic, or post-thrombotic etiologies; patients with the greatest disease burden have involvement of the inferior vena cava (IVC) and/or the iliac veins. In patients with severe chronic venous insufficiency presenting with healed or active venous ulcers, more than one-third have iliocaval obstructions of at least 50%, with about one-quarter having iliocaval obstructions of greater than 80% [32]. In this section, we will describe the clinical characteristics of iliocaval obstructive disease, followed by endovascular management.

7.4.2 Etiologies

There are a broad range of etiologies contributing to iliocaval obstruction. Malignant caval obstructions are uncommon and occur secondary to masses that compress or rarely invade the IVC or iliac veins (Fig. 7.11). Various cancers can result in retroperitoneal nodal or direct tumoral involvement that can cause caval obstruction; metastases from distant sites have been described as well [33].

- Patients may present with symptoms of lower extremity pain, swelling, skin changes, or lymphorrhea.
- Endovascular stent placement of unresectable malignancies often provides immediate relief;

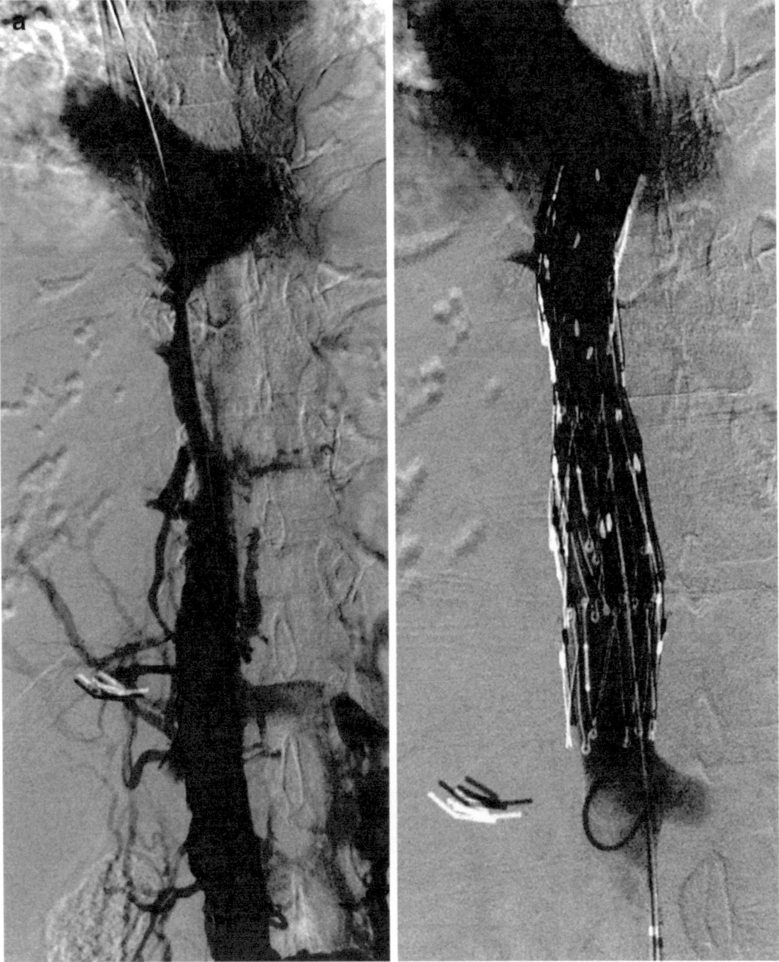

Fig. 7.11 Malignant obstruction of the IVC due to cholangiocarcinoma (Panel **a**). Panel (**b**) Patency restoration following deployment of stents

however, recurrence in symptoms due to stent occlusion or stenosis occurs in more than one-third of patients; thus, intervention should be considered as largely palliative [33].

- Similarly, retroperitoneal fibrosis due to therapeutic radiation or inflammatory processes can cause iliocaval obstruction.

Thrombotic causes of iliocaval obstruction are often a result of deep vein thrombosis (DVT) and subsequent post-thrombotic syndrome (PTS). PTS results from chronic venous reflux and obstruction, combining to result in ambulatory venous hypertension, a potentially debilitating condition characterized by edema refractory to compression, severe pain with extended standing or walking, permanent skin damage, and stasis ulceration [34].

- Some degree of PTS develops in up to 50% of DVT patients [35]; severe PTS, resulting in ulceration, may occur in up to 10% [36].

Perhaps the most common cause of chronic iliocaval obstruction, at least in the United States, is thrombosis secondary to an in situ IVC filter (Fig. 7.12). While there has been increased awareness surrounding long-term complications of IVC filters, retrieval rates remain low [37].

- The prospective, randomized Prevention du Risque d'Embolie Pulmonaire par Interruption Cave (PREPIC) trial demonstrated that patients who received permanent IVC filters had a cumulative incidence of recurrent DVT

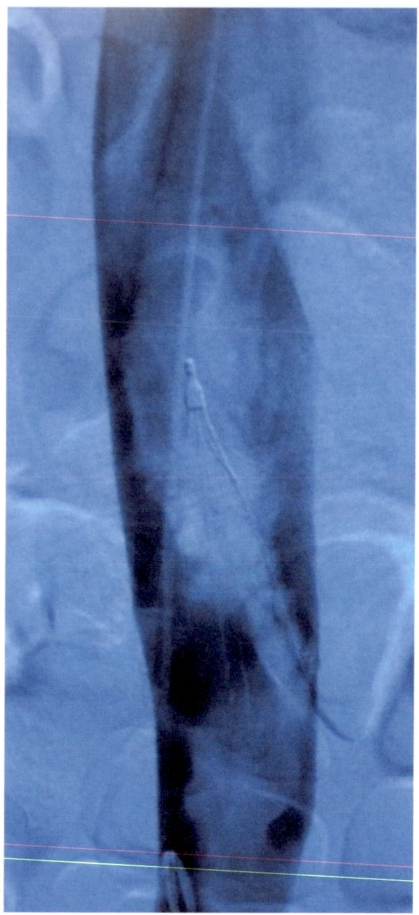

Fig. 7.12 Thrombosis secondary to an in situ filter

7.4.3 Clinical Presentation of Iliocaval Disease

Overall, the symptomatology of chronic iliocaval obstructions varies broadly. Presenting symptoms of pain or swelling and venous claudication are the most common, approaching 100% and 81%, respectively [41].

- The venous CEAP (clinical, etiological, anatomical, pathophysiological) is widely used to broadly classify lower extremity disease [42].
- The clinical severity score (VCSS) and Villalta PTS are more precise in scoring disease severity. In a series of 120 patients with IVC thrombosis, 37% presented with class 3 symptomatology, whereas 26% presented with class 4 and 19% presented with class 6 [43]. Similar distributions have been reported, with clinical class 3 being the most common [44, 45].
  - In a series of 89 patients with non-malignant obstructive iliocaval lesions, the median presenting VCSS score was 9 prior to stenting [44].

7.4.4 Endovascular Management of Chronic Iliocaval Occlusion

Venous stent placement was first described in the late 1980s to address low patency rates following surgical bypass [46]. Since then, it has been recognized that stent placement is safe and can lead to significant improvement in symptoms [47–49]. Despite common practice, the development of dedicated venous stents has lagged behind arterial stents, though several venous-specific designs are now available.

Elgiloy-braided stents have the greatest breadth of experience for venous obstruction [50]. Neglén et al. demonstrated that among 982 femoro-iliocaval veins, primary patency was 57% and assisted-primary patency rates were 80% in thrombotic lesions [49]. In a series of 115 patients undergoing bilateral stenting for iliocaval obstruction, primary patency rates at 4 years

of 8.5% at 1 year, which increased to 20.8% at 2 years and 35.7% at 8 years [38, 39].

- More recently, it has been shown that about 2% of indwelling IVC filters may result in symptomatic iliocaval obstruction. Desai et al. demonstrated in a study of 1582 filter-bearing patients that male sex, central neurologic disease, and implantation time greater than 6 or 12 months were significantly associated with IVC thrombosis [40].
- Causes are likely multifactorial. IVC filters trap thrombus, which may predispose further propagation. Additionally, the type of filter may play a role due to geometric variability resulting in differential flow dynamics and subsequent clot entrapment. Lastly, there may be inherent thrombogenicity of the filter itself as a foreign object.

were demonstrated to be 61% using Wallstents [51].

Contemporary studies have focused on the utilization of dedicated venous stents in the IVC.

- In a series of 59 patients with IVC obstruction, endovascular reconstruction using the Vici Venous Stent (Veniti, Fremont, CA) resulted in primary patency rates of 91.2%, 71.0%, and 24.1% at 1, 3, and 5 years, respectively [52].
- For patients in this cohort presenting with PTS, Villalta scores decreased from 14.2 to 8.1 at 1 year follow-up and 6.8 at 2 years [52].

7.4.5 Pre-procedural Considerations

Successful iliocaval reconstruction is dependent on thorough imaging review. Duplex ultrasound is a noninvasive imaging modality that provides information about the inflow, the degree of obstruction, and the presence of concomitant superficial venous disease.

- When considering endovascular intervention, this is crucial to adequately assess the status of common femoral vein (CFV) inflow and profunda femoris vein to confirm inflow adequacy and ultimately determine whether stents can be supported.
- Axial imaging, including computed tomographic venography (CTV), is very useful in assessing the IVC and iliac anatomy, as well as for the presence of causative factors such as an IVC filter.

Access sites depend on the extent and anatomic location of vascular disease and should be selected to ensure that the inflow can be fully assessed during a procedure, and that a stent can be placed into the CFV should it be significantly compromised. Femoral and popliteal vein access are most common followed by greater saphenous vein. Internal jugular venous access may be helpful in the event adjunctive access is necessary.

7.4.6 Intra-procedural Considerations

Successful venous stent placement requires full consideration of the natural history of venous disease, pathophysiologic processes, and the mechanical properties of veins. Due to the elastic properties of the vein wall, pre-dilation of long-standing occlusions should be done prior to deploying a stent to overcome any fibrous retraction resulting from chronic post-thrombotic material [53].

- When more than one stent is deployed along the vessel, it is necessary to overlap the stents to ensure a stent separation does not occur.
  - Uncovered portions may result in recurrent stenosis in that area [51].
- The cranial and caudal ends of the venous stent should be placed in "healthy" venous segments, ensuring adequate inflow and outflow. Intraprocedurally, intravascular ultrasound (IVUS) is an adjunct imaging technique that should be employed to determine cranial and caudal landing zones. IVUS is also helpful in determining the size of the vessel, degree of obstruction, and can also provide information on the chronicity of clot based on echogenicity.

For patients that require bilateral stent placement, various techniques may be used including a "double-barrel" method, inverted Y stenting (requiring fenestration), and apposition (Fig. 7.13). It has been suggested that the double-barrel technique results in superior patency rates and the lowest re-intervention rates [51]. In most cases, a 14-mm double-barrel stent extending into single 14 mm stents in each iliac vein may be used.

- Lastly, while placing stents across the inguinal ligament is controversial in arterial lesions, venous stents can safely be deployed over this region; indeed, it is frequently required if there is an inflow/CFV lesion [54].
- When crossing the ligament, a 12-mm stent is used.

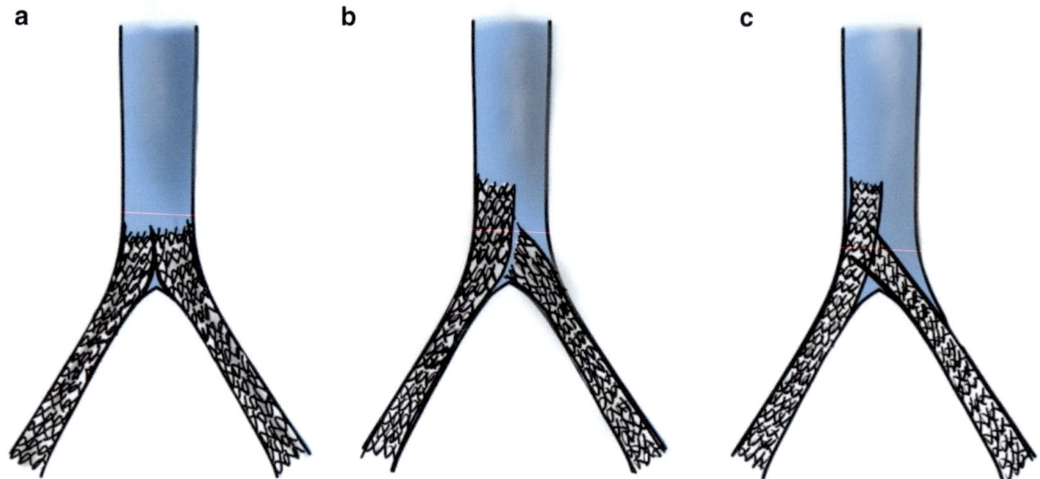

Fig. 7.13 (Panel **a**) The double-barrel technique involves the deployment of two parallel stents in the IVC, extending into the iliac veins. (Panel **b**) The apposition technique involves a stent extending into the ipsilateral iliac vein, with the contralateral stent deployed with the proximal end adjacent to the ipsilateral stent. (Panel **c**) In the fenestration technique, the contralateral limb penetrates through the ipsilateral stent

7.4.6.1 IVC Filter Management

The presence of an IVC filter in the vessel may pose a unique challenge as it may be difficult to retrieve the filter; the predominant approach had been stent placement across a chronic IVC filter; this technique is further described below:

- Neglén et al. demonstrated that patency rates at 54 months are 32% with this technique; early stent occlusion within 30 days occurred in 12% of patients [55].

More recent data, however, suggests that removal of the IVC filter whenever possible is favored. Single-session IVC filter removal, recanalization, and endovascular reconstruction has been shown to result in excellent early patency rates, with 96% of patients maintaining iliocaval stent patency at 1–3 months (Fig. 7.14).

- This technique has demonstrated improvement in VCSS edema and pain subscores by 1.4 and 0.6, respectively [56].
- At 1-year follow-up, primary, primary-assisted, and secondary patency by limb is 94%, 96%, and 100%, respectively; at 2 years it is 91%, 95%, and 100%, respectively [56].

- Thus, antecedent removal of IVC filters prior to recanalization demonstrates high rates of durable clinical success and is encouraged when possible.

7.4.6.2 Stenting Across Filters

In filters that cannot be removed, stenting across the filter is one approach to treat filter-related IVC thrombosis. This is done by crossing the obstructed area with a guidewire, followed by dilating with a balloon. This either displaces or flattens the filter against the vessel wall to allow for the deployment of the stent. There are several considerations when stenting through IVC filters, although most published studies have reported overall feasibility, safety, and efficacy with this method.

- Neglén et al. published a series suggesting that primary and secondary patency following IVC stenting is not influenced by the presence of an IVC filter, even at 54 months (32% and 75%, respectively) [55].
- However, there was a significant association between patency and the extent of disease (occlusive vs. non-occlusive) [55].

Reports of retroperitoneal hemorrhage, back pain, and IVC perforation with stent placement

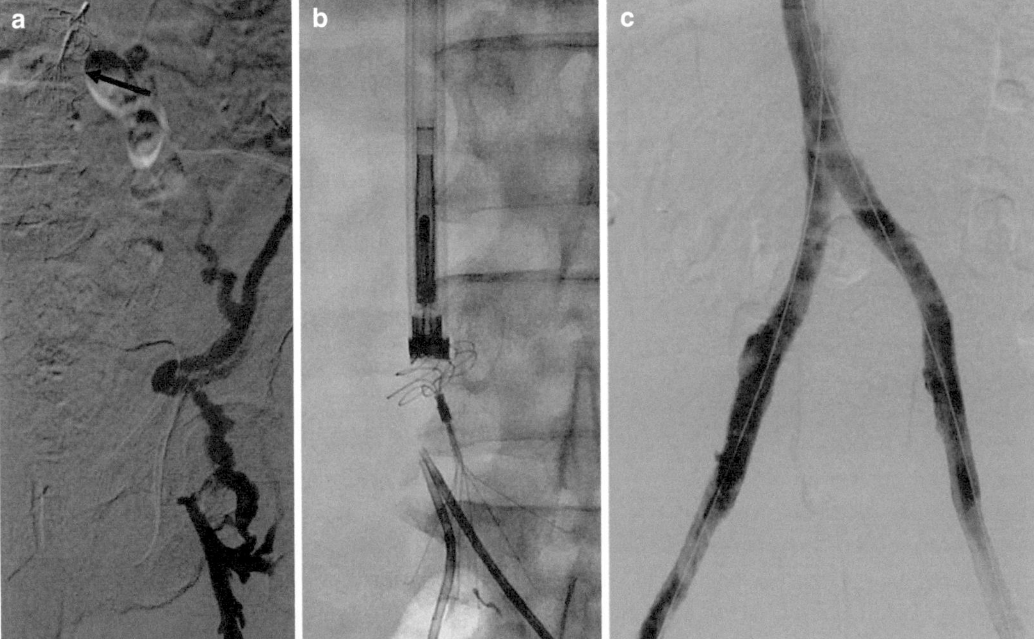

Fig. 7.14 (Panel **a**) Example of extensive IVC thrombus secondary to a permanent inferior vena cava filter (arrow). (Panel **b**) Retrieval of IVC filter using foreign body retrieval device and photothermal ablation with a 14 Fr excimer laser sheath. (Panel **c**) Completion venogram demonstrating restored patency throughout the IVC and common iliac veins

across IVC filters are limited [57]. However, there are numerous hypothetical risks associated with this method include deformity or fracture of the filter that theoretically may penetrate the IVC, although this has not been definitively supported by the literature [56]. Another concern is whether displacement of the filter impacts patency of the stent by precluding complete stent expansion [55]. Renal vein thrombosis is another rare but reported complication [57].

7.4.6.3 Advanced Recanalization Techniques

In iliocaval occlusions that cannot be traversed with standard wire/catheter technique, advanced recanalization techniques including sharp recanalization and radiofrequency guidewires may be used.

- There is a risk of damage to adjacent structures, particularly arteries, and familiarity with the technique, preparedness for intraprocedural complications, correlation with pre- and intraprocedural imaging are key to limiting the risk of these procedures.

For sharp recanalization, a balloon or snare can be placed distal to the occlusion via a separate access site, to serve as a target. A sheath is employed close to the occlusion and a needle is carefully advanced under direct visualization.

- Sharps including the stiff end of a 0.035″ guidewire, straight needles, trans-septal needles, or Rosch-Uchida needles may be used [58].
- In a retrospective review of central venous occlusions, outcomes for sharp recanalization include a 90–95% technical success rate with minimal adverse effects (2–3%) [59, 60]. Prior stenting or length of occlusion is not significantly associated with the probability of technical success [59].

– Long-term patency data is further promising, with 79% of reconstructions remaining patent following sharp recanalization [59].

RF wires have also been described as another option for traversing vessel obstructions. The PowerWire RF Guidewire (Baylis Medical, Montreal, Quebec) is the most reported in the literature. RF wires have a technical success of crossing and resolving the occlusion ranging from 69 to 100% [61–64].

Post-procedural Management and Pharmacotherapy

There is no consensus on anticoagulation following iliocaval reconstruction of chronic obstructions. Dual antiplatelet therapy with clopidogrel and aspirin may be used in the short term, with indefinite use of aspirin [65]. It is noted, however, that there is a paucity of randomized-controlled data that supports the use of dual antiplatelet therapy [66–68]. In patients with extensive occlusions, thrombophilia, and a history of long-term anticoagulation, warfarin or direct oral anticoagulants may be efficacious following endovascular treatment. The length of treatment remains at the providers' discretion, although it generally varies between 6 and 12 months for patients with a single DVT episode [68]. For all patients, compression stockings should be continued post-operatively along with continued ambulation and exercise recommendations [66].

7.4.6.4 Conclusion

Iliocaval obstruction can result in severe symptoms secondary to venous stasis and significantly impact the quality of life. Contemporary treatment involves endovascular stent placement. Current techniques and devices allow for relatively immediate symptom relief, although high rates of re-intervention remain an ongoing concern. In patients with IVC filters, removal of the filter is favored and may be associated with improved patency. In complex recanalizations, where the obstruction cannot be traversed with standard technique, advanced techniques using

sharp recanalization or RF wires may be necessary. Robust pre-procedural planning, familiarity with the array of endovascular devices needed to perform such procedures, and diligent follow-up are essential to maintaining good long-term outcomes.

7.5 Surgical Options

Jordan C. Tasse

In the current era, surgical approaches to venous obstructive disease are extremely limited, and often mostly historically described due to the growth of endovenous success. Of note, surgical venous bypass is mostly reserved for possible fem-fem surgical bypass known as the Palma procedure, using saphenous vein conduit. Other options include PTFE and or addition of arteriovenous fistula creation to increase the venous inflow as the low-pressure flow can be prone to early or recurrent thrombosis.

Interestingly completely percutaneous common femoral to common femoral vein prosthetic stent graft bypass creation has been performed, with long-term success. Due to the limited sample size, it is reserved for extreme situations only and is soon to be published.

7.6 Compression Therapy

Griffin Mcnamara, Jillian Drogin, and Keith Pereira

7.6.1 Compression Therapy in Wound Care: Why and How

Compression therapy is essential in the treatment of edema secondary to both venous insufficiency and lymphedema. Generally, these therapies are required for patients with CEAP of 3–6 and patients with symptomatic lymphedema. Though this treatment is relatively straightforward, providers must consider the benefits and risks of different forms of compression therapies. The minimum tolerable compression pressure tailored to the patient's requirement should be ensured to maximize compliance. The most efficacious therapy is the one that the patient can tolerate, and time should be spent counseling patients to ensure compliance with these therapies. This chapter will focus on the rationale of compression therapy, available options and their indications, proper use, and contraindications.

7.6.2 Why Compression Therapy?

Optimal wound care and compression therapy will heal most small venous ulcers of short duration. There is Level A evidence showing that venous ulcers heal faster with compression when compared to no compression [69].

- Compression narrows veins, restores valve competence, and reduces ambulatory venous pressure, thus reducing venous reflux.
- It alleviates limb edema by decreasing inflammatory cytokines, accelerating capillary flow, and lowering capillary fluid leakage.
- It also softens lipodermatosclerosis, improves lymphatic flow and function, and enhances fibrinolysis [70].
- Goals of compression therapy are ulcer healing, reduction of pain and edema, and prevention of recurrence [71].

7.6.3 Types of Compression Therapies

Compression therapies are split into broad categories based on static vs. dynamic and elastic vs. inelastic.

- Static therapies maintain compression and shape.
- Dynamic therapies administer intermittent compression.
- Elastic therapies stretch before applying the desired pressure.

- Non-elastic is less pliable and often used as wraps or bandages.

The type of compression therapy for a patient is dependent on many factors, some of which include the etiology (Venous vs Lymphedema), presence of ulcer, and body habitus. Figure 7.15 illustrates a flowchart of the optimal use of compression therapies.

The most common and efficacious options are static and elastic garments such as compression stockings. These are available in numerous lengths and pressures. Most studies recommend a pressure of at least 20–30 mmHg in patients with chronic venous insufficiency [72–74]. Higher pressures of 40–50 mmHg may be used in the treatment of severe chronic venous insufficiency, but 50–60 mmHg is typically reserved for patients with severe lymphedema or burn scars. Variation in length can be utilized to target disease with options ranging from knee-high, which is ideal for most patients, to the top of the thigh which may be required after venous surgery. However, these options still have their limitations.

- Patients with severe obesity or edema may not be able to fit into stockings.
- In addition, chronic lipodermatosclerosis may prevent the stockings from applying pressure due to subcutaneous fibrosis and hardening of the skin.
- When using stockings, it is important to perform ulcer care prior to placement and put them on before getting out of bed in the morning when edema is minimal.

Static inelastic stockings such as the Unna boot, a disposable wrap applied to the lower extremities, rely on muscle contraction to apply pressure [75]. Benefits of this option include low price, disposability, ease of application, antimicrobial properties, and ability to be changed in patients with draining ulcers [76]. Nonetheless, these options are typically less effective than elastic bandages as pressure is dependent on muscle contraction and patients may require frequent dressing changes [75].

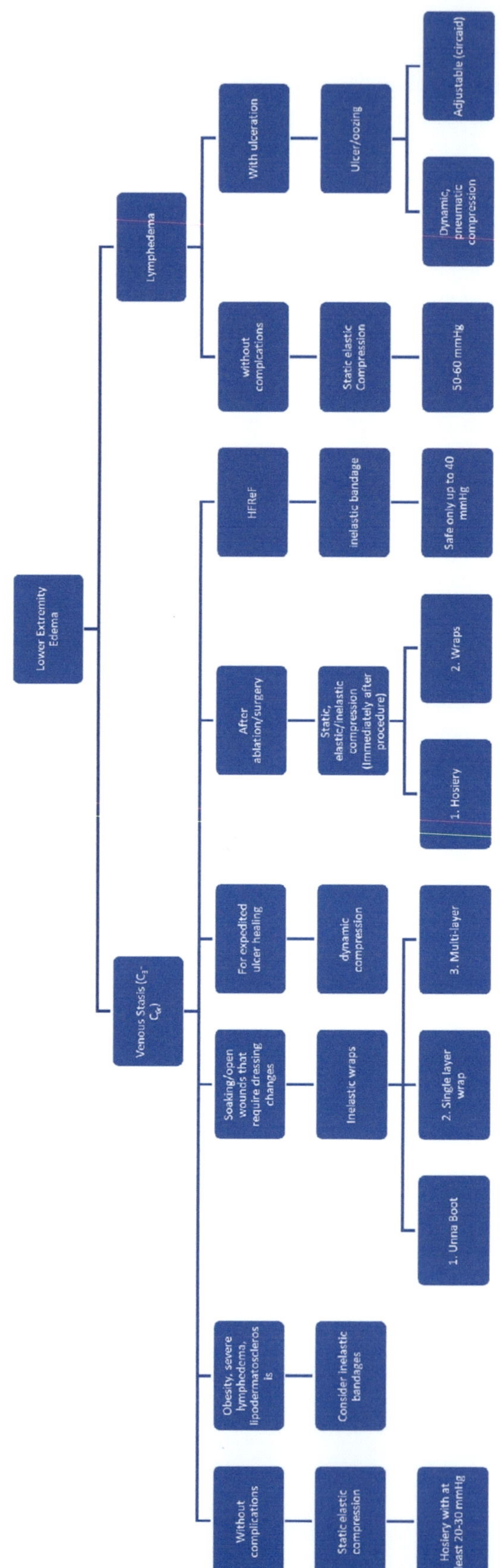

Fig. 7.15 Flowchart illustrating the optimal use of compression therapy

Multilayer dressings are static dressings that combine elastic and inelastic components in up to four layers. These are the most labor-intensive dressings but report similar efficacy to compression stockings when used properly [74].

- The base is a protruding padding layer that offloads compression from high-pressure areas such as bony prominences that are susceptible to developing ischemic changes.
- The next layer, the crepe bandage, is an absorbent layer that smooths the padded layer.
- The third layer is an elastic bandage that can provide significant pressure with stretch and overlap [76, 77].
- Finally, a cohesive elastic bandage is placed for an even greater level of compression. Together, the layers can add up to 40 mmHg of pressure [76].

Dynamic therapies deliver intermittent pneumatic compression via a compression pump or sleeve. These are used in patients with lymphedema and to promote fibrinolysis in patients with chronic ulcers [78–80]. Pneumatic compression is efficacious for patients with stage 1 lymphedema on the ISL staging scale, while stage 2 lymphedema requires additional assistance from healthcare providers to maintain this efficacy [81]. This option, like the other therapies, is heavily dependent on patient compliance [82].

Finally, there are adjustable therapies, e.g., Circaid, that are used primarily for lymphedema. These therapies utilize overlapping and intertwining straps secured by Velcro. They are well tolerated and promote good compliance. Further, compression with adjustable bandages is more effective at 40 mmHg than 60 mmHg, highlighting the importance of patient tolerance and compliance in these therapies [83].

7.6.3.1 Contraindications to Compression Therapy

Compression stockings are only efficacious in the treatment of venous ulceration and lymphedema. Some of the contraindications include:

1. Arterial ulceration and significant peripheral arterial disease (PAD) are absolute contraindications to compression stocking use. The recommended ankle-brachial index (ABI) cutoff for absolute contraindication is an ABI <0.5, however, careful consideration must be taken in patients with any level of PAD [9, 84–86].
   (a) For patients with PAD, studies suggest that up to 40 mmHg of compression is safe if the absolute ankle pressure in extremities is greater than 60 mmHg [87].
2. Superficial and deep venous thrombosis, in patients without current anticoagulation therapy, are contraindications for compression therapy due to the theoretical risk of dislodged clots causing a pulmonary embolism.
3. Chronic heart failure with reduced ejection fraction may be exacerbated by these therapies because of fluid volume shifts. A study that examined the use of inelastic bandages in patients with heart failure demonstrated that ejection fraction was further reduced by 72% when under pressure of 21–30 mmHg and 103% at 31–40 mmHg [87].
4. Cellulitis, infection, or skin necrosis are additional contraindications for compression therapy. Conversely, for patients with recurrent cellulitis, compression therapy may help to prevent future infections [88].

7.6.3.2 Complications from Compression Therapies

Most complications from these therapies stem from improper use. Skin necrosis may occur when bandages are applied too tightly, or necessary padding layers are not placed on high-pressure areas. Due to the location of these bandages, fungal infections may occur when dressings are not changed at proper intervals. Further, fungal infections are more common in patients with exudate accumulation, and this factor should be taken into consideration during wound care planning. Finally, contact dermatitis may occur from the zinc in Unna boots or the latex in elastic wraps and the type of bandage should be changed accordingly.

References

1. Hardman RL, Rochon PJ. Role of interventional radiologists in the management of lower extremity venous insufficiency. Semin Interv Radiol. 2013;30:388–93. https://doi.org/10.1055/s-0033-1359733.

2. Rutherford RB, Padberg FT Jr, Comerota AJ, Kistner RL, Meissner MH, Moneta GL. Venous severity scoring: an adjunct to venous outcome assessment. J Vasc Surg. 2000;31(6):1307–12. https://doi.org/10.1067/mva.2000.107094.

3. Eberhardt RT, Raffetto JD. Chronic venous insufficiency. Circulation. 2005;111(18):2398–409.

4. Gethin G, Cowman S, Kolbach DN. Debridement for venous leg ulcers. Cochrane Database Syst Rev. 2015;9:CD008599.

5. Gohel MS, Heatley F, Liu X, Bradbury A, Bulbulia R, Cullum N, et al. A randomized trial of early endovenous ablation in venous ulceration. N Engl J Med. 2018;378(22):2105–14.

6. Adam DJ, Naik J, Hartshorne T, Bello M, London NJM. The diagnosis and management of 689 chronic leg ulcers in a single-visit assessment clinic. Eur J Vasc Endovasc Surg. 2003;25(5):462–8.

7. Schroeppel DeBacker SE, Bulman JC, Weinstein JL. Wound care for venous ulceration. Semin Interven Radiol. 2021;38(2):194–201.

8. O'Meara S, Cullum N, Nelson EA, Dumville JC. Compression for venous leg ulcers. Cochrane Database Syst Rev. 2012;11:CD000265.

9. Franks PJ, Barker J, Collier M, Gethin G, Haesler E, Jawien A, et al. Management of patients with venous leg ulcers: challenges and current best practice. J Wound Care. 2016;25(Suppl 6):S1–S67.

10. Lippman HI, Fishman LM, Farrar RH, Bernstein RK, Zybert PA. Edema control in the management of disabling chronic venous insufficiency. Arch Phys Med Rehabil. 1994;75(4):436–41.

11. Gibson K, Elias S, Adelman M, Hager ES, Dexter DJ, Vayuvegula S, Chopra P, Kabnick LS. A prospective safety and effectiveness study using endovenous laser ablation with a 400-µm optical fiber for the treatment of pathologic perforator veins in patients with advanced venous disease (SeCure trial). J Vasc Surg Venous Lymphat Disord. 2020;8(5):805–13.

12. Rochon PJ, Vu CT, Ray CE, et al. ACR Appropriateness Criteria Radiologic Management of Lower-Extremity Venous Insufficiency. American College of Radiology; 2009. https://acsearch.acr.org/docs/69507/Narrative/. Accessed 8 April 2022.

13. Tessari L, Cavezzi A, Frullini A. Preliminary experience with a new sclerosing foam in the treatment of varicose veins. Dermatol Surg. 2001;27:58–60.

14. Hamel-Desnos C, Desnos P, Wollmann J-C, Ouvry P, Mako S, Allaert F-A. Evaluation of the efficacy of polidocanol in the form of foam compared with liquid form in sclerotherapy of the greater saphenous vein: initial results. Dermatol Surg. 2003;29(12):1170–5. discussion 1175

15. Hager ES, Washington C, Steinmetz A, Wu T, Singh M, Dillavou E. Factors that influence perforator vein closure rates using radiofrequency ablation, laser ablation, or foam sclerotherapy. J Vasc Surg Venous Lymphat Disord. 2016;4(1):51–6.

16. Van den Bos R, Arends L, Kockaert M, Neumann M, Nijsten T. Endovenous therapies of lower extremity varicosities: a meta-analysis. J Vasc Surg. 2009;49(1):230–9.

17. Jimenez JC, Lawrence PF, Woo K, Chun TT, Farley SM, Rigberg DA, et al. Adjunctive techniques to minimize thrombotic complications following microfoam sclerotherapy of saphenous trunks and tributaries. J Vasc Surg Venous Lymphat Disord. 2021;9(4):904–9.

18. Lessne ML, Bajwa J, Hong K. Fatal reperfusion injury after thrombolysis for phlegmasia cerulea dolens. J Vasc Interv Radiol. 2012;23(5):681–6. https://doi.org/10.1016/j.jvir.2012.02.007.

19. Perkins JMT, Magee TR, Galland RB. Phlegmasia caerulea dolens and venous gangrene. Br J Surg. 1996;83(1):19–23. https://doi.org/10.1002/bjs.1800830106.

20. Kolluri R, Lugli M, Villalba L, Varcoe R, Maleti O, Gallardo F, Black S, Forgues F, Lichtenberg M, Hinahara J, Ramakrishnan S, Beckman JA. An estimate of the economic burden of venous leg ulcers associated with deep venous disease. Vasc Med. 2022;27(1):63–72. https://doi.org/10.1177/1358863X211028298.

21. Kibbe MR, Ujiki M, Goodwin AL, Eskandari M, Yao J, Matsumura J. Iliac vein compression in an asymptomatic patient population. J Vasc Surg. 2004;39(5):937–43. https://doi.org/10.1016/j.jvs.2003.12.032.

22. Oguzkurt L, Ozkan U, Ulusan S, Koc Z, Tercan F. Compression of the left common iliac vein in asymptomatic subjects and patients with left iliofemoral deep vein thrombosis. J Vasc Interv Radiol. 2008;19(3):366–70. https://doi.org/10.1016/j.jvir.2007.09.007.

23. Van Vuuren TMAJ, Kurstjens RLM, Wittens CHA, van Laanen JHH, de Graaf R. Illusory angiographic signs of significant iliac vein compression in healthy volunteers. Eur J Vasc Endovasc Surg. 2018;56(6):874–9. https://doi.org/10.1016/j.ejvs.2018.07.022.

24. Rabinovich A, Kahn SR. How I treat the postthrombotic syndrome. Blood. 2018;131(20):2215–22. https://doi.org/10.1182/blood-2018-01-785956.

25. Pascarella L, Shortell CK. Medical management of venous ulcers. Semin Vasc Surg. 2015;28(1):21–8. https://doi.org/10.1053/j.semvascsurg.2015.06.001.

26. Raju S. Best management options for chronic iliac vein stenosis and occlusion. J Vasc Surg. 2013;57(4):1163–9. https://doi.org/10.1016/j.jvs.2012.11.084.

27. Wolpert LM, Rahmani O, Stein B, Gallagher JJ, Drezner AD. Magnetic resonance venography in the diagnosis and management of May-Thurner syndrome. Vasc Endovasc Surg. 2002;36(1):51–7.

28. Birn J, Vedantham S. May–Thurner syndrome and other obstructive iliac vein lesions: Meaning, myth, and mystery. Vasc Med. 2015;20(1):74–83. https://doi.org/10.1177/1358863X14560429.
29. Grøtta O, Enden T, Sandbæk G, et al. Infrainguinal inflow assessment and endovenous stent placement in iliofemoral post-thrombotic obstructions. CVIR Endovasc. 2018;1:29. https://doi.org/10.1186/s42155-018-0038-9.
30. Bajwa R, Bergin D, O'Sullivan GJ. Aiming for the bottom corner: how to score a field goal when landing venous stents in May–Thurner syndrome. J Vasc Interv Radiol. 2019;30(10):1555–61. https://doi.org/10.1016/j.jvir.2019.04.033.
31. Neglén P, Darcey R, Olivier J, Raju S. Bilateral stenting at the iliocaval confluence. J Vasc Surg. 2010;51(6):1457–66. https://doi.org/10.1016/j.jvs.2010.01.056.
32. Marston W, Fish D, Unger J, Keagy B. Incidence of and risk factors for iliocaval venous obstruction in patients with active or healed venous leg ulcers. J Vasc Surg. 2011;53(5):1303–8.
33. Maleux G, Vertenten B, Laenen A, et al. Palliative endovascular treatment of cancer-related iliocaval obstructive disease: technical and clinical outcomes. Acta Radiol. 2016;57(4):451–6.
34. Johnson BF, Manzo RA, Bergelin RO, Strandness DE Jr. Relationship between changes in the deep venous system and the development of the postthrombotic syndrome after an acute episode of lower limb deep vein thrombosis: a one- to six-year follow-up. J Vasc Surg. 1995;21(2):307–12. discussion 313
35. Vedantham S, Goldhaber SZ, Julian JA, et al. Pharmacomechanical catheter-directed thrombolysis for deep-vein thrombosis. N Engl J Med. 2017;377(23):2240–52.
36. Kahn SR. The post-thrombotic syndrome. Hematology Am Soc Hematol Educ Program. 2016;2016(1):413–8.
37. Sarosiek S, Crowther M, Sloan JM. Indications, complications, and management of inferior vena cava filters: the experience in 952 patients at an academic hospital with a level I trauma center. JAMA Intern Med. 2013;173(7):513–7.
38. Group PS. Eight-year follow-up of patients with permanent vena cava filters in the prevention of pulmonary embolism: the PREPIC (Prevention du Risque d'Embolie Pulmonaire par Interruption Cave) randomized study. Circulation. 2005;112(3):416–22.
39. Decousus H, Leizorovicz A, Parent F, et al. A clinical trial of vena caval filters in the prevention of pulmonary embolism in patients with proximal deep-vein thrombosis. Prevention du Risque d'Embolie Pulmonaire par Interruption Cave Study Group. N Engl J Med. 1998;338(7):409–15.
40. Xiao N, Karp J, Lewandowski R, et al. Inferior vena cava thrombosis risk in 1582 patients with inferior vena cava filters. Radiology. 2022;303(2):300–2.
41. Rollo JC, Farley SM, Jimenez JC, Woo K, Lawrence PF, DeRubertis BG. Contemporary outcomes of elective iliocaval and infrainguinal venous intervention for post-thrombotic chronic venous occlusive disease. J Vasc Surg Venous Lymphat Disord. 2017;5(6):789–99.
42. Lurie F, Passman M, Meisner M, et al. The 2020 update of the CEAP classification system and reporting standards. J Vasc Surg Venous Lymphat Disord. 2020;8(3):342–52.
43. Raju S, Hollis K, Neglen P. Obstructive lesions of the inferior vena cava: clinical features and endovenous treatment. J Vasc Surg. 2006;44(4):820–7.
44. Hartung O, Otero A, Boufi M, et al. Mid-term results of endovascular treatment for symptomatic chronic nonmalignant iliocaval venous occlusive disease. J Vasc Surg. 2005;42(6):1138–44. discussion 1144
45. Jayaraj A, Crim W, Knight A, Raju S. Characteristics and outcomes of stent occlusion after iliocaval stenting. J Vasc Surg Venous Lymphat Disord. 2019;7(1):56–64.
46. Zollikofer CL, Largiader I, Bruhlmann WF, Uhlschmid GK, Marty AH. Endovascular stenting of veins and grafts: preliminary clinical experience. Radiology. 1988;167(3):707–12.
47. Black S, Gwozdz A, Karunanithy N, et al. Two year outcome after chronic iliac vein occlusion recanalisation using the vici venous stent((R)). Eur J Vasc Endovasc Surg. 2018;56(5):710–8.
48. Delis KT, Bjarnason H, Wennberg PW, Rooke TW, Gloviczki P. Successful iliac vein and inferior vena cava stenting ameliorates venous claudication and improves venous outflow, calf muscle pump function, and clinical status in post-thrombotic syndrome. Ann Surg. 2007;245(1):130–9.
49. Neglen P, Hollis KC, Olivier J, Raju S. Stenting of the venous outflow in chronic venous disease: long-term stent-related outcome, clinical, and hemodynamic result. J Vasc Surg. 2007;46(5):979–90.
50. Shamimi-Noori SM, Clark TWI. Venous stents: current status and future directions. Tech Vasc Interv Radiol. 2018;21(2):113–6.
51. Neglen P, Darcey R, Olivier J, Raju S. Bilateral stenting at the iliocaval confluence. J Vasc Surg. 2010;51(6):1457–66.
52. Thulasidasan N, Morris R, Theodoulou I, et al. Medium-term outcomes after inferior vena cava reconstruction for acute and chronic deep vein thrombosis and retroperitoneal fibrosis. J Vasc Surg Venous Lymphat Disord. 2022;10(3):607–16. e602
53. Schwein A, Georg Y, Lejay A, et al. Endovascular treatment for venous diseases: where are the venous stents? Methodist Debakey Cardiovasc J. 2018;14(3):208–13.
54. Neglen P, Tackett TP Jr, Raju S. Venous stenting across the inguinal ligament. J Vasc Surg. 2008;48(5):1255–61.
55. Neglen P, Oglesbee M, Olivier J, Raju S. Stenting of chronically obstructed inferior vena cava filters. J Vasc Surg. 2011;54(1):153–61.

56. Desai KR, Xiao N, Karp J, et al. Single-session inferior vena cava filter removal, recanalization, and endovenous reconstruction for chronic iliocaval thrombosis. J Vasc Surg Venous Lymphat Disord. 2019;7(2):176–83.

57. Chick JFB, Jo A, Meadows JM, et al. Endovascular iliocaval stent reconstruction for inferior vena cava filter-associated iliocaval thrombosis: approach, technical success, safety, and two-year outcomes in 120 patients. J Vasc Interv Radiol. 2017;28(7):933–9.

58. Rivers-Bowerman MD, Lightfoot CB, Meagher RP, Carter MD, Berry RF. Percutaneous sharp recanalization of a membranous IVC occlusion with an occlusion balloon as a needle target. Radiol Case Rep. 2017;12(3):537–41.

59. McDevitt JL, Srinivasa RN, Gemmete JJ, et al. Approach, technical success, complications, and stent patency of sharp recanalization for the treatment of chronic venous occlusive disease: experience in 123 patients. Cardiovasc Intervent Radiol. 2019;42(2):205–12.

60. Cohen EI, Beck C, Garcia J, et al. Success rate and complications of sharp recanalization for treatment of central venous occlusions. Cardiovasc Intervent Radiol. 2018;41(1):73–9.

61. Guimaraes M, Schonholz C, Hannegan C, Anderson MB, Shi J, Selby B Jr. Radiofrequency wire for the recanalization of central vein occlusions that have failed conventional endovascular techniques. J Vasc Interv Radiol. 2012;23(8):1016–21.

62. Sivananthan G, MacArthur DH, Daly KP, Allen DW, Hakham S, Halin NJ. Safety and efficacy of radiofrequency wire recanalization of chronic central venous occlusions. J Vasc Access. 2015;16(4):309–14.

63. Iafrati M, Maloney S, Halin N. Radiofrequency thermal wire is a useful adjunct to treat chronic central venous occlusions. J Vasc Surg. 2012;55(2):603–6.

64. Keller EJ, Gupta SA, Bondarev S, Sato KT, Vogelzang RL, Resnick SA. Single-center retrospective review of radiofrequency wire recanalization of refractory central venous occlusions. J Vasc Interv Radiol. 2018;29(11):1571–7.

65. Notten P, Ten Cate H, Ten Cate-Hoek AJ. Postinterventional antithrombotic management after venous stenting of the iliofemoral tract in acute and chronic thrombosis: a systematic review. J Thromb Haemost. 2021;19(3):753–96.

66. Mahnken AH, Thomson K, de Haan M, O'Sullivan GJ. CIRSE standards of practice guidelines on iliocaval stenting. Cardiovasc Intervent Radiol. 2014;37(4):889–97.

67. Attaran RR, Ozdemir D, Lin IH, Mena-Hurtado C, Lansky A. Evaluation of anticoagulant and antiplatelet therapy after iliocaval stenting: factors associated with stent occlusion. J Vasc Surg Venous Lymphat Disord. 2019;7(4):527–34.

68. Milinis K, Thapar A, Shalhoub J, Davies AH. Antithrombotic therapy following venous stenting: international Delphi consensus. Eur J Vasc Endovasc Surg. 2018;55(4):537–44.

69. O'Meara S, Cullum NA, Nelson EA. Compression for venous leg ulcers. Cochrane Database Syst Rev. 2009;(1):Cd000265.

70. Brem H, Kirsner RS, Falanga V. Protocol for the successful treatment of venous ulcers. Am J Surg. 2004;188(1A Suppl):1–8.

71. Abu-Own A, Scurr JH, Coleridge Smith PD. Effect of leg elevation on the skin microcirculation in chronic venous insufficiency. J Vasc Surg. 1994;20(5):705–10.

72. O'Meara S, Cullum N, Nelson EA, Dumville JC. Compression for venous leg ulcers. Cochrane Database Syst Rev. 2012;11(11):Cd000265.

73. Shi C, Dumville JC, Cullum N, Connaughton E, Norman G. Compression bandages or stockings versus no compression for treating venous leg ulcers. Cochrane Database Syst Rev. 2021;7(7):Cd013397.

74. Mauck KF, Asi N, Elraiyah TA, Undavalli C, Nabhan M, Altayar O, et al. Comparative systematic review and meta-analysis of compression modalities for the promotion of venous ulcer healing and reducing ulcer recurrence. J Vasc Surg. 2014;60(2 Suppl):71S–90S.

75. Moffatt C. Variability of pressure provided by sustained compression. Int Wound J. 2008;5(2):259–65.

76. Moffatt C. Four-layer bandaging: from concept to practice. Int J Low Extrem Wounds. 2002;1(1):13–26.

77. Partsch H. Compression therapy. Int Angiol. 2010;29(5):391.

78. Allenby F, Boardman L, Pflug JJ, Calnan JS. Effects of external pneumatic intermittent compression on fibrinolysis in man. Lancet. 1973;2(7843):1412–4.

79. Tarnay TJ, Rohr PR, Davidson AG, Stevenson MM, Byars EF, Hopkins GR. Pneumatic calf compression, fibrinolysis, and the prevention of deep venous thrombosis. Surgery. 1980;88(4):489–96.

80. Comerota AJ. Intermittent pneumatic compression: physiologic and clinical basis to improve management of venous leg ulcers. J Vasc Surg. 2011;53(4):1121–9.

81. Badger CM, Peacock JL, Mortimer PS. A randomized, controlled, parallel-group clinical trial comparing multilayer bandaging followed by hosiery versus hosiery alone in the treatment of patients with lymphedema of the limb. Cancer. 2000;88(12):2832–7.

82. Ko DS, Lerner R, Klose G, Cosimi AB. Effective treatment of lymphedema of the extremities. Arch Surg. 1998;133(4):452–8.

83. Mosti G, Cavezzi A, Partsch H, Urso S, Campana F. Adjustable velcro compression devices are more effective than inelastic bandages in reducing venous edema in the initial treatment phase: a randomized controlled trial. Eur J Vasc Endovasc Surg. 2015;50(3):368–74.

84. Andriessen A, Apelqvist J, Mosti G, Partsch H, Gonska C, Abel M. Compression therapy for venous leg ulcers: risk factors for adverse events and complications, contraindications - a review of present guidelines. J Eur Acad Dermatol Venereol. 2017;31(9):1562–8.

85. O'Donnell TF Jr, Passman MA, Marston WA, Ennis WJ, Dalsing M, Kistner RL, et al. Management

of venous leg ulcers: clinical practice guidelines of the Society for Vascular Surgery ® and the American Venous Forum. J Vasc Surg. 2014;60(2 Suppl):3s–59s.

86. Wittens C, Davies AH, Bækgaard N, Broholm R, Cavezzi A, Chastanet S, et al. Editor's choice - management of chronic venous disease: clinical practice guidelines of the European Society for Vascular Surgery (ESVS). Eur J Vasc Endovasc Surg. 2015;49(6):678–737.

87. Mosti G, Iabichella ML, Partsch H. Compression therapy in mixed ulcers increases venous output and arterial perfusion. J Vasc Surg. 2012;55(1):122–8.

88. Webb E, Neeman T, Bowden FJ, Gaida J, Mumford V, Bissett B. Compression therapy to prevent recurrent cellulitis of the leg. N Engl J Med. 2020;383(7):630–9.

Timothy E. Yates and Sreekumar Madassery

8.1 Follow-Up Planning

Timothy E. Yates

8.1.1 Scope

Treatment of critical lower limb ischemia or chronic limb-threatening ischemia is challenging and demanding. It is therefore the author's opinion that not all vascular specialists are well-suited for this highly specific branch of vascular medicine. The patient cohort has 54% mortality at 4 years with a terrible quality of life and several comorbid conditions that can make the patient's final years frankly miserable [1].

This subset requires advocacy and physicians committed to following through to the end of a wound, whether this means complete wound healing, minor amputation, or in several unsalvageable cases, major amputation. Physicians not willing to consider the entire spectrum should not take care of these patients. Additionally, while not discussed exhaustively here, not all patients truly SHOULD be treated aggressively. This is for several reasons. For one, in a portion of patients, extensive or angiosomally directed revascularization may be unnecessary. For example, in the *Korean Journal of Radiology*, peroneal-only artery endovascular revascularization resulted in only 7% of major amputations in 104 limbs [2, 3]. Additionally, comorbid conditions and in patients' age, have been associated with significantly worse outcomes, particularly in nonagenarians [4].

Still, consensus recommendations cite revascularization as the optimal treatment for patients with critical lower limb ischemia, given poor prognosis and significant functional and psychological impairment following major amputation [5–7].

One can see that the approach to patients with ischemic wounds is philosophically different than for claudicants. This is also true of follow-up strategies. In the first place, multiple conditions must be managed in a coordinated fashion, and this is typically best done in a multidisciplinary way [8]. Despite this, each patient needs a fervent navigator, so ultimately the vascular specialist is best served by establishing ownership over the patient and helping the patient to see appropriate care partners. Follow-up, therefore, is an extension of your initial consultation, not an intervention [9].

The following sections will share the authors' practice strategy based on a combined 20+ years of practice. This is meant to be practical and

T. E. Yates
Interventional Vascular and Oncologic Radiology,
CLI Vascular Specialists, Del Ray, FL, USA

S. Madassery (✉)
Department of Vascular and Interventional Radiology,
Rush University Medical Center, Chicago, IL, USA

S. Madassery, A. Patel (eds.), *Limb Preservation for the Vascular Specialist*,
https://doi.org/10.1007/978-3-031-36480-8_8

where possible, guideline based. But more important than dogma, is to stimulate thought for WHY we have adopted this approach. The rationale for each aspect will be shared, but any differences of opinion with the reader are welcomed because it is in these differences that learning takes place. Follow up at the authors' practice is as follows:

- Follow up phone call and 2 weeks post-intervention visit: evaluate groin, early thrombosis, and confirm appropriate medical therapy.
- Monthly until healed or 4 months (reassessment of original intervention, consideration of additional intervention, medical optimization, appropriate wound care).
- After healing: 3, 6, and 12 months with duplex (patency less important).
- Minor amputation follow-up
  - Offloading
  - A1c management
  - Medical optimization
  - Risk factor amelioration
- Major amputation follow-up
  - Prosthetic fitting
  - Resources for psychological development
  - Physical therapy
- Death

8.1.2 Initial Follow-Up

It is the author's institutional practice for care coordinators to call patients within one business day of any procedure. This has been an extremely valuable touch point with patients since the practice is entirely office-based and outpatient. Unlike the constant monitoring in a hospital, outpatient centers depend on transport returning the patient home safely and that no overnight untoward events transpire. The initial call is to ensure the patient is safe and recovering appropriately. Any concerns or complications will be dealt with initially by phone but can also be handled in person if issues arise that demand live attention. This phone call makes patients feel more concierge care and allows them to clarify any overhanging questions regarding their procedures. Finally, post-operative medications are confirmed prior to ending the call.

If all proceeds in the typical fashion within the first 24 h, the patient will be seen physically at 2–4 weeks post-op. This short-term follow-up is primarily to assess patient clinical symptoms (resolution of rest pain, reperfusion edema, wound healing), puncture sites, and to perform baseline post-intervention noninvasive studies (ultrasound duplex, ankle-brachial index, and/or pulse-volume recordings). Occasionally insurers will deny payment for duplex this short after index studies, but the clinical and technical information gleaned from this post-procedure duplex is invaluable for subsequent comparison, therefore at the author's practice it is offered to all patients, despite reimbursement status. At this visit, appropriate anticoagulant and/or antiplatelet medications are confirmed. Additional risk factor management including glycemic control and continued smoking cessation are stressed.

8.1.3 Monthly Wound Checks

After initial post-operative evaluation, follow-up is designed to confirm that reperfusion has translated to improvement in wound healing.

- This visit is highly correlated also with additional but separate visits to managing podiatrists or wound physicians. Important checkpoints at this visit include wound photos with measurements (TAKE OFF THE SHOES!) and pulse assessment by handheld Doppler and physical exam.

These visits are carried out monthly to the third-month post-procedure. Duplex is again performed at this 3-month point, to compare pre- and post-procedure imaging. Tibial patency is usually dismal, so making it to this 3-month mark without reocclusion is usually associated with better limb salvage rates.

8.1.4   Assessing Plateaus and Return to Non-healing: Four-Month Visit

In the Reed paper in Annals of Vascular Surgery from 2016 they found that wound healing by 3 months was associated with a significant decrease in major amputations while healing taking greater than 4 months was associated with greater major adverse limb events (MALE—major amputation, surgical endarterectomy, or bypass) [10].

- It is therefore a good target to heal wounds before this 4-month point. The author's group also associates a plateau in healing at 4 months as an indicator for reintervention and reassessment of management, if clinically appropriate.

It is important for the vascular specialist to define that reperfusion is only a part of the wound-healing equation. Hemoglobin A1c management, infection management, and appropriate wound care are of absolutely critical importance to wound healing, and revascularization is NOT a substitute for appropriate multispecialty care. WIfI classification for CLI/CLTI patients has been shown to be of prognostic value as well and should be considered as a tool in the treatment process [11].

8.1.5   Amputations

Most patients do not desire amputation. However, in the world of critical ischemia, minor amputations can be limb- and lifestyle-saving, despite the corporeal disfigurement.

- Minor amputations (digital, ray, transmetatarsal, etc.) may be planned pre-revascularization or may become a necessity after. This conversation should be had prior to any revascularization, to best prepare patients for expected outcomes, aka appropriate informed consent.

Patients are generally much more accepting of minor and major amputations, if they have been appropriately informed and considered before any surgical intervention. Greater preparation also provides patients with resources such as physical therapy, offloading information, and prosthetic company contacts in the case amputations must be performed. Patients will generally also trust and confide in you as their practitioner if they see your predictions come to fruition, as opposed to being surprised by complications.

8.1.6   Minor Amputation Follow-Up

Minor amputations are best coordinated with the orthopedic or podiatric surgeons performing the procedures. Appropriate bandaging, compression wraps, and offloading footwear are vital to rapid healing. The goal is to reduce trauma to the wound bed in the early days of healing.

- Foot surgeons often see these patients weekly, with wound checks and dressing changes. Enzymatic or mechanical debridement may also be necessary.
- In the author's practice, these patients are seen monthly for pulse and wound checks in tandem with their foot surgeons.
- Wounds are documented with disposable rulers in the medical record as a second objective set of data to prove wound healing or stalling.

Additional considerations include excellent glycemic control for diabetics, preferably preemptively arranged with primary or endocrine physicians (<7% targets) [12]. Patients with ESRD will require regular dialysis and hypertension management. Finally, infected wounds may require additional antibiotic management orally or parenterally. This should be also performed prospectively with infectious disease specialists, when possible, as venous access may be required in addition to arrangements for regular infusion therapy.

8.1.7 Major Amputation Follow-Up

Minor amputations are usually the goal for advanced wounds limited to digits and the forefoot. However, in some patients, their disease at presentation is so fulminant that a major amputation (above-knee or below-knee amputations, AKA or BKA, respectively) may be the only lifesaving option. These are most often seen in patients with rapidly spreading infection, extensive tissue loss, and unresolving ischemic rest pain. In this sick patient cohort, time is of the essence.

- The vascular specialist may often be faced with the ethical decision between advancing directly to primary above or below-knee amputation vs the longer and potentially costly option of attempted limb salvage, associated with higher reintervention rates but potentially higher long-term morbidity.
- In the latter group, secondary major amputations are associated with up to 50% 2-year mortality [13].

Additionally, despite appropriate multidisciplinary care, revascularization and medical optimization, wounds, and minor amputations can still progress to major amputations. Patients in these categories still need resources and support, even more than those with limb salvage. Maintaining close relationships with local rehabilitation centers, prosthetic providers, and physiatrists are recommended. Additional considerations include psychosocial services to help patients understand and manage the major life changes associated with major amputation.

- Early mobilization and physical therapy are important to prepare patients for their lives after amputation, since only around 50% of patients will be ambulatory after major amputation [14].

Family members, spouses, and friends should be included in the process, since patients often have a difficult time integrating information comprehensively while concomitantly going through the process. Put yourself in their shoes! Set these sick patients up for success and redirection as much as possible. Their days are significantly more counted than yours. Compassion and consistency are probably the most important responses as a provider while patients embark on an often lonely and stigmatizing path. You can be a true patient advocate for them through this process simply by remaining available.

8.1.8 Life After Healing

Patients with smaller wounds, decreased comorbidities, clear insight into pathology, and appropriate care will often heal their wounds. Several studies have indicated that tibial patency is in fact *not* directly related to wound healing and limb salvage. Additionally, multiple vessel revascularization may not be associated with higher limb salvage rates [15].

- Once a wound is healed, appropriate risk factor modification may be sufficient to prevent reinjury and recurrence of ischemic or diabetic wounds. We, therefore, default to our standard 3-, 6-, and 12-month follow-up protocols for patients once they no longer have true critical ischemia.
- These visits will include both clinical and lower extremity arterial duplex. The role of duplex is often debated and given the absence of clinical symptoms may be omitted if felt more appropriate. This may save patients costs and visit time.

8.1.9 Death

While less common, deaths may occur in the perioperative period or within several weeks to months of the index procedures. This may be procedure related, but it must also be stated that these patients at baseline have dismal mortality rates, as stated previously.

- Patients and family members must be reminded of the gravity of disease *before* interventions.

It is the author's office practice to maintain contact with family members through these unfortunate events and where feasible, flowers or cards are a humane gesture to these families that often frequent our offices. It is also recommended that physicians speak with family members to convey condolences if possible. Remember the "if this was my relative" approach and it will serve you well.

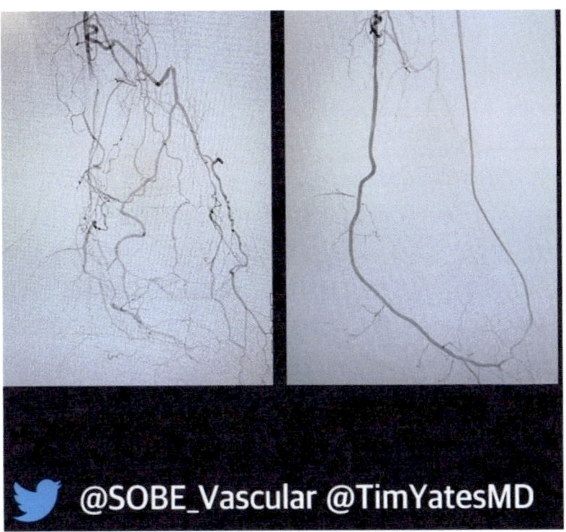

Fig. 8.1 Example of angiogram images celebrated on Twitter (images from author)

8.2 Monitoring the Wound

Timothy E. Yates

Wound monitoring after revascularization, wound care, and/or amputation should be consistent and regular. Wound care follow-up can be performed solely by the vascular specialists or in a multidisciplinary with involved consultants. Basic components include regular documentation of the wound photographically with wound measurements at predetermined intervals. Additionally, some ancillary technologies and techniques may improve wound healing and patient outcomes.

8.2.1 Angiography Is Not Enough

Many vascular specialists in modern times celebrate their angiograms with images, Twitter posts, and well-edited referral talks (Fig. 8.1).

And while there may be technical merit and even educational value to this process (or shameless plugging), this is only the beginning for wound patients. For true limb salvage, the vascular specialist is called to a higher standard and a significantly more involved process. Follow-up and wound monitoring provide objective evidence of wound healing and progress. In another section, titled "Follow-up Planning" I lay out our practice's approach to follow-up after consultation and revascularization. These steps will there-

fore not be rehashed here. Instead, we will focus on our approach to wound monitoring with reference to some additional clinical practices in the literature, as performed by a variety of specialties from internal medicine, podiatry, infection disease, and vascular specialties. The approach is simple: regular monitoring with photo documentation and measurements is done at every visit. These basic steps will provide the lion's share of necessary data to make additional clinical decisions.

8.2.2 Approaches to Wound Monitoring

Wound monitoring can be both direct and indirect. The process can also be very simple or more complex, depending on the structure of the involved practices. Whatever style is adopted, consistency, and sustainability are important. It is our recommendation that the revascularization specialist either become proficient in wound care or have competent partners/colleagues that can serve this purpose. Vascular surgeons typically include wound care as part of their training and practice. However, for interventional radiologists or cardiologists, this discipline may be more unfamiliar. In some scenarios, it may behoove the IR or IC to learn basic or advanced wound care.

This may provide a more comprehensive approach for their patients and allow them to build a stronger referral stream. This potential should be measured against the necessary time required to become proficient and a true assessment of long-term return on investment (ROI) [16]. Not all vascular specialists will have the desire to spend this time and effort. And yes, this is OK. It is *not* the author's suggestion that physicians try to master every skill related to their specialty. In fact, in modern medicine, this is usually time, cost, and psychologically prohibitive. If direct wound care is infeasible, then relationships with local wound care physicians, orthopedists, and podiatrists can prove to be invaluable. These specialists will invariably be more attuned to different varieties of debridement, offloading, wound cleaning, and additional therapies. Some will also have access to hyperbaric oxygenation, stem cell therapy, or other complementary strategies. When it comes to wound healing and limb salvage, consideration should be given to *all* options, at least initially. Each patient will have different tolerance in terms of time, finances, and clinical status.

There may also be significant benefits to developing community and hospital partnerships for wound care. Specialized wound centers can spend the time and resources needed to manage these patients. In fact, some studies have shown that these specialized locations can more efficiently treat wounds than larger and busier tertiary care centers and this attention is associated with decreased incidence of major amputations [17]. Timing of revascularization and wound care can usually be coordinated effectively once these relationships are established.

From the patient's perspective, early-stage wound care usually implies more time in physician offices. In the direct post-procedure period, it is beneficial to regularly assess wound healing and overall progress. This should be coupled with regular wound checks in the vascular specialty offices as well. This level of follow-up ensures patient buy-in, appropriate progress, and early correction for the occasional mishap. Wound monitoring should be photo documented at every visit, with measurements included in the photographs to provide objective evidence of wound healing or stalling. Additionally, with modern telecommunication technology, HIPAA-compliant images can be shared in addition to real-time video between providers to assess postoperative progress. Overall, this will give patients more confidence that their providers communicate effectively, in addition to taking their healing seriously. These steps normalize the process and create metrics to judge limb salvage and wound healing objectively.

8.2.3 Our Approach

Simply put, to heal a wound, you must look at it. It must not be an afterthought, but an integral part of the process. We do not have a wound care center in our office, but instead, we work very closely with a group of highly skilled and aggressive reconstructive podiatrists in the community, as well as some local hospital-based and freestanding wound care centers. We find the IR-podiatry relationship to be the best for our patients. This is simply because the two specialties can convene in rapid fashion on correcting pathological states but are also well equipped to perform adequate follow-up. Cardiologists can also benefit from this structure. Vascular surgeons, in contrast, may be able to manage all aspects from revascularization to wound care. Regardless, because we as IRs have excellent podiatry partners, our in-office exams are simple and to the point. Every time the patient comes after revascularization, we examine the wound. We see our wound patients 2 weeks after revascularization and then monthly until either the wound is healed, or additional revascularization is deemed necessary and/or feasible. Our medical assistants unwrap the wound each visit and document the wound photographically while taking measurements for longitudinal comparison. Physicians then examine pulses and the wound bed for signs of progress. All final documentation is then immediately faxed to the wound care physicians. Evidence of secondary infection, wound dehiscence after amputation, or new wounds/gangrene will usually be picked up early using this technique. It is also not uncommon for our physicians to connect with wound partners via video chat at the time of examination, to confer on progress and further treatment planning. We find this open loop of communication engenders trust between the patient and all care providers. Overall, we find this decreases unnecessary redundancy and wasted time with phone calls between offices.

8.2.4 Additional Considerations

A variety of more complex and comprehensive wound monitoring techniques exist. Each practice must calculate a ROI for implementing these technologies on a case-by-case basis. Important considerations include benefits to patients, start-up and maintenance costs, reimbursement, and time investment. Various technologies have proven beneficial in the wound-healing process. A representative but non-exhaustive list of some of these technologies is included below:

- Patient empowerment and self-monitoring: Psychosocial factors can be the most important obstacles to wound healing in patients with chronic disease [18]. Often there is a disconnect between current state and causal factors. Patient knowledge and empowerment have been shown to increase capacity for self-monitoring and care. The establishment of reasonable timelines can help the patient maintain and expand progress by reviewing self-monitored goals, targets, and achievements [19]. It has been demonstrated that thoughtful planning of lifestyle changes, endovascular intervention, and wound care increase patient motivation and treatment compliance [20, 21]. Through these empowerment methods, the physician–patient interaction is firmly established, and a coordinated attack can be launched to prevent amputation.
- Smart dressings [22]: This is a class of wound dressings containing a variety of microelectronic sensors, designed for real-time monitoring of the wound environment and can apply required actions to support the healing prog-

ress. Newer and more flexible microelectronic sensors enable next-generation wound dressing substrates or "electronic skin," for real-time monitoring of physiochemical markers in the wound environment.
- Hyperspectral imaging in small studies has been shown to be complementary to ABI measurements [23]. This technique can be used to assess local tissue oxygenation throughout healing and may serve as a troubleshooting option, particularly for wounds that stall in the healing process. This technology quantifies tissue perfusion and viability via the absorption of visible light in hemoglobin molecules over an ulcer. Tissue oxyhemoglobin, deoxyhemoglobin, and oxygen saturation can all be determined with this technique.
- Transcutaneous oximetry ($TcPO_2$) has been shown to be predictive of healing after amputation—a value less than 40 mmHg results in a 24% increased risk of healing complication compared to over 40 mmHg and the risk further increases as the TcPO2 decreases [24].
- Debridement: As mentioned in previous chapters, this technique involves removal of dead, damaged, or infected tissue, resulting in improved healing potential of the remaining healthy tissues. Even nonviable tissue, debris, calluses, or thickened skin surrounding ulcers can result in non-healing in the periphery. Removal of this tissue has been shown to improve wound-healing rates [9]. There are five major categories of debridement, which will only be listed here to be concise. The BEAMS acronym lists them all [25]:
  - Biological
  - Enzymatic
  - Autolytic
  - Mechanical
  - Surgical sharp
- Antibiotic therapy: WIfI staging system has robustly demonstrated that infection is an independent predictor of major amputation [26]. Incorporating the scale into the wound-monitoring process, therefore, is logical. It is made easier by incorporating tools like the Society for Vascular Surgery smartphone app, which can be used at each visit.

8.3 Summary

Irrespective of the method used, the basic approach to wound monitoring is to regularly inspect and evaluate the wound. Generally, best outcomes are associated with wound healing prior to 3 months, with major adverse limb events associated with healing times greater than 4 months. It is therefore our recommendation that the 4-month period after vascular reconstruction and limb-sparing amputation be more visit/follow-up intensive. This will allow involved parties to best optimize this process with the intent to recover early and decrease reintervention. Simple follow-up techniques include regular wound checks with photo documentation and longitudinal measurements. Additional technologies can be employed to assess tissue perfusion and wound healing, as delineated above.

References

1. Mustapha JA, Katzen BT, Neville RF, Lookstein RA, Zeller T, Miller LE, Jaff MR. Disease burden and clinical outcomes following initial diagnosis of critical limb ischemia in the Medicare population. J Am Coll Cardiol Intv. 2018;11(10):1011–2.
2. Bae JI, Won JH, Han SH, Lim SH, Hong YS, Kim JY, Kim JD, Kim JS. Endovascular revascularization for patients with critical limb ischemia: impact on wound healing and long term clinical results in 189 limbs. Korean J Radiol. 2013;14(3):430–8.
3. Faglia E, Clerici G, Clerissi J, Mantero M, Caminiti M, Quarantiello A, et al. When is a technically successful peripheral angioplasty effective in preventing above-the-ankle amputation in diabetic patients with critical limb ischaemia? Diabet Med. 2007;24:823–9.
4. Takeji Y, Yamaji K, Tomoi Y, Okazaki J, Tanaka K, Nagae A, Jinnouchi H, Hiramori S, Soga Y, Ando K. Impact of frailty on clinical outcomes in patients with critical limb ischemia. Circ Cardiovasc Interv. 2018;11(7):e006778.
5. Norgren L, Hiatt WR, Dormandy JA, Nehler MR, Harris KA, Fowkes FG, TASC II Working Group. Inter-society consensus for the management of peripheral arterial disease (TASC II). J Vasc Surg. 2007;45(Suppl. S):S5–67.
6. Jones WS, Patel MR, Dai D, Vemulapalli S, Subherwal S, Stafford J, Peterson ED. High mortality risks after major lower extremity amputation in Medicare patients with peripheral artery disease. Am Heart J. 2013;165:809–15. 815.e1
7. Suckow BD, Goodney PP, Cambria RA, Bertges DJ, Eldrup-Jorgensen J, Indes JE, Schanzer A, Stone DH, Kraiss LW, Cronenwett JL, Vascular Study Group of New England. Predicting functional status following amputation after lower extremity bypass. Ann Vasc Surg. 2012;26:67–78.
8. Armstrong EJ, Alam S, Henao S, Lee AC, DeRubertis BG, Montero-Baker M, Mena C, Cua B, Palena LM, Kovach R, Chandra V. Multidisciplinary care for critical limb ischemia: current gaps and opportunities for improvement. J Endovasc Ther. 2019;26(2):199–212.
9. Mustapha JA, Katzen BT, Neville RF, Lookstein RA, Zeller T, Miller LE, Jaff MR. Determinants of long-term outcomes and costs in the management of critical limb ischemia: a population-based cohort study. J Am Heart Assoc. 2018;7(16):e009724.
10. Reed GW, Salehi N, Giglou PR, Kafa R, Malik U, Maier M, Shishehbor MH. Time to wound healing and major adverse limb events in patients with critical limb ischemia treated with endovascular revascularization. Ann Vasc Surg. 2016;36:190–8.
11. van Haelst ST, Teraa M, Moll FL, de Borst GJ, Verhaar MC, Conte MS. Prognostic value of the Society for Vascular Surgery Wound, Ischemia, and foot Infection (WIfI) classification in patients with no-option chronic limb-threatening ischemia. J Vasc Surg. 2018;68(4):1104–13.
12. Fesseha BK, Abularrage CJ, Hines KF, Sherman R, Frost P, Langan S, Canner J, Likes KC, Hosseini SM, Jack G, Hicks CW. Association of hemoglobin A1c and wound healing in diabetic foot ulcers. Diabetes Care. 2018;41(7):1478–85.
13. Ogaki T, Iida O, Hata Y, Yamauchi N, Yokoi C, Takahara M, Terashi H, Mano T, Asada Y. The perioperative and long-term fates of patients with chronic limb-threatening ischaemia who underwent secondary major amputations. Int Wound J. 2022;19(1):36–43.
14. Chopra A, Azarbal AF, Jung E, Abraham CZ, Liem TK, Landry GJ, Moneta GL, Mitchell EL. Ambulation and functional outcome after major lower extremity amputation. J Vasc Surg. 2018;67(5):1521–9.
15. Hater H, Halak M, Sunoqrot H, Khaitovich B, Raskin D, Silverberg D. Revascularization of multiple tibial arteries is not associated with improved limb salvage. J Vasc Surg. 2021;74(1):170–7.
16. Asche CV, Kim M, Brown A, Golden A, Laack TA, Rosario J, Strother C, Totten VY, Okuda Y. Communicating value in simulation: cost–benefit analysis and return on investment. Acad Emerg Med. 2018;25(2):230–7.
17. Flores AM, Mell MW, Dalman RL, Chandra V. Benefit of multidisciplinary wound care center on the volume and outcomes of a vascular surgery practice. J Vasc Surg. 2019;70(5):1612–9.
18. Olivieri B, Yates TE, Vianna S, Adenikinju O, Beasley RE, Houseworth J. On the cutting edge: wound care for the endovascular specialist. Semin Intervent Radiol. 2018;35(05):406–26. Thieme Medical Publishers

19. Koenigsberg MR, Corliss J. Diabetes self-management: facilitating lifestyle change. Am Fam Physician. 2017;96(06):362–70.
20. Kavitha KV, Tiwari S, Purandare VB, Khedkar S, Bhosale SS, Unnikrishnan AG. Choice of wound care in diabetic foot ulcer: a practical approach. World J Diabetes. 2014;5(04):546–56.
21. Koenigsberg MR, Bartlett D, Cramer JS. Facilitating treatment adherence with lifestyle changes in diabetes. Am Fam Physician. 2004;69(02):309–16.
22. Farahani M, Shafiee A. Wound healing: from passive to smart dressings. Adv Healthc Mater. 2021;10(16):2100477.
23. Grambow E, Sandkühler NA, Groß J, Thiem DG, Dau M, Leuchter M, Weinrich M. Evaluation of hyperspectral imaging for follow-up assessment after revascularization in peripheral artery disease. J Clin Med. 2022;11(3):758.
24. Arsenault KA, Al-Otaibi A, Devereaux PJ, Thorlund K, Tittley JG, Whitlock RP. The use of transcutaneous oximetry to predict healing complications of lower limb amputations: a systematic review and meta-analysis. Eur J Vasc Endovasc Surg. 2012;43(3):329–36.
25. Broadus C. Debridement options: BEAMS made easy: learn how the various debridement methods promote wound healing. Wound Care Advisor. 2013;2(2):15–9.
26. Beropoulis E, Stavroulakis K, Schwindt A, Stachmann A, Torsello G, Bisdas T. Validation of the Wound, Ischemia, foot Infection (WIfI) classification system in nondiabetic patients treated by endovascular means for critical limb ischemia. J Vasc Surg. 2016;64(1):95–103. https://doi.org/10.1016/j.jvs.2016.01.040. Epub 2016 Mar 16

When Is the Wound Closed?

9

Timothy E. Yates and Sreekumar Madassery

9.1 Should I Reintervene?

Timothy E. Yates

Endovascular procedures are associated with minimally invasive approaches, decreased recovery time, as well as decreased complication rates compared to open surgical bypass [1]. However, compared to open surgical alternatives, endovascular procedures are plagued by the need for more frequent reinterventions and recurrence of ulcers [2, 3]. On the other hand, surgical revascularizations may not be possible in many patients, due to lack of suitable targets, and small arterial disease (SAD), seen in diabetic and renal failure patients. In the treatment of critical lower limb ischemia, multiple factors influence wound healing, including:

- Infection
- Extent of tissue loss
- Ischemia
- General cardiovascular status [4]

Many of the factors cross over into different areas of medicine and therefore, a team-oriented multidisciplinary approach is associated with best outcomes, like oncological care [5]. While the goal of tissue loss prevention is at the core of vascular reconstruction and wound care, the order in which this occurs will vary between differing patients. Some patients may be completely spared of amputation by timely intervention and wound care, while others may require a staged approach of revascularization and minor amputation, with recovery spanning months.

- The 3–4 month period post-revascularization is the "goldilocks" zone for healing wounds in most patients [6].
- After this period, the initial intervention, current clinical status, and wound care strategies must be reconsidered.
- Tibial patency is usually poor and if reocclusion or elastic recoil is present, a second-stage reintervention or alternate revascularization bed may need to be considered.

A "less is more" approach to revascularization is often used in the author's practice, which is in line with recent papers suggesting multivessel revascularization is in fact not associated with improved wound healing. Additionally, patients with diabetes demonstrate reduced primary

T. E. Yates
Interventional Vascular and Oncologic Radiology,
CLI Vascular at Palm Vascular Centers of Florida,
Fort Lauderdale, FL, USA

S. Madassery (✉)
Department of Vascular and Interventional Radiology,
Rush University Medical Center, Chicago, IL, USA

patency rates after percutaneous intervention, which may be secondary to more advanced disease states at presentation [7]. This will typically require higher reintervention rates.

- Despite this, Armstrong et al. found that diabetic patients typically can attain short-term primary patency, and limb salvage rates equivalent to non-diabetics, speaking in favor of rcintervention in appropriately chosen patients [5].

While there is often dispute in the revascularization approach across specialties, the author will focus on our practice-specific approaches. Geography, individual skill set, and patient characteristics must always be considered first. This guide is meant to be practical, to help you when the data does not fit directly into your decision-making. Factors in favor of reintervention in our practice include:

- Reasonable revascularization targets.
  - Angiosomal or angiographosomal targets are a *starting point* for index and subsequent revascularization, but direct targets may be technically infeasible. First, we consider patency of the original revascularization zone [8].

    In situation a, the prior revascularization remains patent. Consideration is given to additional tibial revascularization (i.e., pedal-plantar loop reconstruction) IF medical factors have been appropriately optimized (i.e., HgA1c, CHF, wound care, and control of infection). While the literature does not support multivessel revascularization in a single setting as advantageous, it is unclear if a staged approach with secondary patency measures has the same outcome [7].

    In situation b, the original revascularization zone is reoccluded. It is our practice to assess potential causes with extravascular ultrasound, angiography, and intravascular ultrasound, for technical defects (dissection, recoil, and/or thrombosis).

We generally recommend revascularization of the original target vessel(s) when feasible, with correction of any technical complication, if feasible. Indirect revascularization may still be a feasible alternative when direct targets are lacking, including peroneal-only revascularization [9, 10]. This may be related to evidence suggesting that tibial patency post-revascularization is not directly related to wound healing.

- While endovascular treatment for CLI is associated with acceptable limb salvage and wound healing rates, certain patient factors may predict poor outcomes. Some of these include renal failure, pedal disease (SAD), or isolated peroneal runoff. In this subset with failure of wound healing, additional revascularization approaches should be considered (i.e., deep venous arterialization) [11].
- Reasonable expectation of positive outcome/prognosis—clinical status and comorbidities are major factors in our practice's original decision to intervene. Reassessment of previously mentioned comorbid conditions still must be a priority when a second procedure is considered. It cannot be understated that critical limb ischemia patients have poor prognosis at baseline, up to 54% mortality by 4 years.
  - If the patient's status has declined considerably from one procedure to another, abstaining from intervention may be the best clinical decision, in line with the Hippocratic oath, *primum non nocere.*
  - Occasionally, major amputations are still unavoidable despite best clinical practices, which underscores the importance of presurgical patient education and informed consent. This will increase the likelihood that all outcomes have been reasonably considered.
- Patient insight and buy-in.
  - Though third on our list, this is probably the most important consideration for both index and secondary revascularization. Wound healing can require months, particularly with more advanced Rutherford/

WIfI stages. This should be clear to the patient prior to any intervention. If the patient is truly averse to lower extremity major amputation and desires all attempts at limb salvage, then the most likely clinical outcomes need to be described and considered. Finally, patients with improved insight and engagement in clinical education have overall improved outcomes in disease states such as coronary artery disease, diabetes, and wound care [12]. But in the end, the patient's desire is the priority. If they ever desire to stop treatment, we support them with resources for physical/psychological care and planning for prosthesis including referral to appropriate limb-replacement services and physical therapy.

- Social support.
  - Patients with critical limb ischemia have significant functional decline [13]. Social support has been linked to both improved clinical outcomes and quality of life in oncology patients [14, 15]. Because of the parallels of functional and clinical impairment with poor prognosis in CLI patients, similar value should be placed on adequate social support, particularly in the perioperative timeframe. This will help the patient in keeping follow-up appointments, manage in-home wound care, and to ensure appropriate medical management.
- Primary care and specialist referral buy-in.
  - As noted in previous sections, revascularization is only one of the many important factors associated with complete wound healing. Multidisciplinary care has been shown to be associated with improved outcomes in these patients. As such, frequent and clear communication with the primary physicians managing medical treatments and podiatry/orthopedic/vascular surgical services should be a priority. Timing revascularization with wound healing and additional amputation should be highly coordinated, with a preference to perform revascularization first [14].

9.2 To Stage or Not to Stage, That Is the Question

The appropriate order of revascularization can be challenging. Patient factors may limit the time a patient can be on the angiography table in a single session. An office-based laboratory is hyperaware of this given that outcomes are dependent on good patient selection. Occasionally, patients may require more extensive revascularization than is permissible with one intervention. Because of this, the interventionist may choose to stage a patient. In our practice it is our policy to maximize treatment efficacy. This can be accomplished by thorough preprocedural evaluation including pulse/wound examination and duplex or cross-sectional angiography. This type of anatomical evaluation will decrease the time the patient is on the table by better-understanding patient-specific anatomy, planning an approach to revascularization via plaque morphology, and deciding on the required equipment. This preprocedural planning can be likened to the process performed in planning of endovascular aortic aneurysm repair. In this way, in our practice, we usually can maximize treatment in one session. In selected cases where additional revascularization is deemed appropriate, appropriate recovery should be ensured for puncture sites and comorbid conditions (such as renal function).

9.3 Summary

Reintervention rates are typically higher in endovascular revascularization compared to open bypass, likely due to the increased complexity of disease patterns and/or comorbidities in the intervention-focused cohorts. Typically, outcomes are poorer if wound healing is incomplete past 4 months. Assessment for the need for additional revascularization should be tailored to patient tolerance and status, in addition to coordination with primary care and amputation/wound care specialists.

- Approach to revascularization (single session vs staging) is both provider- and patient-dependent, but in general, our practice is "less is more" considering multivessel tibial revascularization may not be associated with improved limb salvage, and in select patients, peroneal only revascularization may result in limb salvage.

Above all, patient understanding is vital to appropriate insight, and their desire ultimately should be weighed heavily against comorbid conditions and overall life expectancy when considering additional revascularization.

References

1. Fukunaga M, Kawasaki D, Nishimura M, Yamagami M, Fujiwara R, Nakata T. Clinical effects of planned endovascular therapy for critical limb ischemia patients with tissue loss. J Atheroscler Thromb. 2019;26(3):294–301.
2. Iida O, Nakamura M, Yamauchi Y, Fukunaga M, Yokoi Y, Yokoi H, Soga Y, Zen K, Suematsu N, Inoue N, Suzuki K. 3-Year outcomes of the OLIVE registry, a prospective multicenter study of patients with critical limb ischemia: a prospective, multi-center, three-year follow-up study on endovascular treatment for infrainguinal vessel in patients with critical limb ischemia. Cardiovasc Intervent. 2015;8(11):1493–502.
3. Meloni M, Izzo V, Giurato L, Del Giudice C, Da Ros V, Cervelli V, Gandini R, Uccioli L. Recurrence of critical limb ischemia after endovascular intervention in patients with diabetic foot ulcers. Adv Wound Care. 2018;7(6):171–6.
4. Ciocan RA, Bolboacă SD, Drugan CR, Gherman CD. The pattern of risk factors in patients with critical limb ischemia. Acta Med Transilvanica. 2018;23(3):52–5.
5. Armstrong EJ, Alam S, Henao S, Lee AC, DeRubertis BG, Montero-Baker M, Mena C, Cua B, Palena LM, Kovach R, Chandra V. Multidisciplinary care for critical limb ischemia: current gaps and opportunities for improvement. J Endovasc Ther. 2019;26(2):199–212.
6. Reed GW, Salehi N, Giglou PR, Kafa R, Malik U, Maier M, Shishehbor MH. Time to wound healing and major adverse limb events in patients with critical limb ischemia treated with endovascular revascularization. Ann Vasc Surg. 2016;36:190–8.
7. Hater H, Halak M, Sunoqrot H, Khaitovich B, Raskin D, Silverberg D. Revascularization of multiple tibial arteries is not associated with improved limb salvage. J Vasc Surg. 2021;74(1):170–7.
8. Shackles C, Herman, K, Gallo V, Rundback JH. Angiographosome-directed revascularization. Endovascular Today. 2018;17(5): 52–7.
9. Bae JI, Won JH, Han SH, Lim SH, Hong YS, Kim JY, Kim JD, Kim JS. Endovascular revascularization for patients with critical limb ischemia: impact on wound healing and long term clinical results in 189 limbs. Korean J Radiol. 2013;14(3):430–8.
10. Faglia E, Clerici G, Clerissi J, Mantero M, Caminiti M, Quarantiello A, et al. When is a technically successful peripheral angioplasty effective in preventing above-the-ankle amputation in diabetic patients with critical limb ischaemia? Diabet Med. 2007;24:823–9.
11. Fernandez N, McEnaney R, Marone LK, Rhee RY, Leers S, Makaroun M, Chaer RA. Predictors of failure and success of tibial interventions for critical limb ischemia. J Vasc Surg. 2010;52(4):834–42.
12. Adams RJ. Improving health outcomes with better patient understanding and education. Risk Manag Healthcare Policy. 2010;3:61.
13. McDermott MM. Medical management of functional impairment in peripheral artery disease: a review. Prog Cardiovasc Dis. 2018;60(6):586–92.
14. Chiang N, Wang J, Marie N, Wu A, Ravindra R, Robinson D. Evaluation of clinical outcomes following minor amputations in australia–an important consideration for timing of revascularisation. Ann Vasc Surg. 2021;76:389–98.
15. Seiler A, Jenewein J. Resilience in cancer patients. Front Psych. 2019;10:208.

Long-Term Imaging

10

Philip T. Skummer, Matthew J. Scheidt,
Parag J. Patel, and Sreekumar Madassery

10.1 How to Follow Arterial Wounds?

Philip T. Skummer, Matthew J. Scheidt,
and Parag J. Patel

10.1.1 Long-Term Imaging Follow-Up

Imaging follow-up is one component of comprehensive patient care prior to and after any arterial or venous intervention. Routine surveillance and subsequent treatment plan frequently depend on locoregional practices, patients' clinically relevant symptoms, and status of wound healing. Imaging follow-up can be divided into arterial and venous procedures from a practical standpoint, with further granular details depending on the progression along the disease pathway, as well as the condition treated and by what technique. This chapter will primarily focus on peripheral arterial disease (PAD) and deep venous disease.

P. T. Skummer · M. J. Scheidt · P. J. Patel
Department of Interventional Radiology, Froedtert
Memorial Lutheran Hospital - Medical College of
Wisconsin, Milwaukee, WI, USA
e-mail: Pskummer@mcw.edu; Mscheidt@mcw.edu;
Papatel@mcw.edu

S. Madassery (✉)
Department of Vascular and Interventional Radiology,
Rush University Medical Center, Chicago, IL, USA

10.1.2 Arterial

10.1.2.1 Peripheral Arterial Disease

Peripheral arterial disease exists on a spectrum from asymptomatic to claudication to limb-threatening ischemia, both chronic and acute. The annual incidence of new lesions on duplex ultrasound and claudication symptoms in patients previously diagnosed with asymptomatic PAD occurs at 35% and 26%, respectively [1]. A position statement by the Society of Vascular Surgery (SVS) states there is no data on benefit or harm for routine surveillance in asymptomatic PAD, particularly with ankle brachial index (ABI) testing. Overall, the clinical benefit of screening all asymptomatic patients is unclear, as well as the significance of any findings related to that screening.

- The standard of care is to only perform invasive PAD treatment on patients with clinically significant lifestyle limiting claudication or limb-threatening ischemia, which can be performed through open bypass or endovascular therapy (EVT) [2].

Modalities for follow-up include routine clinical evaluation with history and physical, ABI measurements, and duplex ultrasound (DUS). Computed tomography (CT) or magnetic resonance (MR) angiography is not recommended for routine surveillance given cost, radiation, use of iodinated contrast, and/or procedural risks [3].

© The Author(s), under exclusive license to Springer Nature Switzerland AG 2023
S. Madassery, A. Patel (eds.), *Limb Preservation for the Vascular Specialist*,
https://doi.org/10.1007/978-3-031-36480-8_10

There have been several articles published on the routine surveillance follow-up of open lower extremity re-vascularization with physical exam, ABI, and DUS for at least 2 years [4]. Surgical bypass arterial anastomoses are particularly prone to stenoses, and over time, there may be progression of atherosclerotic disease resulting in hemodynamically significant stenoses of the native arteries. Early critical graft stenosis has been found to result in lower patency rates and a higher incidence of amputation [5].

- DUS allows for the accurate evaluation of all aspects of arterial reconstruction. Surveillance of lower extremity bypass grafts routinely includes immediate post-procedure follow-up with subsequent exams at 1 month, 6 months, 12 months, and then annually with multiple authors also including a 3-month follow-up examination [6, 7].

Early repair of graft stenoses has demonstrated improved long-term patency prior to complete occlusion [8]. Stone et al. developed ultrasound criteria using peak systolic velocity (PSV) of a stenosis and velocity ratio (Vr), which is the velocity at the stenosis relative to the non-stenotic segment [9]. These authors followed patients every 6 months after the baseline examination and determined:

- PSV >300 cm/s and Vr >3.5 are predictive of >70% stenosis. Patients with >70% stenosis were then considered for repair or angiography [9].
- Patients with PSV 180–300 cm/s and Vr >2–3.5 were considered to have stenosis between 50% and 70% and underwent short-term interval follow-up in 2–3 months [9].
- A similar follow-up and treatment protocol was implemented by Landry et al., who also included uniformly low PSV <45 cm/s throughout the graft as indication for arteriography. Lesions resulting in 50% or more stenosis on angiography were treated [7].

There is a relative paucity of high-quality research on an optimal imaging follow-up plan for EVT compared to the more defined guidelines and evidence supporting recommended surveillance and re-intervention on asymptomatic bypass graft stenoses. Technically successful EVT of PAD has been defined as residual stenosis of 30% or less [10]. There have been a variety of studies evaluating DUS in concert with clinical follow-up; many of which have been limited by sample size, inconsistencies with follow-up, and relative historical data compared to more modern technology and procedural techniques. Furthermore, many studies have heterogenous patient populations regarding arteries treated, techniques used (angioplasty with or without stenting), and indication for treatment (claudication, chronic limb-threatening ischemia, or acute limb ischemia).

DUS findings from de novo stenoses or infrainguinal vein bypass grafts have been extrapolated and applied to EVT. Baril et al., reported DUS successfully predicted in-stent stenosis within the superficial femoral artery (SFA), which was subsequently confirmed with angiographic findings. Baril et al., followed patients at 1 month, 3 months, and then every 6 months with DUS, ABI, and clinical evaluation [10].

- They determined the combination of PSV >275 cm/s and Vr >3.5 was the most specific and predictive for in-stent stenosis of >80%.
- These authors noted that symptomatic patients had a mean PSV >360 cm/s and Vr >3.6, suggesting that earlier angiography with clinically appropriate intervention could be considered when in-stent stenosis was 80%.
- Similar findings were reported by Shrikhande et al., with PSV > 204 cm/s having a 98% sensitivity and 95% specificity for detecting a 70% or greater SFA stenosis; as well as PSV >223 cm/s having 94% sensitivity and 95% specificity for detecting a 70% or greater femoropopliteal (FP) stenosis [11].

Re-intervention when clinically appropriate could result in improved assisted patency rates, given that patients who present with complete occlusion have lower rates of technically successful restoration of flow, and increased risk of distal embolization [10]. Contrary to the predictive value of DUS for above-the-knee inflow lesions, there are contradictory results on tibial surveillance.

Shrikhande et al. reported tibial DUS results poorly correlated to angiographic findings, while Saqib et al. reported the opposite. It should be noted that many of these patients were symptomatic with re-stenosis and presented with nonhealing or worsening wounds and/or rest pain. Only 10% of patients were asymptomatic in the setting of recurrent stenosis [11, 12].

While DUS may be able to accurately diagnose recurrent stenoses, there have been overall conflicting results on the value of screening DUS on long-term patency.

- Mewissen et al. reported significantly high clinical failure at 1 year in those patients with at least 50% stenosis of FP EVT at 30-day follow-up DUS [13].
- Humphries et al. reported abnormal DUS for any infrainguinal EVT at 30 days was associated with increased major amputation risk, but did not correlate with primary patency rates [14].
- Troutman et al. found 58% of patients with abnormal screening ultrasound with PSV >300 cm/s, Vr >3.0, or diffuse PSV <50 cm/s went on to occlusion, which was significantly more than the 3% of patients who occluded with normal screening DUS [15].
- Bui et al. demonstrated mixed results with DUS after FP disease treated with EVT and concluded questionable benefit of DUS surveillance [16]. In patients with normal DUS on baseline examination 1 week after EVT, approximately 60% remained normal during the observation period. While patients with abnormal baseline DUS after EVT, approximately 40% remained stable or improved without intervention. It should be noted, re-intervention was dependent predominantly on recurrent symptoms or nonhealing wounds, rather than DUS findings.

Early failure within the first 6 months after EVT is predictive of poor primary and secondary patency of repeat EVT intervention [17]. Early EVT failure was found to be associated with critical limb ischemia as the indication for re-intervention compared to claudication; this is possibly related to disease burden at time of presentation, as well as the remaining burden at the end of the procedure [13].

- It should be noted that below-the-knee interventions may suffer from repeat interventions as there are limited options other than atherectomy and angioplasty for treatment in this space, although many newer tools are being developed. Additionally, small artery disease (SAD) pattern in diabetics and renal failure patients can limit successful outflow for EVT or Surgical interventions.

It is difficult to predict which patients with stenoses on DUS are going to progress given limited data on the pathophysiology, and temporal course of residual or recurrent stenoses after EVT. These imaging endpoints have been considered within the context of the patient and any symptoms [18].

- There is a paucity of data regarding when to intervene in asymptomatic re-stenosis. Some authors have suggested re-intervening if ABI decreased by greater than 0.15 from post-procedure baseline or if greater than 70% stenosis on DUS to improve long-term absolute patency, particularly in intermediate or long-length stenoses [19].

10.1.3 Conclusion

- A screening DUS can be included with comprehensive routine clinical follow-up involving history, physical exam, and hemodynamic measurements; however, should not function as the sole follow-up method given the dependence on operator technique and possible imaging limitations related to body habitus, prior surgery, or dense calcifications.
- Intervening on residual or recurrent stenosis after EVT may improve limb salvage rates [19].

- No high-quality randomized control trials exist comparing DUS to other screening modalities nor evaluating the benefit and long-term outcomes of prophylactic intervention after EVT. A threshold of recurrent severe stenosis (>70%) has been suggested for re-intervention on asymptomatic patients to avoid the potential risk of intervening on a smaller area of stenosis that may have had an otherwise benign course [19].
- Patients who may benefit most from close surveillance and early re-intervention include those with failed prior open or surgical interventions, as well as patients presenting with severe ischemia, persistent wounds/tissue loss, new stenotic lesions post-intervention, poor runoff, and/or long-segment treatments [3, 19, 20].

10.1.4 Bypass Follow-Up

The official suggestion from SVS is patients who were treated for intermittent claudication are part of a clinical surveillance program that consists of an interval history to detect new symptoms, ensure compliance with medical therapies, record subjective functional improvements, pulse examination, and measurement of resting and, if possible, post-exercise ABIs [2].

- Arterial disease treated with bypass should be evaluated with physical examination, ABI, and DUS within the first month of treatment to establish a baseline, then again at 6 months, 12 months, and annually if there are no new symptoms [8].
- A 3-month follow-up should be included with infra-inguinal vein bypass grafts. Angiogram with possible intervention should be performed should PSV >300 cm/s or Vr >3.5 [3].
- Cross-sectional imaging should be performed if there is a decrease in ABI >0.15 or mid-graft velocity decrease to PSV <45 cm/s without obvious cause on DUS. Closer follow-up

should be performed within 6–12 weeks in patients with moderately elevated PSV (200–300 cm/s) or Vr (3.5 > Vr > 2) [3, 21].
- Patients with a worsening clinical vascular examination, return of rest pain, nonhealing wounds, or new tissue loss should undergo DUS at any time point.

10.1.5 EVT Patients

- Post-EVT patients should be evaluated with physical examination, ABI, and DUS within the first month of treatment to establish a baseline, 6 months, 12 months, and then annually if there are no new symptoms [8].
- Continued surveillance at 3 months and then every 6 months is indicated for the endovascular interventions using stents because of the potential increased difficulty of treating an occlusive or stenotic in-stent lesion [8].
- Also, 3 and 6 months follow-up is recommended for those who have undergone angioplasty or atherectomy to treat critical limb ischemia because of an increased risk of recurrent rest pain or tissue loss should the intervention fail as well as those who have had any tibial artery intervention [8].
- Those patients with a worsening clinical vascular examination, return of rest pain, nonhealing wounds, or new tissue loss should undergo repeated DUS or possible cross-sectional arterial imaging (6, 3), especially if decrease in ABI >0.15 [8].
- Angiogram with re-intervention should be considered in patients with DUS-detected restenosis >70%, as defined as PSV >300 cm/second or PSV ratio >3.5 [3, 14].
- Recurrence of symptoms such as rest pain or new/worsening wounds should prompt DUS, regardless of time from intervention. Suggested follow-up intervals with DUS and recommended next steps based on DUS findings are summarized in Tables 10.1 and 10.2.

Table 10.1 Follow-up intervals

	Baseline (within 1 month)	3 months	6 months	Every 12 months	Every 6 months
Peripheral arterial disease					
Intermittent claudication				x	
Lower extremity bypass	x	x	x	x	
Endovascular therapy[a]	x	x	x		x
Treatment with critical limb ischemia	x	x	x		x
Deep venous disease					
Pharmaco-mechanical catheter-directed thrombolysis	x	x	x	x	
Left iliac vein stenting/Iliocaval reconstruction	x	x	x	x	

[a]Consideration can be given to annual surveillance in patients with stable examinations, particularly in those without stent grafts

Table 10.2 Abnormalities on DUS or Exam (Peripheral Arterial Disease)

Elevated PSV (200–300 cm/s) or Vr (3.5 > Vr > 2)	Repeat DUS in 6–12 weeks, resume surveillance timing if no significant change or angiogram with possible intervention if worsen
PSV > 300 cm/s or Vr > 3.5	Angiogram with possible intervention
ABI decrease >0.15	Correlate with DUS, if no evident abnormality, then further work-up with CT or MR angiogram or catheter angiogram with possible intervention
PSV < 45 cm/s in bypass graft	Correlate with DUS, if no evident abnormality, then further work-up with CT or MR angiogram or catheter angiogram with possible intervention
Change in vascular examination, rest pain, nonhealing wounds, or new tissue loss	Perform DUS then treatment based upon findings as described above
PAA stent narrowing 50% or more	Catheter angiogram

DUS Duplex ultrasound, *PSV* peak systolic velocity, *VR* velocity ratio, *ABI* Ankle brachial index, *CT* computed tomography, *MR* magnetic resonance

10.2 How to Follow Venous Wounds?

Philip T. Skummer, Matthew J. Scheidt, and Parag J. Patel

10.2.1 Venous

10.2.1.1 Deep Venous Diseases

Deep venous disease exists on a spectrum regarding the presence and extent of thrombus, type of intervention required, and chronicity of thrombus. Venous DUS, CT/MR venography, and Direct Catheter Venography can play an important role in pre-procedure planning and follow-up in select cases. Surgical or endovascular intervention for deep venous thrombosis (DVT) is primarily driven by the location of the thrombus, with the main goal of prevention, or reducing severity of post-thrombotic syndrome (PTS). The Acute Venous Thrombosis: Thrombus Removal with Adjunctive Catheter-Directed Thrombolysis (ATTRACT) Trial was a major multi-centered, prospective, randomized, assessor-blinded clinical trial evaluating the relationship between endovascular therapy for acute (14 days or less) proximal (femoral through iliac vein) DVT, that included evaluation of PTS, and quality of life [22].

- This study demonstrated that pharmaco-mechanical catheter-directed thrombolysis resulted in lower clot burden at 1 month and common femoral vein non-compressibility was associated with greater incidence and severity of PTS.

- The follow-up imaging regimen in this trial included DUS at baseline, 1 month, and 12 months post-procedure with reflux DUS at 12 months.
- Post-procedure success can be defined with objective scoring to grade residual thrombus, such as the Venous Clinical Severity Scoring, Villalta scoring system, or venous registry index, with post-procedure success considered >50% clearance of luminal clot burden [23].

Similar to PAD, there is a paucity of high-quality studies to evaluate the optimal timing of imaging follow-up on patients after intervention. Long-term patient-centered outcomes such as quality of life scores and absence of PTS symptoms, are key components of post-intervention follow-up [23].

- One potential metric to be considered with long-term imaging follow-up is the presence of venous reflux on DUS.
- Comparison between both lower extremities can be used as a functional surrogate measure for presence of clinically relevant PTS [23].
- New/worsening symptoms or wounds should prompt DUS, regardless of time from intervention.
- Suggested follow-up intervals with DUS and recommended next steps based upon DUS findings are summarized in Tables 10.1 and 10.3.

Table 10.3 Abnormalities on DUS or Exam (Deep Venous Disease)

Unable to evaluate iliac vein patency	CT or MR venogram
In-stent stenosis or thrombus >50%	Catheter venogram
Recurrent symptoms	Perform DUS then treatment based upon findings as described above

DUS Duplex ultrasound, *CT* computed-tomography, *MR* magnetic resonance

10.2.1.2 May-Thurner Syndrome

May-Thurner Syndrome (MTS), also known as iliac vein compression syndrome, is secondary to extrinsic compression of the left common iliac vein by the right common iliac artery, resulting in luminal narrowing, which can potentially lead to acute thrombosis. Patients with acute thrombosis often undergo catheter-directed thrombolysis as this can lead to chronic, more difficult to treat, occlusion when not addressed. The standard of care for treating patients with clinically relevant iliac vein compression syndrome pathology is stenting of the left common iliac vein, particularly now with dedicated venous stents. Several studies have evaluated the efficacy of treatment protocols for MTS, both in the acute and chronic setting, as well as if DVT is present.

In May-Thurner syndrome, routine clinical follow-up consists of a physical exam, screening DUS, and determining CEAP (clinical, etiological, anatomical, and pathophysiological) classification, venous clinical severity score (VCSS), and venous claudication score. Particular attention on post-treatment surveillance DUS is made for any extrinsic stent compression, in-stent stenosis, and stent integrity.

- Various follow-up schedules were proposed by different authors with most agreeing on early post-procedure clinic visits and DUS at 2–6 weeks, then 6 months, 12 months, and annually [24, 25]. Evidence of flow limiting in-stent stenosis or thrombosis on DUS, as well as worsening symptoms, should prompt diagnostic venography with possible intervention.

10.2.2 Iliocaval Stent Reconstruction

Iliocaval Stent reconstruction serves as an adjunct to iliocaval or iliofemoral thrombosis and as part of the treatment of MTS. Most studies regarding follow-up for iliocaval reconstruction are institution dependent, reported as part of publications describing the technical factors related to the procedure, with a heterogenous patient population involving both acute and chronic thrombus, as well as thrombosis secondary to an inferior vena cava filter. Imaging follow-up should not happen in isolation and patients should be clinically evaluated at similar time points, to determine symptomatic improvement. Clinical evaluation includes:

- Obtaining objective data points such as CEAP classification.
- Physical exam to evaluate for skin changes or ulceration.
- Leg circumference measurements.
- Record of patient compliance regarding the use of compression garments and medication adherence [26].

The Cardiovascular and Interventional Radiological Society of Europe (CIRSE) developed practice guidelines for iliocaval stenting and recommended post-procedural monitoring with physical examination and assessment of CEAP classification, as well as DUS to identify stent thrombosis or in-stent stenosis requiring intervention.

- Suggested surveillance intervals by CIRSE were 1 month, 3 months, 6 months, and 12 months post-procedure then annually afterward [27].
- Hage et al. conducted a survey of providers performing iliocaval reconstruction with approximately 95% of responders performing imaging follow-up with either DUS or CT venogram within the first month then a majority repeating relevant imaging at 6 months intervals afterward [28].
- This follow-up regimen was similar to many of the published articles at individual institutions, with early acquisition of baseline examination with DUS obtained immediately post-procedure through the first month, at 6 months, and then annually [29, 30].
- Recurrent luminal obstruction of greater than 50% on post-intervention imaging warrants further evaluation with dedicated catheter-directed venography. Catheter-directed intervention is warranted for stent thrombosis or in-stent stenosis of at least 50% [26].

10.2.3 Chronic Venous Disease

Chronic venous disease is typically the sequela of DVT resulting in venous insufficiency, reflux, and hypertension. Endovenous thermal ablation (EVTA) can be utilized to treat these incompetent veins and re-distribute blood through more functional venous drainage pathways. Successful treatment can be documented by DUS showing acute venous wall thickening then complete occlusion and ultimately obliteration of the treated venous segments [26].

- One study had a seven visit, 8-month follow-up schedule to assess treated veins at 2 days, 1 week, 2 weeks, 1 month, 3 months, 5 months, and 8 months [31]. Such a detailed follow-up program may not be required for all patients as the average time to essential venous obliteration is less than 6 months [31].
- A multi-society consensus statement on superficial venous insufficiency with EVTA defined the endpoint in DUS surveillance as the time when the treated vein is no longer sonographically visualized.
- In addition, follow-up DUS should be performed if new varicosities develop to determine if recurrent reflux in a previously treated vein or a new venous pathway is responsible for the clinical symptoms [32].

References

1. Mohler ER 3rd, Bundens W, Denenberg J, Medenilla E, Hiatt WR, Criqui MH. Progression of asymptomatic peripheral artery disease over 1 year. Vasc Med. 2012;17(1):10–6.
2. Society for Vascular Surgery Lower Extremity Guidelines Writing Group, Conte MS, Pomposelli FB, Clair DG, Geraghty PJ, McKinsey JF, et al. Society for Vascular Surgery practice guidelines for atherosclerotic occlusive disease of the lower extremities: management of asymptomatic disease and claudication. J Vasc Surg. 2015;61(3 Suppl):2S–41S.
3. Conte MS, Bradbury AW, Kolh P, White JV, Dick F, Fitridge R, et al. Global vascular guidelines on the management of chronic limb-threatening ischemia. Eur J Vasc Endovasc Surg. 2019;58(1S):S1–S109. e33.

4. Norgren L, Hiatt WR, Dormandy JA, Nehler MR, Harris KA, Fowkes FG, et al. Inter-Society Consensus for the Management of Peripheral Arterial Disease (TASC II). J Vasc Surg. 2007;45 Suppl. S:S5–67.

5. Mofidi R, Kelman J, Berry O, Bennett S, Murie JA, Dawson AR. Significance of the early postoperative duplex result in infrainguinal vein bypass surveillance. Eur J Vasc Endovasc Surg. 2007;34(3):327–32. (25)

6. Armstrong PA, Bandyk DF, Wilson JS, Shames ML, Johnson BL, Back MR. Optimizing infrainguinal arm vein bypass patency with duplex ultrasound surveillance and endovascular therapy. J Vasc Surg. 2004;40(4):724–30. discussion 730-1

7. Landry GJ, Moneta GL, Taylor LM Jr, Edwards JM, Yeager RA, Porter JM. Long-term outcome of revised lower-extremity bypass grafts. J Vasc Surg. 2002;35(1):56–62. discussion 62-3

8. Zierler RE, Jordan WD, Lal BK, Mussa F, Leers S, Fulton J, et al. The Society for Vascular Surgery practice guidelines on follow-up after vascular surgery arterial procedures. J Vasc Surg. 2018;68(1):256–84.

9. Stone PA, Armstrong PA, Bandyk DF, Keeling WB, Flaherty SK, Shames ML, et al. Duplex ultrasound criteria for femorofemoral bypass revision. J Vasc Surg. 2006;44(3):496–502.

10. Baril DT, Rhee RY, Kim J, Makaroun MS, Chaer RA, Marone LK. Duplex criteria for determination of in-stent stenosis after angioplasty and stenting of the superficial femoral artery. J Vasc Surg. 2009;49(1):133–8. discussion 139

11. Shrikhande GV, Graham AR, Aparajita R, Gallagher KA, Morrissey NJ, McKinsey JF, et al. Determining criteria for predicting stenosis with ultrasound duplex after endovascular intervention in infrainguinal lesions. Ann Vasc Surg. 2011;25(4):454–60.

12. Saqib NU, Domenick N, Cho JS, Marone L, Leers S, Makaroun MS, et al. Predictors and outcomes of restenosis following tibial artery endovascular interventions for critical limb ischemia. J Vasc Surg. 2013;57(3):692–9.

13. Mewissen MW, Kinney EV, Bandyk DF, Reifsnyder T, Seabrook GR, Lipchik EO, et al. The role of duplex scanning versus angiography in predicting outcome after balloon angioplasty in the femoropopliteal artery. J Vasc Surg. 1992;15(5):860–5. discussion 865-6

14. Humphries MD, Pevec WC, Laird JR, Yeo KK, Hedayati N, Dawson DL. Early duplex scanning after infrainguinal endovascular therapy. J Vasc Surg. 2011;53(2):353–8.

15. Troutman DA, Madden NJ, Dougherty MJ, Calligaro KD. Duplex ultrasound diagnosis of failing stent grafts placed for occlusive disease. J Vasc Surg. 2014;60(6):1580–4.

16. Bui TD, Mills JLS, Ihnat DM, Gruessner AC, Goshima KR, Hughes JD. The natural history of duplex-detected stenosis after femoropopliteal endovascular therapy suggests questionable clinical utility of routine duplex surveillance. J Vasc Surg. 2012;55(2):346–52.

17. Robinson WP 3rd, Nguyen LL, Bafford R, Belkin M. Results of second-time angioplasty and stenting for femoropopliteal occlusive disease and factors affecting outcomes. J Vasc Surg. 2011;53(3):651–7.

18. Tielbeek AV, Rietjens E, Buth J, Vroegindeweij D, Schol FP. The value of duplex surveillance after endovascular intervention for femoropopliteal obstructive disease. Eur J Vasc Endovasc Surg. 1996;12(2):145–50.

19. Connors G, Todoran TM, Engelson BA, Sobieszczyk PS, Eisenhauer AC, Kinlay S. Percutaneous revascularization of long femoral artery lesions for claudication: patency over 2.5 years and impact of systematic surveillance. Catheter Cardiovasc Interv. 2011;77(7):1055–62.

20. Gerhard-Herman MD, Gornik HL, Barrett C, Barshes NR, Corriere MA, Drachman DE, et al. 2016 AHA/ACC Guideline on the Management of Patients With Lower Extremity Peripheral Artery Disease: a Report of the American College of Cardiology/American Heart Association Task Force on Clinical Practice Guidelines. J Am Coll Cardiol. 2017;69(11): e71–e126.

21. Mills JLS, Wixon CL, James DC, Devine J, Westerband A, Hughes JD. The natural history of intermediate and critical vein graft stenosis: recommendations for continued surveillance or repair. J Vasc Surg. 2001;33(2):273–8. discussion 278-80

22. Weinberg I, Vedantham S, Salter A, Hadley G, Al-Hammadi N, Kearon C, et al. Relationships between the use of pharmacomechanical catheter-directed thrombolysis, sonographic findings, and clinical outcomes in patients with acute proximal DVT: results from the ATTRACT Multicenter Randomized Trial. Vasc Med. 2019;24(5):442–51.

23. Vedantham S, Grassi CJ, Ferral H, Patel NH, Thorpe PE, Antonacci VP, et al. Reporting standards for endovascular treatment of lower extremity deep vein thrombosis. J Vasc Interv Radiol. 2009;20(7 Suppl):S391–408.

24. Bozkaya H, Cinar C, Ertugay S, Korkmaz M, Guneyli S, Posacioglu H, et al. Endovascular treatment of iliac vein compression (May-Thurner) syndrome: angioplasty and stenting with or without manual aspiration thrombectomy and catheter-directed thrombolysis. Ann Vasc Dis. 2015;8(1):21–8.

25. Rollo JC, Farley SM, Oskowitz AZ, Woo K, DeRubertis BG. Contemporary outcomes after venography-guided treatment of patients with May-Thurner syndrome. J Vasc Surg Venous Lymphat Disord. 2017;5(5):667–676.e1.

26. Kurklinsky AK, Bjarnason H, Friese JL, Wysokinski WE, McBane RD, Misselt A, et al. Outcomes of venoplasty with stent placement for chronic thrombosis of the iliac and femoral veins: single-center experience. J Vasc Interv Radiol. 2012;23(8):1009–15.

27. Mahnken AH, Thomson K, de Haan M, O'Sullivan GJ. CIRSE standards of practice guidelines on iliocaval stenting. Cardiovasc Intervent Radiol. 2014;37(4):889–97.

28. Hage AN, Srinivasa RN, Abramowitz SD, Cooper KJ, Khaja MS, Barnes GD, et al. Endovascular iliocaval reconstruction for the treatment of iliocaval thrombosis: from imaging to intervention. Vasc Med. 2018;23(3):267–75.

29. Chick JFB, Srinivasa RN, Cooper KJ, Jairath N, Hage AN, Spencer B, et al. Endovascular iliocaval reconstruction for chronic iliocaval thrombosis: the data, where we are, and how it is done. Tech Vasc Interv Radiol. 2018;21(2):92–104.

30. Hage AN, Srinivasa RN, Abramowitz SD, Gemmete JJ, Reddy SN, Chick JFB. Endovascular iliocaval stent reconstruction for iliocaval thrombosis: a multi-institutional international practice pattern survey. Ann Vasc Surg. 2018;49:64–74.

31. Yang CH, Chou HS, Lo YF. Incompetent great saphenous veins treated with endovenous 1,320-nm laser: results for 71 legs and morphologic evolvement study. Dermatol Surg. 2006;32(12):1453–7.

32. Khilnani NM, Grassi CJ, Kundu S, D'Agostino HR, Khan AA, McGraw JK, et al. Multi-society consensus quality improvement guidelines for the treatment of lower-extremity superficial venous insufficiency with endovenous thermal ablation from the Society of Interventional Radiology, Cardiovascular Interventional Radiological Society of Europe, American College of Phlebology and Canadian Interventional Radiology Association. J Vasc Interv Radiol. 2010;21(1):14–31.

Long-Term Medical Management 11

Ian Del Conde and Sreekumar Madassery

11.1 Arterial Disease Management

Ian Del Conde

Peripheral arterial disease (PAD) is highly prevalent in the general population, and these patients are at elevated risk of cardiovascular morbidity and mortality.

- With decreasing ankle-brachial indices below 0.9, the event rate of cardiovascular endpoints rapidly rises.
- In patients with an ankle-brachial index below 0.7, the 5-year risk of major cardiac events is approximately 19%, which is higher than the highest risk category of the Framingham risk score [1] (Fig. 11.1).
- At 5 years, mortality rates of PAD are similar to those seen in more readily recognized lethal conditions such as colorectal cancer or Hodgkin's disease. Even with contemporary medical management, patients with PAD have high rates of major cardiovascular events.

In addition to high cardiovascular morbidity and mortality, patients with PAD and claudication have a markedly diminished quality of life. Using validated tools such as the SF 36 questionnaire, patients with intermittent claudication have a quality of life that is at par with conditions such as congestive heart failure or chronic lung disease. Additionally, PAD patients experience major adverse limb events, such as amputation. In a recent study, 6.8% of real-world patients with PAD underwent amputation [2]. In 2009, the hospital costs associated with amputation or staggering totaled over $8.3 billion [3].

11.1.1 Medical Management of PAD

The management of patients with PAD follows a three-pronged approach focused on:

- The prevention of major adverse cardiac events, including myocardial infarction, stroke, and death.
- Improving function and quality of life.
- Preventing limb loss (Fig. 11.2).

Every patient with peripheral arterial disease should be prescribed:

- Complete smoking cessation
- Antithrombotic therapy
- Aggressive lipid management

I. Del Conde
Miami Cardiac and Vascular Institute, Baptist Health South Florida, Miami, FL, USA
e-mail: iand@baptisthealth.net

S. Madassery (✉)
Department of Vascular and Interventional Radiology, Rush University Medical Center, Chicago, IL, USA

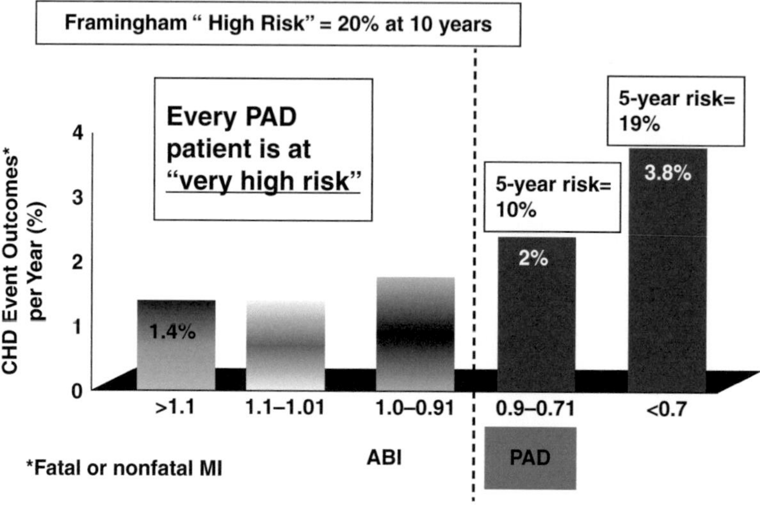

Fig. 11.1 Coronary heart disease (CHD) outcomes plotted against ankle: brachial index (ABI)

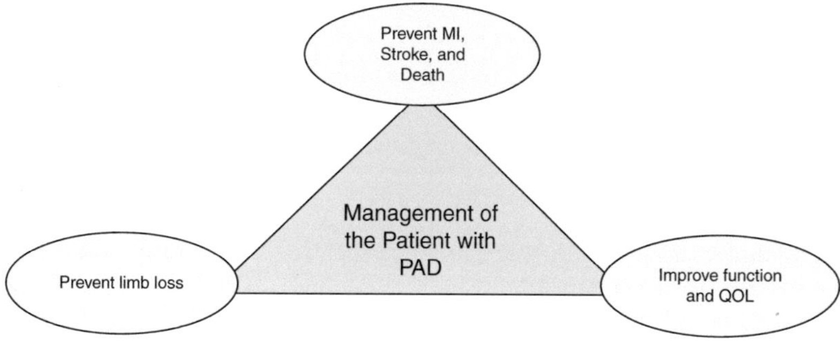

Fig. 11.2 Three-pronged approach to the medical management of patients with PAD

- Blood pressure control
- Diabetes control
- Regular exercise
- Foot care

11.1.2 Walking Program

There is ample evidence that a walking or exercise program improves the ability to walk in patients with claudication, even to a greater degree compared to drug therapies such as cilostazol. In a meta-analysis, an exercise program led to 120% increase in walking distance among patients with claudication, which was superior compared to all other noninvasive interventions [4].

The current PAD guidelines provide a class Ia recommendation for a supervised exercise program to improve functional status and quality of life and to reduce leg symptoms [5]. It should be noted that as of May 2017, the Centers for Medicare and Medicaid Services have approved reimbursement for supervised exercise training, only if the therapy meets specific criteria, such as sessions lasting 30–60 min delivered by certified personnel.

11.1.3 Antithrombotic Therapy in Stable PAD

Even though antiplatelet therapy is widely accepted as a standard in patients with peripheral arterial disease, in a well-performed meta-analysis, Berger et al. found little data to support the use of aspirin for the prevention of major adverse cardiac events among patients with PAD [6].

- Notwithstanding, antiplatelet therapy receives a class Ia recommendation in the current PAD guidelines and should be used in all patients with peripheral arterial disease.

There are reasons to believe the ADP receptor antagonist **Clopidogrel** may be superior to aspirin. In the CAPRIE trial, in which aspirin and clopidogrel were compared head-to-head amongst patients with a prior history of stroke, myocardial infarction, or PAD, the PAD subgroup derived particular benefit from clopidogrel with a 24% relative risk reduction in the occurrence of stroke myocardial infarction or cardiovascular death [7].

- Despite the absence of data replicating these findings, some clinicians have interpreted the CAPRIE study as an indication that clopidogrel should be the preferred antiplatelet drug in patients with PAD. Although there were hopes that the third-generation P2Y12 inhibitor ticagrelor would be superior to clopidogrel in patients with peripheral internal disease in the prevention of cardiovascular endpoints, the EUCLID trial failed to demonstrate any outcomes advantage of ticagrelor over clopidogrel [8].

There is limited data to support the use of dual antiplatelet therapy in patients for the medical management of stable peripheral arterial disease (i.e., excluding patients with recent endovascular revascularization).

- In the CHARISMA study, dual antiplatelet therapy with aspirin and clopidogrel resulted in slightly lower rates of myocardial infarction and hospitalization compared to aspirin alone, at the cost of increased minor bleeding [9].

Vorapaxar is an antiplatelet drug that blocks the thrombin receptor on the platelet surface as well as on endothelial cells. It is not an anticoagulant. Thrombin is the most potent platelet agonist known and is particularly relevant in in vivo platelet activation and aggregation.

- In a large, randomized control trial looking at secondary prevention of cardiovascular

disease, vorapaxar led to a lower risk of hospitalization for acute limb ischemia as well as for peripheral revascularization compared to placebo among patients with PAD [10].

More recently, the combination of aspirin plus ultra-low-dose rivaroxaban at 2.5 mg twice daily has been studied in patients with stable CAD or PAD in the COMPASS trial.

- The combination of low-dose rivaroxaban and aspirin led to a 28% relative risk reduction in the composite endpoint of cardiovascular death, myocardial infarction, or stroke compared to aspirin alone, and was also associated with a 46% relative reduction in the composite of major adverse limb events comprised of acute limb ischemia, critical limb ischemia, and amputation [11].
- Additionally, the combination arm was associated with a statistically significant 18% decreased risk of all-cause mortality compared to aspirin.

11.1.4 Antithrombotic Therapy Post-Revascularization

The optimal duration of dual antiplatelet therapy in patients who have undergone endovascular revascularization for lower extremity peripheral arterial disease has not been well defined. Several factors contribute to the difficulty in establishing an optimal antithrombotic regimen, including a broad range of complexity and anatomical considerations of the peripheral arterial disease itself, and the various devices, procedures, and technologies used to treat the disease. For example, tibioperoneal disease treated with a coronary drug-eluting stent carries a higher risk of stent thrombosis than a large stent used in the iliac segments.

- In practice, the duration of dual antiplatelet therapy in patients undergoing endovascular revascularization is guided by the manufacturers of the revascularization devices themselves, which in turn is extrapolated from the coronary literature.

- Most instructions for use (IFUs) recommend anywhere from 1 to 6 months of dual antiplatelet therapy following revascularization.

One of the most recent investigations to help define the duration of dual antiplatelet therapy after endovascular revascularization was led by Choo and colleagues [12]. The study involved 693 patients who received dual antiplatelet therapy for either less than 6 months or over 6 months.

- Dual antiplatelet therapy for over 6 months duration was associated with decreased 5-year major adverse cardiovascular and major adverse limb events, with no signal toward increased major bleeding.
- Major adverse cardiac events occurred less frequently in the DAPT group for ≥6 months group than in the DAPT for <6 months (17.3% vs 31.3%; hazard ratio, 0.44; 95% confidence interval, 0.3–0.65; $P < 0.001$). Major adverse limb events also occurred less frequently in the DAPT for ≥6 months group than the DAPT for <6 months group (21.5% vs 43.7%; hazard ratio, 0.42; 95% CI, 0.3–0.58; $P < 0.001$).
- One important caveat of this study is that it looked at patients who were treated between 2008 and 2013, thereby not fully reflecting current devices and adjunct pharmacotherapies that have become standard in the management of PAD.

As mentioned earlier in the chapter, a more recent large PAD randomized controlled trial, the COMPASS trial, suggested that the addition of ultra-low dose rivaroxaban may decrease the rate of serious limb events following revascularization compared to the standard of care. The multicenter VOYAGER PAD trial tested the efficacy and safety of low-dose rivaroxaban (2.5 mg twice daily) compared to placebo on a background of aspirin therapy in 6564 patients who had previously undergone surgical (35%) or endovascular

(65%) revascularization for symptomatic peripheral artery disease within the past 10 days [13]. Use of clopidogrel on top of aspirin/rivaroxaban or aspirin/placebo was allowed at the discretion of the investigators for up to 6 months. The primary outcome (a composite of cardiovascular death, acute limb ischemia, major amputation, myocardial infarction, or stroke) occurred in 15.5% of the rivaroxaban + aspirin arm compared to 17.8% of the placebo + aspirin arm, representing a 15% relative risk reduction in the primary outcome ($p = 0.009$). Although the rate of major bleeding occurred more frequently among patients in the combination arm of rivaroxaban + aspirin (1.9% vs. 1.35%, $P = 0.07$), there were no excess events of intracerebral hemorrhage or fatal bleeding.

- The findings of VOYAGER PAD confirm the notion of the role of very low-dose anticoagulation (specifically with rivaroxaban) added on top of antiplatelet therapy with aspirin in patients with atherosclerotic peripheral arterial disease, both in the stable phase as well as post-revascularization.

11.1.5 Putting It Together

- A reasonable general antithrombotic strategy in patients following endovascular revascularization is to treat with dual antiplatelet therapy with aspirin and clopidogrel per IFU of the device used, which is generally for 1–3 months, and possibly longer (up to 6 months) with more complex disease at higher risk of thrombosis.
- If the patient is considered to have an acceptable bleeding risk profile (without specific risk factors for life-threatening bleeding), then rivaroxaban 2.5 mg twice daily can be added to the regimen. Once clopidogrel is stopped, the risk-benefit of long-term aspirin 81 mg daily plus rivaroxaban 2.5 mg twice daily can be considered.

11.1.6 Medication Failure Versus Non-responders

Resistance to aspirin and clopidogrel has been well studied and documented. Although the phenomenon is real, occurring in up to 30–40% of patients, the mechanisms behind such resistance are varied [14]. In some instances, the resistance is due to pharmacokinetic factors limiting the absorption, metabolism, and bioavailability of the drug. In other instances, however, there does appear to be a true genetically determined resistance to the antiplatelet drug, mostly by altered metabolism of the drug. Despite the intellectual appeal of testing for clopidogrel and aspirin resistance to guide therapy, the results of such strategies have been mixed and there is no consensus on how to best manage these patients.

- From a clinical standpoint, when encountering a patient in whom clinical failure or resistance is suspected, it is critical to first confirm complete adherence to the antiplatelet medication.
- If clinical failure is determined, it is reasonable to measure clopidogrel or aspirin resistance using commercially and clinically available platelet function analyzers to help identify an appropriate regimen.
- Treatment decisions must be individualized and may include the various antithrombotic drugs approved for clinical use and described in this chapter.

11.1.7 Statin Therapy

All patients with peripheral arterial disease should receive high-intensity statin therapy [15]. Per current lipid guidelines, patients should be treated with a minimum of atorvastatin 40 mg daily or rosuvastatin 20 mg daily, ideally targeting an LDL level less than 100, and possibly less than 70 mg/dL.

11.1.8 Cilostazol

The mechanism of action of cilostazol has not been fully elucidated, but it is clear that it improves claudication symptoms. In a meta-analysis of 8 randomized control trials involving over 2700 patients with moderate-to-severe claudication, cilostazol lead to a 50% and a 67% increase in mean walking distance and pain-free walking distance, respectively [16].

- Cilostazol should be started at 50 mg twice daily and after 3–4 weeks the dose should be increased to the target dose of 100 mg twice daily. It should be taken on an empty stomach.
- In real-life registries, over 50% of patients stop the drug after 36 months due to side effects, such as diarrhea, headaches, palpitations, or dizziness.
- There is a black box warning against the use of cilostazol in patients with a history of congestive heart failure or an ejection fraction lower than 40%.

11.1.9 PCSK9 Inhibitors

The role of PCSK9 inhibitors in patients with PAD has been highlighted in the FOURIER trial. PAD patients who received the PCSK9 inhibitor Evolocumab (Repatha) had a 27% risk reduction in the composite of cardiovascular death, myocardial infarction, or stroke compared to placebo. In a PAD subanalysis [17], the number needed to treat to prevent major adverse cardiac events was 29 patients over 2.5 years.

11.1.10 Hypertension Management

Patients with peripheral arterial disease and hypertension should be treated to achieve a goal of blood pressure less than 130/85 mmHg, preferably with an ACE inhibitor. In the landmark HOPE trial, patients with atherosclerotic vascular disease had a 22% reduction in the relative risk of myocardial infarction, stroke, or cardiovascular death compared to placebo [18].

11.2 Venous Disease Management

Ian Del Conde

Although a comprehensive review of the medical management of patients with acute deep vein thrombosis (DVT) is beyond the scope of this chapter, readers are referred to the most recent update of the American College of Chest Physicians update on the management of venous thromboembolism [19]. For the purpose of the interventionalist treating patients with acute DVT, the discussion will be focused on the acute management of patients with DVT as it relates to endovascular therapy.

- Most patients with lower extremity deep vein thrombosis can be managed medically (usually in the ambulatory setting) using a target-specific oral anticoagulant, such as apixaban or rivaroxaban, which do not require parenteral heparin products at treatment initiation.
- As discussed in prior sections, catheter-directed therapies are often considered in patients with more extensive lower extremity DVT, such as DVT involving the inferior vena cava or the iliofemoral segments. These patients generally require hospitalization and should be treated with either a low molecular weight heparin at a therapeutic dose, or an unfractionated heparin drip.

The duration of anticoagulation in patients with acute proximal lower extremity DVT depends on the presentation. There are three clinical factors obtained by history that identify patients as having an increased risk of recurrent venous thromboembolism:

1. Patients with active cancer.
2. Those with a prior history of venous thromboembolism.
3. Those with unprovoked DVT (i.e., without preceding major transient risk factors, such as surgery or immobilization).

Patients at increased risk of recurrent venous thromboembolism usually complete 3–6 months of therapeutic anticoagulation (generally with a target-specific oral anticoagulant) and are subsequently considered for extended treatment for the prevention of recurrent venous thromboembolism. Extended treatment is accomplished with a reduced dose of rivaroxaban [20] or apixaban [21], which has been shown to have a favorable risk: benefit profile.

References

1. Leng GC, Fowkes FG, Lee AJ, et al. Use of ankle brachial pressure index to predict cardiovascular events and death: a cohort study. BMJ. 1996;313(7070):1440–4.
2. Jones WS, Patel MR, Dai D, et al. High mortality risks after major lower extremity amputation in Medicare patients with peripheral artery disease. Am Heart J. 2013;165(5):809–15. 815.e1
3. Ziegler-Graham K, MacKenzie EJ, Ephraim PL, et al. Estimating the prevalence of limb loss in the United States: 2005 to 2050. Arch Phys Med Rehabil. 2008;89(3):422–9.
4. Gandhi S, Weinberg I, Margey R, Jaff MR. Comprehensive medical management of peripheral arterial disease. Prog Cardiovasc Dis. 2011;54(1):2–13.
5. Gerhard-Herman MD, Gornik HL, Barrett C, et al. 2016 AHA/ACC guideline on the management of patients with lower extremity peripheral artery disease: executive summary: a report of the American College of Cardiology/American Heart Association Task Force on Clinical Practice Guidelines. Circulation. 2017;135(12):e686–725.
6. Berger JS, Krantz MJ, Kittelson JM, Hiatt WR. Aspirin for the prevention of cardiovascular events in patients with peripheral artery disease: a meta-analysis of randomized trials. JAMA. 2009;301(18):1909–19.
7. CAPRIE Steering Committee. A randomised, blinded, trial of clopidogrel versus aspirin in patients at risk

of ischaemic events (CAPRIE). CAPRIE Steering Committee. Lancet. 1996;348(9038):1329–39.

8. Hiatt WR, Fowkes FG, Heizer G, et al. EUCLID Trial Steering Committee and Investigators. Ticagrelor versus Clopidogrel in Symptomatic Peripheral Artery Disease. N Engl J Med. 2017;376(1):32–40.

9. Cacoub PP, Bhatt DL, Steg PG, Topol EJ, Creager MA. CHARISMA Investigators. Patients with peripheral arterial disease in the CHARISMA trial. Eur Heart J. 2009;30(2):192–201.

10. Bonaca MP, Scirica BM, Creager MA, Olin J, et al. Vorapaxar in patients with peripheral artery disease: results from TRA2{degrees}P-TIMI 50. Circulation. 2013;127(14):1522–9. 1529e1-6

11. Anand SS, Bosch J, Eikelboom JW, et al. COMPASS Investigators. Rivaroxaban with or without aspirin in patients with stable peripheral or carotid artery disease: an international, randomised, double-blind, placebo-controlled trial. Lancet. 2018;391(10117):219–29.

12. Cho S, Lee Y, Ko Y, et al. Optimal strategy for antiplatelet therapy after endovascular revascularization for lower extremity peripheral artery disease. J Am Coll Cardiol Intv. 2019;12(23):2359–70.

13. Bonaca MP, Bauersachs RM, Anand SS, et al. Rivaroxaban in peripheral artery disease after revascularization. N Engl J Med. https://doi.org/10.1056/NEJMoa2000052.

14. Schwartz KA. Aspirin resistance: a clinical review focused on the most common cause, noncompliance. Neurohospitalist. 2011;1(2):94–103.

15. Stone NJ, Robinson JG, Lichtenstein AH, American College of Cardiology/American Heart Association Task Force on Practice Guidelines, et al. 2013 ACC/AHA guideline on the treatment of blood cholesterol to reduce atherosclerotic cardiovascular risk in adults: a report of the American College of Cardiology/American Heart Association Task Force on Practice Guidelines. Circulation. 2014;129(25 Suppl 2):S1–45.

16. Thompson PD, Zimet R, Forbes WP, Zhang P. Meta-analysis of results from eight randomized, placebo-controlled trials on the effect of cilostazol on patients with intermittent claudication. Am J Cardiol. 2002;90(12):1314–9.

17. Bonaca MP, Nault P, Giugliano RP, et al. Low-density lipoprotein cholesterol lowering with evolocumab and outcomes in patients with peripheral artery disease: insights from the FOURIER trial (further cardiovascular outcomes research with PCSK9 inhibition in subjects with elevated risk). Circulation. 2018;137(4):338–50.

18. Heart Outcomes Prevention Evaluation Study Investigators, Yusuf S, Sleight P, Pogue J, Bosch J, Davies R, Dagenais G. Effects of an angiotensin-converting-enzyme inhibitor, ramipril, on cardiovascular events in high-risk patients. N Engl J Med. 2000;342(3):145–53.

19. Stevens SM, Woller SC, Kreuziger LB, Bounameaux H, Doerschug K, Geersing GJ, Huisman MV, Kearon C, King CS, Knighton AJ, Lake E, Murin S, Vintch JRE, Wells PS, Moores LK. Antithrombotic therapy for VTE disease: second update of the CHEST guideline and expert panel report. Chest. 2021;160(6):e545–608. https://doi.org/10.1016/j.chest.2021.07.055. Epub 2021 Aug 2. Erratum in: Chest. 2022 Jul;162(1):269.

20. Weitz JI, Lensing AWA, Prins MH, Bauersachs R, Beyer-Westendorf J, Bounameaux H, Brighton TA, Cohen AT, Davidson BL, Decousus H, Freitas MCS, Holberg G, Kakkar AK, Haskell L, van Bellen B, Pap AF, Berkowitz SD, Verhamme P, Wells PS, Prandoni P, Investigators EINSTEINCHOICE. Rivaroxaban or aspirin for extended treatment of venous thromboembolism. N Engl J Med. 2017;376(13):1211–22. https://doi.org/10.1056/NEJMoa1700518. Epub 2017 Mar 18

21. Agnelli G, Buller HR, Cohen A, Curto M, Gallus AS, Johnson M, Porcari A, Raskob GE, Weitz JI, AMPLIFY-EXT Investigators. Apixaban for extended treatment of venous thromboembolism. N Engl J Med. 2013;368(8):699–708. https://doi.org/10.1056/NEJMoa1207541. Epub 2012 Dec 8

Correction to: Venous Interventions

Syed Samaduddin Ahmed, Adam Said,
Osman Ahmed, Patrick Lee,
Sreekumar Madassery, Ron Winokur,
Brian P. Holly, Mark Lessne, Shin Mei Chan,
Kush R. Desai, Jordan C. Tasse, Griffin Mcnamara,
Jillian Drogin, and Keith Pereira

Correction to:
Chapter 7 in: S. Madassery, A. Patel (eds.), *Limb Preservation for the Vascular Specialist*, https://doi.org/10.1007/978-3-031-36480-8_7

The original version of Chapter 7 was inadvertently published with incorrect city and state for the author Dr. Mark Lessne. The correct city is "North Carolina" and this has been updated in the revised publication.

The updated version of this chapter can be found at https://doi.org/10.1007/978-3-031-36480-8_7

Index